Evidence-based public health

Evidence-based public health

effectiveness and efficiency

Edited by

Amanda Killoran and Michael P Kelly

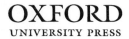

OXFORD

UNIVERSITY PRESS

OXFORD

UNIVERSITY PRESS

Great Clarendon Street, Oxford OX2 6DP

Oxford University Press is a department of the University of Oxford.
It furthers the University's objective of excellence in research, scholarship,
and education by publishing worldwide in

Oxford New York

Auckland Cape Town Dar es Salaam Hong Kong Karachi
Kuala Lumpur Madrid Melbourne Mexico City Nairobi
New Delhi Shanghai Taipei Toronto

With offices in

Argentina Austria Brazil Chile Czech Republic France Greece
Guatemala Hungary Italy Japan Poland Portugal Singapore
South Korea Switzerland Thailand Turkey Ukraine Vietnam

Oxford is a registered trade mark of Oxford University Press
in the UK and in certain other countries

Published in the United States
by Oxford University Press Inc., New York

British Library Cataloguing in Publication Data

Data available

Library of Congress Cataloging-in-Publication Data

Evidence-based public health : effectiveness and efficiency / edited by
Amanda Killoran and Mike Kelly.
      p. ; cm.
   Includes bibliographical references and index.
   ISBN 978–0–19–956362–3 (alk. paper)
  1. Public health—Research—Methodology. 2. Evidence-based medicine.
3. National Institute for Health and Clinical Excellence (Great Britain)
4. Public health administration—Great Britain—Evaluation.
5. Evidence-based medicine—Great Britain—Evaluation. I. Killoran,
Amanda. II. Kelly, Michael P. (Michael Patrick), 1953-
  [DNLM: 1. Public Health Administration—Great Britain. 2. National
Institute for Health and Clinical Excellence (Great Britain)
3. Evidence-Based Practice—Great Britain. 4. Program Evaluation—Great
Britain. WA 540 FA1 E93 2009]
   RA440.85.E95 2009
   362.10972—dc22   2009032939

Typeset in Minion by Cepha Imaging Private Ltd., Bangalore, India
Printed in Great Britain by CPI Antony Rowe

ISBN 978–0–19–956362–3

10 9 8 7 6 5 4 3 2

Foreword

Much is made of the differences between the evidence—and the studies which generate it—for public health practice and interventions used in clinical practice. The standard research paradigm, commonly assumed to be the 'gold standard' in clinical practice using randomization, is uncommon in public health research. And the use of economic modelling has been much more common in appraising interventions in clinical practice, although now it is now applied in public health. These and other differences are sometimes used to support the contention that there is an unbridgeable divide between the two disciplines, which makes it unfeasible to consider the application of the evaluative techniques used by one to the other.

These arguments were extensively rehearsed when the Health Development Agency merged with NICE, in 2005. Concerns were expressed that NICE's perceived reliance on randomized controlled trials, would be applied to its new public health function, forcing an impractical evaluative approach onto the available evidence. Instead, the Centre for Public Health Excellence established at NICE after the merger, continued to use the best of the methodology developed by the Health Development Agency but also began to explore the extent to which some of the approaches used by the other teams inside NICE might add value to conventional assessment and appraisal in public health. And this worked both ways. The groups in NICE responsible for preparing guidance on clinical practice started to look at the way in which field work, for example, long used in the preparation of public health guidance, might help to improve knowledge about the application of guidance in day-to-day practice. This approach is being used in the new NICE quality standards, which will be introduce from early 2010. However, it has been in the field of economic analysis that the most obvious developments have taken place. Initially by the Public Health Interventional Advisory Committee and then by the public health Programme Development Groups, the application of cost-effectiveness analysis and where appropriate and possible the use of quality-adjusted life years as the metric of choice, has led to a fundamental change in the way the argument for investing in public health interventions has been put forward. By using economic analysis, the already persuasive case for prevention has been enhanced by a compelling analysis of value for money, allowing comparisons between approaches both within public health and with clinical practice.

This new book, edited by Amanda Killoran, public health analyst, and Mike Kelly, the Director of the Centre for Clinical Practice at NICE, draws on the pioneering work which he has led both before and since the merger of NICE and the Health Development Agency. It brings this experience together with insightful pieces from some of the best thinkers, practitioners, and methodologists working in health in the United Kingdom and internationally. It is an outstanding piece of work of which the authors should feel rightly proud.

Andrew Dillon and Sir Michael Rawlins
Chief Executive and Chair
The National Institute for Health and Clinical Excellence (NICE)

Foreword

The growing policy focus on health improvement and wellbeing is placing an ever-greater emphasis on the need for sound evidence-based public health. At the same time, public services are heading for turbulent waters as the economic downturn takes its toll on their future funding and growth. The risk of public health once again being seen as an easy target when it comes to cutting investment is all too real. The only way to prevent public health budget raids, which have occurred all too readily during previous economic hard times, is to be able to put forward strong and convincing business cases for investment. It hardly needs stressing that these will need to be underpinned by sound evidence although it alone will not be sufficient to ensure that public health is spared the worst over the coming years.

This book is therefore both welcome and timely as it deals with a set of issues which a strong evidence base must address. There are two areas where the evidence base is especially weak. First, there remains a dearth of good studies investigating the costs and benefits of interventions. Yet, without such information it becomes difficult to persuade cost-conscious managers to invest (or not to disinvest), especially when the impact of such investment on improved health outcomes might not be realised for many years. Encouraging health economists to turn their attention from health care to health remains a key issue. It is therefore heartening to see a section of the book devoted to the contribution of health economists to public health and resource allocation.

Second, while there are important gaps in the evidence base as many observers have noted over the years, there is already strong evidence in some areas that fails to get acted upon. Arguably, then, the priority for public health practitioners is to give more attention to the vexed issue of knowledge transfer—or exchange to those who prefer to see the issue as one involving a two-way dialogue among co-equals in preference to pearls of wisdom being handed down from on high by academics who then, for the most part, withdraw from the process leaving it to practitioners and others to act on the evidence as best they can. Often such evidence is de-contextualised which can reduce its value and make its application problematic. We also know from various studies that such a linear, rational process in respect of the uptake of evidence is misconceived and fails to reflect the barriers which exist. Yet, incentives for academic researchers to focus on knowledge exchange are few and the academic career is still largely shaped by securing peer-reviewed research publications in reputable outlets. Important though these are, they are insufficient by themselves to bring about an evidence-based culture in health improvement and wellbeing. Initiatives from the National Institute for Health Research, such as the five centres of excellence in public health research established in England, Wales and Northern Ireland in 2008 (Scotland has its own equivalent research collaborative) and mentioned in the book, are therefore welcome and will hopefully have an impact on such biases although tensions and contradictions remain, not least in academe. Moreover, public health is not confined to the NHS and other agencies, in particular local government, need to raise their game and become more literate when it comes to the uses and limits of evidence since they must also take an increasingly hard-nosed approach to investment issues. Indeed, when it comes to tackling the social determinants of health and health inequalities, local government has a more wide-ranging and significant role than the NHS especially in respect of education and housing.

The importance of NICE being responsible for advising on best evidence for public health through the work of its Centre of Public Health Excellence cannot be overstated as increasingly, at a policy level, links are made between acute care and health. Almost uniquely, given its remit, NICE straddles the two domains. At the same time, it is devoting more attention to the use made of research in practice and to overcoming the barriers to its uptake. Of course, all stages of research—from generating evidence, through its synthesis, to its impact on policy and practice—are linked (or should be) and, for the impact of research to be maximised, those consuming it also need to be actively engaged from the outset in its genesis, helping to identify the key questions and shape the methods used to address them.

It goes without saying that research will never be perfect or beyond contestability. Nor will evidence by itself ever solely determine the outcome of policy—as Michael Marmot put it, we shall continue to have policy-based evidence as distinct from evidence-based policy. It is in any case unlikely that research could ever be so conclusive and unequivocal that it can afford to disregard any dissenting voices. In a democracy, evidence can only ever be one ingredient in the policy mix which is as it should be.

There is also the issue of complexity and evidence. Public health has been characterised as a set of complex 'wicked issues' which defy simple or straightforward answers. We need research evidence that can help us to ask the right questions and not simply provide the answers. There is unlikely to be a single answer in any case. What is important is that research is 'good enough' to inform policy and practice and at least allow progress to be made which can subsequently be evaluated so that the policy or its implementation can either be strengthened and continued or modified or discontinued. If, as in the case of Sure Start for example, the evidence fails to give a clear-cut answer but yet seems to suggest that the intervention, at least in some places, is resulting in benefits that may impact on health longer term, then policy-makers must decide whether to continue investing in it or whether funds should be diverted elsewhere.

The various contributions and contributors to this collection go far in covering many of the key issues that demand urgent attention if public health evidence is truly to come of age and play a much more critical part in decision-making than has been the case hitherto. Nonetheless, major challenges remain, among them how evidence and good (as opposed to bad) science can be made more accessible to the media without it being distorted to create attention-grabbing headlines and sound bites. Then there is the use of evidence as advocacy to bring about policy change perhaps, though not solely, through the creation of a social movement in thinking about, and acting on, health. The public too often receives mixed messages about public health interventions and whether they work or not, and most of these are directed at individual lifestyle changes. The upstream social determinants get little attention in terms of their wider societal impact if we continue to allow the health gap to widen. Indeed, they are often dismissed as being associated with the political left and as ideologically rather than evidence-driven. What has been termed 'lifestyle drift' has become pervasive throughout health policy in recent years, a point also made in the book. No matter how well-intentioned governments may be and how committed they appear to be to tackling the social determinants of health, when it comes to the detail of actions to be taken they struggle and seem unable to translate societal-level factors which cause distress at an individual level to societal-level solutions. Quite the reverse since the solutions advanced are instantly reducible to what individuals need to do to alter their behaviour or to what producers should do to make healthier choices easier and better informed. Such measures may have a place but they can hardly be said to amount to what is required to narrow the health gap on the scale needed to make significant inroads.

If nothing else, this book will have served a valuable purpose if it prompts readers to reflect upon such issues and perhaps also to act on them. It will be all too easy over the next few difficult years in public policy to allow public health to be overshadowed by what are seen to be more important issues, such as securing future economic growth and maintaining a sickness service. That would be a serious mistake and there are welcome signs that both ministers and their officials understand this risk. But if doing something about the social determinants of health is to remain high on the political agenda, then having the evidence to justify the case for change will be more essential than ever. Hopefully this book can assist in this endeavour.

David J Hunter
Professor of Health Policy and Management
Durham University
September 2009

Acknowledgements

The editors wish to thank Andrew Dillon and Sir Michael Rawlins respectively Chief Executive and Chair of the National Institute for Health and Clinical Excellence (NICE), for the immense commitment they have given to the development of the public health at NICE since 2005, and their support for the production of this book. The development of public health at NICE has generated many challenging questions relating to the application of the evidence-based approach, originally devised in clinical medicine, to the broader field of public health. The Chief Executive and Chair and the NICE Board have encouraged and supported wholeheartedly this scientific and practical endeavour.

We also wish to acknowledge the outstanding contributions made by the authors of the chapters, in sharing their experience and expertise on the diverse set of topics encompassed in this volume.

Finally our special thanks go to Emma Doohan (née Stewart) who has managed this project through all its stages with dedication and commitment as well as immense good humour.

Contents

Contributors

Dr Laurie M Anderson
Senior Scientist, Washington State
Institute for Public Policy

Nick Baillie
Programme Manager, Implementation,
NICE

Prof Jacqueline Barnes
Director of Local Context Analysis,
National Evaluation of Sure Start,
Birkbeck University of London

Prof David Barnett
Chair of Appraisals Committee,
Technology Appraisals, NICE;
Professor of Clinical Pharmacology,
University of Leicester

Prof Mel Bartley
Professor of Medical Sociology,
University College London

Prof Adrian Bauman
Centre for Physical Activity and Health,
University of Sydney

Prof David Blane
Professor of Medical Sociology,
Imperial College London

Prof Jay Belsky
Research Director National
Evaluation of Sure Start,
Birkbeck University of London

Prof Virginia Berridge
Professor of History, Centre for
History in Public Health, London School
of Hygiene and Tropical Medicine

Prof Lyndal Bond
Associate Director, MRC Social and
Public Health Sciences Unit,
University of Glasgow

Meindert Boysen
Programme Director Technology
Appraisals, NICE

Prof Fiona C Bull
School of Population Health,
University of Western Australia

Helen Butler
Senior Lecturer, School of Education,
Australian Catholic University Limited

Chris Carmona
Analyst, Centre for Public Health
Excellence, NICE

Dr Kalipso Chalkidou
Director of Policy Consulting, NICE

Dr Richard Cookson
Senior Lecturer, Department of
Social Policy and Social Work,
University of York

Annie Coppel
Associate Director, Implementation,
NICE

Peter Craig
Programme Manager, MRC Population
Health Sciences Research Network,
University of Glasgow

Dr Hugo Crombie
Analyst, Centre for Public Health
Excellence, NICE

Prof Anthony Culyer
Ontario Research Chair in Health
Policy & System Design, University of
Toronto and Professor of Economics,
University of York

Dr Steven Cummins
Senior Lecturer and NIHR Fellow,
Queen Mary University of London

Prof Melanie Davies
Professor of Diabetes Medicine,
University of Leicester

Prof Nancy Devlin
Director of Research,
Office of Health Economics

Prof Paul Dieppe
Professor Nuffield Department of
Orthopaedic Surgery,
University of Oxford

Nick Doyle
Clinical and Public Health
Analyst, NICE

Dr Jane E Ferrie
Senior Research Fellow on Whitehall II
Study, University College London

Dr Klaus Gebel
Centre for Physical Activity and Health,
University of Sydney

Prof Hilary Graham
Professor of Health Sciences,
University of York

Susan Griffin
RCUK Academic Fellow, Centre for
Health Economics, University of York

Jane Huntley
Associate Director, Centre for Public
Health Excellence, NICE

Prof Roger Ingham
Director, Centre for Sexual Health
Research, University of Southampton

James Jagroo
Analyst, Centre for Public Health
Excellence, NICE

Prof Michael P Kelly
Director of the Centre for Public Health
Excellence, NICE

Prof Kamlesh Khunti
Professor of Primary Care, Diabetes and
Vascular Medicine, University of Leicester

Dr Amanda Killoran
Analyst, Centre for Public Health
Excellence, NICE

Prof Mika Kivimäki
Professor of Social Epidemiology,
University College London; UK and
Finnish Institute of Occupational Health

Lord Krebs
Principal of Jesus College,
Oxford University

Prof Catherine Law
Professor of Public Health and
Epidemiology, MRC Centre of
Epidemiology for Child Health,
UCL Institute of Child Health
Chair, Public Health International
Advisory Group (NICE)

Prof Peter Littlejohns
Clinical and Public Health Director NICE

Prof Anne Ludbrook
Health Economics Research Unit,
University of Aberdeen

Dr Carole Longson
Director Centre for Health Technology
Evaluation, NICE

Prof M Judith Lynam
Director Culture, Gender & Health
Research Unit, University of British
Columbia

Prof Sally Macintyre
Director MRC Social and Public Health
Sciences Unit, University of Glasgow

Prof Sir Michael Marmot
Director UCL Institute for Society and
Health, University College London

Prof David V McQueen
Associate Director for Global Health
Promotion, Centre for Chronic Disease
Prevention and Health Promotion,
Centres for Disease Control and
Prevention, Atlanta US

Prof Edward Melhuish
Executive Director, National Evaluation of Sure Start, Birkbeck University of London

Prof Susan Michie
Director, Centre for Outcomes Research and Effectiveness, University College London

Val Moore
Director of Implementation, NICE

Antony Morgan
Associate Director, Centre for Public Health Excellence, NICE

Prof Stephen Morris
Reader, Research Department of Epidemiology and Public Health, University College London

Dr Bhash Naidoo
Health Economist, Technology Appraisals, NICE

Prof Irwin Nazwreth
Director, MRC General Practice Research Framework

Dr Lesley Owen
Health Economist, Technology Appraisals, NICE

Prof David Parkin
Professor of Economics, City University, London

Prof Ray Pawson
Professor of Social Research Methodology, University of Leeds

Dr Steven D Pearson
President of the Institute for Clinical and Economic Review, Harvard Medical School, US

Prof Mark Petticrew
Professor, Department of Public Health and Policy, London School of Hygiene and Tropical Medicine

Prof Chris Power
Professor of Epidemiology and Public Health, MRC Centre of Epidemiology for Child Health, UCL Institute for Child Health

Prof Nigel Rice
Professor of Health Economics, University of York

Julie Royce
Associate Director, Implementation, NICE

Harald Schmidt
Assistant Director, Nuffield Council on Bioethics

Prof Mark Sculpher
Professor of Health Economics, University of York

Dr Lion Shahab
Research Psychologist University College London

Dr Debbie Smith
Research Associate Health Psychology, University College London

Dr Sanjeev Sridharan
Associate Professor Health Policy, University of Toronto

Prof Andrew Stevens
Chair of Appraisals Committee, Technology Appraisals, NICE
Professor of Public Health, University of Birmingham

Dr Margaret Stone
Senior Research Fellow, University of Leicester

Dr Catherine Swann
Associate Director, Centre for Public Health Excellence, NICE

Jacqui Troughton
Senior Researcher, Department of Diabetes, University Hospitals of Leicester NHS Trust

Prof Robert West
Cancer Research UK Health Behaviour
Research Centre, University College
London

Clare Wohlgemuth
Analyst, Centre for Public Health
Excellence, NICE

Prof Jeremy Wyatt
Professor of Health Informatics,
University of Dundee

Dr Thomas Yates
Senior Researcher, Department of
Cardiovascular Sciences, University of
Leicester

Introduction: effectiveness and efficiency in public health

Amanda Killoran and Michael P Kelly

Aims and objectives

In 1972 a seminal text was published. This was Archie Cochrane's *Effectiveness and Efficiency: Random Reflections on Health Services* (Cochrane 1972). Cochrane's attack on the self-serving and complacent nature of clinical medicine marked one of the earliest pleas for taking an evidence-based approach to medicine. We deliberately recall this concern with 'Effectiveness and efficiency' in the subtitle of our book and in this introduction. In nearly forty years things have moved on, and the evidence-based approach is well established in clinical medicine. It is making significant inroads in public health. Our aim is much more modest than Archie Cochrane's. We seek not to bring about a revolution, but to plot, in a systematic and decidedly non-random way, a guide to an evidence-based approach to public health, including the public health role of the UK's National Institute for Health and Clinical Excellence (NICE).

The objectives are:

- to describe the role of evidence-based public health in addressing the health challenges of the 21st century;
- to set out frameworks for evaluating the effectiveness and cost-effectiveness of policies and interventions that improve health equity;
- to examine use of evidence in understanding variations in health within the population, and its role in design and implementation of interventions and evaluating equity of health outcomes;
- to document the approaches and methods to generating and synthesizing evidence on what works in changing individual health behaviours and wider social determinants; and
- to describe the development of evidence-based public health guidance and standards, and their role in changing policy and practice to improve health equity, with particular reference to the experience of NICE.

Public health challenges

At the start of the 21st century inequalities in health between different social groups are an important concern in all developed countries (CSDH 2008). While the overall health of populations has continued to improve in developed societies, social inequalities in health have remained an enduring feature. This social patterning is expressed in immediate concerns.

Smoking, obesity, misuse of drugs and alcohol, high rates of teenage conception, stress, and poor mental health are disproportionately concentrated among the less well-off. It is depicted epidemiologically in the burden of disease. Those who are socially disadvantaged can expect to experience greater ill health and die younger. This applies on the global canvas as well.

Policy makers and practitioners seek effective strategies that can reduce these health inequalities while sustaining overall health improvements. The importance of an evidence-based approach to public health is acknowledged by governments. Research attention has increasingly focused on explaining the causes of inequalities as the basis for defining the opportunities to secure improvement through effective interventions. Furthermore, the evidence on the effectiveness and cost-effectiveness of different public health policies and interventions, although comparatively underdeveloped, is growing. Public health researchers now have a sound set of 'evaluation frameworks' of theory, approaches and methods, and experience, to generate and synthesize evidence of what works and inform and change policy and practice. This book sets out this evidence-based approach to public health.

Health equity and the social gradient of health inequalities

The concept of health equity is fundamental to public health, and a precise definition is a prerequisite for measurement, evaluation, policy, and accountability. Health equity is an ethical principle related to human rights and social justice; and involves a judgement that most health inequalities are unnecessary, avoidable, unfair, and unjust. Health inequity is not synonymous with health inequalities. Health inequalities are the measurement of differences in health, and not all differences will be avoidable or unfair.

Health equity can be defined as:

> The absence of systematic disparities in health (or in the major social determinants of health) between social groups with different levels of underlying social advantage/disadvantage—that is different positions in a social hierarchy . . . Examples of more and less advantaged social groups include socioeconomic groups, racial/ethnic or religious groups, or groups defined by gender, geography, age, disability, sexual orientation and other social characteristics.

(Braveman and Gruskin 2008)

The causes of health inequalities are complex and multi-factorial. However, the evidence demonstrates that many health inequalities are systematically linked to social determinants (Blas et al 2008). In most societies the distribution of health across social groups takes the form of a gradient: the lower an individual's socio-economic position, the worst their health. This gradient is the product of the unequal distribution of social determinants ie of power, resources, goods, and services (Graham and Kelly 2004).

Rights and opportunities to be healthy

The pursuit of health equity is a central concern of policy makers internationally. Explicit policy goals and strategies commit governments to actions on health inequalities (as discussed further below).

The concept of health equity is closely linked to human rights and social justice. The right to health is incorporated within international human rights legislative frameworks. Sen's work has been influential in helping translate the theory of social justice into policy. Notions of equal opportunity to be healthy, to enjoy substantive freedoms and capabilities recognize that health is a prerequisite for full individual agency and freedom and inequalities in social conditions arising from social position can profoundly compromise freedom.

> Capabilities are substantive human freedoms or real opportunities (such as the ability to avoid premature mortality, to be adequately nourished, to have access to adequate health, social services and education, to participate in and to influence public life and to enjoy self respect) that people value and have reasons to value.

(Sen 2004; 2005)

Importantly, this perspective recognizes that individuals and groups have differential needs and vulnerabilities and that positive measures are required to secure equality of opportunity. This capability approach can help ensure pursuit of health equity is integrated within legislative mechanisms and analysis.

A model of social determinants of health

The report *Closing the gap in a generation* prepared by the WHO Commission on Social Determinants of Health (CSDH 2008) provides an important international lead for countries faced with the common concern of reducing health inequalities. The aim is to achieve health equity and social justice, defined as 'improving the average health of countries and abolishing avoidable inequalities in health within countries . . . the aim should be to bring the health of those worse off up to the level of the best'. The Commission conducted a comprehensive review of existing evidence on both the theories relating to social inequalities in health as well as evaluation research on the effectiveness of policies and interventions. Social determinants are explained as the causes of health inequalities and the focus for action.

Importantly the Commission's conceptual framework (Figure I.1) builds on previous work to define the causal pathways that generate marked differences in health status.

The causes of social inequalities in health encompass the structures and processes at global and national levels which shape the conditions of daily life: 'the conditions in which people grow, live, work and age'. These, in turn, determine individuals' experiences and behaviours that are either health enhancing or health damaging. Figure I.1 shows the linking of societal structures, conditions of daily living, behaviours, and biological and psychosocial factors operating at the individual level.

'Social position' and the everyday experience of that social position, provides the critical interface between the wider societal structures and individuals' experience of disadvantage and health outcomes. An individual's social position may be defined according to indicators that include socio-economic status, ethnicity, and gender, and is the product of the process of social stratification operating in societies. It serves to advantage or disadvantage individuals in ways that impact on an individual's daily life and their

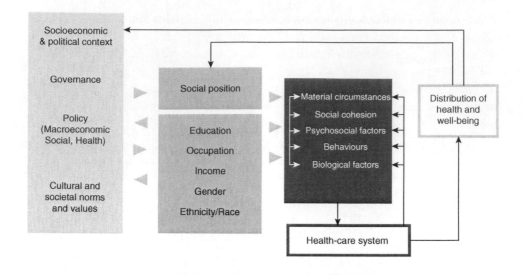

Fig. I.1 Commission on Social Determinants of Health conceptual framework
Source: Amended from Solar and Irwin 2007

experiences throughout life. It produces differential exposures to influences that increases their risk of disease and vulnerability to poor health. It helps explain how the impact of disadvantage is reflected in the social patterning of health behaviours and disease at a group and population level.

Evidence-based public health

Evidence-based public health is the process involved in providing the best available evidence to influence decisions about the effectiveness of policies and interventions and secure improvements in health and reductions in health inequalities.

There is now considerable understanding of what this process involves as a scientific discipline. We draw heavily on the experience in England in this book, and specifically the learning of the Centre for Public Health Excellence at NICE, as well as the work of the Commission of Social Determinants of Health.

Evidence-based public health has a number of key features:

◆ conceptual plausibility: an understanding of causal pathways defining the factors influencing health and the potential for intervention;

◆ use of different types of evidence to determine *what works for whom in what circumstances*;

◆ translation of evidence into practical guidance for policy and practice, taking account of ethical issues and social values, and understanding the conditions necessary for local implementation;

- relevance to and engagement with governance mechanisms to integrate evidence-based guidance within policy; and

- advancement of understanding of what policies and interventions are effective and cost-effective, and directing strategic investment in research and evaluation to address gaps in the evidence base.

The process of evidence-based public health provides the structure of this book. The sections and chapters demonstrate these features. Figure I.2 below (adapted from Kelly et al 2007) maps the components of the process.

English experience of an evidence-based public health

The experience of England over the last decade provides a country-level example of development of evidence-based public health: 'a process of review of evidence, setting targets, developing a comprehensive strategy and monitoring progress' (DH 2008, Eurothine 2007). It is important to acknowledge that in England certain conditions have proved supportive to the development of this evidence-based approach. These are described below.

Political ideology and values

The social model of health and understanding of the role of social determinants in addressing health inequalities was compatible with the Labour Government's *political ideology and values*, and wider policy agenda of reducing social exclusion and deprivation.

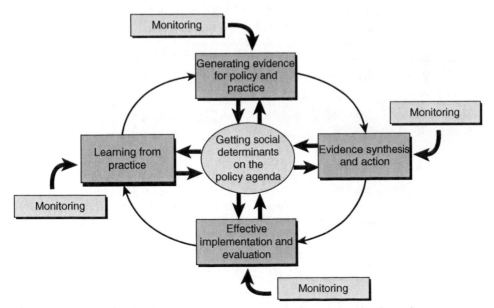

Fig. I.2 Framework for developing, implementing, monitoring, and evaluating policy

Governance

Use of evidence was integral to the Government's *governance mechanisms*, and particularly the performance management and accountability system across the public sector (Public Service Agreements). Long term 'outcome-based' targets are set for government departments. Locally the NHS and local government are expected to meet national standards. In principle these quality standards are based on evidence of what works and are used as measures for interim monitoring of progress towards long term outcomes. Public health became increasingly integrated within this governance system.

In 2001 targets for reducing health inequalities were set for the first time. The target was:

> By 2010 to reduce inequalities in health outcomes by 10% as measured by infant mortality and life expectancy at birth.

This followed the *Independent Inquiry into Inequalities in Health* (the Acheson Inquiry) which reviewed the scientific evidence on health inequalities. The aim was to reduce the social gradient of inequalities in health across the population, rather than only targeting those who are worst off and experiencing the worst health. Achieving the target would be dependent on a faster rate of improvement among those worst off relative to more affluent groups. *Tackling Health Inequalities: A Programme for Action 2003* set out a plan of cross-government commitments to meet the national target. These encompassed a comprehensive range of specific strategies and programmes that addressed both upstream and downstream social determinants of health.

The subsequent national health strategy *Choosing health: making healthier choices* (2004), however, appeared to shift the focus of action from upstream to downstream; emphasizing personal responsibilities for health and promoting individual behavioural approaches to achieving healthy lifestyles. Government's role was defined as supporting individuals making healthier choices. This meant working with industry and the media 'to create the conditions for adopting healthier lifestyles'. Nevertheless, this was set within the broader cross-government strategy tackling the wider social determinants.

Investing in public health research and evidence

There has been increased Government investment in strengthening the evidence base to inform decisions on improving health and reducing health inequalities. Treasury-led reviews of the cost-effectiveness of action for improving health and reducing health inequalities (Wanless 2003, 2004) proved influential in giving impetus to the development of the evidence base. It stated:

> evidence based principles still needed to be established for public health expenditure decisions . . . and that a great deal more discipline is needed to ensure problems are clearly identified and tackled and multiple solutions frequently needed are sensibly coordinated and that lessons are learnt which feed back directly into policy.
>
> (Wanless 2004)

Government investments have sought to strengthen the academic and research infrastructure to provide evidence on the effectiveness of strategies and interventions for improving health and reducing health inequalities. This included the establishment in 2005 of the Centre for Public Health Excellence within the National Institute for Health and Clinical Excellence (through the merger of the Health Development Agency with NICE).

Another development was the establishment of the Public Health Research Consortium in 2005 which brought together researchers from 11 UK institutions to work on an integrated programme of research. The aim was to strengthen the evidence base for interventions to improve health, with a strong emphasis on tackling socio-economic inequalities in health, funded by the Department of Health Policy Research Programme. Since then new arrangements have been put in place for the strategic coordination of UK healthcare research funding, following a major review (Cooksey 2006).

In 2008 five Centres of Excellence in public health were set up designed to strengthen public health research in the UK. The Centres are supported by a partnership of funders including the Economic and Social Research Council (ESRC), the Medical Research Council (MRC), the Wellcome Trust, and other major health charities. The designated Centres are based at five universities in Newcastle, Cardiff, Belfast, Cambridge, and Nottingham.

In addition, many of the specific national strategies concerned with public health priorities have been underpinned by national evaluation programmes. *The Programme for Action* on health inequalities has been subject to regular monitoring based on twelve cross-government national headline indicators covering a combination of disease outcomes (cancer and heart disease), health behaviours (teenage pregnancy, smoking, healthy eating, physical activity), and wider social determinants (housing, educational attainment, children living in low-income households).

The most recent (and final) *Tackling health inequalities: 2007 status report on the programme for action* increases understanding of complex issues involved in monitoring and evaluating the effectiveness of actions to reduce health inequalities (Department of Health 2008). The report demonstrates the major challenges involved in pursuing the dual goals of improving overall health and reducing health inequalities. It showed the relative gap in life expectancy between England as a whole and the areas with the worst health and deprivation indicators (about 28% of the total population) was wider than at the baseline (1995–97). The different target indicators showed different impact on the health gap. This was attributed in part to lag times between actions and health outcomes. The long term trend of widening inequalities in many of the social determinants of health (including smoking, educational attainment, and income) had yet to be reversed. More attention needed to be given to the wider determinants of health (beyond the NHS) and programmes should be extended beyond targeted disadvantaged areas and groups.

The overall approach of a target-driven strategy was supported as part of a European-based review of evidence on the effectiveness of policies and interventions (Eurothine project 2007). Despite conceptual, technical, and implementation issues, use of a range of indicators to monitor progress towards goals was viewed as crucial in assessing effectiveness and securing government accountability for action.

Most recently (May 2009) the document *Tackling health inequalities: 10 years on—a review of developments in tackling health inequalities in England over the last 10 years* has been published by the Department of Health (Department of Health 2009). This examined the changes in policies, social and behavioural determinants, and outcomes that have influenced the pattern of health inequalities since the 1998 Acheson Inquiry. It documented in detail the cross-government policy response across different social determinants and included analyses of differential exposures, vulnerabilities, and consequences (such as health-related behaviours) and differential outcomes in health. This report was intended to be the context for a strategic review that will look forward to 2020 and beyond.

Audience

This book will be of interest to all those concerned with advancing an evidence-based approach to public health and tackling health inequalities; including policy makers, researchers, organizations, and individuals with a public health remit. The book will be a key reference source for students and academics engaged in public health and related disciplines concerned with research and evidence on the effectiveness and cost-effectiveness of programmes and interventions. The book will also be of interest to a range of professionals and policy makers with a public health remit (working across different sectors including health, local government, and education).

Structure of the book

The different parts of the book are designed to cover the main features of evidence-based public health as discussed above.

Part 1 Public health challenges of 21st century: This part sets the context for an evidence-based approach to public health focusing on the experience of the UK. It introduces central themes: a focus on the social determinants of health, the relationship between policy and evidence, and ethical dimensions relating to an evidence-based approach.

Part 2 Evidence-based frameworks: This part sets out a range of conceptual, theoretical, and methodological frameworks that inform the design of public health policies and interventions, and the evaluation of their effectiveness and cost-effectiveness.

Part 3 Generating evidence: This part demonstrates the approaches and methods involved in developing and evaluating complex interventions, through a series of examples of evaluations of different types of public health programmes and interventions.

These represent a range of possible intervention options for improving health and reducing inequalities in health: interventions designed to address the structural, environmental, organizational, social, and behavioural causes of health risk and disease.

Part 4 Synthesizing evidence and developing guidance: This part is concerned with the processes and methods of synthesis of evidence and developing guidance on the effectiveness and cost-effectiveness of public health interventions. Ways of securing implementation of the guidance are also outlined. It draws on the experience of the National Institute for Health and Clinical Excellence (NICE).

Part 5 Knowledge, evidence, and policy: A set of reflections on epistemological, historical and practice issues, relating to the development of an evidence-based approach to public health, are presented here. In particular various schools of thought on how and whether evidence matters are considered. It may be that the real impact of evidence is through 'enlightenment': a process of gradual inculcation of new scientific knowledge and evidence within policy, academic and public discourse and debate, rather than any immediate specific actions.

References

Blas, E, Gilson, L, Kelly, MP, Labonte, R, Lapitan, J, Muntaner, C, Ostlin, P, Popay, J, Sadana, R, Sen, G, Schrecker, T, Vaghri, Z (2008) 'Addressing social determinants of health inequities: what can the state and civil society do?' *The Lancet*, 372: 1684–9

Cochrane, AL (1972) *Effectiveness and efficiency: random reflections on health services.* London: British Medical Journal/Nuffield Provincial Hospitals Trust

CSDH (2008) *Closing the gap in a generation: health equity through action on the social determinants of health.* Geneva: WHO

Cooksey, D (2006) *A review of UK health research finding.* London: Stationery Office

CSDH (2008) *Closing the gap in a generation: health equity through action on the social determinants of health. Final report of the Commission on Social Determinants of Health.* Geneva: WHO

Braveman, P and Gruskin, S (2003) 'Defining equity in health' *J Epidemiol. Community Health*, 57: 254–8

Department of Health (2003) *Tackling health inequalities: a programme for action.* London: Department of Health

Department of Health (2004) *Choosing health: making healthy choices easier.* London: Department of Health

Department of Health (2008) *Tackling health inequalities: 2007 status report on the Programme for Action.* London: Department of Health

Department of Health (2009) *Tackling health inequalities: 10 years on: a review of developments in tackling health inequalities in England over the last 10 years.* London: Department of Health

Eurothine project (2007) *Tackling health inequalities in Europe: an integrated approach.* Rotterdam: Eurothine

Graham, H and Kelly, MP (2004) *Health inequalities: concepts, frameworks and policy.* London: Health Development Agency

Independent Inquiry into Inequalities in Health (Acheson Inquiry) (1998) *Report of the Independent Inquiry into Inequalities in Health.* London: TSO

Kelly, M, Morgan, A, Bonnefoy, J, et al (2007) *The social determinants of health: developing an evidence base for political action.* Geneva: CSDH/WHO. Available at: <http://www.who.int/social_determinants/resources/mekn_final_report_102007.pdf>.

Sen, A (2004) 'Elements of a theory of human rights' *Philosophy & Public Affairs* 32/4: 315–56

Sen, A (2005) 'Human rights & capabilities' *Journal of Human Development* 6/2: 151–66

Solar, O and Irwin, A (2007) *A conceptual framework for action on the social determinants of health.* Geneva: CSDH/WHO

Wanless, D (2003) *Securing our future health: taking a long-term view.* London: HM Treasury

Wanless, D (2004) *Securing good health for the whole population: final report.* London: HM Treasury

Vizard, P and Burchardt, T (2007) *Developing a capability list: final recommendations of the equalities review steering group on measurement.* London: Centre for Analysis of Social Exclusion

Part 1

Public health challenges of the 21st century

Chapter 1

Trends and scenarios in public health in the UK

Mel Bartley and David Blane

Introduction

This chapter considers the nature of future public health challenges in the UK based on an assessment of the socio-economic and demographic context that determines health and disease.

It explores the lessons and implications arising from:

- past trends in social, economic, and demographic influences on health including social and health policy developments;
- current trends in health behaviour risk factors and mortality across social groups; and
- demographic shifts relating to life expectancy particularly at middle age.

Based on this analysis we indicate that understanding of future public health challenges will require extending the scope of the evidence base. Further evidence is needed to understand more precisely the interrelationship between key elements of the social context and behavioural risk factors, and health outcomes. It is clear that public health strategies that focus solely on behavioural risk factors are unlikely to be effective in securing future health improvement and reductions in health inequalities.

Lessons of the past

A decade ago the Office for National Statistics published an authoritative review of the health of the British population during the previous 150 years (Charlton and Murphy 1997). In the first section of this chapter we draw heavily on this work to identify the major socio-economic and demographic influences on past improvements in health and to suggest ways in which the same factors may remain relevant to future trends. Some readers might prefer examples that differ from those offered below, but the range of factors indicated by the sub-headings is worth considering whenever future trends and scenarios are analysed. It is important to consider the big picture in this way because it gives due weight to the factors shaping the more proximal issues within public health such as teenage pregnancy, obesity, tobacco smoking, physical exercise, nutrition, alcohol consumption, and health inequalities.

Changing roles of women Change in the birth rate demonstrates clearly the importance of women's changing roles and expectations—in this case, the desire to limit family size. Between the 1870s and the 1930s in England and Wales the crude fertility rate fell from around 36 to 14 births per 1,000 population (Coleman and Salt 1992). The reduction in family size was achieved in the absence of effective contraceptive aids and despite limited lay knowledge of the subject and the opposition of the medical profession and most other established opinion. Sexual abstinence, *coitus interruptus* and, to a lesser extent, abortion probably were the means by which the fall in birth rate was achieved, with an increase in the age at marriage perhaps also contributing (Burnett 1989). This autonomous change in behaviour coincided with, and probably was generated by, a change in the demographic and socio-economic context of family life. Child death rates were falling, so fewer births were required to ensure inheritance and financial and practical support at older ages. Compulsory education meant that children became an expense rather than a source of household income. And industrialization generated factory jobs for women, with relatively high wages paid year round, increasing the potential income foregone due to raising children. Concurrently, women's organizations had begun to disseminate knowledge about contraception. Lower birth rates and consequent smaller families improved health by increasing household per capita consumption and reducing the number of pregnancies and levels of residential crowding and domestic labour (Bartley et al 1997).

Today, as in most rich countries, the UK birth rate has fallen below replacement levels. Several aspects of socio-economic development are relevant. Women's employment has become more central to economic life. The shift from manufacturing to service industries has removed men's physical advantage. It is no longer possible to denigrate women's earnings as *pin money*; instead these earnings are essential to keep a large proportion of children above the poverty line. The combination of few children, negligible maternal mortality and long female life expectancy makes paid employment a realistic option for most women for most of their lives. Tertiary education followed by professional training mean that a large proportion of a woman's reproductive life has passed by the time they become financially independent and established in a career; and that what remains of their reproductive life coincides with a world of work where long hours are a precondition for career advancement. Any substantial change in this situation is likely to require a shift in *men's* social roles and expectations comparable to that responsible for the initial fall in birth rates. Most men have responded to women's involvement in paid employment by doing more of the household's domestic labour, but as yet there is little sign that most men are prepared to work half-time when raising children. Until this shift in role expectations occurs, it is likely that the birth rate will remain below replacement which, among other things, means a future shortage of family members to provide informal care when kith and kin are sick, disabled, or infirm.

Standard of living The years 1870–1910 in Britain deserve attention because the crude death rate fell by an unprecedented amount, from around 23 to 14 deaths per 1,000 population (Blane 1988; Blane 1989; Blane 1990). Two-thirds of the way through this transition, medical examination of volunteer recruits to the Army for the Boer War screened much of the young male population in Britain during 1897 and 1902, rejecting some 40% as physically or medically unfit (Bartley et al 1997). These young men were part of a society where hard poverty was endemic, particularly during childhood, parent-hood, and old age (Rowntree 1901). Thirty shillings per week were required to support adequate family nutrition (Oddy 1970; Dingle 1972), so protein and calorie malnutrition would have been normal among the families of casual and unskilled workers, such as agricultural labourers, seamen, wool-spinners, cotton-spinners and weavers, engineering workers, and compositors (Bowley 1900). Astonishingly, these levels of hardship were the result of 25 years of rising real wages (Phelps-Brown and Browne 1968), due to the rela-tive movement of prices and money wages and to a shift in industrial employment from casual work in workshops to more regular work in factories (Wood 1909). Unemployed people were excluded from these improvements; instead their situation worsened with the introduction of Able-Bodied Test Workhouses, Stoneyards and Labour Yards (Webb and Webb 1929). The Boer War army volunteers, in consequence, grew up at a time of rising real wages but increased privation for the unemployed, when perhaps half of the working class, which itself comprised some three-quarters of the total population, was at risk of poverty and protein and calorie malnutrition.

Future trends in health and mortality may be similarly influenced by change in real wages, patterns of employment, and the social distribution of disadvantage. Material affluence in UK, as measured by gross domestic product per person, increased from around £3,000 in the mid 1940s to over £8,000 (at constant prices) in the mid 1990s (Bartley et al 1997). Health benefits followed the near universal spread of refrigerators (food hygiene; fresh food), washing machines and bathrooms (personal hygiene), central heating (residential warmth), telephones (social participation), holidays away from home (health) and more varied nutrition (health). Over the same period of time, motor car ownership increased from around 50 to 450 per 1,000 population, with more contradic-tory health effects; the growth of suburbs and commuting from rural areas allowed less residential crowding, but motor vehicle accidents rose and the demise of more energetic forms of travel contributed to rising levels of obesity. Future trends are likely to be influ-enced by whether material affluence continues to increase in a world of globalization, new industrial powers, and global warming; and by the level of success in containing the health-damaging effects of affluence (motor vehicle accidents, obesity, and so on). Population-wide trends obscure social distributions which also are important, particu-larly to health inequalities. Recent estimates, based on the best scientific evidence, of the minimum income for healthy living for a single young man (Morris et al 2000) and a retired single person and couple (Morris et al 2007) found sizeable discrepancies. The minimum income for healthy living for a young man was more than the statutory minimum wage for 40 hours per week and considerably more than welfare benefits if unemployed. Similarly, the minimum income for healthy living for retired people was greater than the pension credit guarantee and considerably more than the state retire-ment pension. Progress on reducing health inequalities may be influenced by whether these discrepancies are addressed.

Technology During the whole of the first half of the twentieth century, around 30 daily train journeys were made per 1,000 population in Britain, made possible by high levels of track laying during the late nineteenth century (Bartley et al 1997). The application of rail technology to the mass transportation of commuters allowed population density to fall in the great cities and industrial towns, where by the 1911 Census some 80% of the population lived. Suburbs, linked by rail to city centre, were built on the marginal land of brick-fields, market gardens, and stables. More affluent employees from the professions, administration and management and clerical grades commuted between city centre and suburbs, where the air was cleaner and housing more spacious. Decanting the more afflu-ent from city centres increased the space available to the manual workers who remained, although such improvements were modest (parents, for example, gaining a separate bed-room from their children)—cooking and food storage remained rudimentary and toilet and washing facilities mostly were shared between households.

Falling population density benefited health through reduced crowding (spread of infectious diseases), access to basic facilities (nutrition and hygiene), greater quiet (education), and privacy (psychological and sexual development). Technologies with comparable impact in future might include information technology, which offers the prospect of new knowledge through linking medical records, a more medically informed lay population through use of internet inquiry, and medical consultation and prescribing at a distance.

Social policy During the latter two-thirds of the nineteenth century, receipt of welfare benefit in Britain was conditional on entry to a workhouse where the regime was intended to deter claimants by, for example, separating husbands, wives, and children and provid-ing conditions worse than those of the poorest labourer (*principle of less eligibility*). The workhouse's primary function of deterring the able-bodied poor through privation and stigma was undermined by urbanization which moved many people from their village origins where the extended family had a duty of care. The workhouse for many urban residents became the only source of shelter or care when ill, old, or orphaned. In an attempt to separate such 'deserving poor' from the unemployed ('able-bodied poor'), workhouses increasingly established first sick wards and then separate infirmaries, which later were incorporated as hospitals into the National Health Service (Bartley et al 1997).

Two features of the workhouse system continue to the present day; namely, attempts to distinguish between the 'deserving poor' and those seen as claiming benefit through idleness or immorality and, second, attempts to motivate paid employment by keeping welfare benefits below wage levels in the unskilled labour market, with the resultant 'poverty trap' where claimants moving into paid employment lose 80–90p in benefit for every £1 they earn as wages, making them in effect the most highly taxed people in the country. The 'deserving poor' largely are people in poor health. Traditionally, their com-bination of poverty and chronic morbidity has been associated with relative neglect by health care services, which is likely to worsen if such care is opened further to market forces.

Health policy One of the most effective health policies was the nineteenth century response to urbanization in Britain. Previously, sewers were designed to drain surface water; in dry spells they allowed stagnant sewage to seep into the ground water and pollute drinking supplies. This ill-designed system was swamped by rapid urbanization, leading to endemic diarrhoea and epidemic typhoid and cholera (Smith 1979). A series of Acts of Parliament established health boards in the most unhealthy areas to improve sewage disposal and water supply (Public Health Act 1848), prohibited the extraction of drinking water from sources highly polluted by sewage (Metropolitan Water Act 1852) and empowered local authorities to raise funds for the construction of sewers and piped water (Local Government Act 1888). In 1865 Bazalgette completed his London sewage works which still deals with up to 400 million gallons of sewage each day (Flinn 1965).

The separation of sewage from drinking water quickly reduced death from enteric infection. The last epidemic of cholera in Britain took place in 1866 and typhoid mortality fell from 1.2 deaths per 1,000 population in 1847–1850 to 0.07 in 1906–1910 (Parliamentary Papers 1916 vol V, in Smith 1979). A contemporary issue of comparable importance is obesity. The consensus view is that greater amounts of daily physical exercise will be part of the solution, but will financial investment on the scale that produced urban sewers be forthcoming for bicycle tracks, footpaths, swimming pools, and playing fields?

Economic development The British economy during the nineteenth century shifted from one that was primarily rural and agricultural to one that was urban and industrial. Some of the health consequences of this shift were beneficial, if slow in coming, such as the increase in living standards (see *standard of living* section above). Others were newly created and eventually solved, such as inadequate sewage disposal (see *health policy* section above). In addition, new industrial diseases (byssinosis, asbestosis, pneumoconiosis, and so forth) appeared that were identified eventually, although effective treatments never emerged.

A comparable transition occurred in the late twentieth century in Britain when de-industrialization eliminated mass production in many industries; coalmining, steel making, shipbuilding, ceramics, textiles, motor car production, and trawler fishing are examples. Nevertheless, the number of jobs in the economy continued to increase in the longer term, with office jobs in, for example, call centres, administration, and finance replacing those in industry. The health consequences of the new economy are unclear as yet. Will living standards continue to improve? Are new problems being created (obesity perhaps) that eventually will be solved? Are new occupational diseases emerging?

Summary When predicting future trends and scenarios in public health it is sensible to consider the lessons of the past. The preceding brief discussion has suggested that such analyses should include consideration of subjective factors, standard of living, technology, social policy, health policy, and economic development. All have profoundly influenced the health of the British population in the past; and are likely to do so in the future.

Current trends

Evidence for the effectiveness of health education aimed at behavioural change can be taken from the trend data in two ways. First, it is possible to examine changes in tobacco smoking over a long period of time (Jarvis 1997) and changes in other lifestyle factors over the past two decades (Bartley et al 2000). Second, it is possible to relate changes in the behaviour of different socio-economic groups to group-specific trends in their health. Taking account of both types of trend, time and social class, adds to the relevance of the evidence for policy.

Time trends Explanations for more recent health trends have focused on the role of health-related behaviors. Improvements in life expectancy have been due to a very large degree to reductions in mortality from heart disease. Since the publication of the reports on the hazards of tobacco smoking by the UK Royal College of Physicians in 1962 and the US Surgeon-General in 1964, tobacco smoking has become the main target for health education and health promotion, directed initially at lung cancer. These policies have had a large degree of success in reducing rates of smoking. By the late 1980s, smoking prevalence in the UK had reduced during the previous decade from over 50% to around 35% in men and from 41% to 31% in women (Pierce 1989).

When other studies indicated that sedentary lifestyles and high fat diets were also implicated in the aetiology of heart disease, health education messages extended to these areas, although nationally representative data were not collected on these topics until the 1980s. In 1984 the first national survey to include a comprehensive list of risk factor measurement, the Health and Lifestyle Survey, was carried out in Great Britain (Blaxter 1990). No other similar studies followed for a decade, until the inception in 1993 of the annual Health Surveys for England (Bennet 1995); joined later by similar surveys in Scotland and Wales.

These surveys made it possible from the mid 1980s to begin to trace changes in health behaviours over time in representative samples of the British population, which can be compared with the American National Health and Nutrition Surveys (NHANES). Although it is not possible to investigate changes in risk factor profiles over the period when the sharp decline in heart disease mortality and associated increase in life expectancy began during the 1970s, it is possible to examine changes in risk factors from the mid 1980s.

Social class trends Bartley and colleagues (Bartley et al 2000) examined social class-specific changes in a wide range of risk factors for cardiovascular disease between 1984 and 1993, using respectively the Health and Lifestyle Survey and Health Survey for England. The risk factors examined were: body mass index, waist–hip ratio, blood pressure, diabetes, diet, physical inactivity, and social support. From the data on social class differences in smoking over the decade 1974–1984, it had been expected that health education would have had the perverse consequence of increasing health inequality by leading to faster uptake of health advice in those in the more advantaged social classes, who tend to have higher education levels and more leisure time (Jarvis 1997). The results of the study showed, surprisingly, that although overall levels of some risk factors had declined, they had done so in a similar manner in all social classes (Figure 1.1). For example, smoking fell from 25% to 20% over the period in men in higher managerial and professional social classes, and from 51% to 42% in semi- and unskilled manual classes; a difference in the rate of change that was not statistically significant. Similar results were seen for eating fruit less than once a day, drinking high-fat milk, and non-participation in active sport. The proportions eating vegetables less than once a day actually increased to a similar extent across the social scale. Although the rates of less healthy behaviour remained higher in semi- and unskilled manual groups, the gap between the more and less advantaged social classes did not change significantly when a formal statistical test was carried out.

Another unexpected finding was that apparent improvement in sport participation and diet (although caloric intake was not measured) had been accompanied by an increase in body mass index which was similar in all social classes. Interestingly, the prevalence of angina pectoris had declined, but the proportions of men with diabetes or some other long-standing illness had increased. One reason for this may have been the major increase in the proportions being treated for high blood pressure—treatment may have reduced the social difference in measured blood pressure, which did decline although not significantly, at the cost of increasing the number of men who regarded themselves as having a chronic illness (Bartley et al 2000).

The exception to the rule of no significant change in the degree of social inequality in risk factors and health behaviours was seen in a measure of psychological well-being—the General Health Questionnaire, which is used widely in population surveys to measure psychological health (a high GHQ score indicates a high probability that a clinical interview would yield a diagnosis of depression or anxiety). In men in the semi- and unskilled manual social classes, the prevalence of psychological distress, as measured by GHQ

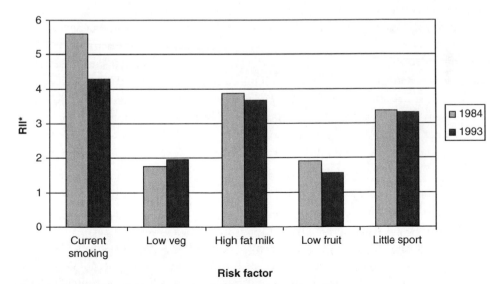

Fig. 1.1 Change in social inequality in CHD risk factors 1984–1993
* Relative Index of Inequality (RII) gives the size of the difference between the least and most advantaged social classes, taking into account levels of risk in all intermediate classes.

score, reduced sharply between 1984 and 1993, whereas in higher level managers and professionals it fell far less. Thus, at a time when inequalities in mortality were increasing, inequalities in mental health according to this measure were decreasing (Bartley et al 2000).

Although these results were unexpected, they are consistent with the rather scant literature on the topic from the same time period. Social gradients in risk factors did not increase in USA (Irrbarren et al 1997) or Australia (Bennett 1995). In Finland, where uniquely at present it is possible to link changes in health behaviour to mortality of the same individuals, an even more relevant finding emerged. This confirmed a decrease in many forms of health risk behaviours, but also showed that the same decrease across different social classes was associated with a greater decline in mortality risk among the more advantaged than among the less advantaged social classes (Vartiainen et al 1998).

Summary Time trend data give some support for an evidence-based public health decision to focus on health behaviours and risk factor change. The relationship between tobacco smoking's falling prevalence and the reduction in lung cancer mortality is persuasive, although the lag time between this cause and its effect remains under-researched and somewhat contentious. Other evidence is less supportive; for example, falling ischaemic heart disease mortality at a time of rising obesity and reduced physical exercise. Such reservations become stronger when social class trends in risk factor change are considered, because social class differences in mortality have increased despite most risk factors changing at similar rates in all social classes.

Future challenges

We are living through an extraordinary demographic transition in Britain. Life expectancy at middle age increased more during the final three decades of the twentieth century than during its first 70 years. The change was more striking among men, but also affected women. The actuarial profession and life insurance industry are concerned by its implications for the financial soundness of pension schemes and the market in annuities. Health care planners anticipate more patients with the diseases of old age and increased demand for their care. The implications for public health depend on assumptions about its cause. If it is assumed to be a one-off gain from tobacco smoking cessation, then the rate of increase in middle age life expectancy should return to its earlier levels. If it is assumed to be due to medical innovation, then the present rate of increase is likely to continue into the future. This section examines the phenomenon in a little more detail.

Life expectancy at middle age Male life expectancy at age 50 years during 1901–1971 increased by an average of 0.6 years per decade, while during 1971–2001 the mean increase per decade was 1.8 years. The equivalent figures for women were 1.0 and 1.2 years per decade (Government Actuary's Department). So, middle-aged life expectancy for both men and women increased decade on decade throughout the whole twentieth century; for most of the century the male increase was only 60% of the female rate; after 1970 the male rate jumped from 60% to 150% of the female rate. Which poses the questions: what happened to men in 1970; and was the cause contemporaneous or earlier, with lagged effects? The specific diseases contributing to the change offer some clues.

To date most attempts to understand the fall in mortality rates at middle age have concentrated on coronary heart disease, which is the most prevalent cause of death (Unal, Critchley, and Capewell 2004; Unal et al 2005). This focus on one cause of death has distracted attention from the bigger picture, in which the change in cause-specific mortality rates has been similar for all of the most prevalent causes of death (Figure 1.2). During 1971–2002, among men in England and Wales, ischaemic heart disease mortality fell by 53.0%, cerebrovascular disease by 55.2%, lung cancer 47.5%, chronic obstructive pulmonary disease 57.9%, pneumonia 57.8%, stomach cancer 65.3%. Within this broadly similar reduction in rates, three patterns of decade change can be seen. An accelerating rate of fall, as illustrated by ischaemic heart disease mortality which fell by 4% during 1971–1981, 18% during 1981–1991 and 40% during 1991–2002. Second, a U-shaped fall, as illustrated by chronic obstructive pulmonary disease, with a 28% fall during 1971–1981, 11% during 1981–1991, and 35% during 1991–2002. Finally, a hump-backed fall, illustrated by pneumonia's 14% fall during 1971–1981, 62% during 1981–1991, and 2% during 1991–2002 (Office for National Statistics 2003).

The hunt for causes It is challenging to fit such observations to explanations of the fall in mortality. In some cases, such as cerebrovascular disease and stomach cancer, the recent fall is part of a long term trend stretching back to the early twentieth century (Charlton and Murphy 1997), while in other cases like ischaemic heart disease the recent fall follows several decades of explosive growth. Also, it is difficult to see how one factor could account for similar rates of fall in the different diseases. Tobacco smoking is associated with the six prevalent diseases mentioned in the previous paragraph, but its aetiological role is greatest for lung cancer, which has fallen least, and probably smallest for stomach cancer

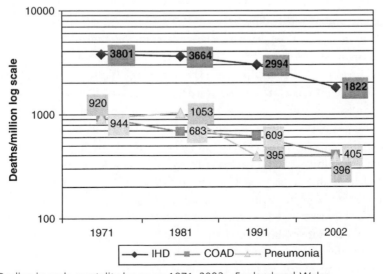

Fig. 1.2 Decline in male mortality by cause 1971–2002—England and Wales

which has fallen most. Further, the cumulative decline in the prevalence of tobacco smoking does not fit easily with either the U-shaped or the hump-backed pattern of decade-by-decade mortality decline. The same arguments apply to medical innovations. While it can be argued that the clinical treatment of hypertension has contributed to the fall in mortality from cerebrovascular disease and that the modern battery of medical and surgical interventions has affected mortality from ischaemic heart disease, it is more difficult to suggest which clinical responses to lung cancer, chronic obstructive pulmonary disease, and stomach cancer could have produced a proportionately similar fall in their mortality rates, let alone their decade-by-decade heterogeneity.

At first sight it is tempting to ask whether wider social change, specifically an unanticipated consequence of de-industrialization in the 1970s and 1980s, might have been at least partly responsible for the change in mortality rates which started in 1970 and had a bigger impact on men than women. The change in mortality by social class does not fit this picture, however, because de-industrialization would have had a greater impact on manual than white-collar workers. In fact the changes were greater for the more advantaged social classes. Male life expectancy at age 65 years in social classes I and II increased by, respectively, 3.3 years and 3.4 years between the early 1970s and the late 1990s, compared with 1.1 year and 1.8 years in social classes IV and V; the comparable figures for women were 1.5 years and 2.8 years versus 0.6 years and –0.1 years (Hattersley 1997). This social class distribution of mortality improvement is part of a longer term trend where, it is sobering to recall, the mortality rate of men aged 55–64 years in 1991 was higher than that of social class I men of the same age in 1921; 2484 versus 2247 deaths per 100,000 (Blane, Bartley, and Davey Smith 1997).

Future research The proper response undoubtedly is to recognize the intellectual challenge posed by the current demographic shift in life expectancy at middle age. We need to research its causes if we are to make informed predictions of future trends. Predictably the actuaries are ahead of public health in this respect. A recent small scale survey by a leading actuary found widely differing estimates among senior epidemiologists of trends to Year 2015 in some of the drivers of heart disease and cancer mortality, including tobacco smoking, systolic blood pressure, total cholesterol, obesity, heart disease treatments, and breast cancer and other cancer treatments (Willets 2008). A range of possibilities needs to be investigated. Could artefactual processes, such as a change in coding rules, account for the difference between pneumonia's hump-backed mortality change and the U-shaped pattern of chronic obstructive pulmonary disease? Does the timing of the introduction and spread of medical interventions for the acute treatment of myocardial infarction and the prevention of hypertension match the fall in mortality from ischaemic heart disease and cerebrovascular disease? What is the lag time between tobacco smoking cessation and the return to near-normal risk of death from lung cancer and ischaemic heart disease; and how well does the fall in tobacco smoking prevalence match the lagged change in mortality from these diseases? Is it possible to estimate the increase in resilience to disease that might be expected from such factors as a more varied diet, longer holidays, and a working life which is shorter because labour force entry is delayed by prolonged education and exit is brought forward by early retirement? Better diet would improve immune function, the body's ability to fight infection. Less time spent in the labour force would mean that people's exposure to physical and psychosocial risks increasingly took place at the healthiest period of the life course. Answering these component questions is a precondition to an evidence-based understanding of future trends in public health.

Conclusions

The present chapter has offered an account of public health that (1) is based in the socio-economic and demographic context of the processes and behaviours which produce health and disease and (2) uses mortality data, and their distribution by social class and gender, to identify major changes and test ideas about their cause.

The chapter started by examining the lessons of the past and thereby identified a number of interesting questions, by no means exhaustive, that are likely to be relevant to future trends and scenarios in public health. The questions included the following:

- What would be required for men, as a matter of course, to work part-time when their children are young?

- Is it possible to ensure for all citizens the minimum income for healthy living?

- Can the potential contribution of information technology to health research, lay knowledge, and medical consultation be enhanced and integrated?

- What will be the intended and unintended consequences for public health of ongoing policy initiatives in relation to chronically sick and disabled people of working age?

- How can a major expansion of investment in bicycle tracks, footpaths, swimming pools, and sports fields be achieved?

- What are the health consequences of the new, de-industrialized economy, in terms of living standards, endemic pathology, and occupational disease?

Emphasis on the socio-economic and demographic context runs somewhat counter to public health's current concerns, which largely focus on the behaviours that may be proximal to health and disease. The second section of the present chapter can be read as a caution against sole reliance on this risk factor approach. Recent change in the prevalence of the main cardiovascular disease risk factors are found to vary by social class in a way that does not match easily with recent class-specific change in coronary heart disease mortality. For some risk factors, such as tobacco smoking, the social class distribution of risk factor change is in the same direction as, and contemporaneous with, the class distribution of change in coronary heart disease mortality. For other risk factors, such as social support, the relationship is in the opposite direction; the risk factor worsens among all social classes at the same time as mortality improves, particularly among the middle class. Finally, there is a third category where risk factor and mortality can only be seen as matching if a lag period is accepted between cause and effect. One benefit of these analyses is to give attention to the idea of a lag between risk factor change and health change. At present the idea tends to be used opportunistically, as a *post hoc* explanation when inconsistencies are found in the evidence, and inconsistently, in the sense that no consensus exists on the length of the lag time between change in specific risk factors and their health outcomes. A more scientific approach to lag times should be part of evidence-based public health. Of equal importance, the lack of a simple and straightforward match between change in cardiovascular disease risk factors and change in coronary heart disease mortality suggests it would be premature for public health to concentrate exclusively on risk factor change.

The third section of the present chapter uses the major demographic shift of our time to illustrate the need for the scientific basis of public health to incorporate both risk factor change, for example tobacco smoking, and changes in the socio-economic context, such as earlier retirement from paid employment, together with new concepts such as resilience which can allow public health to reclaim the health part of its title. This broader approach is evidence-based and promises an effective public health.

Acknowledgement

The authors acknowledge with gratitude the support of UK Economic and Social Research Council award number RES-596-28-00.

Bibliography

Bartley, M, Blane, D, and Charlton, J (1997) 'Socioeconomic and demographic trends 1841–1994', in J Charlton and M Murphy (ed), *The Health of Adult Britain 1841–1994*. Volumes 1 and 2, pp 74–92. London: The Stationery Office

Bartley, M, Fitzpatrick, R, Firth, D, and Marmot, M (2000) 'Social distribution of cardiovascular disease risk factors: change among men in England 1984–1993' *Journal of Epidemiology and Community Health* 54: 806–14.

Bennett, S (1995) 'Cardiovascular risk-factors in australia—trends in socioeconomic inequalities' *Journal of Epidemiology and Community Health* 49: 363–72

Blane, D (1990) 'Real wages, the economic cycle and mortality in England and Wales' *International Journal of Health Services* 20: 43–52

Blane, D (1988) 'Labour theory of value and health', in G Scambler (ed), *Sociological Theory and Medical Sociology*, pp 8–36. London: Tavistock

Blane, D, Bartley, M, and Davey Smith, G (1977) 'Disease aetiology and materialist explanations of socioeconomic mortality differentials' *European Journal of Public Health* 7: 385–91

Blane, D (1989) 'Preventive medicine and public health: England and Wales 1870–1914', in C Martin and D McQueen (ed), *Readings for a New Public Health*, pp 7–12. Edinburgh: Edinburgh University Press

Blaxter, M (1990) *Health and lifestyles*. London: Tavistock

Bowley, A (1900) *Wages in the United Kingdom in the nineteenth century*. Cambridge: Cambridge University Press

Burnett, J (1989) *Plenty and want: a social history of diet in England from 1815 to the present day*. 3rd edn. London: Routledge

Charlton, J and Murphy, M (1997) *The health of adult Britain 1841–1994*. Volumes 1 and 2. London: HMSO

Coleman, D and Salt, J (1992) *The British population*. Oxford: Oxford University Press

Dingle, A (1972) 'Drink and working class living standards in Britain 1870–1914' *Economic History Review* 25: 608–22

Drever, F and Whitehead, M (1997) *Health inequalities*. London: HMSO

Flinn, M (ed) (1965) *Chadwick's 1842 Report on the Sanitary Condition of the Labouring Population of Great Britain*, with introduction by Flinn. Edinburgh: Edinburgh University Press

Government Actuary's Department (n.d.) *English life tables: life expectancy 1901–2001*. <http://www.gad.gov.uk/Demography%20Data/Life%20Tables/Historic_interim_life_tables.html>.

Hattersley, L (1997) 'Expectation of life by social class', in F Drever and M Whitehead (ed), *Health inequalities*, pp 73–82. London: TSO

Irbarren, C, Luepker, RV, McGovern, PG, Arnett, DK, and Blackburn, H (1997) 'Twelve-year trends in cardiovascular disease risk factors in the Minnesota Heart Survey. Are socioeconomic differences widening?' *Archives of Internal Medicine* 157: 873–81

Jarvis, M (1997) 'Patterns and predictors of smoking cessation in the general population', in C Bolliger and K Fagerstrom (ed), *Progress in respiratory research: the tobacco epidemic*, pp 151–64. Basel: S Karger

Morris, JN, Donkin, AJM, Wonderling, D, Wilkinson, P, and Dowler, EA (2000) 'A minimum income for healthy living' *Journal of Epidemiology and Community Health* 54: 885–9

Morris, JN, Wilkinson, P, Dangour, A, Deeming, C, Fletcher, A (2007) 'Defining a minimum income for healthy living (MIHL): older age, England' *International Journal of Epidemiology* 36: 1300–7

Oddy, D (1970) 'Working class diets in nineteenth century Britain' *Economic History Review* 23: 314–322

Office for National Statistics (2003) 'Deaths: selected causes' *Health Statistics Quarterly* 20: 58–9 (Table 6.3)

Phelps-Brown, E and Browne, M (1968) *A Century of Pay*. London: St Martin's

Pierce, J (1989) 'International comparisons of trends in cigarette smoking prevalence' *American Journal of Public Health* 79: 152–7

Rowntree, S (1901) *Poverty*. London: Macmillan

Smith, F (1979) *The People's Health*. London: Croom Helm

Unal, B, Critchley, JA, and Capewell, S (2004) 'Explaining the Decline in Coronary Heart Disease Mortality in England and Wales Between 1981 and 2000' *Circulation* 109: 1101–7

Unal, B, Critchley, JA, Fidan, D, and Capewell, S (2005) 'Life-years gained from modern cardiological treatments and population risk factor changes in England and Wales, 1981–2000' *American Journal of Public Health* 95: 103–8

Vartiainen, E, Pekkanen, J, Koskinen, S, Jousilhati, P, Salomaa, V, and Puska, P (1998) 'Do changes in cardiovascular risk factors explain the increasing economic difference in mortality from ischaemic heart disease in Finland?' *Journal of Epidemiology and Community Health* 52/7: 416–9

Webb, S and Webb, B (1929) *English poor law history, Part II: the last hundred years. English local government*, Volumes 8–9. London: Cass

Willets, R (2008) *Obtaining the views of epidemiologists on future mortality change*. London: Paternoster

Wood, G (1909) 'Real wages and the standard of comfort since 1850' *Journal of the Royal Statistical Society* 72: 91–103

Chapter 2

Policy and evidence-based public health

Catherine Law

Introduction

In the 1999 *Modernising Government* white paper, the UK Government, then newly in power, noted that it 'must produce policies that really deal with problems, that are forward-looking and shaped by evidence rather than a response to short-term pressure' (Great Britain Cabinet Office 1999). A recent 'Google' search for the phrase 'evidence-based policy' returned almost 16,000 hits from UK Government websites, suggesting widespread practical as well as official acceptance of the need for evidence-based policy. However, this acceptance has been followed by increasing recognition of the challenges of using evidence to shape policies. As the DEFRA website notes, 'all policies are based on evidence—the question is more whether the evidence itself, and the processes through which this evidence is put to turn it into policy options, are of sufficiently high quality' (Department for Environment, Food and Rural Affairs 2006).

The term 'evidence-based policy' also begs a question: what counts as 'evidence'. Researchers tend to see this as deriving from research—in short, to be scientific knowledge (Porta 2008). However, in reflecting on the processes of policy making, Lomas describes the use of 'information', which can include not only research but also anecdote, experience, and even propaganda (Lomas 2000). This chapter will concentrate on the role of scientific research in evidence-based public health policy. This is neither to downplay the importance of other types of information in a democratic process nor to ignore legitimate influences on policy making other than information, such as social, electoral, ethical, cultural, and economic considerations (Black 2001). Rather, the chapter focuses on the usefulness and potential of scientific knowledge amongst the many influences on the complex process of policy making.

Coupled with the recognition of the use of evidence in health policy is the current climate of support for research. Research funding has increased considerably in recent years (HM Treasury 2007). Whilst this has been partly to enhance commercial competitiveness, research for public good has also been prominent in recent strategic documents highlighting the value (financially and otherwise) of applied health research (Cooksey 2006; Department of Health 2006).

Yet despite this positive recent history, the use of research evidence in public health policy poses many challenges. This chapter will introduce these challenges, drawing on examples from international, national, and local policy making. It will first consider the need for evidence within policy processes and then go on to discuss the usefulness of the current evidence base, highlighting some of the gaps. It will discuss some of the challenges in using and developing the evidence base, illustrating the clashes between research and policy cultures and processes, and where progress is being made. Finally it will consider how policy influences research and how this field may develop in the future.

The need for evidence

Public health is 'the science and art of preventing disease, prolonging life and promoting health through the organized efforts of society' (Acheson 1988). As well as valuing information other than science, this definition also implies that policy making for public health will be carried out by a range of organizations within society—government departments (including but not limited to health), other public bodies, commercial enterprises, and voluntary organizations—and that this policy making operates at different levels: international, national, and local. Health care policy is an important element in the fight to promote public health, but policy for health will be made by most policy-making organizations, even though many will not categorize or even recognize it as such.

Policy making is not a discrete event but a continuous process, often depicted as a cycle (Davies et al 2000; HM Treasury 2003). This may be described as starting with a description of the problem for which policy is desired, and then being followed by a cycle of policy development and specification, implementation, assessment of impact, learning from the experience, and then contributing that learning to further policy development. Each stage of this cycle (as well as the description of the problem) can either be informed by evidence (which can be derived from theoretical or empirical sources, and through a variety of methods), or generate new evidence. Of course policy making can also be prosecuted without reference to the evidence. But using the evidence carries with it a number of potential advantages. First, it allows policy makers to learn from the successes and failures of others. For example, international experience of banning tobacco advertising informed the development of similar policies in the UK (Action on Smoking and Health 2006). Second, research can be used to assess whether or not a policy actually achieves its desired outcomes. The evaluation of the Sure Start programme, described elsewhere in this book, is a good example of this (National Evaluation of Sure Start 2008). However, policies are not infrequently introduced either without any intention to assess their impact or with the assumption that an evaluation will show that the policy was beneficial, often by demonstrating activity rather than effectiveness (Judge and Bauld 2006). Third, use of the evidence should promote efficiency, for example by identifying groups of people most in need or for whom a policy would be ineffective. Fourth, assessment of impact and the development of policy learning should make future policy making easier. Set against these seemingly obvious advantages are the costs of evidence generation and gathering in terms of time and money, commodities of critical importance to policy makers, and the political risk of promoting a policy which is subsequently proven to be unsuccessful or harmful.

Usefulness of current evidence base

A challenge to the greater use of evidence in public health policy is the current state of the evidence base. Numerous academic and policy commentators have commented not only on the small size of the body of knowledge but also its nature and specific gaps (Department of Health 1999; Independent Inquiry into Inequalities in Health 1998; Wellcome Trust Public Health Sciences Working Group 2004). For example, much research illuminates the scale of the problems in public health, or describes their nature, but less is focused on interventions to change those problems (Millward et al 2003; Petticrew et al 2004). Whilst description of public health problems can inform policy development, and so should not be undervalued, it is insufficient for informed political action. Furthermore, studies of interventions tend to be focused on relatively small scale actions, and much less frequently test complex interventions or policies. Health economics research is a particular gap in the evidence. Sir Derek Wanless's 2004 report, *Securing Good Health for the Whole Population*, considered that 'the major constraint to further progress on the implementation of public health interventions is the weakness of the evidence base', noting particularly the lack of information about cost-effectiveness (Wanless 2004).

Arguably, development of the evidence base in public health has been both hindered and promoted by the parallel rise to prominence of evidence-based medicine. On the one hand, evidence-based medicine has established the value of evidence in the minds of many practitioners and managers, leading to greater sophistication in the health system workforce. On the other hand, the perceived dominance of particular research designs, particularly the randomized controlled trial, in evidence-based medicine, may have focused attention towards public health research on the proximal rather than distal causes of public health problems. This in turn may have led to a preponderance of simple, individual level interventions delivered in the health care system rather than complex interventions directed at the wider determinants of health that more closely resemble the actions of policy making. For example, one of the main direct causes of inequalities in adult health and life expectancy is the social patterning of smoking and smoking-related diseases. Though research has shown that pharmacological therapies and smoking cessation services are effective in helping individual cigarette smokers to quit (National Institute for Health and Clinical Excellence 2008a), the links between disadvantage and smoking are deeply entrenched in society and it is unlikely that health service interventions alone will break those links (Graham et al 2006).

It is often said that policy makers need to know 'what works, for whom, in what circumstances' (Pawson et al 2005; Pawson and Tilley 1997). A dissection of the research needed to inform such an apparently reasonable request reveals why the current evidence base is so limited. Few intervention studies are large enough to be able to study differential effectiveness, nor do they often include all target groups of interest. For example, there are few studies of interventions to promote the health of marginalized groups such as people who are homeless (Power et al 1999) or children in the care of public authorities (Cocker and Scott 2006). Understanding the influence of different circumstances on effectiveness implies comparative research across a range of settings as well as the need to employ qualitative and quantitative research methods. And many of the answers to 'what works, for whom and in what circumstances' can only be derived from syntheses of studies, bringing a wide range of evidence and study designs together.

Challenges in developing and using the evidence base

Synthesizing evidence

Striking historical examples demonstrate the potentially tragic consequences of ignoring the evidence. A cumulative meta-analysis of the relationship of infant sleeping position and sudden infant death syndrome (SIDS) showed that, although research studies indicated that prone sleeping was a risk factor for SIDS from 1970 onwards, the evidence was not collated to demonstrate this in a convincing way. Advice (from Governments, professionals, and others) in the 1970s and 1980s that babies should or might sleep on their fronts was contrary to this publicly available, but dispersed, evidence. As a result, it is estimated that this 'preventive' advice may have contributed to the deaths of over 10,000 babies in the UK alone (Gilbert et al 2005).

It is an irony that, small though the existing evidence base for public health is, it is almost certainly underused. Policy makers are clear that they value a 'mixed economy' of evidence (Petticrew et al 2004) and researchers have described bringing this together as akin to assembling a jigsaw of evidence (Whitehead et al 2004). Yet such assembled syntheses are thin on the ground. The reasons for this are complex and probably relate to both the capacity and interest in carrying out such work and to methodological development. Systematic review and meta-analysis have developed enormously in recent years, and initiatives such as the Campbell and Cochrane collaborations (Campbell Collaboration 2008; Cochrane Collaboration 2008) are making welcome progress in bringing together what we know in some fields. However, methodology for synthesizing information across different research designs—the 'mixed economy' of research favoured by policy makers—is much less advanced (Dixon-Woods et al 2005). Furthermore, policy makers often ask broad questions, which challenge some of the traditional features of systematic review.

Interpreting evidence

Science is popularly seen as absolute—sound or flawed, right or wrong. That the same research can be interpreted differently implies misunderstanding. But political ideology may determine how facts are interpreted. Under previous Governments, the socio-economic differentials in smoking were seen to reflect individual responsibility (Department of Health 1992). After New Labour came to power in 1997, these same differentials were interpreted as a matter of social injustice, to which the state had a duty to respond (Department of Health 1999).

Related to this, as Marmot has discussed, the willingness to take action may influence decision makers' view of the evidence as much as the evidence influences their willingness to take action. Marmot highlights two reports, published in 2004, on the reduction of alcohol related harm. One report, authored by a group of scientists, came to the conclusion that an important component of a harm reduction strategy was to reduce the average level of consumption of alcohol in the general population (Academy of Medical Sciences 2004). The other report, from the Prime Minister's strategy unit, concluded that this was not viable because the main mechanisms of achieving it, reducing access and increasing price, had unwanted side effects (Prime Minister's Strategy Unit 2004). Both considered the same evidence and came to opposite conclusions on the desirability of a specific action, presumably related to both explicit and implicit values (Marmot 2004).

A further barrier to interpreting the evidence is that researchers and policy makers tend to operate in separate worlds, and may be in relative ignorance of each other's culture, methods, processes and needs. For example, policy makers' needs are often not taken into account when reporting research, whilst they find the importance that researchers place on the uncertainties and ambiguities of research findings unhelpful. In particular, policy makers have highlighted their wish for researchers to draw out the policy implications of research, although to achieve this is likely to require further academic training and joint working across research and policy communities (Black 2001; Petticrew et al 2004; Wellcome Trust Public Health Sciences Working Group 2004; Whitehead et al 2004).

Taking evidence-based decisions

As already noted, challenges to taking evidence-based decisions include the nature of the evidence base, the need to use many sources of evidence, and the different interpretations that can be made of evidence. For nearly all decisions and plans, the evidence base is incomplete. How much evidence is needed before a decision can be made will vary according to the nature of the evidence gaps but is also likely to be influenced by the political imperative to tackle a problem. This, in turn, is driven by other influences such as culture, public opinion, and ideology. Policy makers are cost conscious, risk averse, and often need to demonstrate achievement in short periods. Consequently, the long timescales of research and the lack of health economics evidence are particular barriers to their use of evidence (Petticrew et al 2004; Wanless 2004). Few studies are designed to examine all possible health outcomes, let alone other outcomes of interest to policy makers. Faced with lack of research, policy is sometimes developed on the basis of so-called 'good practice' (Department of Health 2007), but as Judge and Bauld have noted, 'simply documenting activity which is frequently demanded and regularly served up is not evidence of good practice and the growing tendency to pretend it does yields little more than propaganda' (Judge and Bauld 2006). Whilst the experiences and wishes of service users, patients and the public, and the conduct of public health practice are important components of the development and implementation of policy, it is important not to confuse either preference or innovation with effectiveness.

Both science and public policy strive towards change. But scientific work focuses on changing knowledge whereas policy making tries to change everyday lives. Whilst both scientists and policy makers would like proof that something will work, they may place different burdens of proof before they are willing to take decisions. Thus, policy makers may decide that an intervention is likely to be beneficial whereas a researcher will decline to make a judgement until further information is gathered.

Evidence-based policy would also be aided if both policy makers and researchers were explicit that there are some questions that cannot be answered by research, and that hiding behind lack of evidence is sterile, because such evidence will never be forthcoming. For example, the UK has high rates of child poverty compared to many of its European neighbours (UNICEF Innocenti Research Centre 2007), and the Government has pledged to eliminate child poverty by 2020 (Department for Work and Pensions 2006). One of its main strategies is to alleviate family poverty by encouraging one or both parents into paid employment. In the Nordic countries, child poverty is tackled primarily through comprehensive income, tax, and social transfers (Li et al 2008). Which of these strategies is the more effective is impossible to prove through research because a direct comparison is impossible and because the context in which any policy of this kind is implemented is likely to be highly influential on its effectiveness. However, research evidence can still be useful. In a synthesis of evidence commissioned by the Joseph Rowntree Foundation, Hirsch and colleagues used literature review, qualitative research, policy analysis, and economic modelling. They conclude that a focus only on employment in disadvantaged families is unlikely to achieve the Government's targets in reducing child poverty and discuss the different direct and indirect policy options that may be helpful (Hirsch 2006). This report is compelling because it fulfils the requirements articulated by policy makers—a 'mixed economy' of research, relevance to policy, and a focus on evaluation and economics (Petticrew et al 2004).

Using evidence at different levels

How evidence is used in the development of policy is also a function of the level of the policy making. At international level, the multitude of settings and circumstances makes achievement of evidence-based consensus challenging, because of the importance of context in interpreting evidence for policy. Perhaps as a consequence, the recent report of the Commission on Social Determinants of Health makes quite general recommendations across a broad range of actions (Commission on Social Determinants of Health 2008). For example, it calls to international and national policy makers to 'commit to and implement a comprehensive approach to early life, building on existing child survival programmes and extending interventions in early life to indicate social/emotional and language/cognitive development'. Whilst this could be seen as an expression of 'motherhood and apple pie', underneath this general recommendation are detailed and powerful recommendations and argument linked to a full description of the underpinning evidence. Implementing these recommendations will challenge many governments around the world: linking them to the evidence gives ammunition to those who will push for change (Davey Smith and Krieger 2008).

At the opposite end of the scale, local policy makers often lack resource or capacity to collate and interpret evidence. Development of evidence-based methods such as health impact assessment for typical local decision making—planning of housing or industrial projects, for example—have had to be pragmatic in order to be relevant to the policy-making context (Health Development Agency 2002; Joffe and Mindell 2002). In other cases, local interpretation of evidence is inappropriate, because there is no plausible influence of local context. The assessment of cost-effectiveness of new medical technologies by the National Institute for Health and Clinical Excellence (NICE) is a good example. The evidence on effectiveness and cost-effectiveness of a specific new medicine for a given condition in a particular patient is not dependent on where that patient lives, so the decision on whether or not to provide it in the health service does not need to consider the local context. In this case, it is efficient, as well as justifiable and equitable, for a national body such as NICE to review the evidence and take an evidence-based decision which then applies to the whole country (National Institute for Health and Clinical Excellence 2008b).

In other cases, local context, including social, political, and cultural contexts, may be critical to the interpretation of the evidence. For example, under the Water Act 2003, public consultation must precede a request by health authorities to fluoridate the water supply. Water fluoridation is controversial—because evidence of its benefits and harms is uncertain and incomplete, and because it may be seen as mass medication when there are alternative ways of preventing dental caries in those at risk. Proponents and opponents both cite strongly stated evidence-based arguments but both cannot be true. As decisions need to balance evidence on harms and benefits together with social values and individual rights, local debate and decision making seem essential. However, such debate can only be well informed if the evidence, and, in particular, uncertainties in the current and future evidence base, are made explicit and accessible. For example, assurance on the absolute safety of water fluoridation can never be given, because small but important risks, particularly for chronic conditions, would be unlikely to be detectable after water had been fluoridated (Cheng et al 2007).

Policy influences on research

The phrase 'evidence-based policy' implies a linear relationship between evidence and policy, whereby a problem is identified and evidence drives the policy solution. However, many commentators believe that, in practice, such linear relationships are rare, and that an enlightenment model is more prevalent. Under this type of model, described by Weiss amongst others (Weiss 1977), research sets out issues, agendas, and accompanying arguments (Black 2001; Nutley et al 2003; Petticrew et al 2004). In such a model, policy inevitably changes research as well as the reverse.

Policy making is full of checks and balances, and the priorities of policy makers in one government department do not necessarily match those of a colleague in another. For example, public health research requires data gathered at population level. The development of information technology has enhanced statistical analysis but at the same time has increased public demand for greater individual data protection. Policy makers have to balance the public good that may come from population health research against the wishes of millions of individuals about the security of their personal detail. Similarly, reasonable demands in clinical studies to require informed consent for the use of medical records in research may become an intolerable burden for accessing uncontroversial data for whole populations (Wellcome Trust Public Health Sciences Working Group 2004).

However, on other occasions, the influence of policy making on research seems not so much a reflection of pragmatic checks and balances but deliberately perverse. A recent report studied the example of exercise referral schemes. It noted how government policy had promoted exercise referral schemes in the absence of evidence of effectiveness and under the implicit assumption that government commissioned research which was being conducted would show that the schemes were effective. Most independent commentators, including NICE, have remained unconvinced that exercise referral schemes are cost-effective. However, their continuing promotion by the Department of Health means that further research evidence is now extremely difficult to collect, because they are too prevalent to make any kind of controlled comparison possible (Sowden and Raine 2008). On the other hand, insisting that health practitioners only provide services or treatments whilst gathering further evidence can result in disinvestment by health commissioners, which also limits the opportunity to gather further evidence (Chalkidou et al 2007).

One of the most obvious influences of policy on public health research is funding. In the UK, Government or Government funded bodies such as the research councils are important funders of much public health research. Given this, it is perhaps surprising that more research funding is not focused on government priorities (Hawkins and Law 2005; National Cancer Research Institute 2002) and to inform the development of effective policy. For example, not all government initiatives have funded evaluation built in at the outset. The recent change from the Welfare Food Scheme to Healthy Start to improve early years nutrition amongst disadvantaged families has been rolled out without any evaluation of effectiveness (Healthy Start 2008). By contrast, the Sure Start initiative, also focused on the early years and in disadvantaged communities, was accompanied by a planned long running evaluation, albeit constrained by the lack of standardization in the programme and without the benefits of random allocation (National Evaluation of Sure Start 2008). The fact that government both designs policies and funds their evaluations affords a unique (but underused) opportunity for development of the evidence base by introducing new policies in ways which would facilitate assessment of effectiveness. And, as Macintyre argues, randomization would be a more equitable method of resource allocation as well as increasing the evidence base. Describing the policy of Health Action Zones, which were piloted in a limited number of areas, she notes 'if funds are available for only 10 Health Action Zones, and who gets them depends partly on the advocacy skills of the local residents, perhaps it would be fairer, as well as more informative, not to choose the 10 poorest or most vociferous areas but the poorest 20, and then randomize them to intervention and comparison arms and monitor the impact' (Macintyre 2003).

However, despite the importance of public funding in the UK, policy makers cannot turn research on and off like tap. Researchers operate within their own spheres, with pressures, rewards and constraints which may not be closely aligned to those of policy makers or even the funders of research. For example, academic promotion or even survival under assessment schemes such as the Research Assessment Exercise depends on prosecuting particular types of research or achieving certain research outputs. In academic public health, this may act as a disincentive towards carrying out multi-disciplinary or evaluative studies or secondary research such as evidence synthesis. Furthermore, tools for measuring the social impact of research are under-developed (Smith 2001), despite social impact being a logical measure of success for applied health research. Perhaps as a result, capacity for public health research is severely lacking. Recent attempts to increase capacity are welcome but require sustained funding, given the long training periods in academic careers (National Institute for Health Research 2008; UK Clinical Research Collaboration Public Health Research Strategic Planning Group 2008; Wellcome Trust Public Health Sciences Working Group 2004).

The future of evidence-based public health policy

In discussing the challenges that face both policy makers and researchers, it is tempting to conclude that the picture of the use of evidence in policy making is one of idiosyncrasy and misuse, ignorance, and frustration. This would not be an accurate conclusion. There has been huge progress in the development of the evidence base, in its use by policy makers, and in the awareness of all stakeholders—policy makers, researchers, practitioners, and the public—that evidence is and should be a critical influence on policy making. Funding for the generation of policy relevant evidence has increased, and the National Institute for Health Research is making progress on coordinating applied research for health (Anon 2008). Evidence is no longer considered to be an obscure, technical topic, considered by faceless experts in the corridors of power, but something in which all have an interest and on which all may comment. For example, the Department of Health funds INVOLVE, an organization committed to patient and public participation in health and social care research (INVOLVE 2008). NICE holds extensive public consultations on all its guidance and has recently started holding its advisory committee meetings in public, something now common amongst public bodies (National Institute for Health and Clinical Excellence 2008b).

But the task in developing evidence-based public health policy is enormous. It requires more primary and secondary research, informed policy, practice and funding communities, and researchers who understand and act on the need for their research to be useful and used. Both public health researchers and public health policy makers aspire to improve the population's health. If they work together, there is no reason why their aspirations should not be realized.

Bibliography

Academy of Medical Sciences (2004) *Calling time: the nation's drinking as a major health issue*. London: Academy of Medical Sciences

Acheson, D (1988) *Public health in England: the report of the committee of inquiry into the future development of the public health function (Cm 289)*. London: HMSO

Action on Smoking and Health (2006) *Factsheet No 19: tobacco advertising and promotion*. Available at: <http://old.ash.org.uk/html/factsheets/html/fact19.html> (accessed 23 September 2008)

Anon (2008) 'In rude health' *Nature* 454: 1–2

Black, N (2001) 'Evidence based policy: proceed with care' *British Medical Journal* 323: 275–9

Campbell Collaboration (2008) *The Campbell Collaboration*. Available at: <http://www.campbellcollaboration.org/> (accessed 23 September 2008)

Chalkidou, K, Hoy, A, and Littlejohns, P (2007) 'Making a decision to wait for more evidence: when the National Institute for Health and Clinical Excellence recommends a technology only in the context of research' *Journal of the Royal Society of Medicine* 100: 453–60

Cheng, KK, Chalmers, I, and Sheldon, TA (2007) 'Adding fluoride to water supplies' *British Medical Journal* 335: 699–702

Cochrane Collaboration (2008) *The Cochrane Collaboration.* Available at: <http://www.cochrane.org/> (accessed 23 September 2008)

Cocker, C and Scott, S (2006) 'Improving the mental and emotional wellbeing of looked after children: connecting research, policy and practice' *Journal of the Royal Society of Health* 126: 18–23

Commission on Social Determinants of Health (2008) *Closing the gap in a generation: health equity through action on the social determinants of health.* Geneva: WHO

Cooksey, D (2006) *A review of UK health research funding.* London: TSO

Davey Smith, G and Krieger, N (2008) 'Tackling health inequities' *British Medical Journal* 337: a1526

Davies, HTO, Nutley, SM, and Smith, PC (2000) *What works? Evidence-based policy and practice in public services.* Bristol: The Policy Press

Department for Environment, Food and Rural Affairs (2006) *Evidence based policy making.* Available at: <http://www.defra.gov.uk/science/how/evidence.htm> (accessed 23 September 2008)

Department for Work and Pensions (2006) *Making a difference: tackling poverty—a progress report.* London: Department for Work and Pensions

Department of Health (1992) *The health of the nation—a strategy for health in England.* London: HMSO

Department of Health (1999) *Saving lives: our healthier nation.* London: TSO

Department of Health (2006) *Best research for best health. A new national health research strategy.* London: Department of Health

Department of Health (2007) *Review of the health inequalities infant mortality PSA target.* London: Department of Health

Dixon-Woods, M, Agarwal, S, Jones, D, Young, B, and Sutton, A (2005) 'Synthesising qualitative and quantitative evidence: a review of possible methods' *Journal of Health Services Research & Policy* 10: 45–53

Gilbert, R, Salanti, G, Harden, M, and See, S (2005) 'Infant feeding position and the sudden infant death syndrome: systematic review of observational studies and historical review of recommendations from 1940 to 2002' *International Journal of Epidemiology* 34: 874–87

Graham, H, Inskip, HM, Francis, B, and Harman, J (2006) 'Pathways of disadvantage and smoking careers: evidence and policy implications' *Journal of Epidemiology and Community Health* 60: 7–12

Great Britain Cabinet Office (1999) *Modernising government (Cm 4310).* London: TSO

Hawkins, SS and Law, C (2005) 'Patterns of research activity related to government policy: a UK web based survey' *Archives of Disease in Childhood* 90: 1107–11

Health Development Agency (2002) *Health Impact Assessment.* London: Health Development Agency

Healthy Start (2008) *Healthy Start.* Available at: <http://www.healthystart.nhs.uk/index.asp> (accessed 23 September 2008)

Hirsch, D (2006) *What will it take to end child poverty? Firing on all cylinders.* York: Joseph Rowntree Foundation

HM Treasury (2003) *The Green Book: appraisal and evaluation in central government.* 3rd edn. Available at: <http://www.hm-treasury.gov.uk/data_greenbook_index.htm> (accessed 23 September 2008)

HM Treasury (2007) *Meeting the aspirations of the British people: 2007 pre-budget review and comprehensive spending review (Cm 7227).* London: TSO

Independent Inquiry into Inequalities in Health (1998) *Report of the Independent Inquiry into Inequalities in Health.* London: TSO

INVOLVE (2008) *INVOLVE: promoting public involvement in NHS, public health and social care research.* Available at: <http://www.invo.org.uk/index.asp> (accessed 23 September 2008)

Joffe, M and Mindell, J (2002) 'A framework for the evidence base to support Health Impact Assessment' *Journal of Epidemiology and Community Health* 56: 132–8

Judge, K and Bauld, L (2006) 'Learning from policy failure? Health Action Zones in England' *European Journal of Public Health* 16: 341–4

Li, J, McMurray, A, and Stanley, F (2008) 'Modernity's paradox and the structural determinants of child health and well-being' *Health Sociology Review* 17: 64–77

Lomas, J (2000) 'Connecting research and policy' *Isuma Canadian Journal of Policy Research* 1: 140–4

Macintyre, S (2003) 'Evidence based policy making' *British Medical Journal*, 326: 5–6

Marmot, MG (2004) 'Evidence based policy or policy based evidence?' *British Medical Journal* 328: 906–7

Millward, LM, Kelly, MP, and Nutbeam, D (2003) *Public health intervention research—the evidence*. London: Health Development Agency

National Cancer Research Institute (2002) *Strategic analysis 2002: an overview of cancer research in the UK directly funded by the NCRI partner organisations*. London: National Cancer Research Institute

National Evaluation of Sure Start (2008) *National Evaluation of Sure Start*. Available at: <http://www.ness.bbk.ac.uk/> (accessed 23 September 2008)

National Institute for Health and Clinical Excellence (2008a) *NICE Public Health Guidance 10: Smoking cessation services in primary care, pharmacies, local authorities and workplaces, particularly for manual working groups, pregnant women and hard to reach communities*. London: National Institute for Health and Clinical Excellence

National Institute for Health and Clinical Excellence (2008b) *National Institute for Health and Clinical Excellence*. Available at: <http://www.nice.org.uk/> (accessed 23 September 2008)

National Institute for Health Research (2008) *National Institute for Health Research*. Available at: <http://www.nihr.ac.uk/> (accessed 23 September 2008)

Nutley, S, Walter, I, and Davies, H (2003) 'From knowing to doing: a framework for understanding the evidence-into-practice agenda.' *Evaluation* 9: 125–48

Pawson, R, Greenhalgh, T, Harvey, G, and Walshe, K (2005) 'Realist review—a new method of systematic review designed for complex policy interventions.' *Journal of Health Services Research & Policy* 10 (suppl 1): 21–34

Pawson, R and Tilley, N (1997) *Realistic evaluation*. London: Sage Publications

Petticrew, M, Whitehead, M, Macintyre, SJ, Graham, H, and Egan, M (2004) 'Evidence for public health policy on inequalities: 1: the reality according to policymakers.' *Journal of Epidemiology and Community Health* 58: 811–6

Porta, M (ed) (2008) *A Dictionary of Epidemiology*. 5th edn. New York: Open University Press USA

Power, R, French, R, Connelly, J, George, S, Hawes, D, Hinton, T et al (1999) 'Health, promotion, and homelessness.' *British Medical Journal* 318: 590–2

Prime Minister's Strategy Unit (2004) *Alcohol harm reduction strategy for England*. Available at: <http://www.cabinetoffice.gov.uk/media/cabinetoffice/strategy/assets/caboffce%20alcoholhar.pdf> (accessed 23 September 2008)

Smith, R (2001) 'Measuring the social impact of research.' *British Medical Journal* 323: 528

Sowden, SL and Raine, R (2008) 'Running along parallel lines: how political reality impedes the evaluation of public health interventions. A case study of exercise referral schemes in England.' *Journal of Epidemiology and Community Health* 62: 835–41

UK Clinical Research Collaboration Public Health Research Strategic Planning Group (2008) *Strengthening public health research in the UK: Report of the UK Clinical Research Collaboration Public Health Research Strategic Planning Group*. London: UK Clinical Research Collaboration

UNICEF Innocenti Research Centre (2007) *An overview of child well-being in rich countries: a comprehensive assessment of the lives and well-being of children and adolescents in the economically advanced nations*. Florence: UNICEF

Wanless, D (2004) *Securing good health for the whole population*. London: TSO

Weiss, CH (1977) 'Research for policy's sake: the enlightenment function of social research.' *Policy Analysis* 3: 531–47

Wellcome Trust Public Health Sciences Working Group (2004) *Public health sciences: challenges and opportunities*. London: Wellcome Trust

Whitehead, M, Petticrew, M, Graham, H, Macintyre, SJ, Bambra, C, and Egan, M (2004) 'Evidence for public health policy on inequalities: 2: assembling the evidence jigsaw.' *Journal of Epidemiology and Community Health* 58: 817–21

Chapter 3

Ethics and evidence in health promotion

David V McQueen

Introduction

> Hygiene is the corruption of medicine by morality. It is impossible to find a hygienist who does not debase his theory of the healthful with a theory of the virtuous. The whole hygienic art, indeed, resolves itself into an ethical exhortation... This brings it, in the end, into diametrical conflict with medicine proper. The true aim of medicine is not to make men virtuous, it is to safeguard and rescue them from the consequences of their vices.
>
> (HL Mencken, *Prejudices,* Third Series (1922))

This chapter seeks to make explicit the ethical dimensions underlying pursuit of an evidence-based approach in the field of health promotion. The field of health promotion is eclectic and multi-disciplinary; a great strength being that it values pragmatism but rejects narrow approaches. Part of the ethos of the field is to value that which is participatory, cross-cutting and partnership enhancing. Similar to most fields of practice, analogous to medicine itself, there is both an art and a science base to the practice. While most in health promotion desire to prove that there is evidence, even considerable evidence, that supports the work of those in the field of health promotion, one cannot escape the view that the notion of evidence rests uncomfortably with many of the concepts and principles of health promotion. Part of that discomfort lies in the realm of ethics. Ethical issues arise in all areas of health promotion, but the particular area of evidence presents special challenges, five of which will be considered in this chapter.

The Ottawa Charter argued for multiple approaches to improve health, reorient health care systems, and empower people (WHO 1986). Many of the principal activities of health promotion pertain to advocacy, partnerships, and coalition building, areas considered more an art than a science, actions more characteristic of a practice rather than a discipline (McQueen 2007). Despite the many conceptual challenges, health promotion is established in many quarters; there are foundations, centres, institutes, schools, departments, buildings, professorships, and programmes labelled with the term 'health promotion'. Thus there is a significant institutionalization of the field. Ultimately, like any institutionalized effort, those who practice and work in such institutions must come to grips with the underlying values and ethos of their practice and as a result confront the ethical challenges that arise.

A discussion on the general ethics of health promotion and practice is not our subject; the topic is far too broad; rather, the purpose here is to address the role of ethics in the search for evidence and effectiveness in health promotion. Many of the ethical considerations rest with the theoretical underpinning of the field, an area only lightly explored in health (McQueen and Kickbusch 2007). Health promotion is not alone in theoretical weakness; both public health and health promotion are theoretically weak and practice strong. This is the product of their historical development. Health promotion, like public health shares in the ongoing debate of whether they are, or should be, rooted in the bio-medical or in the social sciences. The outstanding feature that would distinguish health promotion from public health is the stronger implied foundation of theory and practice based in the social sciences, whereas the biomedical model, best evidenced in epidemiology, strongly underpins much of the practice of public health.

Complicating the picture on assessing evidence and effectiveness for health promotion is the history of health promotion itself. As it developed in the last third of the 20th century, health promotion took on different perspectives in different countries. Notable was the difference between the United States and the European Continent. In Europe health promotion was largely framed by concerns with the social, economic, and political roots of health and offered a strong focus on the sociopolitical environment as the place for health promotion action. The current emphasis on the so-called 'social determinants' of health is an element of this way of thinking about public health and health promotion. This was also the primary experience of Canada as witnessed by the elements and importance of the Ottawa Charter. This focus remains a strong component in European health promotion (McQueen 1994). In the USA, health promotion developed largely by extension of the traditional scope of health education, an area of work and academia that was quite well developed institutionally. Given its roots in education and socio-psychology it was logical that the primary focus of health promotion action should be on the individual and on changing attitudes, opinions, beliefs, and behaviours (Daniel and Green 2002). Whether or not modern health promotion, that is the health promotion practised globally now, has fully integrated these two traditions remains the subject of historical analysis and not of this chapter. Nonetheless, these two health promotion traditions will and do influence the meaning and scope of ethics as it relates to evaluation, evidence, and effectiveness in health promotion.

Health promotion is a field of action, largely premised on a concept of 'doing good', improving and promoting health. Because of this orientation it is far more difficult to set the boundaries of ethical containment for the field. It provides a broad and loosely bounded continuum. Some in health promotion might argue on ethical grounds for the strictest boundaries for action; that is by asserting the absurdity and wrongness of changing anything with values, models, and priorities that stem from outside those held by persons in that chosen area to be changed. For example, taking communities as the chosen area for interventions, the values and priorities for change must derive from inside the community itself and not be imposed values from the change agents, particularly if those change agents are from outside the community in question. A more relaxed belief, current in health promotion, is the sanctification of 'context' as being a most relevant operational principle. That is, the present context of any peoples and/or environment to be changed must be taken into sympathetic account in any intervention. At the other end of the change spectrum are those who practise health promotion with models, derived largely from their own views and epistemology, who believe that the change they intend to make to or for individuals or populations are correct and for a greater good. For example, cigarette smoking is regarded by many in health promotion as an unacceptable behaviour without socially mitigating value under any circumstances or contexts and therefore efforts to stop smoking are ethical *sui generis*. Each of these perspectives and the many positions along this continuum present different ethical challenges. There are always ethical costs of doing nothing, doing a little, or doing a lot.

Within the dimensions of the ethics discussion with regard to evidence, I focus on five areas that are particularly critical to health promotion. These areas are:

1 consideration of concepts and values;

2 insufficient evidence;

3 complexity and contextualism;

4 reflexivity-motivations and personal ethics; and

5 causality pitfalls, harm, and blame.

Consideration of concepts and values of health promotion

In a monograph on evidence and information, Robert Butcher (1998) defined evidence in a fashion that is most pertinent to health promotion. He wrote: 'A piece of evidence is a fact or datum which is used, or could be used, in making a decision or judgment or in solving a problem. The evidence, when used with the canons of good reasoning and principles of valuation, answers the question why, when asked of a judgment, decision, or action.' The challenge for the notion of evidence from a health promotion perspective is on the role of judgements in assessing evidence of effectiveness to determine action. The process of interpreting the evidence and judgement of evidence is often unclear and confounded with issues of expert opinion and bias. The underlying rationale for why the action will achieve the desired outcomes is rarely made explicit. However, evaluation of effectiveness demands definition of what constitutes 'success' and specification of criteria for gathering and collecting the evidence.

To illustrate, consider the area of healthy public policy, a key concern of contemporary health promotion. Globally, there is a large literature about health policy, but in terms of content it is full of assertions and opinions about what constitutes good policy, a largely hortative literature. In addition it is largely analytical and prescriptive. As a result of such an approach the analyses rarely deal with the evidence for the evaluation of effectiveness of policies. For one thing, in the policy arena there are often many competing expert views on what policy should be as well as the methods to attain it. However, in the real world of policy decision taking, few policy decisions are made in the terms that any single expert or policy advocate specifies. In general, policies that are taken up are a mixture of many different opinions and the result of complex political and administrative decisions.

Thus, to trace the evidential source of a particular policy approach becomes a monumental if not impossible task. And yet, we are still in need of knowing or estimating whether there is evidence that a particular policy has been effective. The conundrum faced by the search for evidence of effectiveness in some areas of health promotion is illustrated here in evaluating public health policy. That is, the degree of uncertainty assessing effectiveness is high; that is, there are almost always added layers of ethical considerations that radically increase the complexity of deciding what 'right' policy is. Evidence in this area is not simply one of a 'science' of assessing effectiveness.

In many topic areas in modern health promotion practice the search for evidence of effectiveness must turn to questions relating to the role of experts, or put another way, who are those that have earned the right for their opinion to be so considered. Furthermore, once the expert academics, lay leaders, practitioners, decision makers, etc, have been identified how can we assess whether their judgement is correct or adequate with regard to assessing effectiveness? A clear difficulty here is that models for assessing such judgemental ability either do not exist or are not as clearly specified and established as those for assessing evidence of effectiveness in 'scientific' areas.

As values enter into the debate around methodology and evidence the concept of harm rises in importance. Despite noble efforts to find evidence of the effectiveness of an intervention or a class of interventions we are often left with the conclusion that there is 'insufficient evidence' to recommend the intervention(s). This does not mean that the intervention is not effective; it means that, at this point in time, using the methods applied, the interventions cannot clearly demonstrate that effectiveness. This common finding in health promoting type interventions heightens need for the 'value' that the intervention does at least not do any harm to the public's health. Despite the considerable importance of this idea of no harm, there is little in the way of methodological guidance as to how to assess it. Human judgement remains the key approach. Further attention will be given to this critical area below.

Building evidence, methodologies, and values

Much of the discussion in the search for evidence centres on methodology. It can be argued that the type of methodology used will determine the kind and nature of evidence that we will find. One realization comes hard for many working on evidence and that is that evidence is not a 'thing in itself', but is a created entity. The creation of evidence is a product of the methodology used to make it. Because it is the product of human actions, it is not freed from human values. It is not the purpose here to go into great depth on this fundamental epistemological question regarding the nature of evidence; however, it is important to see how methodological concerns create their attendant ethical problems. Too often, those seeking methods for evidence are mired in the intricate details of constructing abstracting forms, analyses of research designs, and assessing whether an intervention has drawn an appropriate statistical sample. In reality, methodology begins with a careful conceptual consideration of how one is to develop the evidence in a particular area of intervention. Health promotion approaches would argue that this conceptual consideration must incorporate values and hence ethical points of view.

The concepts and principles of health promotion directly impact on the methodological debate on evidence and evaluation. As discussed in considerable detail in the book *Evaluation in health promotion* (Rootman et al 2001) health promotion is an area of involvement that stems largely from some underlying values that relate public health actions to health. Evaluation efforts and their underlying methodological approaches are informed by and transformed by these values. Thus, one cannot separate the concepts and principles of the field of health promotion from the methodologies that are appropriate to its evaluation. Indeed, it is a value that evaluation itself should, in the general case, be health promoting.

This value component of evaluation raises a peculiar issue for health promotion and the search for evidence. In most of the 'classic' literature on assessing evidence, scientific-based methodology is at the forefront. Thus the literature in this 'classic' approach debates issues such as random controlled trials versus comparison studies. The approach is clearly one of what is the appropriate 'scientific' methodology. However, in much of the search for evidence in public health the insistence on 'scientific' methodology, eg the RCT or other traditional designs, gives a secondary and less acceptable role to methodologies based on judgement. Even less attention may be paid to the role of values in the methodological approach. Nonetheless, operationalizing judgement and developing approaches that emphasize health promotion values is a key methodological problem in the health promotion evaluation literature.

The issue of insufficient evidence

Health promotion prides itself in taking an ethical stance that it is concerned with values such as equity, empowerment, participation, etc. Given that, it is remarkable how little attention the evidence debate has placed on the notion of 'harm'. Perhaps this is because, in the early days, it was not easily perceived that one might do harm by 'doing good'. However, it is easy to make the case that interventions may have negative side effects. Change, whether at the individual or social level, always implies that something else is given up. When change is made in a highly complex system it becomes much more difficult to see what exactly is exchanged. What is remarkable is that most groups that work with the question of evidence invariably turn to the problem of harm. In the most obvious case the notion of harm is a consequence of a common finding of evidentiary review groups. That finding is that, following extensive reviews of a particular intervention, the review group can only conclude that there is 'insufficient evidence' to make a recommendation of whether or not the intervention is effective. Unfortunately this is a very common outcome. Why it is so is the meat of an extensive discussion, but it remains a fact. The finding of 'insufficient evidence' is particularly troubling because of the need to make a recommendation. Should one encourage the continuation of this type of intervention until we can conclusively say it is effective or not? Or, should one take up the question of potential harm done by the continuation of such interventions. In fact there are at least two highly credible harms to consider: 1. the harm to the individuals, community, etc being intervened upon, and 2. resources that are taken away from other important intervention areas by the continuation of an intervention considered to lack evidence.

Complexity and contextualism

Since Ottawa health promotion has self-identified as being multidisciplinary, multi-sectoral, and eclectic. A major by-product of this broad focus is the emphasis on complexity. This topic is covered in detail in McQueen and Kickbusch (2007). In many respects the notion of complexity is the product of postmodernism, in that modernism argued that the world was understandable through science, whereas post modernistic thinking developed the idea that not only was the world complex, but possibly more complex than we could understand. Many now recognize the complexity of social systems, social change, and the complex infrastructures that are implied in health promotion practice.

With regard to assessing evidence and effectiveness, complexity makes the effort extremely difficult. Several factors are pertinent. First, causal relationships which may indeed be operating in a complex situation cannot be 'seen'. That is, the methodological skills to analytically 'pull out' or identify true relationships either do not exist or may be inaccessible to most practitioners in the field. In fact, it may be argued that we simply do not have the methodological knowledge base to disentangle incredibly complex relationships between variables and variable clusters. Second, few practitioners can imagine and/or construct a complete model of the complexity. That is, when the system is very complex so many variables are operating that the researcher/practitioner cannot possibly anticipate all those that should be included in a relevant model. In fact, the history of models is one of reducing complexity rather than describing it in full. Third, measurement of many important variables remains problematic (Campostrini 2007). In fact, measurement assumptions in statistics are rarely satisfied in data collection and research. From an ethical perspective complexity challenges the idea that those in health promotion practice can ever make a decision that is not fraught with the probability of doing some harm. This could lead to inaction; nonetheless the denial of complexity is a challenge for health promotion. Simplicity is easier to argue than complexity because: a) cognitively, people want single direct causal connection to an outcome; b) most causal models are conceived of as linear with discreet interconnecting causes; and c) traditionally science tends to be reductionist in its relationship between theory and proof, stripping away complexity to understand the 'true cause'. Further, the placement of health promotion institutionally has generally been in places with traditional approaches to science and public health, particularly schools of public health. Complexity is a real problem because it masks what many would like to see as the real or main reason why something happens. Further, there seems to be an innate need in people to understand precisely why something succeeds or fails. In short, simple answers are preferable for many who practice health promotion; simple answers, however, may mask potential harmful aspects that are bound up in complexity.

Coterminous with the development of the complexity idea in health promotion is the notion of 'contextualism'. Contextualism is a philosophical view that emphasizes the *context* in which an action, utterance, or expression occurs, and asserts the action, utterance, or expression can only be understood relative to that context. Largely arising out of late 20th century scepticism, it is the second theoretically-based idea that impacts on the search for evidence in health promotion. However, contextualism as a concept also has implications for ethics that parallel the concerns for evidence.

To begin with contextualism in many ways is an idea that is anathema to theory building because it goes against the grain of the search for standards, universality, comparability, and best practice. Obviously all human activity takes place in contexts; exploring the idea more deeply only adds layers to that observation and reveals how social actions are related to the context. The challenge is trying to grasp the meaning of contextualism when we want to understand evidence and the ethical dimensions.

Contextualism reveals the limitations of a science related to logical positivism, the view that reason alone may lead to an understanding of society. This view, of course has been severely challenged by recent thinking in the philosophy of science that more or less parallels the modern thinking leading to health promotion. The philosophy of science has moved relatively seamlessly from the logical positivism of the Vienna school (Suppe, 1997) to embrace those ideas of Kuhn and followers. Further, contextualism has allowed cynicism, scepticism, relativism and deconstructionism to be seen as appropriate approaches to understanding the human condition. It adds many challenges to interpreting the ethics associated with human actions. For health promotion, a field of action steeped in practice that occurs in a context, contextualism provides an approach to excuse the idea that there is any easy way to link practice to observation or observed effects that can be generalized. Indeed, the principle effect of contextualism as an idea is not scepticism or hopeless complexity but its attack on the notion of generalizability. Further, it argues that reality is directly in the context and not in a more abstract notion derived from theory. In turn this notion implies that it is the context itself in which consensus can be found. Many health promoters, practicing 'in the field' have this notion almost as a mantra. If one argues that a health promotion programme that works in Chicago couldn't possibly work in Jakarta because of contextualism, then it is *ipso facto* difficult to come up with a common theory of a health promotion programme for large cities. Thus so-called evidence of best practice and notions of 'effectiveness' are seriously compromised. But so are the ethical considerations.

Reflexivity and ethics in the search for evidence

The third theoretically based idea that impinges on the search for evidence in health promotion is the notion of reflexivity. In contrast to contextualism, whose locus lies mainly in the social fabric, the notion of reflexivity lies primarily within the individual. My view of reflexivity is largely an elaboration of a concept developed by the sociologist Gouldner and others. Essentially the argument is that we frame or construct our theories based on our own biography. For example, if one develops a theory that is based on dynamism, accenting change over time, it is in response to a deep-seated inner need to understand why change occurs. Furthermore, and most pertinent for health promotion, deep seated opinions and beliefs may be highly emotional and even based in moral consciousness. But Gouldner makes another linkage on reflexive sociology that is relevant to this evidence: '... those who supply the greatest resources for the institutional development of sociology are precisely those who most distort its quest for knowledge. And a Reflexive Sociology is aware that this is not the peculiarity of any one type of established social system, but is common to them all' (Gouldner 1970, p 498). The parallel to the development of health promotion as a field and its institutions is clear. Health promotion, as a field of action, often fails to be reflexive and reveal the parameters of individual motivations for its work. The work is largely viewed as good on its own merits; that is, it is based on personal 'ethical' principles that are good in themselves. For evidence, this is a threat of prejudice and error; for ethics, it represents the triumph of personal views.

Evidence of health promotion effectiveness, ethics, and issues

Few topics in the field of health promotion have engendered as much heated debate as that of evidence. The importance of evidence for health promotion practice should be seen in a larger context of discussions on evidence-based medicine taking place in much of the world, a debate which cannot be dismissed as pertinent only to medicine. Health promotion is also challenged by the debate (Adrian 1994; Allison and Rootman 1996; Macdonald et al 1996; Nutbeam 1998; Sackett 1996). Today, proponents of public health, health promotion practitioners, and health researchers are urged to base their work on evidence. In May 1998, the 51st World Health Assembly urged all Member States to 'adopt an evidence-based approach to health promotion policy and practice, using the full range of quantitative and qualitative methodologies' (WHO 1998).

Nonetheless, it is clear that when applying ideas of contextualism and reflexivity to notions such as 'evidence', and 'effectiveness' that these notions are Western derived, European-American, and in many ways European language notions. Most of those who have written and write about evidence have Western approaches that are derived from Western scientific training. These approaches and the biases inherent in them developed largely out of philosophical conjectures of the past two centuries, mainly from British and continental 18th and 19th century philosophers and culminating in debates around logical positivism (Bhaskar, 1997; Suppe, 1977). Logical positivism operates on the tenet that meaning is only verifiable through rigorous observation and experiment. In this context the word evidence has a very strict analytic meaning. Similarly, the randomized controlled clinical trial (RCT) and the quasi-experimental approach are largely creations of a Western literature and reflect a reification of the positivist notion. Many social sciences, particularly anthropology and sociology, have alternative, but none the less Western-derived approaches to assessing evidence and the effectiveness of interventions. The important thing to note is that these Western-derived ideas are contextual and not free of the ethical biases within that context. One cannot argue that ethics derive from philosophy and religion and not recognize the biographical nature of those philosophies and religions.

Western causality, pitfalls, harm, and blame

When one asserts that a causal relationship exists between one variable and another, the strength and validity of that assertion is evidence that the relationship is real. In another sense evidence is the strength of the knowledge base for what works. In any case, evidence remains a highly conceptual word and is used when we have knowledge that something highly relates to something else. In positivistic science this 'evidence' can often be precisely stated, in many cases modelled, and in some cases even expressed in a deterministic mathematical formulation. In empirical science this 'evidence' is usually the end statement that results after a large number of observations that two or more variables always, the deterministic case, or in general, the probabilistic case, relate to each other in a highly predictable way. An example of each of these will suffice. In the first case when an object falls from a height, it will fall to the ground in a fashion that is almost entirely described by a deterministic mathematical formula; in the second case the presence of dark cumulus clouds in the sky precedes a very high chance that there will be rain. However, there is a third case of contextual probability that also exists. If a person discharges a pistol into a crowd, there is an expectation of harm. In each case there is a conceptualization of evidence and one would argue that in each case there is a reasonably high expectation of the outcome. Nonetheless, the reader will immediately recognize that these are simple, not complex, examples of the concept of evidence. By changing the context in any of the examples, the notion of evidence becomes more problematic as does the identifiable path of causality. Nonetheless, evidence is usually thought to have a strong theoretical base in logical positivism. The reality is that the base in logical positivism is more rigid than types of causality generally found in health promotion.

Only rarely in practice is there a simple causality, that is where one active discreet variable causes something to happen in another discreet variable, the classic A causes B, where A and B are clearly defined on a metric scale. Almost always in practice the simplest causation is mediated through another variable or variables. In the reality of day-to-day community interventions we have multiple causes, multiple outcomes and multiple so-called intervening variables. Furthermore, many of these variables may be very loosely defined and measured. Not only are many interventions complex, but in many cases the intervention and its related outcomes are so complex and so distal that we can only hope to understand a small piece of the underlying causality. This is analogous to the topic of 'unexplained variance' in traditional multivariate statistics. Nonetheless, many practitioners are unhappy with any amount of unexplained variance. The reality of health promotion practice is that causality is almost always too complex to describe with much degree of probability, let alone determinism.

How do ethics enter into this discussion of causality? First and foremost, to attribute causality where it is not proven is not only wrong and bad science, but it may lead to harm. One could argue that doing bad science is not morally wrong, but it is difficult to make a justifiable case for doing harm. Thus the high causality expectation of evidence is an ethical burden for any activity or intervention undertaken when there is even the slightest possibility of harm. It needs to be recognized that harm itself is a causal outcome. However, it is a problematic outcome because generally harm would be an unanticipated outcome of an intervention in health promotion. This is in contrast to some classical research designs in pharmaceutical research where harm, eg negative side effects, is an anticipated outcome.

There is, of course, another serious ethical dimension of causality. What if there is a strong, well-proven causal relationship between a single variable and another single variable. In public health we have many such cases in the infectious disease area that appear to meet this criterion, eg the smallpox virus causes smallpox. There are fewer such straightforward causalities in the chronic diseases area. For example, we can assert that smoking causes lung cancer, but we are already on probabilistic grounds because it doesn't inevitably lead to lung cancer. We have to be satisfied with a population-based probability statement that we can, with a good degree of certainty, predict that a bounded percentage of regular smokers out of 1000 will get lung cancer and we are reasonably comfortable with the notion that if a smoker gets lung cancer it was probably caused, in full or in part, by smoking. In any case this reputed causal relationship is one of the strongest in the armoury of behavioural risk factors leading to deleterious health effects. Surely it would be difficult to make a case that a population reduction in smoking could cause any harm.

However, harm is also a broad concept and once you start to deconstruct its meaning the relation to causality becomes a question of ethics. Even with the extreme example of smoking one can imagine a harm scenario. Take the case of the earlier common practice of providing free cigarettes to people on the street; this is now regarded as 'wrong doing' and frowned upon. But what of providing cigarettes to soldiers just before they are to land at Omaha Beach in Normandy during WWII? In that case the probabilistic causal relationship to lung cancer is not only distal, but hardly seems relevant in the context. Context, causality, harm, and ethics are bound up in many ways beyond this simple example. In the case of harm, the notion of blame and its relation to causality is highly related. This becomes most apparent in the so-called identification of the 'causes of the causes', a phrase so well articulated in the work of the WHO Commission (CSDH). Again, even in the ideal case of smoking, blame is difficult to assess. Cigarettes are, after all, a product of an agricultural industry that is condoned and supported worldwide by subsidies, taxpayers, industrialists, politicians, and many other constituencies. In reality there is no apparent good reason to have the tobacco plant regarded as anything other than a noxious weed; yet, it is a widely accepted commercial product in much of the world. Can you have cigarette smokers without tobacco is a question of causality, harm, blame, and ethics? Those soldiers in Normandy had cigarettes the same as they had shoes. From the standpoint of health promotion practice, where is the cause of lung cancer and where should be the intervention? Where is the blame and where is the harm?

The preceding scenario might seem to be an extreme example. However, it illustrates how a deconstruction of the relationships among the notions of harm, causality, complexity, and context impinge on questions of ethics. Ultimately, most complicated health promotion interventions, when fully deconstructed, will present ethical challenges.

Conclusion: the dilemma of complexity

In the real world, whether events, are physical, biological, social, or a combination of these, complexity is the operating principle. Events take place in a context that consists of the impact and relationship of many variables. In the classical, notably positivist, approach to science, experimentation often follows a methodology that calls for the reduction of complexity in a multivariate situation. This is the classical case one tries to 'control' for all variables other than those directly in the causal relationship you want to observe. The RCT is an example of this classical reductionist approach, but most other experimental designs, including quasi-experimental designs, are also reductionist. The underlying assumptions are that, by holding constant all other variables that might interfere or mask a 'true' causal relationship that does exist, one can see the primary relationship that one desires to prove. Essentially, reductionism is a simplifying process; a wonderful, but now largely archaic idea.

The acceptance of complexity leads one away from such reductionist methodologies. There are a number of reasons for this. First, the real world of events consists of phenomena that are made up of many elements (variables) which interact in a mixture of orderly and chaotic ways that are the parts of the whole phenomenon. Second, the whole is more than the sum of the parts; that is why simple reductionism, or deconstruction, does not always work as a methodology. Third, it is entirely possible that changes in parts of the whole are dependent on the properties that bind all the different components of the whole. Fourth, the argument is also made that change can occur in complexity primarily because of forces within the whole and not due to any external forces or agents. Fifth, the relationships of component parts may not be simply deterministic or definably probabilistic, but in fact highly random or chaotic, which leads to grave problems in assigning or seeing causal relationships. Finally, complexity makes the idea of knowledge very problematic, particularly how one creates knowledge. There are other important elements of complexity that go beyond these six issues, but these alone present many challenges to those concerned with the ethical implications of actions.

For the assessment of evidence as it relates to health promotion effectiveness, the position one takes on the continuum of absolute reductionism to total complexity determines not only an investigator's methodological approach, but also one's view of how evidence is created. Clearly evidence is easier to agree upon in situations where complexity is minimized; where very clear causal pathways operate and variation among very few variables is limited, linear, and highly deterministic. As the health promotion interest or intervention becomes more multivariate, less metric and measurable, and highly contextual, that is as complexity increases, evidence of effectiveness becomes difficult to explain in positivistic terms and the more one turns to judgement as a form of evidence. It is this dependence on judgement that introduces ethical dilemmas that need to be made more explicit.

What then is the future for evidence-based health promotion that takes account of these multiple ethical concerns? It is clear that evidence-based health promotion needs to move forward with an underlying ethical posture that accounts for the special challenges introduced by the ethos of the field. First and foremost it needs to place its values at the heart of its methodological approach. For example, the value of equity should guide not only the assessment of the effectiveness of interventions, but also the methodological approach undertaken. To be concrete, evaluations of evidence of effectiveness should include equity considerations as an inclusive part of any intervention analysis and these must be assessable, measureable variables to assess if equity has been addressed, ie improved or at least maintained by the intervention. Thus, an intervention that apparently improves population health but increases inequity in the same or contingent populations is a) not a health promoting intervention and b) is not meeting the ethical expectations of health promotion practice.

Second, as difficult as it may be to increase the role for 'judgement' in the assessment of evidence, it cannot be ignored as a critical approach. The effect of 'complexity' in interventions has, among other concerns, challenged all the more traditional 'scientific' models of assessment of evidence. There is, simply stated, no model that provides a level of 'scientific' certainty that frees the evaluator from 'judgement' entering into the assessment of evidence. It is a role for health promotion to make this need for 'judgement' explicit and to note the 'ethical' mandate that is raised by 'judgement' as a methodological tool.

Finally, health promotion is the most likely 'home' for evaluation of the effectiveness of those interventions that address the so-described social determinants of health. Its underlying social science theoretical orientation is the obvious choice for evaluation in this area. Health promotion as a field is now coming to grips with its social science theoretical base in a way that allows a new sense of what is evidence and how to evaluate the effectiveness of complex, population-based interventions to improve and promote the health of the public.

The conclusions in this paper are those of the author and do not necessarily represent the official views of the Centers for Disease Control and Prevention.

Bibliography

Adrian, M et al (1994) 'Can life expectancies be used to determine if health promotion works?' *American Journal of Health Promotion* 8/6: 449–61

Allison, K and Rootman, I (1996) 'Scientific rigor and community participation in health promotion research: are they compatible?' *Health Promotion International* 11/4: 333–40

Bhaskar, R (1997) *A Realist Theory of Science*. 2nd edn. New York: Verso

Butcher, Robert B (1998) 'Foundations for Evidence-Based Decision Making' in *Volume 5: Evidence and Information, Canada Health Action: Building on the Legacy*. Quebec: Editions MultiMondes

Campostrini, Stefano (2007) 'Measurement and effectiveness: methodological considerations, issues and possible solution' Chapter 18 in David V McQueen and Catherine M Jones (eds), *Global Perspectives on Health Promotion Effectiveness*. New York: Springer Science & Business Media

CDC, Internet site for the Community Guide: <http://www.thecommunityguide.org/index.html>.

Daniel, M and Green, LW (2002) 'Health promotion and education' in Lester Breslow et al (eds), *Encyclopedia of Public Health*, pp 541–7. New York: MacMillan

Doyle, J, Waters, E, Yach, D, McQueen, D, De Francisco, A, Stewart, T, Reddy, P, Gulmezoglu, AM, Galea, G, and Portela, A (2005) 'Global priority setting for Cochrane systematic reviews of health promotion and public health research' *J Epidemiol Community Health* 59: 193–7

EWG, European Working Group on Health Promotion Evaluation (1998) *Health Promotion Evaluation: Recommendations to Policymakers*, Pamphlet. Ottawa: WHO(EURO), Health Canada

Gouldner, Alvin W (1970) *The Coming Crisis of Western Sociology*. New York: Basic Books

IUHPE (1999) *The evidence of health promotion effectiveness: a report for the European Commission by the International Union for Health Promotion and Education* Brussels—Luxembourg: ECSC–EC–EAEC

Jones, C and McQueen, D (2005) 'The European region's contribution to the global programme on health promotion effectiveness (GPHPE)' *Promotion and Education* Suppl 1: 9–10

Killoran, A, Swann, C, and Kelly, M (2006) *Public health evidence: tackling health inequalities*. Oxford: Oxford University Press

MacDonald, G et al (1996) 'Evidence for success in health promotion: suggestions for improvement' *Health Education Research: Theory and Practice* 11/3: 367–76

McQueen, DV (1989) 'Thoughts on the ideological origins of health promotion' *Health Promotion International* 4: 339–42

McQueen, DV (1994) 'Health promotion in Canada: a European/British perspective with an emphasis on research' in AP Pederson, M, O'Neill, and I Rootman (eds), *Health promotion in Canada: provincial, national and international perspectives*, pp 335–47. Toronto: WB Saunders

McQueen, David V (2003) 'The evidence debate broadens: three examples' Editorial, *Social and Preventive Medicine* 48/5: 275–6 [Editor of Special Issue on Evidence-based health promotion.]

McQueen, DV (2002) 'The evidence debate' invited editorial in. *Journal of Epidemiology and Community Health* 56: 83–4

McQueen, DV (2001) 'Strengthening the evidence base for health promotion' *Health Promotion International* 16/3: 261–8

McQueen, DV and Anderson, L (2001) 'What counts as evidence? Issues and debates' Chapter 4 in Rootman et al (2001) *Evaluation in health promotion: principles and perspectives*, pp 63–83. WHO Regional Publications, European Series, No 92. (Reprinted in M Sidell et al (ed), Debates and dilemmas in promoting health: a reader. 2nd edn. Milton Keynes: Open University Press, 2002.)

McQueen, DV, Kickbusch, I, Potvin, L, Pelikan, J, Balbo, L and Abel, T (2007) *Health and modernity: the role of theory in health promotion*. New York: Springer Publishing

McQueen, David V and Jones, Catherine M (eds) (2007) '*Global perspectives on health promotion effectiveness*' New York: Springer Science & Business Media

Nutbeam, D (1998) 'Evaluating health promotion - progress, problems, and solutions' *Health Promotion International* 13/1: 27–44

Poland, B (1996) 'Knowledge development and evaluation in, of and for healthy community initiatives. Part I: guiding principles' *Health Promotion International* 11/2: 237–47

Rootman, I, Goodstadt, M, McQueen, D, Potvin, L, Springett, J, and Ziglio, E (eds) (2000) 'There is a shortage of evidence regarding the effectiveness of health promotion' Chapter 24 in *Evaluation in health promotion: principles and perspectives*. Copenhagen: WHO (EURO)

Sackett, D et al (1996) 'Evidence-based medicine: What it is and what it isn't' *British Medical Journal* 150: 1249–5

Suppe, F (ed) (1977) *The Structure of Scientific Theories*. 2nd edn. Urbana, IL: University of Illinois Press

Task Force on Community Preventive Services (2000) 'Introducing the Guide to Community Preventive Services: methods, first recommendations and expert commentary' *American Journal of Preventive Medicine* 18/1 (supplement 1)

Tones, K (1997) 'Beyond the randomized controlled trial: a case for "judicial review"' *Health Education Research* 12/2: 1–4

World Health Assembly (1998) *Resolution WHA 51.12 on Health Promotion*. Agenda Item 20, 16 May 1998. Geneva: WHO

WHO, EURO (1984) *Health promotion: a discussion document on the concepts and principles*. Copenhagen: WHO, EURO. Published also in Health Promotion International (1986) 'A discussion document on the concept and principles of health promotion' Health Promotion International 1: 73–6

WHO (1986) *The Ottawa Charter*. WHO/HPR/HEP/95.1. Geneva: WHO

WHO, EURO (1998) *Health promotion evaluation: recommendations to policymakers report of the WHO European Working Group on Health Promotion Evaluation*. EUR/ICP/VST 05 01 03. Copenhagen: WHO/EURO

WHO (1998) *WHO Health Promotion Glossary*. WHO/ HPR/HEP/98.1. Geneva: WHO

Zaza, S, Briss, P, and Harris, K (2005) *The Guide to Community Preventive Services*. Oxford: Oxford University Press

Part 2

Evidence-based frameworks

Chapter 4

Theory-driven evaluation of public health programmes

Ray Pawson and Sanjeev Sridharan

Introduction: the idea in a nutshell

This chapter provides an introduction to the use of theory-driven approaches in the evaluation of public health programmes.

It commences with some core ideas and principles, and then sets out the main research strategies and designs associated with the approach. It concludes with an indication of some noteworthy benefits and tangible limitations.

Research on the anticipatory health care policy in Scotland (emphasizing preventive medicine and care in the community) is then used to illustrate some details of the application of the method. This case study highlights the role of the theory as the competent but fallible driver of the programme, with evaluation design and methods playing the role of the modest but astute navigator.

Public health programmes can be conceptualized in many ways. To the auditor they are flows of expenditure. To the politician they are ideological flagships. To the administrator they are responsibilities in need of staffing and management. To the practitioner they are a means of earning a living. To the public they are but one of scores of daily episodes clamouring for their attention. Whilst all of these perceptions are justifiable, this chapter commences with a different standpoint, one that we believe is vital to evaluation—namely, that programmes are theories.

In what sense can public heath interventions be considered as theories? To grasp the idea it is useful to consider the passage of interventions from birth to adulthood. They spark into life in the heads of policy architects, pass into the hands of practitioners and, hopefully, into the hearts and minds of programme subjects. That journey is an 'if-then' proposition. The preliminary idea, ambition, expectation, hypotheses, or 'programme theory' is that *if* certain resources (sometimes material, sometimes social, sometimes cognitive) are provided *then* they will insinuate peoples' reasoning to a sufficient extent that a change to healthier behaviour will follow.

Like all hypotheses, these speculations turn out to be true or false (or, more usually, a bit of both). These eventualities provide the underlying logic for theory-driven evaluation. Research begins by eliciting the key theories assumed in the construction of programmes and then goes on to test their accuracy and scope—the programmes are supposed to work out like this but what happens in practice? Empirical work is conducted with the task of discovering where the prior expectations have proved justified and where have they been dashed—and why? These investigations, moreover, end with theory, that is to say a better understanding of how interventions really work. If the evaluation has gone to plan, it should lead to development, a more discriminating theory, specifying for whom and in what circumstances and in what respects a programme works. Theories, unlike programmes and populations, are portable—with the further potential benefit that many of the findings of theory-driven inquiry are transferable.

To encapsulate this abstract vision in a nutshell, and to see how it can be adopted as a method of evaluation, consider the tale of one of our favourite programme theories. In the 90s in the UK, a group of health educators became taxed with the idea that the unhealthy life styles of many adolescents, girls most especially, were shaped by popular culture and, most especially, by the less than wholesome pastimes of film, soap, and rock stars. This led to the programme theory of trying to insinuate equally attractive but decidedly healthy role models, most especially sports stars, into the pages and onto the airwaves of the teen media. The editors of these outlets needed little encouragement and so a brave conjecture, known amongst denizens of health education as 'Dishy David Beckham theory', sprang into life.

Evaluation methodology enters the scene as follows. A good way to test the programme in question is to test the core theory. Readers might like to follow the detailed investigations on this score in Mitchell (1997). Suffice it to say here that the evidence indeed attests to a besotted enthusiasm for poring over pictures of Beckham and friends in the teen magazines. But, alas, this pastime continued to exercise girls' minds rather than their bodies. Few respondents reported any renewed interest in sport and exercise. We thus witness the failure of the 'role model theory' as implemented in this instance—although the possibility remains that it might still work in other circumstances and in other respects. Beckham's image continues to be used to sell perfume and underpants, but as health education his only use was to score an own-goal. We leave our health educators back at the drawing board and pass on to consider how to design a programme theory evaluation.

Designing a theory-driven evaluation

We offer a simple, five-stage overview of the method in this section. Readers will note that the model follows fastidiously the classic cycle of scientific investigation, namely hypothesis-building, data collection, data analysis, and theory revision (Franklin and Ebdon 2005). In practice of course, investigations are never as linear and orderly as this and evaluators find themselves fidgeting back and forth before the circuit is completed.

Eliciting and surfacing the underlying programme theories

Programme theories are easily spotted. Read any public health discussion, debate, manifesto, guideline, advisory leaflet and they fight to the surface. Their propositional form is readily deciphered. Public health theories tend to run along these lines:

A. An attempt to comprehend the social and institutional problems that give rise to unhealthy behaviour or to inequalities of health.

B. This is followed by conjectures on what changes must be made to these systems to reduce ill health, which then gives rise to . . .

C. Ideas for bringing fresh resources to individuals and/or communities in the hope of changing behaviour for the better.

Readers will be able to recite their own versions of ABC, but for illustration's sake we begin with a miniature example:

Deaths from house fires are still significant:

A. Because people give low priority to fire danger, are unaware of the utility of alarms in early escape, and find them awkward to install and maintain.

B. The solution lies in overcoming lack of motivation, increasing knowledge of the dangers, dealing with penny-pinching, and making battery replacement easier.

C. A programme combining information, free distribution, and the hard-wiring of alarms will increase usage and reduce danger.

The substance of such theories will, of course, be different, according to whether the chain of conjectures ends in 'carrots' (such as alarm giveaways), 'sticks' (eg smoking bans), or 'sermons' (eg dietary advice). Their form, however, is much the same—conjectures about the problem, what to do about it, and how to go about it. This way of thinking gives theory-driven evaluation its first and defining task, namely eliciting and surfacing the underlying programme theories.

Theories are best elicited from their procreators and this may involve either:

1 Reading and close analysis of programme documentation, guidance, regulations etc on how the programme will go on achieve its ends

2 Interviews with programme architects and/or managers and/or practitioners on how their intervention will generate the requisite change

Programme theories normally flow quite readily from these inquiries, though a couple of related difficulties should be noted. The first, located at the higher levels of the political greasy pole, is a tendency to ambiguity or even amnesia in policy discourse (Shackley and Wynne 1997; Pollitt 2000). These authors note that promised solutions to the world's problems may gain a wider currency if they maintain a deliberate imprecision. This may assist initially in gathering more leery participants to the policy table. Further down the line a certain obscurity or forgetfulness in regard to the original aims may help when the time comes to proclaim success. The second problem, located nearer the daily grind of programme practice, occurs when the core theory is either seemingly so obvious or buried tacitly in the minds of the programme workers that it can fail to surface in the interview. In these situations, a little persuasion is sometimes required to encourage practitioners to spell out how their actions worm their way into participants' choices (Pawson and Tilley 1997, Ch 6).

These problems aside, theory elicitation is relatively simple. Indeed, given that there is no shortage of ideas for reform in the policy-making classes, we should also issue the advice that it can be too simple. What invariably happens in such exercises is that theory elicitation operates in the plural, culminating in the discovery of not one but scores of potential programme theories. A second, preparatory phase is thus required before bringing them to investigation.

Mapping and selecting the theories to put to research

The programme theory perspective has the huge advantage of penetrating into the black box of an intervention. It rapidly takes us beyond the 'one problem—one cure' view of social programmes. Having found a means of eliciting the programme theories at work, the next stage is to begin to codify or to map them. A confusing array of techniques is available for this task, known variously as concept mapping, logic modelling, system mapping, theories-of-change, problem and solution trees, scenario building, configuration mapping, and so on (Trochim 1989: Kaplan and Garrett 2005; Snowden et al 2008). All of them involve trying to render, usually in diagrammatic form, the process through which the programme achieves its ends. These maps may concentrate on identifying: the various causes of the problem, the administrative stepping stones to be achieved, the unfolding sequence of programme activities and inputs, the successive shifts in dispositions of participants, the progressive targeting of programme recipients, the sequence of intervention outputs and outcomes. We make no attempt to describe all such pathways here. Rather we pursue a core and prior issue.

Producing the requisite list, chart, or diagram of the levers of the potential change in a programme is never a straightforward task. Even in our nascent example on smoke alarms above, readers will have noted three or four separate ideas on the boil about the problem and about its resolution. If one examines a complex, multi-agency, multi-objective intervention such as the UK Health Action Zones, researchers are immediately confronted with an overabundance of programme theories (Judge and Bauld 2001). This particular initiative encouraged community-based solutions to local health problems. Many stakeholders thus had the opportunity to become programme theorists and multiple strands of activities immediately sprung up rendering it impossible to capture the intervention in terms of a single model.

The supreme exemplification of complexity mapping is the famous 'spaghetti diagram' developed for the 'Foresight Tackling Obesities' project. The authors attempted to provide comprehensive mapping of the multiplicity of factors contributing to the obesity epidemic as a prelude to mounting a comprehensive counter attack. Behind the simple observation that waistbands are growing lies a complex web of reinforcement ranging across individual psychology and physiology, attitudes toward physical activity, norms on body shapes, cultures of food consumption, economics of food production, structures of the built environment, and so on (Vandenbroek et al 2007). In all 108 factors—'the drivers of obesity'—are depicted as lines of influence on the map.[1]

---

[1] Several versions of the 'obesity systems model' are available and can viewed at:<http://www.foresight.gov.uk/Obesity/12.pdf> and <http://www.visualcomplexity.com/vc/project_details.cfm?index= 622&id=622&domain=>.

Public health programmes work by persuading subjects to change and the theory-driven approach gets the evaluator closer to the ideas that do so. We trust we have demonstrated, however, that there is never a single theory to be put to the test. There are always multiple theories built into any intervention and these will indeed change as the programme matures, learns from others, changes hands, suffers rivalries, becomes fatigued, and so on. A crucial, and in our view underemphasized, initial step in the programme theory evaluation is thus to sift though the map of ideas and select the subset of theories to be put to test.

The warrant for the strategy is never the claim that *the* programme theory is being put to the test. Rather, the logic of inquiry is that *a* subset of current and significant programme theories will be interrogated. A judgement call is involved at this point. Researchers come to the decision that they have identified some of the dominant ideas that infuse a particular area of programming and that they are worthy of evaluating in their own right, without assuming they are exemplified perfectly in any specific application. This justification is all the more pertinent given that the end point of the exercise is to refine programme theory rather than pass a verdict on any particular episode.

So how does theory-driven evaluation concentrate its fire? Much good advice exists on this score (Stame 2004: Pawson, 2006b), including Weiss's (2000) aptly titled '*Which links in which theories should we evaluate?*'. There is no one formula for making the judgement call, the following list giving only a preliminary indication of potential priorities:

- It might be that a particular intervention is drawn up with a clear legislative framework—in which these ordinances about who-should-do-what-to-whom constitute the theory to be tested.

- Programme theories are much imitated, the same ideas fetching up in different policy sectors—in which case it is the 'big idea' that needs clarification and refinement by comparing its efficacy in different domains.

- It might be that there is a clash of ideas about how a particular programme should and does work—in which case the theory dispute or programme hotspot might be put to adjudication.

- It might be that the programme flows through many different hands—in which case the consistency of the theories applied by different stakeholders is the theme to be addressed.

- Given the 'performance measurement' culture, it might be that the programme comes with set timetables and targets—in which case these can inform the theories under test.

- It might be that a policy maker or sponsor has key but limited responsibilities in mounting a programme—in which case a heavy dose of pragmatism might infuse the choice of hypotheses up for inspection.

Theory-driven evaluation is driven by conceptual clarity and, by whatever route, the selection of the theoretical framework for investigation must be made and must be made clearly.

Formalizing the theories to put to test

This objective is much aided by the final leg of what is still the preparatory stage of inquiry. After electing, mapping, and selecting programme theories, the time comes to formalize them. They need to be transformed into a propositional form, rendering them as hypotheses suitable for empirical research. Programme theories come to life as insights, brain waves, bright ideas, and informed guesses. Sometimes they turn out to be wishful thinking and pipe dreams. What evaluation research requires, by contrast, are testable propositions.

Once again it is the case that there are a number of ways of setting up programme theories as hypotheses for empirical investigation. We distinguish two main forms here, beginning with an account of what unites them before spelling out the differences. The various models are illustrated in Figure 4.1. The theory-driven approach attempts to get inside the black-box of interventions and get away from black-box methods of investigating them. In the classic experimental trial the programme is regarded as a singular treatment (X) and the singular hypothesis under investigation (Figure 4.1) is about whether this treatment brings about an intended outcome (Y). Such a proposition is tested by an experimental and control group comparison, examining the difference in outcomes under the presence and the absence of the treatment. We refrain from covering the by-now, standard critiques of this strategy, other than to note that even if outcome differences are apparent in favour of the treatment, that this particular method cannot tell us anything about why the treatment works. There is hardly need to add that the 'why?' question is the *raison d'être* of the theory-driven approach.

In Figure 4.1, we distinguish between 'theories-of-change' (Connell et al, 1995) and 'realist' hypotheses (Pawson and Tilley, 1997). Both are attempts to investigate the internal process operating within a programme. Both approaches remind us that programmes work by persuading subjects (individuals or communities) to change. And subjects, from the very beginning, will be relatively recalcitrant or willing. Subjects on the threshold of a programme will ponder, wait, figure, investigate, and change their minds. Subjects over the threshold will dive in, tread warily, pull out, dawdle, support, sabotage, take over, malinger, proselytize, and so on. Programme theories plan to shift the tide, moving sufficient numbers of the marginal and refractory into compliance and commitment with the intervention goals.

Theories-of-change hypotheses try to capture such a sequence (Figure 4.1, Diagram 2) as a set of 'stepping stones'. Programme plans are quite literally put to paper and then become the hypothesis to be tested. Typically, this might involve mapping the decisions made about the inputs or resources on which the programme should be built, and how they are translated into activities or outputs for programme participants, and how these embed themselves into subjects' actions, firstly through some immediate understanding to programme ideas, then to some intermediate compliance with its activities, and then in the long-term behavioural change. The precise make-up of the 'mile posts' in the sequence will differ according to the type of intervention and the set of sub-theories

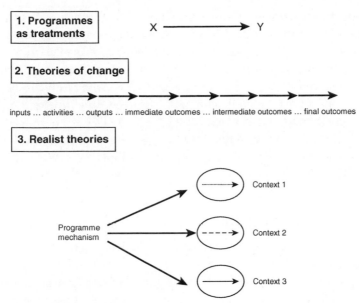

Fig. 4.1 Formalizing programme theories

selected for investigation. The key point is that subsequent investigation interrogates this process and thus comes to an understanding of why the programme has worked to plan or why it has unravelled.

Realist hypotheses (Figure 4.1, Diagram 3) begin with the selection and identification of a key programme 'mechanism'. A mechanism is not the programme, the name of the programme or the presence or absence of the programme. A mechanism describes what goes on within the programme to change behaviour—what is on offer that might persuade people to change? Mechanisms take many forms in public health interventions. They may offer incentives or giveaways in the hope that people continue using the gift. They may offer instruction in the hope that people learn the lessons. They may offer advice or mentoring in the hope that people follow the guidance. They may impose legislation and policing in the expectation that people will comply.

Reconceptualizing the active ingredient of programme as an 'offer' (or even an injunction) immediately gives rise to the possibility that some people will reject the offer (or disobey the injunction). Realist hypotheses thus attempt to differentiate programme subjects and their circumstances (normally abbreviated as 'contexts') in respect to how they might respond to the programme mechanism. Figure 4.1, Diagram 3 illustrates such a proposition in which the same mechanism is postulated as generating contrasting outcomes (designated by the different arrow styles) in three different contexts. Programmes are always targeted and realist hypotheses attend to theories on why particular targets may be appropriate. As a simple example, consider again for whom and in what circumstances a smoke alarm giveaway might reduce fire fatalities. In context one, the alarm may go to a house already fitted with the devices—in which case the giveaway may become a throw-away. In context two, say a pensioner household, the alarm may offer protection only if help is given with installation and fiddly battery changes. In context three, the newly built house, protection would be up and ready for new residents with plenty of other things on their minds. Programmes are built with many more eventualities in mind and such hypothesies raise the opportunity to test them.

It is quite possible, of course, to run these two modes of hypothesis building together (Blamey and Mackenzie 2007). But, by whatever formula, theory-driven evaluation expends considerable effort in teasing out and setting down formally key conjectures on why programmes work.

Data collection and analysis

We now turn to the collection and analysis of the data to interrogate the chosen pro-gramme theories. Despite these being major activities in the research cycle we run them together and indeed in reverse order here, better to reveal the core principles. Whilst it is appropriate to follow custom and refer to this stage as 'theory testing', these approaches prefer the designation 'theory refinement'. The objective is not to accept or reject pro-gramme theories. The mission is to improve them, a cause we illustrate in Figure 4.2.

A theory-of-change analysis inspects the 'stepping stones' of the programme imple-mentation chain in the expectation that some will wobble, their spacing will prove irregu-lar and there is a danger of them being covered in a policy swell. Less metaphorically, the presumption is that the programme theories will always be achieved imperfectly. They will face ambivalence or resistance, they will generate unintended consequence, other priorities and programmes will intervene. The purpose of the analysis is thus to inspect

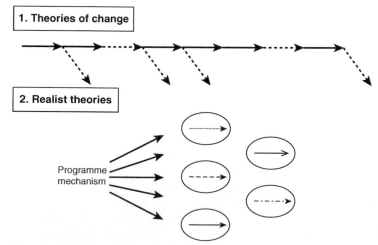

Fig. 4.2 Refining programme theories

the fidelity of the hypothesized implementation chain (Figure 4.1, Diagram 2) in order to uncover its flows, blockages, and leakages (as represented in Figure 4.2, Diagram 1).

Such analysis may be developed in two ways. The first is as an explanatory adjunct in summative evaluation. If the purpose of the evaluation is to discover 'what works', then attention is concentrated on the final outcomes of the theories-of-change sequence. A comparison of the expected and actual outcomes provides a measure of success. But just as significantly, the empirical exploration of the earlier pathway will provide a detailed explanation of that relative success and failure. Successful programmes will have established a strong activity base, generated quick wins, met intermediate outcomes, and so on; struggling programmes will have faced a rockier ride.

The other usage of theories-of-change analysis is in programme planning or formative evaluation. Here the logic map provides the architectural diagram for the construction of the programme. Rather than building a programme with the broad ambition that it will generate the requisite behavioural change, the theories-of-change map demands justification for every step and decision along the way. Such planning should cover the feasibility, plausibility and testability of each component theory. The latter feature is particularly important for it allows for some trial and error in constructing the programme, correcting progressively for the looming leaks, emerging blockages and unintended consequences as envisioned in Figure 4.2, Diagram 1.

Attention now shifts to realist analysis and to Figure 4.2, Diagram 2. The goal is the same—to refine the initial programme theory (Figure 4.2, Diagram 3). In this case attention is paid to learning more about the scope and targeting of an intervention. Realist analysis starts with the idea that the programme on offer will have varying appeal. Deepening the understanding of the programme involves a better understanding of the contours of that appeal. Certain subgroups will have been hypothesized as optimal targets in the original programme theory and the purpose of analysis is to check the range finding. Some expectations will be confirmed, some will prove misguided, and the end product of the analysis will be an improved picture of programme efficacy and inefficacy (crudely represented by the revised fivefold outcome configuration in the diagram).

It is important to point out that this process of contextual specification applies to individuals, their histories, and characteristics, but also to their institutions, localities, and communities. The mantra of realist evaluation is about learning 'for whom, in what circumstances, over what duration, and in what respects' a programme works—and the analysis of context can be sensitive to all of these dimensions. The other realist objective, of course, is to understand 'why' the programme works and this involves close understanding of the programme mechanism and its precise utility and appeal in the different quarters of an intervention. Public health programmes do not work passively, they work only with the acquiescence of participants. Knowing why a programme works rests on the ability to explain the making of that decision.

Having demonstrated the objectives of data analysis, we now step backwards to see what form the data take and how they are collected. Much depends, of course, on the policy concern, the intervention details, and the precise programme theory. However, some broad principles may be established, the most fundamental of which is that theory-driven analysis demands a multi-method evidence base. A brief glimpse back at Figures 4.1 and 4.2 enables us to grasp the necessity for mixed methods. The theories-of-change map is based on the simple, unimpeachable sociological truth that actions have consequences. It depicts the development of a programme in which a particular set of activities drives an intervention output, another process will generate a further outcome, and so on The realist diagram follows another irreproachable idea, namely that the same process does not always lead to the same outcome. A programme that works in one context will not necessarily succeed in another.

Here then are the basic and active ingredients of social change. How does one trace them? Well, data on process is generated, broadly speaking, using *qualitative* methods; outputs and outcomes are measured via *quantitative* approaches; contextual information requires *comparative* observation and measurement. Testing any programme theory requires the conjunction or *triangulation* of all three.

Beneath these broad data collection strategies lies a whole raft of potentially useful techniques. Researching decision-making processes might rely on observation, participation, interviewing, self-report, focus groups, document analysis, and so on. Measuring outcomes might rely on attitude testing, scaling, behavioural outcomes, administrative records, and so on. Comparative information might be compiled through any of these techniques and be based on case studies of particular subgroups and subsections of an intervention across its different trials. Perhaps the most significant alternative in this palette of methods is that the data may not only be gleaned live and *in situ* but also retrospectively by synthesizing the evidence from existing evaluations. Pawson (2006a) can be consulted for examples of how systematic review can be conducted in both theories-of-change and realist modes. What connects all approaches, and what remains the core principle of evidence gathering, is that the choice of data collection technique should be theory-driven rather than method-given.

From theory to practice: 'Have a Heart Paisley'

The programme

Our example of the theory-driven method in practice is drawn from a recent evaluation of a Scottish national demonstration project called *Have a Heart Paisley* (HaHP). In line with recent Scottish health policy, HaHP promoted a shift towards a health service with an emphasis on preventive medicine (Scottish Executive 2005a and 2005b). The immediate goals were to deliver a targeted programme for the working age population, those aged 45 to 60 at risk of heart disease, and those of any age with heart disease in Paisley. It was recognized that additional effort would be required to attract those individuals who were typically least likely to engage with health services, notably those living in one of the most deprived areas of Scotland. The long-term aim of HaHP was to reduce the total burden and levels of inequality of coronary heart disease (CHD) in the town of Paisley through an integrated programme of secondary and primary prevention (Blamey et al 2004).

HaHP was designed as a 'testing ground for national action' which would provide 'a learning resource for the rest of Scotland'. It was hoped that local successes would inspire national change.

Planning and implementing interventions to address problems of health inequalities in poor communities provides multiple conceptual and operational challenges—fallible theories are involved from the outset. For example, even 'deprived communities' are heterogeneous; both the destitute and the tolerably well-off might reside in such a locality. It is feasible that an initiative intended to address problems of inequalities might end up exacerbating them; one mechanism through which this may happen is if the relatively well-to-do in the poor communities are the ones who engage at higher rates with the intervention. There may be many other contextual reasons why a programme intended to address health inequalities might not work as intended. Earlier we described programmes as 'offers' and the offer to engage in a CHD intervention may not be perceived with the same level of attractiveness by all programme recipients: obstacles might include rigid health routines marked by family and gender; psychological constructs such as lack of confidence; political scepticism towards the role of government in solving health problems; and access limitations due to the impairments of some recipients.

Against this background, practical decisions on how to implement the programme have to be made. Box 4.1 describes the key phases involved in the primary prevention dimension of HaHP. As the programme unfolded, activities were developed in four key areas: screening, health coaching, and micro-interventions. Recall our earlier discussion of the internal complexity of public health programmes and note the accumulation of subprocesses at each stage.

Box 4.1 HaHP primary prevention measures

Reach

HaHP targeted individuals aged 45–60 years old through delivery of a tailored primary prevention system. The Central Data Repository, a centralized data base that linked data from general practices, laboratories, hospital and national datasets, was used to support the delivery of primary prevention and acted as a sampling frame for the intervention. All eligible individuals (ie those aged 45 to 60, without a history of heart disease, living in Paisley, and enrolled with a Paisley GP) were sent a personal invitation through the mail to attend a 'heart health check'. Mailing was targeted at the most deprived post-code sectors in the first instance. Subsequent post-code sectors were then offered the intervention. Recipients who accepted the offer to attend a heart health check were required to contact a call centre number provided in the invitation letter.

Screening

All those who accepted this offer were screened by HaHP's nurses. This enabled their risk of developing coronary heart disease in the next ten years to be calculated (Framingham Risk Score), and individuals were informed of their risk status (low, moderate, or high).

Health Coaching

All screening participants were then offered an opportunity to meet with a HaHP 'Health Coach'. The planned function of 'Health Coaching' in HaHP phase 2 was as a method to engage the target population, to provide one-to-one, client-led support and individualised guidance to empower individuals to make positive lifestyle changes aimed at reducing risk of developing CHD.

Micro-interventions

Additionally, health coaches had the option of also 'signposting' individuals either to HaHP's own 'micro-interventions' or to other appropriate community services identified during a local mapping exercise. Health coaches utilized a web base to guide their consultations and to capture details of services for use in 'signposting' suitable individuals.

Design and delivery of the evaluation

Our account now follows the actual investigation (Sridharan et al, 2008), beginning with what we can only describe as the wrestle to elicit, surface, and formalize the HaHP programme theories. The evaluation team worked closely with the programme staff and policy planners in developing the programme theory for HaHP. Note, first of all, a fit with what was described earlier as the preliminary ABC (what's the problem, what to do about it, how to go about it) of problem logic. In this instance we have:

A. Individuals in multiple disadvantaged situations often give low priority to their health and do not use available resources (eg NHS) to monitor and prevent disease/chronic conditions.

B. The solution lies in providing a complex set of services including screening, health coaching, additional interventions to inform and empower individuals living in high levels of multiple deprivation.

C. A programme combining information from screening and support from a health coach as well as additional information and services from other interventions will lead to improved lifestyles and reduced risks to CHD in the target population. This, in turn, can lead to reduced health inequalities.

The clarification of programme logic emerged by stages, the next of which was to render programme logic into a theories-of-change map as in Figure 4.3. Note that the choice of black boxes in this figure emphasises the point that not only is the program itself a black box, the components of the intervention (eg reach, screening or health coaching) can themselves be black boxes. An important goal of theory-driven evaluation is to 'unpack' each of the black boxes in turn.

Let us begin with the seemingly simple business of making contact and reaching out to the community. In practice this depends on a somewhat shakier hypothesis about the efficacy of letters received through the post. Is there not a risk that this is too blunt an instrument to reach some of the most deprived? Will the message be lost amidst the junk mail? How many people actually respond to written communications? Is the message conveyed appropriately? Should mailed letters be combined with other promotional methods? Is there a chance that the 'worried well' or the 'healthy deprived' are more likely to engage with the offer to participate?

At the screening stage, individuals were informed of the risk of developing coronary heart disease in the next ten years (the Framingham Risk Score was calculated), and individuals were informed of their risk status (low, moderate, or high). Again, there is nothing straightforward and automatic about such a process. Clearly, the ability of the screening to trigger change in individuals depended critically on the ability of those carrying out the screening to effectively communicate the individual's risk, and to explain the basic changes that could be made to lower this risk. Additionally, this method of screening relies entirely on the validity of the Framingham risk score. Recent work has suggested that socio-economic status may be an independent risk factor for cardiovascular disease (Hippisley-Cox et al 2007; Lyratzopoulos et al 2006; Tunstall-Pedoe and Woodward 2006) and socio-economic status is not accounted for in the Framingham scale.

Health coaching was another key aspect of the HaHP intervention. Basic assumptions on how the health coaching would work were not clear at the start of the intervention. How was the health coaching framework modified to target deprived individuals? How exactly did health coaching empower individuals? The relationship between coach and client is important in effecting change; however it can also result in a reliance on the coach for continued support, which is not practical as a long-term solution. This relationship may also interfere with the clients' relationships with doctors, as coaching relationships may be more personal while GP interaction may be more clinical. If individuals

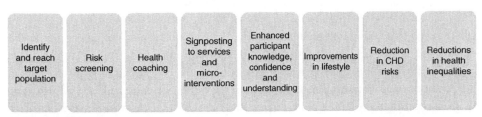

Fig. 4.3 HaHP programme logic

refer to their coaches preferentially and not feel the need to discuss topics with their GPs, this in turn could interfere with the doctor's ability to provide effective medical care.

There is a small forest of issues in the above three paragraphs and even these raise only a small subset of questions that can emerge when one puts the microscope to the causal logic of the programme. As explained in the first part of the paper, one can always dig more deeply for programme theories. Given the centrality of 'reach' in addressing problems of health inequalities, we return to stage one and spell out the working theory in further, minute detail. A key trigger to the intervention is the intended recipient deciding to call the telephone number provided to enrol for screening. The following activities must occur before such a call is made:

Letter of invitation is mailed → letter delivered (a number of letters, especially in the poorer communities were returned undelivered) → letter is opened and read → a decision is made that the HaHP scheme might provide benefit, despite the time involved → a decision is taken to make the phone call → the phone call is actually made.

All of these stages might attract a differential response. Poorer individuals may be less likely to receive the letter of invitation due to inadequate registration with services and censuses, higher rates of transitions between addresses, periods of homelessness, and so on. They may be less likely to read and digest the material given disparities in literacy rates and in familiarity with the contents of the communication. Finally, poorer individuals might lack the means, experience, and confidence to contact the call centre.

All of these 'micro-theories' and more emerged in discussion with programme staff. Recall that in our earlier discussion we pointed out that programme theories also lie in more general policy considerations. Our field here is public health and the success of the programme in reaching the target population can be said to rest on two opposing and long-standing sets of theories. The 'optimistic' theory sees public health as a lifeline to the poor. In the present context the poorest individuals would see in the initial communication a recognition of their significant needs and would thus self-select into the intervention at higher rates. The underlying idea is that deprived individuals are very aware of their often long-standing health problems and they would view the intervention as a rare opportunity to address them. Moreover, the earliest sets of letters were directed to the poorest areas. The initial programme plan was that the poorest individuals living in the poorest areas would self-select into the intervention and enrol into the programme at high rates. (Note that there was no formal programme mechanism to provide the services based on socio-economic need.)

A second theoretical view is pessimistic. In general terms this argument goes that, without a formal mechanism to restrict services to the poorest, the 'worried well' and the 'better off' are generally more likely to self-select into health programmes. Not only do the worried well have a heightened understanding of their health needs but they are smarter in making the most of a 'free' opportunity to improve their health. Other forces add to this less optimistic scenario. The health inequalities literature reports extensively on the 'hard-to-reach' and the failure of many programmes to engage the homeless and illiterate or those in transient or unstable situations. For instance, Velupillai et al (2008, p134) uncover a repeated pattern in which 'the "worried well" and "healthy deprived" would preferentially volunteer'.

Hopefully, the above has proved the reader with a taste of how some of the HaHP programme assumptions were elicited, formalized, and prioritized. We now move to the data and give an indication of how the theories were tested. Dozens of conjectures were interrogated and for the purposes of this exposition we stay with the issues concerning the programme's reach. Inquiry focused on the following three questions:

- How did the programme staff view the programme's ability to address problems of health inequalities?

- How did intended recipients react to the reach efforts of the primary prevention intervention? This required interviews with individuals who responded to the invitation to engage with the intervention as well as those who declined to participate. This aspect of the study was limited because ethical clearance was granted only for individuals who were willing to engage with the intervention.

- Was the programme successful in reaching individuals with multiple disadvantages (eg the poorest individuals living in the poorer areas)? Administrative data collected on characteristics of individuals (where they lived, socio-economic status as measured by the council tax band of the home, age, gender) at the multiple stages of the intervention (see Figure 4.2) allowed the examination of whether the programme was successful in reaching individuals with multiple disadvantages.

Table 4.1 summarizes the research questions, data collection methods, and the analysis that followed. Note the avowedly mixed-methods focus of a theory-driven approach. Findings are organized by question order in Table 4.1.

Did the intervention have the leverage to impact health inequalities?

Programme staff felt that the recruitment strategy had failed largely to engage the target 'hard-to-reach' population and had resulted in an over-representation of the 'worried well.' Key evidence laid in the fact that many clients reported being aware of the need to make changes before receiving the invitation letter and thus being prompted to take part because of that existing awareness.

A number of practitioners provided feedback to help develop a more nuanced method of targeting. Key ideas included the need for a targeting approach that was both multi-tiered and multilevel, and also the need to pay special attention to the sampling frame and the specific prompts required to impact on hard-to-reach populations.

What was it about the intervention that made it attractive for targeted individuals to engage with the intervention?

The analyses from the intended recipients were limited because ethical clearance was granted only for individuals who had consented to be on the study. The individual life circumstances, constraints, and views of those who did not respond to the invitation,

Table 4.1 Data collection and analysis for exploring reach activities

Data source	Research questions	Data collection/analysis
Programme stakeholders	Did the intervention have the leverage to impact health inequalities? Did the programme have the ability to reach individuals with multiple disadvantages who normally do not engage with the health system? How should the programme have been implemented to maximize reach?	15 in-depth semi-structured interviews with key stakeholders involved in the planning and early implementation of HaHP.
Intended programme recipients	What was it about the intervention that made it attractive for targeted individuals to participate in the intervention? Why was this intervention different from the normal health service intervention? Was this intervention likely to appeal to individuals with multiple disadvantages?	Semi-structured interviews were carried out with primary prevention clients who came for screening. Ethical clearance was only obtained to interview individuals who were willing to participate in the intervention.
Administrative data	Were individuals living in poor areas (as measured by the Scottish Index of Multiple Deprivation) more likely to engage with HAHP? Were poorer individuals (as measured by council tax band of the house they lived in) more likely to engage with HAHP?	Letters of invitation were sent to a total of 11,277 individuals. Data on engagement at the multiple stages of the intervention was collected by the programme's internal evaluation team. Multivariate multilevel models were implemented to address the questions.

or who did not participate in the intervention was not known. This limits our ability to address the question but we can still learn about the reasons why individuals participated in the intervention.

All of the ten participants interviewed expressed some degree of readiness to change. Many clients were aware of health issues before taking part, claiming to have responded to the invitation because they wanted to get fitter, to lose weight, or stop smoking. Other reasons included a perception of their own aging and associated deteriorating health, or of a family history of heart disease.

The personal invitation seemed to be important to clients, with some recognizing that they were unlikely to have addressed their health needs without the invitation. Two clients reported having noticed posters in their GP surgery for health interventions and had considered them, but did not take action until invited directly. Taking part was also tied to the idea that 'someone was interested'; this applied to the invitation to health screening but more particularly to the ongoing support from health coaches.

Relationship between area-level poverty, socio-economic status, and participation in the intervention

Multilevel models were developed to assess the impact of area and individual level measures of deprivation on engagement with the intervention. If the programme was successful in reaching the hard-to-reach, then one would expect individuals in lower socio-economic groups and poorer areas to be engaged with the intervention at higher levels. This pattern was not obtained and a somewhat paradoxical finding emerged.

The area level measure of deprivation was not predictive of those who engaged with the intervention. After controlling for differences in individual levels of deprivation, individuals living in poorer areas were not any more likely to engage with the intervention than those living in more affluent areas. However, individual level measures of deprivation were strongly predictive of engaging with the intervention. Poorer individuals had a substantially reduced likelihood of enrolling into the programme.

Implications and conclusions

In these closing remarks we consider the implications and utilization of the findings presented above, using them to reflect on one of the bolder claims for the method, namely that there is 'nothing as practical as a good theory' (Weiss 1995; Pawson 2003). Theory-driven evaluation does not aim to provide verdicts on interventions. It seeks to explain success and failure, both being highly relevant to the business of programme development.

As often happens in the fevered world of policy making, within about a year of the HaHP evaluation starting, another set of interventions called 'Keep Well' began to be implemented in multiple communities in Scotland. Keep Well has since become the central plank of Scotland's anticipatory care policy. Although the two interventions differed in important ways, they had in common a focus on preventive medicine and impacting health inequalities. Accordingly, the lessons on reach, as summarized above, were able to be fed into the planning efforts for Keep Well.

The challenge for interventions attempting to address problems of health inequalities is to identify specifically how individuals who fall within the intersections of disadvantage at the individual and community levels are identified and reached. The enormous advantage of a theory-driven approach for problems of health inequalities is the attention it brings to *who* engages with the intervention. Assessing effectiveness for complex interventions focused on health inequalities, without paying attention to who is treated, might not be very helpful.

In this respect the 'negative' findings from HaHP find immediate use. A programme with a broad brush approach on 'poor areas' may only be a start—other more focused approaches are needed to target poor people in poor areas. Individuals with the greatest need, such as those with multiple disadvantages or co-morbid conditions, may not be identified through standard sampling frames, such as a central data repository. In this respect the HaHP research conjoins with a rich literature beginning to emerge on sampling techniques required to reach hard-to-reach population (Heckathorn 1997, 2002; Salganik and Heckathorn 2004).

Some of the more 'positive' findings of HaHP evaluation also found immediate use. Interviews with the intervention staff indicated the need for tailor-made approaches to reach those who are most deprived, stressing the use of personal invitation followed by personal contact. These lessons on the dynamics of reach were disseminated widely through a series of 'Anticipatory Care' reports that were targeted at the policy and practice community, and in a presentation at the Anticipatory Care Policy organized by the Health Department of the Scottish Government. A notable aspect of these dissemination efforts was that the results were shared while the evaluation of Have a Heart Paisley was still ongoing and outcomes data were still being collected.

Coming finally to broader claims for the methods, we conclude by highlighting one of the real strengths of the theory-driven approach, namely its dynamic view of learning. Programmes unfold through a complex chain of steps—an evaluation learning system similarly needs to follow the causal chain dynamically.

One of the more interesting aspects of the external validity/generalizability literature is how little this literature has dealt with the challenges of generalizing from evaluations of complex interventions. Often the business of learning from evaluations is almost entirely focused on the results of the impact evaluation—usually obtained at the end of the study that may take up to five years. The reality, given the complexity of many interventions, is a need for a richer body of learning that can highlight the complexity of planning, implementation, and pathways by which the interventions work. As described by Sanderson, other functions of evaluations can include 'influencing the conceptualisation of issues, the range of options considered and challenging taken-for-granted assumptions about appropriate goals and activities' (Sanderson 2003, p 333). Theory-driven evaluation can help create a road map that is often missing at the start of an intervention.

Theory-driven evaluations also help raise questions on what incentives are provided by programmes in order to reach their long-term goals—as here on reaching individuals with multiple disadvantages. In an output-driven culture ('you must serve 500 individuals this month'), there are strong incentives to treat the worried well and the healthy poor because they are typically easier to engage. As described above, theory-driven approach brings much needed clarity on a simple issue—who actually participates in interventions aimed at reducing health inequalities and *why*.

Acknowledgements

The evaluation team for Have a Heart Paisley Phase Two was commissioned by Health Scotland and was co-funded by Health Scotland and the Scottish Government's Public Health and Health Improvement Directorate.

Bibliography

Blamey, A, Ayana, M, Lawson, L, Mackinnon, J, Paterson, I, Judge, K (2004) *Final report of the independent evaluation of the National Health Demonstration Project Have a Heart Paisley (Phase One)*. Glasgow: Public Health and Health Policy, University of Glasgow. Available at <http://www.scotland.gov.uk/Publications/2005/03/20836/54354>

Blamey, A and Mackenzie, M (2007) 'Theories of change and realistic evaluation: peas in a pod or apples and oranges?' *Evaluation* 13/4: 439–55

Connell, J, Cubish, A, Schorr, L, and Weiss, C (eds) (1995) *New approaches to evaluating community initiatives*. Volume 1. Washington DC: Aspen Institute

Franklin, A and Ebdon, C (2005) 'Practical experience: building bridges between science and practice' *Administrative Theory and Praxis* 27/4: 628–49

Heckathorn, D (1997) 'Respondent-driven sampling: a new approach to the study of hidden populations' *Social Problems* 44: 174–99

Heckathorn, D (2002) 'Respondent driven sampling II: deriving valid population estimates from chain-referral samples of hidden populations' *Social Problems* 49: 11–34

Hippisley-Cox, J, Coupland, C, Vinogradova, Y, Robson, J, May, M, and Brindle, P (2007) 'Derivation and validation of QRISK, a new cardiovascular disease risk score for the United Kingdom: prospective open cohort study' BMJ 335: 136

Judge, K and Bauld, L (2001) 'Strong theory, flexible methods: evaluating complex community-based initiatives' *Critical Public Health* 11/1: 19–38

Kaplan, S and Garrett, G (2005) 'The use of logic models by community based initiatives' *Evaluation and Programme Planning* 28/2: 167–72

Lyratzopoulos, G, Heller, P, McElduff, M, Hanily, M, and Lewis, P(2006) 'Deprivation and trends in blood pressure, cholesterol, body mass index and smoking among participants of a UK primary care-based cardiovascular risk factor screening programme: both narrowing and widening in cardiovascular risk factor inequalities' *Heart* 92: 1198–206

Mitchell, K (1997) 'Encouraging young women to exercise: can teenage magazines play a role?' *Health Education Journal* 56/2: 264–73

Nestle, M (2003) *Food politics: how the food industry influences nutrition and health*. Berkeley: University of California Press

Pawson, R (2003) 'Nothing as practical as a good theory' *Evaluation* 9/4: 471–90

Pawson, R (2006a) *Evidence based policy: a realist perspective*. London: Sage

Pawson, R (2006b) 'Simple principles for the evaluation of complex programmes' in A Killoran, C Swann, and M P Kelly (eds), *Public health evidence*. Oxford: Oxford University Press

Pawson, R and Tilley, N (1997) *Realistic evaluation*. London: Sage

Pollitt, C (2000) 'Institutional amnesia: a paradox of the "information society"' *Prometheus* 18/1: 5–12

Sanderson, I (2003) 'Is it "what works" that matters? Evaluation and evidence-based policy making' *Journal of Research Papers in Education* 18/4: 329–43

Salganik, M and Heckathorn, D (2004) 'Sampling and estimation in hidden populations using respondent-driven sampling' *Sociological Methodology* 34: 193–239

Scottish Executive (2005a) *Delivering for health*. <http://www.scotland.gov.uk/Resource/Doc/76169/0018996.pdf>

Scottish Executive (2005b) *Building a health service fit for the future*. <http://www.scotland.gov.uk/Resource/Doc/924/0012113.pdf>

Shackley, S and Wynne, B (1997) 'Global warming potentials: ambiguity or precision as an aid to policy?' *Climate Research* 8/1: 89–106

Snowdon, W, Schultz, J, and Swinburn, B (2008) 'Problem and solution trees: a practical approach for identifying potential interventions to improve nutrition' *Health Promotion International* 23/4: 345–53

Sridharan, S, Gnich, W, Moffat, V, Bolton, J, Harkins, C, Hume, M, Nakaima, A, MacDougall, I, and Docherty, P (2008) *Evaluation of Primary Prevention Intervention: Have a Heart Paisley Phase 2*. Glasgow: NHS Health Scotland. Available at: <http://www.chs.med.ed.ac.uk/ruhbc/evaluation/hahpfinal>

Stame, N (2004) 'Theory-based evaluation and types of complexity' *Evaluation* 10/1: 58–76

Trochim, W (1989) A special issue of *Evaluation and Program Planning* on concept mapping for planning and evaluation 12

Tunstall-Pedoe, H and Woodward, M (2006) 'By neglecting deprivation, cardiovascular risk scoring exacerbate social gradients in disease' *Heart* 92: 307–10

Vandenbroek, P, Gossens, J, and Clemens, M (2007) *Tackling obesities: future choices—building the obesity systems map*. Government office for Science, Foresight Programme. London: Department of Innovation, Universities and Skills

Velupillai, N, Packard, C, Batty, G, Bezlyak, V, Burns, H, Cavanagh, J, Deans, K, Ford, I, McGinty, A, Millar, K, Sattar, N, Shiels, P, and Tannahill, C (2008) 'Psychological, social and biological determinants of ill health (pSoBid): study protocol of a population-based study' *BMC Public Health* 8: 126. Available at: <http://www.biomedcentral.com/1471-2458/8/126>

Weiss, C (1995) 'Nothing as practical as a good theory' in Connell, J et al (eds), *New approaches to evaluating community initiatives*. Volume 1. Washington DC: Aspen Institute

Weiss, C (2000) 'Which links in which theories should we evaluate?' in P Rogers et al, *Program theory in evaluation: challenges and opportunities*. New Directions for Evaluation No 87. San Francisco: Jossey Bass

Chapter 5

Equity, risk, and the life-course: a framework for understanding and tackling health inequalities

Hilary Graham and Chris Power

Introduction

The opportunity to live a long and healthy life remains unequal. This is true even in high-income countries with the highest levels of life expectancy. In the UK, as in other rich societies, there are persisting socio-economic differences in health, with those in more advantaged circumstances enjoying better health over longer lives than those in poorer circumstances. These socio-economic differences are captured using a range of indicators of people's circumstances, including their educational level, the occupation of the family's main earner, and the income of the household. The indicators reveal pronounced health differences at all stages of life. For example, children from poorer backgrounds are less likely to survive into adulthood (Wagstaff 2000) and more likely to grow up with health problems (Emerson et al 2006). In adulthood, the ageing process starts earlier and happens more quickly for those in poorer circumstances, bringing with it a higher risk of physical and cognitive impairment in middle and older age (McMunn et al 2003; Melzer et al 2006).

Such health differences are commonly referred to as health inequalities; in the US, the term 'health disparities' is preferred (see Graham 2007). Over the last decade, these inequalities and disparities have become a focus of policy. New public health policies have been launched with reductions in health inequalities as a core goal in the four constituent nations of the UK (England, Northern Ireland, Scotland, and Wales), Canada, Norway, New Zealand, Sweden, and the US. The goal is proving to be very challenging. It requires lifting levels of health in poorer groups closer to those enjoyed by better-off groups. For this to happen, the health of poorer groups has to improve more rapidly than better-off groups. However, in high-income societies, the rate of health gain has tended to be greater in better-off groups, a trend that widens rather than narrows health inequalities (Mackenbach 2005). Further, the diseases which underlie the trend, like coronary heart disease and cancer, typically develop over long time periods and in response to factors operating from childhood and across adulthood. This means that tackling inequalities in adult health requires policies which address their childhood antecedents.

Policy makers are therefore turning their attention to the childhood influences on adult health. In many ways, it is not a new policy focus. The long-term effects of childhood disadvantage have been of intermittent political concern across the 20th century (Kuh and Davey Smith 1993; Finch 1993). In recent decades, evidence has accumulated that childhood conditions do indeed have long-term effects on adult health. However, because this evidence is both extensive and complex, it can remain out of reach of policy makers and practitioners. This chapter aims to make it accessible to those working to tackle health inequalities.

The chapter begins by looking at three concepts which underpin research and policy to promote people's health: inequalities, equity, and risk. It then discusses how childhood conditions influence adult health, pointing to the importance of a set of interconnected pathways which operate from before birth and across the life-course. Next, we present a framework which captures these processes. Finally, we apply the framework to UK policies to illustrate how it can inform policy review and development.

Inequality, inequity and risk

Inequality and inequity The concept of *inequalities* is a descriptive one. It tells us that people's life chances and health chances are linked to broader inequalities in their social position but passes no moral judgement about this fact. The concept of *inequity* is widely used to signal that these inequalities are unfair and unjust. This judgement rests on the principle that we are morally equal: that no one individual or group has an inherent right to a better life or better health than another. This principle of moral equality is applied particularly to children. There is a widely-held view that 'every child matters' and that societies have a collective responsibility to ensure that all children, regardless of the circumstances into which they are born, have an equal chance of a fulfilling and healthy life (HM Treasury 2003).

The work of Amartya Sen has been particularly important in informing thinking about how to build a society which levels up people's life chances and health chances (Sen 1980; 1999). He notes that pre-existing inequalities between people mean that a fairer society can not be achieved simply by ensuring that everyone has the same basic resources: for example, children have the same educational opportunities or that adults have the same income. Inequalities in people's circumstances mean that they will require different quantities and different combinations of resources to achieve equality in what they can be and do. He gives the example of two people with and without impairments, noting that the person with impairments may require greater educational opportunities to achieve the same life chances as the person without impairments and a higher income to secure the same standard of living (Sen 1999). Similarly, a child born to parents who themselves were disadvantaged as children—for example, who were poor and struggled to gain educational qualifications—is likely to require more by way of educational resources, financial help, and professional support to have the same life chances as a child born to parents who, when they were young, grew up in an economically secure family and did well at school. Through examples such as these, Sen argues that what societies should be striving for is equality in what he calls 'capabilities', which he defines as 'the substantive freedoms to choose a life one has reason to value' (Sen 1999, p 74). It is a concept which puts the emphasis on giving every child the resources they need to influence, and make genuine choices about, the future direction of their lives. Informed by Sen's capabilities' perspective, international agencies like the United Nations Development Programme are advocating strong equity-oriented policies, particularly in the early years of life (UNDP 2005).

Risk When describing health inequalities, those in the most advantaged circumstances are often taken as the reference group against which other groups are compared. The focus is on the risk of an outcome, like poor health, in less advantaged groups relative to the risk in the most advantaged group. In other words, it is on *relative risk*. Low birth weight (<2500g) and small for gestational age, the major causes of death in the first year of life, provide examples. Evidence for Britain suggests that a baby born into an unskilled manual family (social class V) is twice as likely to be low birth weight and to be small-for-dates as a baby born to parents in professional occupations (social class I) (Fairley and Leyland 2006). As this example suggests, the use of relative risk can succinctly convey the magnitude of health inequalities. By comparing other groups with those who enjoy the highest standards of health, it also underlines the scope for levelling up health for all children closer to the level attained by the best-off group.

Knowing the relative risk of an outcome tells us nothing about how common the outcome is, either in disadvantaged or advantaged groups. In high-income countries, many adverse outcomes are not common even in the poorest groups. The *absolute risk* is therefore low. In the study cited above, 6 in 100 babies born to parents in social class V were low birth weight. However, in social class I, the proportion was 3 in 100 (Fairley and Leyland 2006). Compared to the reference group, the relative risk of low birth weight was twice as high for the most disadvantaged children. A similar pattern was found for the proportion of babies who were small for gestational age.

As the example of low birth weight illustrates, relative risk and absolute risk capture different dimensions of health inequalities. It is important to be aware of the difference when investigating, and seeking to address, the association between poor circumstances and poor health (Lynch et al 2006).

Childhood circumstances matter for adult health

There is increasing evidence that adult health is influenced by circumstances earlier in life, with childhood disadvantage increasing the risk of premature death in adulthood. This pattern is found across countries and ethnic groups, for men and women and for both younger and older cohorts (Galobardes et al 2007). The pattern is illustrated in Figure 5.1. Based on the British 1946 birth cohort, it tracks survival from age 26 (when almost all children were still alive) to age 54. As it indicates, the absolute risk of death is higher among adults born into manual households (6 per 100) than among adults who grew up in non-manual households (3 per 100), and their death rates are twice as high. A similar pattern is apparent for specific causes of death, with adults from poorer childhood backgrounds at greater risk of early death from 'big killers' like coronary heart disease, stroke, and respiratory disease than those from more advantaged backgrounds (Davey Smith et al 2001; Galobardes et al 2007).

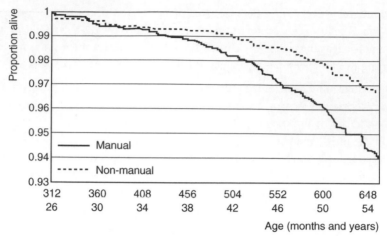

Fig. 5.1 Cumulative death rates age 26 to 54 by father's social class at birth among men and women in the 1946 birth cohort study

Source: Reproduced from Kuh et al 2002 with permission from BMJ Publishing Group Ltd

Low household income is often used to identify children growing up in poor circumstances. One widely-used measure defines a child as poor if she or he lives in a household with an income which, after account is taken of its size and composition, is less than 60% of median household income. Figure 5.2 takes this measure and compares the proportion of children living in poverty in countries which are broadly similar in their overall levels of wealth, with the US significantly richer than the rest. The figure points to marked national differences in the absolute risk of a child living in poverty, from nearly 1 in 3 in the US to less than 1 in 10 in Denmark, Finland, Sweden, and Norway. The figure suggests, too, that in most countries children are at greater risk of poverty than the population as whole: in other words, their relative risk is higher. However, in the Nordic countries, child poverty rates are appreciably below the overall poverty rate.

Why childhood circumstances matter for adult health

Knowing that childhood circumstances matter for adult health does not tell us why they matter. An important starting point is an appreciation that childhood is a period of development—particularly rapid in the early years of life but continuing through adolescence—which is shaped by the child's environment. Developmental processes embrace physical and emotional development and the acquisition of cognitive and social skills; they include, too, the development of health-related behaviours like cigarette smoking. The concept of 'developmental health' has been coined to capture these broad dimensions of children's health, with children's opportunities to reach their potential facilitated or impeded by their social and material environment (Hertzman and Keating 1999).

There is considerable evidence that the conditions in which children are conceived, born, and grow up influence adult health through a set of interlocking pathways. Three pathways have been identified as particularly important, with a child's circumstances

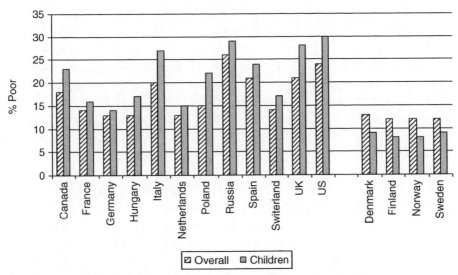

Fig. 5.2 Percentage of children and the total population living in poverty 2000
Source: Luxembourg Wealth Study 2008
Note: poverty defined as a household income <60% of median income adjusted for household size and composition

impacting on adult health by influencing (i) their health in childhood (ii) their pathways into adulthood and their adult socio-economic circumstances (iii) their health-related behaviours. We discuss these pathways separately: in reality, they work alongside and through each other.

(i) Childhood circumstances and child health From the moment of conception, the development process is genetically regulated but not genetically determined (Halfon and Hochstein 2002). Instead, it is stimulated and shaped by the child's environment. As a result, experiences which are physically and emotionally nurturing become embedded in body structures and functions in ways which promote future health. Conversely, environmental adversity in the early years of life—chronic disadvantage, for example—has been found to induce long-term patterns of physical, cognitive, and emotional development which leave children vulnerable to poor health in later life.

One example is physical development in early life. Children born to mothers whose own developmental health was constrained by disadvantage come into the world in poorer health than the children of mothers who have led more privileged lives. Evidence on birth weight and child-to-adult growth trajectories point to marked socio-economic gradients in infant health and child development (Dezateux et al 2004; Li et al 2004). Both birth weight and growth trajectories are, in turn, associated with risk factors for cardiovascular disease, like blood pressure, blood lipids, and blood glucose levels in adulthood (Li et al 2007; Thomas et al 2007; Cooper and Power 2008).

A second example is cognitive development. Children are born with a rich network of brain cells already in place. But this neural network is activated and sculpted by the conditions into which infants are born. Early cognitive ability lays the foundation for self-confidence at school entry and for praise from teachers, for high test scores and exam grades through school, and for future entry into non-manual occupations which secure a place on the higher echelons of the socio-economic hierarchy (see Graham 2007). Social disadvantage can put barriers in the way of children's cognitive development, leaving them more vulnerable to developmental difficulties than children growing up in more advantaged circumstances (Yeung et al 2002; Emerson et al 2006).

Socio-economic inequalities in cognitive skills are evident at a very young age. At age three, the children of parents with high levels of education and high incomes achieve higher scores in cognitive assessments (naming objects presented in pictures, naming colours, recognizing shapes and letters etc) than children from less advantaged backgrounds (George et al 2007). Figure 5.3 captures inequalities in cognitive development from age 7 to age 16 as measured by children's scores in mathematical tests (at each age, a z-score of 0 is average for that age). Parental social class is based on father's occupation, with the figure focusing on the highest occupational groups (professional: social class I; managerial: social class II) and lowest groups (semi-skilled manual: IV; unskilled manual: V). As it suggests, social advantage is associated with above-average scores and social disadvantage with below-average scores, with the cognitive trajectories of children diverging as they progress through primary and secondary school (Jefferis et al 2002). It appears that children from professional families gain more from what schools are teaching and tests are assessing than children from poorer backgrounds, a finding confirmed by wider research on children's progress through the UK education system (Reay 1998; Cassen and Kingdom 2007).

Children growing up in disadvantaged circumstances also face stresses and challenges that children from more affluent backgrounds can avoid. They are more likely to grow up in families with serious financial worries, to be cared for by parents who are under strain and to experience major family change (parental separation and divorce, for example) (Yeung et al 2002). These stresses and challenges can take a toll on children's emotional well-being, with elevated rates of emotional and behavioural problems (finding it hard to be self-confident, to concentrate and to contain anxiety and aggression, for example) found among children from poorer families (Power and Matthews 1997; Meltzer et al 2000).

(ii) Children's circumstances and adult circumstances If all children had the same life chances, then the circumstances in which they grew up would not predict their socio-economic circumstances in adulthood. However, studies demonstrate that children's social backgrounds exert a powerful influence on their future socio-economic position. Thus, children born to parents with high status and well-paid jobs are more likely to have high status and well-paid jobs when they grow up than children born to parents restricted to low paid and insecure work. The evidence suggests that this pattern is stronger in the UK than in other European countries and has become more marked over time (Breen 2004; Blanden et al 2005).

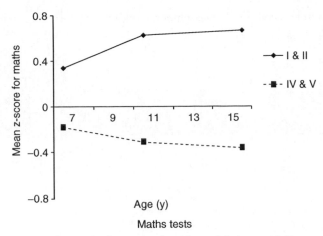

Fig. 5.3 Average z scores for maths from ages 7–16 by social class at birth among participants in the 1958 birth cohort study

Source: Reproduced from Jefferis et al 2002 with permission from BMJ Publishing Group Ltd
Notes:
1. A child with a score of 0 is about average relative to other children of that age. An increasing z-score with age signals improvement in relative achievement.
2. Social class I and II (professional and managerial occupations; social class IV and V (semi-skilled and unskilled manual occupations and children with no male head of household).
3. Low birthweight children excluded.

These intergenerational continuities in socio-economic circumstances mean that childhood disadvantage increases the risk of disadvantage across the life-course. This matters for health because poor adult circumstances increase the risk of poor health and premature death, and do so over and above the effect of conditions earlier in life (Kuh et al 2002). It matters for health, too, because rates of poor health and premature mortality rise in line with duration of exposure to poor circumstances. Rates are lowest among adults who avoid disadvantage from birth and across their lives; they are highest among those who never escape it (Power et al 1999; Davey Smith et al 1997).

Education is central to the process through which privilege and disadvantage are transmitted across the generations (Gangl et al 2004). In high-income countries like the UK, educational qualifications are increasingly required to enter the labour market, and high levels of qualifications are needed for careers which offer fulfilling work, job security, and high pay. Parents who have educational qualifications and successful careers are well-placed to ensure that their children 'follow in their footsteps'. Figure 5.4 takes the example of higher education to illustrate the influence of parental background on children's educational trajectories in Britain. While higher education participation rates have increased for all income groups, a steep socio-economic gradient remains. Further, the figure suggests that the gradient has steepened since the 1970s (Machin 2003). As a recent

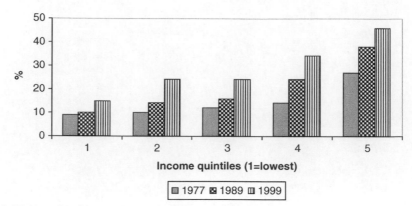

Fig. 5.4 Higher education participation among 19-year-olds by parental income (in quintiles) in Britain in the late 1970s, 1980s, and 1990s
Source: Machin 2003, Table 2

study concludes 'the expansion of higher education in the UK has benefited those from richer backgrounds far more than poorer people' (Blanden et al 2005, p 12).

Facing greater barriers to educational success, children from disadvantaged backgrounds are more likely to become disaffected by school and to invest in identities which do not rely on doing well at school and in the labour market (Graham 2007). For example, they are more likely to take on parental responsibilities early and outside a cohabiting relationship. Figure 5.5 maps the educational and domestic patterns among young women by parental social class based on the UK's official classification, the National Statistics Socio-economic Classification (NS-SEC). As it indicates, only a minority had no educational qualifications, was a mother by the age of 22, or was a lone parent. However, the proportions are lowest among women from advantaged backgrounds and highest among those from disadvantaged backgrounds. Early motherhood can offer a self-affirming route into adulthood, but also leaves young women vulnerable to continuing disadvantage in adulthood (Graham and McDermott 2006). As this suggests, a disadvantaged start in life can constrain a child's life-course both directly, by limiting their educational opportunities, and indirectly, by shaping the life choices that they make within their constrained circumstances.

(iii) Children's circumstances and health-related behaviours Everyday activities—what we eat and with whom, whether and what we smoke, whether and how we take exercise—are integral to our identity and to affirming our sense of belonging, both within our families and within the communities which matter to us. At the same time, these behaviours influence our health (Cavill et al 2006; Government Office 2007; Khaw et al 2008). There is evidence that at least some health-related behaviours are socially patterned, with children from poorer backgrounds more likely to develop and sustain behaviours which take a toll on their current and future health.

Children from poorer households are less likely to consume fresh fruit and vegetables and to take part in sport and exercise (swimming, football, gymnastics, etc). For example,

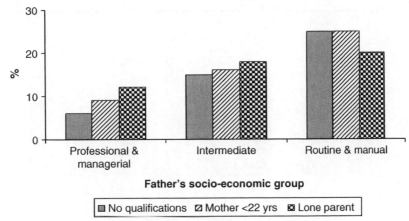

Fig. 5.5 Educational and domestic trajectories by childhood socio-economic circumstances (based on father's occupation), women aged 22 to 34, Britain, 1998–2002
Source: unpublished data reproduced with permission of Southampton Women's Survey

the consumption of the recommended five or more portions a day of fresh fruit and vegetables rises from 15% in the poorest fifth of households to over 30% in the richest income quintile (Craig and Mindell 2008). In turn, behaviours established in childhood tend to continue ('track') into adult life, as seen for example for levels of physical activity (Parsons et al 2006).

Energy intake (diet) and energy expenditure (physical activity) are the major determinants of body mass index (BMI), with a BMI of $\geq$ 30 defining someone as obese. Inequalities in obesity were largely absent among children growing up in the 1960s (Power et al 2003). But as rates have increased, inequalities in childhood obesity have strengthened, with rates increasing fastest among children from poorer backgrounds (Stamatakis et al 2005). As children grow up, patterns of BMI track into adulthood (Serdula et al 1993).

In the UK, there is also evidence that poorer childhood circumstances are associated with higher rates of adult smoking in the white population. The majority of smokers take up the habit in their teenage years—and then continue to smoke in adulthood (Goddard 2008; Jefferies et al 2004). As Figure 5.6 suggests, young people from poorer backgrounds are more likely to become regular smokers and to smoke heavily. In turn, poorer childhood circumstances and heavier smoking in adolescence reduce the chances of quitting in adulthood and increase the chances of remaining a smoker into middle age (Jefferies et al 2003).

Building the framework

The section above has reviewed evidence linking childhood circumstances and adult health. While the evidence is extensive, it is not without limitations. In the UK, the major longitudinal studies were established when Asian and African-Caribbean families made up a small proportion of the population. They can therefore shed light on how childhood

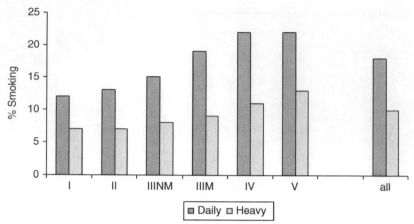

Fig. 5.6 Prevalence of daily and heavy smoking (>35 cigarettes a week) among young people aged 15 by parental social class, Scotland, 1999
Source: Sweeting and West 2001, Table 1

disadvantage can compromise future health among white children. However, they can say little about how a child's cultural background and their exposure to, or protection from, racism mediates the effects of childhood disadvantage on health in adult life. Further, birth cohort studies, like other surveys, collect quantitative information on individuals and the families they live in. It is an approach which, to date, reveals little about children's perspectives on their lives (Redmond 2008). It also cannot capture how the operation of broader social institutions—like the education system, the labour market and welfare agencies for example—maintains or moderates inequalities in people's circumstances and in their health.

While the evidence is incomplete, it suggests that links between childhood disadvantage and poor adult health can be broken down into the constituent elements discussed in this chapter: poor childhood circumstances, a set of interconnecting child-to-adult pathways, poor adult circumstances, and poor adult health. Figure 5.7 captures these elements. It needs to be emphasized that the figure is a schematic representation of dynamic and interconnected processes. But the figure includes both the core factors and underlying relationships highlighted in the more complex models developed by epidemiologists (see, for example, Kuh et al 2004).

The starting point is childhood disadvantage. This stems from parental disadvantage and has its effects from before birth and across childhood. Childhood disadvantage shapes the pathways that link childhood disadvantage to poor adult health. The pathways include the development of physical and emotional health, and health behaviours: these are seen to affect adult health directly. But the pathways also range across cognitive development and educational progress, and investment in identities like young parenthood. Educational and social pathways shape adult health primarily through their impact on adult circumstances; additionally, they exert an influence on key health behaviours which persist into adulthood.

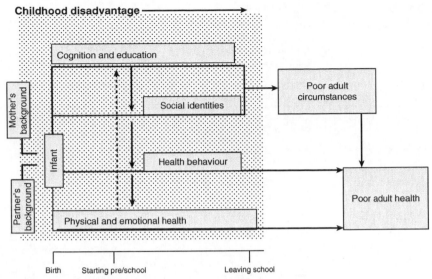

Fig. 5.7 Lifecourse framework linking childhood disadvantage to poor adult health
Source: Graham and Power 2004

A framework for policy review and development

The evidence on which the framework is built suggests that children's unequal circumstances leave them unequal in their opportunities of living a long and healthy life: unequal in what Sen terms 'capabilities'. To give every child the chances and choices available to those growing up in advantaged circumstances, governments need to act on the sequence of factors through which childhood circumstances influence adult health. Specifically, policies are required which narrow inequalities in the lives of parents, present and future, in the material and social conditions of poor children, their developmental health (physical, emotional, and cognitive) and health behaviour, their educational and social trajectories, their adult circumstances, and their adult health.

Table 5.1 illustrates how policies can be mapped onto this sequence. It gives examples from the UK where the dominant focus has been on interventions targeted at poorer groups. Over the last decade, a raft of initiatives have sought to improve the employability of young people with few educational qualifications (for example, the New Deal for Young People), raise the incomes of poor families (child poverty strategy), and support poor parents in their parenting role (Sure Start, Teenage Pregnancy Strategy, Healthy Start, Family Nurse Partnership). While important, these initiatives form only part of a much larger system through which resources are distributed between socio-economic groups and across the life-course. The table therefore includes both targeted interventions and the major social institutions, including the education system, the labour market, and the tax system, which govern everyone's lives.

There are three reasons why the process of policy review and development should cover both targeted interventions and mainstream policies.

Table 5.1 Tackling the links between childhood disadvantage and adult health: UK programmes 1997–2008

Tackling inequalities in:	Established systems and policies (examples)	Targeted interventions (examples)
Today's and tomorrow's parents	Education system, employment policies	New Deal for Young People
Circumstances of poor children	Social security system, social housing provision, tax policy	Working Tax Credit, Child Tax Credit
—their developmental health	Pre-school provision, recreational provision	Sure Start, Healthy Start, Family Nurse Partnership
—their health behaviour	Tobacco control and food policies, recreational provision	Sure Start
—their educational and social trajectories	Education system, employment policies, social security system	Teenage Pregnancy Strategy
—their adult circumstances	Social security system, social housing provision, employment and tax policy	New Deal for Communities
—their adult health	Health services, personal social services	Smoking cessation services

Firstly, the life chances and health chances of children from poorer backgrounds are powerfully shaped by macro institutions and the policies which regulate them. The labour market is one example. Even in times of low unemployment, parents who are confined to the low-skilled sector of the labour market are disproportionately affected by wider economic conditions. Compared to parents in professional and managerial jobs, they are much more likely to experience intermittent employment, low pay, and redundancy, and much less likely to have jobs where earnings are reliable and increase in real terms over time (Goldthorpe and McKnight 2006). The social security system is another example. The living standards of poor children are underwritten by the UK's complex structure of welfare benefits and tax credits to a much greater extent than children from richer families. But the value of safety-net benefits like income support, the major benefit for out-of-work households, provide an income well below the poverty line (of 60% median income) (Stewart 2005). Looking beyond the social security system to other parts of the welfare state, the social housing sector (housing rented from local authorities and housing associations) is home to Britain's poorest families. Like the majority of the population, they also rely on publicly-funded schools for their children's education and the National Health Service for their health care (Rickards et al 2004).

Secondly, wider systems and policies mediate the effects of targeted interventions to reduce social inequalities in children's circumstances and life chances. Where the wider systems and policies are contributing to a narrowing of these inequalities, the intervention has a better chance of success; where they are reinforcing them, it is likely that the positive effects of the intervention will be significantly diluted. For example, the UK's goal of eliminating child poverty has relied primarily on targeted financial support for poor families (tax credits and welfare benefits). The reforms introduced since the late 1990s have been progressive, with the proportion of children in poverty (in households below 60% of median income) falling from 1997 to 2005—although there is now evidence that rates are rising again (Brewer et al 2008). But targeted policies can not address wider inequalities in income and wealth. With incomes continuing to rise sharply for the richest households, income inequality has not fallen since 1997: on most measures it has increased (Brewer et al 2008).

Thirdly, focusing on wider systems underlines the importance of equity-oriented strategies which work across them. The Nordic countries have developed strong family policies by integrating policy fields which have traditionally remained separate in the UK. Employment policies support high rates of maternal employment (eg paid and comprehensive parental leave), child care policies provide subsidized or free child care, and social security policies provide a structure of universal benefits and an income for out-of-work families which lift them above the poverty line (Ferrarani and Forssén 2005; Whiteford and Adema 2006; Stewart 2005). Combined with redistributive fiscal policies and delivered through universal rather than targeted policies, the result is a low rate of child poverty (Figure 5.2).

Conclusion

There is increasing evidence that the social conditions in which children spend their early years have long-term effects on their health. Our aim has been to develop a framework which can inform policy by pointing to key pathways linking childhood conditions to adult health.

The framework suggests that policies to reduce inequalities in children's circumstances should be a cornerstone of policies to reduce social and health inequalities. But it also makes clear that early-years policies are not enough. The framework underlines the importance of policies which narrow inequalities not only in children's circumstances but over the life-course and across generations. Its life-course perspective argues for an integrated approach which includes targeted programmes and the mainstream policies in which they are embedded. Without this broad approach, targeted interventions are unlikely to address the inequalities in people's past and current circumstances which underpin health inequalities.

Acknowledgements

The chapter draws on two key sources. Firstly, it updates work funded by England's Health Development Agency prior to its incorporation into the National Institute for Health and Clinical Excellence (NICE) and undertaken by the authors. The report, *Child disadvantage and adult health: a lifecourse framework*, is available at <http://www.nice.org. uk/aboutnice/whoweare/aboutthehda/evidencebase/keypapers/papersthatinformand supporttheevidencebase/childhood_disadvantage_and_adult_health_a_lifecourse_ framework.jsp>; see also Graham and Power 2004. Secondly, the chapter draws on *Unequal Lives: Health and Socioeconomic Inequalities* (Hilary Graham 2007).

Funding support: GOSH/UCL Institute of Child Health receives a proportion of funding from the Department of Health's NIHR Biomedical Research Centres funding scheme and the Centre for Paediatric Epidemiology and Biostatistics benefits from support from the Medical Research Council in its capacity as the MRC Centre of Epidemiology for Child Health.

Bibliography

Blanden, J, Gregg, P, and Machin, S (2005) *Intergenerational mobility in Europe and North America*. London: Centre for Economic Performance, London School of Economics

Breen, R (ed) (2004) *Social mobility in Europe*. Oxford: Oxford University Press

Brewer, M, Muriel, A, Phillips, D, and Sibieta, L (2008) *Poverty and inequality in the UK: 2008*. London: Institute for Fiscal Studies

Cassen, R and Kingdom, G (2007) *Tackling low educational achievement*. York: Joseph Rowntree Foundation

Cavill, N, Kahlmeier, S, and Racioppi, F (eds) (2006) *Physical activity and health in Europe: evidence for action*. Copenhagen: WHO Europe. Available at: <http://www.euro.who.int/document/e89490.pdf>

Cooper, R and Power, C (2008) 'Sex differences in the association between birthweight and lipids in middle-age: findings from the 1958 British birth cohort' *Atherosclerosis* 200/1: 141–9

Craig, R and Mindell, J (2008) *Health survey for England 2006: obesity and other risk factors in children*. London: NatCen for the Information Centre

Davey Smith, G, Gunnell, D, and Ben-Shlomo, Y (2001) 'Lifecourse approaches to socio-economic differentials in cause-specific adult mortality' in D Leon and G Walt (eds), *Poverty, inequality and health*. Oxford: Oxford University Press

Davey Smith, G, Hart, C, Blane, D, Gillis, C, and Hawthorne V (1997) 'Lifetime socioeconomic position and mortality: prospective observational study' *British Medical Journal* 314: 547–52

Dezateux, C, Bedford, H, Cole, T, et al (2004) 'Babies' health and development' in S Dex and H Joshi (eds), *Millennium cohort study first survey: a user's guide to initial findings*. London: Centre for Longitudinal Studies, Institute of Education, University of London

Emerson, E, Graham, H, and Hatton, C (2006) 'Household income and health status in children and adolescents in Britain' *European Journal of Public Health* 14/4: 354–60

Fairley, L and Leyland, AH (2006) 'Social class inequalities in perinatal outcomes: Scotland 1980–2000' *Journal of Epidemiology and Community Health* 60: 31–6

Ferrarani, T and Forssén, K (2005) 'Family policy and cross-national patterns of poverty' in O Kangas and J Palme (eds), *Social policy and economic development in the Nordic Countries*. Basingstoke: Macmillan/Palgrave

Finch, L (1993) *The classing gaze: sexuality, class and surveillance*. Sydney: Allen and Unwin

Galobardes, B, Davey Smith, G, and Lynch, JW (2007) 'Systematic review of the influence of childhood socioeconomic circumstances on risk of cardiovascular disease in adulthood' *Annals of Epidemiology* 17: 511–13

Gangl, M, Muller, W, and Raffe, D (eds) (2004) *Transitions from education to work in Europe*. Oxford: Oxford University Press

George, A, Hansen, K, and Schoon, I (2007) 'Child development' in K Hansen and H Joshi (eds), *Millennium cohort study second survey: a user's guide to initial findings*. London: Centre for Longitudinal Studies

Goddard, E (2008) *Smoking and drinking among adults, 2006*. Newport, Wales: Office for National Statistics

Goldthorpe, JH and McKnight, A (2006) 'The economic basis of social class' in S Morgan, DB Grusky, and GS Fields (eds), *Mobility and inequality: frontiers of research from sociology and economics*. Stanford: Stanford University Press

Government Office for Science (2007) *Foresight: tackling obesities: future choices—project report*. Available at: <http://www.foresight.gov.uk/OurWork/ActiveProjects/Obesity/KeyInfo/Index.asp>

Graham, H (2007) *Unequal lives: health and socioeconomic inequalities*. Buckingham: Open University Press

Graham, H and McDermott, E (2006) 'Qualitative research and the evidence-base of policy: insights from studies of teenage mothers in the UK' *Journal of Social Policy* 35/1: 1–17

Graham, H and Power, C (2004) 'Childhood disadvantage and health inequalities: a framework for policy based on lifecourse research' *Child: Care, Health and Development* 30: 671–9

Halfon, N and Hochstein, M (2002) 'Life course health development: an integrated framework for developing health, policy, and research' *The Milbank Quarterly* 80/3: 433–79

Hertzman, C and Keating, DP (eds) (1999) *Developmental health and the wealth of nations.* London: Guildford Press

HM Treasury (2003) *Every child matters,* Cm 5860. London: The Stationery Office

Jefferis, B, Power, C, and Hertzman, C (2002) 'Birthweight, childhood socio-economic environment and cognitive development in the 1958 British birth cohort' *British Medical Journal* 325: 305–8

Jefferis, BJ, Graham, H, Manor, O, and Power, C (2003) 'Level of cigarette smoking and socio-economic circumstances in adolescence: how do they affect adult smoking?' *Addiction* 98: 1765–72

Jefferis, JMH, Power, C, Graham, G, and Manor, O (2004) 'Effects of childhood socio-economic circumstances on persistent smoking' *American Journal of Public Health*, 94: 279–85

Khaw, K-T, Wareham, N, Bingham, S, et al (2008) 'Combined impact of health behaviours and mortality in men and women: the EPIC-Norfolk prospective population study' *PLOS Med* 5: 1

Kuh, D and Davey Smith, G (1993) 'When is mortality risk determined? Historical insights into a current debate' *Social History of Medicine* 6: 101–23

Kuh, D, Hardy, R, Langenberg, C, Richards, R, and Wadsworth, NEJ (2002) 'Mortality in adults aged 26–54 related to socioeconomic conditions in childhood and adulthood: post war birth cohort study' *British Medical Journal* 325: 1076–80

Kuh, D, Power, C, Blanc, D, and Bartley, M (2004) 'Socioeconomic pathways between childhood and adult health' in DL Kuh and Y Ben-Shlomo (eds), *A life course approach to chronic disease epidemiology.* 2nd edn. Oxford: Oxford University Press

Li, L, Manor, O, and Power, C (2004) 'Early environment and child-to-adult growth trajectories in the 1958 British birth cohort' *American Journal of Clinical Nutrition* 80: 185–92

Li, L, Law, C, and Power, C (2007) 'Body Mass Index throughout the life-course and blood pressure in mid-adult life: a birth cohort study' *Journal of Hypertension* 25: 1215–23

Luxembourg Wealth Study (2008) *Database.* Available at: <http://www.lisproject.org/lwstechdoc.htm> (multiple countries; 2000)

Lynch, J, Davey Smith, G, Harper, S, and Bainbridge, K (2006) 'Explaining the social gradient in coronary heart disease: comparing relative and absolute approaches' *Journal of Epidemiology and Community Health* 60: 436–41

Machin, S (2003) 'Unto them that hath . . . .' *CentrePiece* 8/1: 5–9

Mackenbach, JP (2005) *Health inequalities: Europe in profile.* An independent expert report commissioned by and published under the auspices of the UK Presidency of the EU. Rotterdam: Erasmus MC University Medical Center

McMunn, A, Hyde, M, Janevic, M, and Kumari, M (2003) 'Health' in M Marmot, J Banks, R Blundell, C Lessof, and J Nazroo (eds), *Health, wealth and lifestyles of the older population in England: the 2002 English longitudinal study of ageing.* London: Institute of Fiscal Studies

Meltzer, H and Gatwood, R (2000) *Mental health of children and adolescents in Great Britain.* London: The Stationery Office

Melzer, D, Gardener, E, Lang, I, McWilliams, B, and Guralnik, JM (2006) 'Measured physical performance' in J Banks, E Breeze, C Lessof, and J Nazroo (eds), *Retirement, health and relationships of the older population in England: the 2004 English longitudinal study of ageing (wave 2).* London: Institute of Fiscal Studies

Parsons, T, Power, C, and Manor, O (2006) 'Longitudinal physical activity and diet patterns in the 1958 British birth cohort' *Med Sci Sports Ex* 38: 547–54

Power, C and Matthews, S (1997) 'Origins of health inequalities in a national population sample' *Lancet* 350: 1584–9

Power, C, Manor, O, and Matthews, S (1999) 'The duration and timing of exposure: effects of socio-economic environment on adult health' *American Journal of Public Health* 89/7: 1059–66

Power, C, Matthews, S, and Manor, O (2003) 'Child-to-adult socio-economic conditions and obesity in a national cohort' *International Journal of Obesity Related Metabolic Disorders* 27/9: 1081–6

Reay, D (1998) *Class work: mothers' involvement in children's schooling.* London: University College Press

Redmond, G (2008) *Children's perspectives on economic adversity: a review of the literature,* IDP 2008-01. Florence: Unicef Innocenti Research Centre

Rickards, L, Fox, K, Roberts, C, Fletcher, L, and Goddard, E (2004) *Living in Britain 2002, No 31. Results from the 2002 General Household Survey.* London: The Stationery Office

Sen, A (1980) 'Equality of what?' in S McMurrin (ed). *Tanner lectures on human values.* Cambridge: Cambridge University Press

Sen, A (1999) *Development as freedom.* Oxford: Oxford University Press

Serdula, MK, Ivery, D, Coates, RJ, Freedman, DS, Williamson, DF, and Byers, T (1993) 'Do obese children become obese adults? A review of the literature' *Preventive Medicine* 22: 167–77

Stamatakis, E, Primatesta, P, Chinn, S, Rona, R, and Falascheti, E (2005) 'Overweight and obesity trends from 1974 to 2003 in English children: what is the role of socioeconomic factors?' *Archives of Disease in Childhood* 90: 999–1004

Stewart, K (2005) 'Changes in poverty and inequality in the UK in an international context' in J Hills and K Stewart (eds), *A more equal society? New Labour, poverty, inequality and exclusion*. London: Policy Press

Sweeting, H and West, P (2001) 'Social class and smoking at age 15: the effect of different definitions of smoking' *Addiction* 96: 1357–9

Thomas, C, Hyppönen, E, and Power, C (2007) 'Prenatal exposures and glucose metabolism in adulthood: are effects mediated through birthweight and adiposity?' *Diabetes Care* 30: 918–24

United Nations Development Programme (UNDP) (2005) *Human Development Report 2005*. New York: UNDP

Wagstaff, A (2000) 'Socioeconomic inequalities in child mortality: comparisons across nine developing countries' *Bulletin of the World Health Organisation* 78/1: 19–29

Whiteford, P and Adema, W (2006) 'Combating child poverty in OECD countries: is work the answer? *European Journal of Social Security* 8/3: 235–56

Yeung, J, Linver, M, and Brooks-Gunn, J (2002) 'How money matters for young children's development: parental investment and family processes' *Child Development* 73: 1861–79

Chapter 6

Vulnerability, disadvantage, and sexual health

Roger Ingham and Debbie Smith

Introduction

This chapter aims to define the important role of social context in influencing health behaviours and health. It focuses specifically on the complex interplay between vulnerability, disadvantage, and sexual health among young people—mirroring national and international concerns. We consider:

- what is meant by the term *sexual health* and what are the key public health concerns;
- what is known about factors associated with poor sexual health; and
- what is known about how poor sexual health outcomes might be alleviated.

Each of these issues will be considered somewhat briefly. Nevertheless, the analysis serves to show that effective strategies for improving sexual health must address the underlying causes of vulnerability and risk among young people.

Defining sexual health and concerns

The World Health Organization (WHO) has developed a 'working definition' of sexual health as follows:

> Sexual health is a state of physical, emotional, mental and social well-being in relation to sexuality; it is not merely the absence of disease, dysfunction or infirmity. Sexual health requires a positive and respectful approach to sexuality and sexual relationships, as well as the possibility of having pleasurable and safe sexual experiences, free of coercion, discrimination and violence. For sexual health to be attained and maintained, the sexual rights of all persons must be respected, protected and fulfilled.

(WHO 2006; unofficial)

There are a number of matters to note about this definition. First, it is made clear on the WHO website that this is 'unofficial'. Although the website does not specify why this is the case, it illustrates clearly that the whole area is not without controversy.

Second, the definition mentions positive aspects of sexual activity (note the term 'pleasurable'), an approach that does not feature prominently in many national policy discussions of the area. Third, mention is made of the rights of *all* individuals, again an approach that raises many issues that may not be universally accepted; for example, in countries where women are constitutionally afforded less power than are men, as well as in countries where same sex activity is illegal and severely punishable.

In England, the National Strategy for Sexual Health and HIV adopted a somewhat less controversial definition, with a balance between positive and negative aspects albeit with a slight leaning towards the latter:

> Sexual health is an important part of physical and mental health. It is a key part of our identity as human beings together with the fundamental human rights to privacy, a family life and living free from discrimination. Essential elements of good sexual health are equitable relationships and sexual fulfilment with access to information and services to avoid the risk of unintended pregnancy, illness or disease

> (DH 2001, p 5)

This leaning towards the negative aspects of sexual health is of course quite understandable. Public health concerns focus on the outcomes of unintended pregnancy and sexually transmitted infections (STIs) rather than whether the sexual activity was enjoyable and fulfilling.

The concept of sexual health differs in many ways from other forms of illness and disease covered in this volume. For example, the specific activity that leads to sexual health outcomes of one kind or another is intertwined with a whole range of moral, religious, legal, and other issues. In other words, policy concern about sexual health, especially amongst younger people, may be as much driven by disapproval of sexual activity *per se* than by negative physical health outcomes.

This contrast is neatly illustrated by the relatively dominant approaches taken by the Governments in the USA and England in relation to teenage pregnancies. The former has approached the issue in primarily moral terms, with substantial national funding being available to support increased provision of abstinence-only education programmes. By contrast, the impetus (at least officially) for a new strategy on teenage pregnancy in England came from the angle of social exclusion and has been continued through the children's well-being agenda. Central to this approach is increased provision of sex and relationships education, greater service provision for young people, and greater practical and material support for young parents.

Indices of sexual health

As mentioned above, the major policy concerns regarding sexual health have been directed towards unintended pregnancy and STIs. In relation to pregnancy, greater policy concern is expressed in relation to early conceptions, with the under 18 year-old bracket being highlighted in current target setting in England. Other concerns are additionally expressed in relation to abortion, with the steady increase in rates amongst women of all ages attracting particular attention.

Sexually transmitted infections give rise to further considerable concerns. Rates of sexually transmitted HIV (as opposed to via needle exchange or blood transfusions) continue to rise year-on-year; although male-to-male and heterosexual routes of transmission are both increasing, the latter is doing so at a much faster rate than the former

(AVERT 2008). Likewise, rates of many other STIs are rising at steady rates, although in some cases it is not easy to ascertain to what extent rising rates reflect greater opportunities for being, and willingness to be, tested.

Indices with regards to psychological sexual health are less tangible. Some studies of young people ask about their views on their first sexual experiences, especially intercourse. Generally, regret is expressed by more young women then young men, and is more likely to be reported when first intercourse was experienced at younger ages (Dickson et al 1998; Wight et al 2000). Other studies have looked at sexual satisfaction amongst older people from within a dysfunction agenda; although such problems may be highly upsetting for the individuals and the partners concerned, they have attracted considerably less public policy attention (and support, given the restrictions placed on NHS prescribing of Viagra, for example).

Why does sexual health matter?

There are a number of levels at which this question can be considered. From a psychological perspective, it is often claimed that a satisfactory and fulfilling sexual life is associated with contentment and happiness. However, it is not at all clear how this can be empirically claimed with certainty, since the separation of the sexual element from other aspects of a close relationship poses methodological challenges! Certainly, therapists do claim that where the sexual element is missing from a relationship, then other aspects are likely to suffer too.

Negative psychological reactions to, and associations with, sexual activity amongst young people are a cause for concern. Some argue that regretted early intercourse may lead to lowered self-esteem and control such that a downward spiral is experienced. Certainly, experience of sexual abuse is closely associated with a wide range of negative health and social outcomes (Kendall-Tackett et al 1993; Kirkengen 2001), even including fear during later childbirth (Eberhard-Gran et al 2008). Again, however, causal links are not easy to disentangle both for conceptual reasons as well as due to the methodological challenges involved.

Considerably greater attention has been paid to more easily measurable physical outcomes concerned with sexual health. If infections were inevitably symptomatic and led to early treatment, then there would be less concern; but they are often not. HIV is virtually always asymptomatic and can take a very long time before its effects are obvious through symptoms. Even when its presence is detected there is no cure, just a means of controlling its impact by the use of highly active retroactive therapy, a highly demanding drug regime that is generally affordable on a substantial basis only within richer countries.

Other STIs vary in their impact. In a sense, the most prevalent STI in the UK—Chlamydia (caused by a bacterium called Chlamydia Trachomatis)—ought not to be a major health problem since it responds well to antibiotic treatment. However, again it is asymptomatic in well over half of cases, meaning that the risk of continued spread is extremely high. Numbers of new episodes at GUM clinics of uncomplicated genital chlamydial infection increased in the UK from almost 49000 in 1998 to almost 122000 in 2007, with considerably larger increases amongst the under-25–year-olds (HPA 2008). Untreated, Chlamydia can have very serious impact on women, including pelvic inflammatory disorder and can lead to infertility by causing damage to the fallopian tubes. Among men, lack of treatment can lead to joint inflammation and impotence by causing inflammation in the testicles.

Sexually transmitted infections are examples of physical diseases or illnesses which clearly harm the body in one way or another. Pregnancy, however, is a perfectly natural function; indeed, rather necessary for the survival of the species! So, why then is it a matter of such concern amongst some policy makers and others? There are, to be sure, a number of physical and biological requirements (a healthy diet, no illicit drugs, etc) for a pregnancy that minimise the risk of ill-health for the fetus and the mother, but these issues do not fall under the heading of 'sexual health' as such.

Rather, it is pregnancies that occur amongst certain groups of women that lead to concern, with a particular focus on those occurring to teenage women. Vulnerability and social exclusion increase a woman's risk for dying during pregnancy and early motherhood (CEMACH 2004). Young mothers are likely to be vulnerable and suffer from social exclusion and thus require special attention from health professionals. However, different ages (teenage, under-18, under-16) are cited at different times as the focus of concern. Further, the actual nature of the concerns varies between those emphasizing primarily physical issues (low birth weight, malnutrition, etc) through psychological and emotional issues (immaturity, inability to cope with parenthood, likelihood of being a single mother, likelihood of missing out on education, employment and earning potential, etc) to issues of a more moral nature (irresponsibility, lack of moral fibre, claiming benefits, etc). There are indeed lower limits that control the relative safeness of early childbirth—specific ages will vary across individuals and depend on the development of the cervix, etc—but there are no strong biological reasons why older teenagers should not have babies (Lawlor and Shaw 2002; Fitzpatrick 2003; Drife 2004).

Assessing levels and patterns of sexual health

As mentioned above, STI rates—at least for HIV and Chlamydia—are inevitably underestimates. Recent rises in rates of the latter almost certainly reflect increasing incidence, but also reflect the wider implementation of opportunistic testing; quite how much of the increases are due to one or the other is difficult to ascertain. A further aspect of STI data is that they are recorded and published by clinic rather than by postcode of residence. Since people can attend clinics outside of their own areas, this means that the kinds of analyses carried out to account for variations in teenage pregnancies (see below) are not possible. It is recognized that STI rates are associated with ethnicity and sex amongst teenagers (Low et al 1997; HPA 2008) but more fine-tuned analyses are hard to achieve.

Conceptions are rather easier to monitor. Apart from spontaneous miscarriages which do not require medical attention, all cases are recorded either as a birth or a termination. This means that it is more straightforward to identify rates by areas (via postcodes) and associate these with other information about those areas. Further, area analyses can also be used to explore factors that are linked to the relative likelihood of abortion and childbirth amongst those who conceive. Additionally, a number of longitudinal cohort studies have used early childbirth (but not abortion) in their range of interests and so it has been possible to model both the prediction of occurrences as well as their sequelae.

Because of the different levels of precision of the data available, the remainder of this chapter focuses on teenage conception as an indicator of sexual health. Clearly, however, the same behaviours that lead to this outcome are also implicated in the transmission of infection.

Variations in under-18 conception rates in England

There are close associations between the patterns of under-18 conception rates and the levels of deprivation of the areas in which young people live. Young women resident in most deprived areas (as assessed by the index of multiple deprivation, Noble et al 2004) are considerably more likely to conceive than are those from the least deprived areas (Clements et al 1998; Diamond et al 1999; Griffiths and Kirby 2000; McLeod 2001; Uren et al 2007). This relationship appears to be fairly universal, with a great deal of research in the USA reporting similar patterns (Singh et al 2001), as well as the UNICEF Report Card that presented data from 29 OECD countries (UNICEF 2001).

Further, amongst those who do conceive, there is a considerably higher probability of abortion being selected amongst those in the least deprived areas (Lee et al 2004; Smith 1993; Tabberer et al 2000). Amongst under-18-year-olds, this 'abortion ratio' ranged between higher tier local authorities in 2006, from 32 to 78%, within an overall England and Wales ratio of 48%.

Analyses such as these report associations between data at aggregate levels, but do not enable individual links to be made. Cohort studies do, however, raise the possibility of casting more light on factors at the individual and/or family level that are implicated in early childbirth. Two such studies are the British Cohort Studies that started in 1956 and 1970. All children born in a particular week in those years have been followed up regularly since then. This has enabled the identification of cases of early childbearing amongst the samples; predictor variables can then be identified and relative risks assessed. Due to the relatively low incidence amongst the samples, teenage pregnancies (rather than under-18) are explored. Note that the data obtained are restricted to childbirth (since abortions are not reported) and rely on those in the initial samples who stay involved for at least twenty years.

Hobcraft and Kiernan (2001), Kiernan (2002), and Berrington et al (2005) report similar factors that predict teenage motherhood, with some evidence of cumulative risk arising (in other words, each additional risk factor adds to the probability of motherhood). The latter study also included assessment of factors affecting the probability of becoming a young father (defined as fathering a child under the age of 23). Figure 6.1 shows the relative odds ratios of a number of variables for both young mothers and fathers; it can be seen that, perhaps not surprisingly, very similar factors appear to affect both.

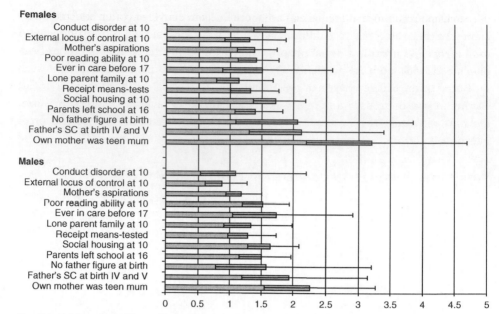

Fig. 6.1 Odds ratios of becoming a teenage (<20) mother and young (<23) father. Adjusted effects (from Berrington et al 2004)

Accounting for variation

These close associations between individual and area characteristics and the incidence of conceptions and their outcomes demand explanation. It may be helpful to think of the processes involved as comprising distinct—but overlapping—components. For a conception to occur, sexual intercourse needs to take place. This event is either adequately protected or not. Once a conception has occurred, then a decision is made as regards the outcome.

The task then becomes one of attempting to identify variation at each of these stages and, where variation is observed, attempting to explain it. In principle, this should be very straightforward; in reality, it is highly challenging! There are no data that reliably point to variations in levels of sexual activity and/or levels of contraceptive use across areas differing in deprivation levels that are sufficiently large to account for the variation in outcomes observed. The British national surveys do report some differences, but these are not substantial (Johnson et al 1994; Wellings et al 2001).

However, some smaller-scale research has attempted to account for variation in a number of aspects that are relevant to sexual activity and outcomes; these are discussed below.

Sexual activity and contraception use

Explanations include both issues relating to future orientation (aspirations and plans for the future) as well as past experiences and established normative structures including those relating to early childbearing as well as wider gender issues.

Teenagers from more affluent areas are more likely to actively avoid a conception by taking the emergency contraceptive pill (Jewell et al 2000). Research in the USA has also found teenagers in more affluent areas are more likely to use contraception effectively than are those in more deprived areas (Alan Guttmacher Institute 1995). Similar results regarding the association between contraceptive use and socio-economic environment was found in a study of five developed countries (Canada, France, Great Britain, Sweden, and the United States) (Singh et al 2001). This study also found that risk of an early pregnancy was increased for young people in deprived areas of the UK, as they were more likely to have sexual intercourse at younger ages.

The level of opportunity available within one's immediate environment may affect the acceptance of teenage pregnancy; for example, Arai argues that structural factors such as educational and occupational opportunities need to be understood for any national targets and prevention programmes to be effective (Arai 2003a; 2003b). An interaction between social class and area has been found, namely on teenage women's future aspirations and under-age sexual intercourse (Smith and Elander 2006). Education is a way to maintain social positioning and attitudes are transmitted within families (Feinstein and Sabates 2006). Educational achievement has been linked to socio-economic environment—young people in more deprived areas of England are more likely than those in more affluent areas to leave school with fewer or no qualifications (Machin et al 2005).

Sexual behaviour and sexual decisions are influenced by socio-economic environment; young people learn normative behaviours from adult role models and through the opportunities directly available to them in their immediate environment (Brewster et al 1993). Career opportunities and visibility may indirectly exert influence on the social representations of teenage pregnancy. In some areas of deprivation there is a seemingly long-standing absence of adult role models to '. . . help keep alive the perception that education is meaningful, that steady employment is a viable alternative to welfare, and that family stability is the norm not the exception' (Wilson 1987, p 56). As a result, teenage pregnancy can be viewed as an alternative and the only accepted 'career' route in such areas.

Gender relations have been discussed fairly extensively in the literature as contributing to the vulnerability of young people to negative sexual health outcomes; much of this has tended to focus on male dominance and the impact of the gendered 'double standard' on decision making with regard to sexual activity and contraceptive use (Holland et al 1998; Crawford and Popp 2003). Other work has focused on the alleged 'crisis in masculinity', whereby the changing roles and opportunities in society have affected all young people, albeit in different ways. For example, working class young men are found to form strong alliances and to create strong male cultures to which they belong (Mac an Ghaill 1994; Willis 1977). Racism has also been reported—with African Caribbean boys being portrayed as highly masculine compared to boys from other ethnic groups (Frosh et al 2002). The important role of sexuality in masculinity and the variation in masculinities due to culture and socio-economic environment means that notions of masculinity contribute to young males' views on sex, conception, and parenthood. Identity confusion in young men has been highlighted as a central component in the current crises in masculinity

(Katz and Buchanan 1999). It has been suggested that this crisis can be attributed to the change in power roles since females were able to work and have more opportunities (Bourke 1994; Whitehead 2002), the focus on young women in research and the suggested 'troublesome reputation' young males are given by the media (Phoenix et al 2003). Hence, gender and relative deprivation appear to interact in affecting vulnerability.

Outcome decisions

Lee et al (2004) explored factors associated with variation in abortion ratios (the proportion of conceptions that end in abortion) amongst under-18-year-olds using a combination of complex statistical analyses on regional and national data through to detailed interviews with young women who had chosen childbirth or abortion. In brief, abortion ratios are statistically predicted by very similar factors to those associated with conception rates; in other words, more deprived areas have higher conception rates but lower abortion proportions. Some notable exceptions to this general pattern are found in some London boroughs which have high conception rates as well as high abortion proportions. These boroughs are also more likely to have high proportions of residents with Caribbean and African ethnicities, although there are no data that enable specific links to be made here.

Personal and community attitudes have been found to influence young women's post-conception decision making (Arai 2007; Lee et al 2004; Tabberer et al 2000). In Britain, acceptance of early heterosexual intercourse is found to be greater in less affluent areas (Thomson 2000). Young people in affluent areas feel they had more to lose from the outcomes of risky sexual behaviour than do those in more deprived areas. Further, since teenage pregnancy is a relatively more frequent occurrence in areas of deprivation it is more likely to be accepted (Thomson 2000). Jewell et al (2000) similarly found that acceptance of abortion was shaped by opportunities linked to socio-economic environment. Teenage women from advantaged areas who had a conception placed greater emphasis on careers, whereas those from more disadvantaged areas emphasized the social acceptability of teenage pregnancy. This may be related to social interactions—friends and peers could exert pressure to abort their pregnancy (Tabberer et al 2000) whilst, on the other hand, young mothers in areas with a high incidence of young pregnancy may function as role models (Whitehead 2001). Abortion decisions appear to be influenced by perceptions of motherhood—which, in turn, are strongly influenced by family and community norms.

In addition, mothers from more deprived areas express a romantic ideology of parenthood and their relationship with their partner pre-birth (Wilson 1995; Allen and Bourke Bowling 1998; Smith 2007)—a romantic ideology where '. . . a baby is part of the dream of marriage and bliss' (Anderson 1991, p 391). This ideology mirrors that of working class women in the 1920s, who wanted marriage and to be a housewife (Bourke 1994)—such would have been an acceptable route to choose when women were less able to have a career than they are today.

In terms of other reasons provided by women for their outcome choices (Lee et al 2004), those from more deprived areas are more likely to talk in terms of fetus-centred issues (for example, 'it's not the baby's fault') whereas those from less deprived areas talked in woman-centred terms (for example, 'I cannot have a baby at this stage of my life'). Education and career plans featured prominently in the latters' decisions (irrespective of their stated attitudes to abortion prior to the pregnancy!). Young women with lower educational aspirations were more likely to accept early motherhood as being somewhat inevitable, as being more accepted in their own communities, and to receive offers of active help of support from their own mothers (although this often came after a short period of anger and disappointment). Many of these young mothers were very content with motherhood, but expressed the wish that they had waited a little longer before having children.

Impact of teenage motherhood[1]

It has been suggested that the difficulties young mothers face have not changed despite the greater level of available support from health professionals and practitioners (Moffit and E-Risk Study Team 2002). These include a three times greater risk for post-natal depression and risk of social exclusion (Ermisch 2003). Liao (2003) used the first ten waves of the British Household Panel Survey (BHPS) to compare the medium to long-term mental health of women in Britain in the 1990s. Results indicated teenage mothers as having a long period of vulnerability to depression (until their children were two years old). One proposed explanation for high rates of depression in young mothers is that the reality does not match '. . . the rosy picture of motherhood that society would have us believe is the norm' (Wilson 1995, p 142). A recent systematic evidence-based review found two major risk factors for post-natal depression; negative life events and lack of social support (Robertson et al 2004).

Young mothers are more likely to live in social exclusion than non-mothers (SEU 1999). However, many predictors are evident before conception and may have increased their vulnerability (see Figure 6.1). For example, those who become teenage mothers are more likely to have dropped out of school before the pregnancy and as a result tend to have no or low qualifications (DCSF 2007), a consequence that results in a large number of teenage parents being unemployed, living on a low wage, or relying on social benefits (UNICEF 2001). Ermisch (2003) used the British Household Panel Survey to explore the association between a mother's age at first birth and the additional impact of a pregnancy; a similar design was used by Berrington et al (2004, 2005) using the British Birth Cohort 1970 sample. Having a birth under the age of 20 was found to limit a woman's chances in the 'marriage market' and any future partners were likely to be unemployed or low earners. In addition, teenage mothers were less likely to be homeowners and their living standard

[1] The focus in this section is on outcomes for young mothers and their children rather than on young fathers. There are a number of reasons for this; first, the ages of fathers of children born to teenage mothers vary considerably; second, there has been little research on the sequelae of early fatherhood; third, when relationship breakdown occurs the fathers may be difficult to trace; fourth, in some cases, there may be economic benefit in a young mother claiming single parent status. In doing this, however, we are not wishing to appear to be ignoring their existence or needs. Increased recent interest in young fathers is exemplified by DCSF (2008a, 2008b).

was 20% lower than the rest of the population. In sum, socio-economic environment had a major influence in predicting young pregnancy which in turn added to the levels of social exclusion. However, when socio-economic environment is controlled, young pregnancy is claimed to have a much lower adverse effect on young people's lives than is often reported (Shaw et al 2006).

However, not all teenage pregnancies result in negative outcomes. Positive meaning and outcomes of teenage pregnancy have been reported; for example, leaving a life of drugs and gangs in a US city to become a mother is reported by Lesser et al (1999). Similarly, the TPSE Interim Report (2004) reports cases of positive outcomes in their evaluation of the England Teenage Pregnancy Strategy and Cater and Coleman (2006) report on a small number of planned teenage births.

Reasons suggested for negative outcomes of teenage pregnancy include being more likely to register the pregnancy late (after 12 weeks) (Allen 2003) and a poor history of antenatal and postnatal attendance (BMJ Health Intelligence 2007). Wiggins et al (2005) reported that 70% of teenagers wanted support during their pregnancy and stated that long-term success for young mothers and their babies can be achieved if support is received during their pregnancy and for a year following the birth. However, to date UK literature on antenatal support and effect on the outcomes of young pregnancy is limited (Swann et al 2003).

Concerns expressed over early motherhood relate to the impact on the child as well as on the mother. Being born into deprivation has a negative impact on the future development and aspirations of children (UNICEF 2007). These include lower birth-weight, higher risk of infant mortality, higher accident rates, and greater risk for a teen pregnancy (Botting et al 1998; Dattani 1999).

Perceived barriers to antenatal care and support services are frequently reported by teenage parents. With young parents reporting feeling judged, intimidated, and dissatisfied with their treatment from health professionals, it should come as no surprise that they do not feel comfortable attending the support services run for them (Hendessi and Dodwell 2002; Wiggins et al 2005). Some young parents may not feel comfortable with the other (often older) people in the class and the content is often seen as irrelevant (Speak 1999). Teenage parents underuse NHS services as they feel unable to ask questions, they feel stigmatized, and lack confidence (Allen 2003; Hendessi and Rashid 2002; Speak 1999). Instrumental barriers to NHS services have been suggested in studies, these include inconvenient surgery hours, lack of female practitioners, inquisitive receptionists (Morgan 2000), and travel costs (Goyder et al 2003). The DH has recently released clear guidelines on commissioning and delivering maternity services for young parents (DCSF/DH/RCM 2008a) and a practical guide for working with young parents (DCSF 2008b); it appears to address many of the barriers highlighted by young parents, so it will be interesting to see the impact this has on teenage parents' maternity attendance and experiences.

The potential value of cross-national comparisons

The data summarized above show clearly that variation in teenage conceptions is associated with geographical region, mainly through associated levels of deprivation and academic achievement. The particular mechanisms through which such broader contextual aspects are translated into actual behaviours are not well understood at present, although some promising leads for further research have been identified.

Looking beyond national boundaries may be fruitful. The initial Social Exclusion Unit report on teenage pregnancy in England was primarily driven by the evidence that England had the highest rate of under 16 and under 18 conceptions in western Europe, and that even the lower rate (relatively affluent) areas in England were higher than those in much of the rest of Europe. The aim was to bring down the rate to nearer the 'European average'. So, attention was drawn to which particular features of other countries had enabled them to achieve lower rates than the UK. This is not an easy question to address, for a number of reasons.

First, data from some countries are of poor quality; this is especially likely to be the case in those countries where teenage sex and/or abortions are more strictly proscribed than in others. Second, age groups used to present national statistics vary from one country to another and, indeed, in countries with low rates, there is no reason why further detailed analyses should be undertaken. For these reasons, data are generally available at national levels on rates of teenage births but little else.

Although birth-rate tables do make for interesting comparisons, it is important to recognize that they only tell a part of the story. For example, the relation between conception rates and birth rates will depend on levels of abortion and, in particular, what proportion of conceptions are terminated. Further, rates are presented per 1000 population of women within a certain age range (15 to 19 years in the case of teenage births) and so will be affected by the proportions of women within this age group having experienced sexual intercourse. Good representative data are simply not available to enable calculation of conception rates amongst just the sexually active population of women; such data would assist tremendously in attempts to ascertain what behavioural processes may account for variation across and within countries (Wellings and Kane 1999; Cheesbrough et al 2002).

Consider one example. From various (reasonably solid but rather dated) surveys, it is possible to ascertain that Sweden, the Netherlands, and England have roughly similar proportions of women (at 85%) reporting having experienced their first intercourse aged 19 years or under. Teenage birth rates, however, vary considerably, from 30.8 per thousand in England, through 6.5 in Sweden to 6.2 in the Netherlands. Such data may encourage us to look for commonalities between Sweden and the Netherlands in order to inform policy responses in England. However, a closer look at available data reveals a somewhat more complex pattern. The abortion proportion (or ratio) and the conception rates vary considerably between countries. In Sweden, 69% of teenage conceptions end in abortion, compared with 42% in England and 33% in the Netherlands. What this means is that the actual teenage conception rate ranges from 11.6 in the Netherlands, 25 in Sweden to 50.9 in England (Ingham 2007).

In other words, just looking at national birth rates provides a false picture that runs the risk of pointing to partially incorrect conclusions. It seems that, although Sweden is more successful at reducing conceptions than is England, the much lower birth rate is achieved through wider availability of, and presumably less stigma associated with, abortion than is the case in England or the Netherlands. Similarly, contraception use is considerably more reliable and consistent in the Netherlands than in these other two countries; this is often attributed to one or more of earlier and more comprehensive sex education in the homes and in schools, greater gender equality, greater acceptance amongst 'adults' that young people need (and have a right) to develop sexually in safe and supportive environments, and other related factors (Ingham and van Zessen 1997).

As well as the conceptual and explanatory potential of cross-national comparisons, there are other factors at work. In terms of policy development, it is commonplace to hear politicians and others referring to 'success' elsewhere and what England can learn from these examples. One such case in recent years has been the decline in the USA of teenage conceptions; some agencies have claimed this is due to the massive increase in funding for, and implementation of, abstinence-only education programmes. Others claim that increases in contraceptive availability and use are primarily responsible and that the decline has occurred despite the abstinence-only movement.

A number of attempts have been made to address this issue (Darroch et al 2001; Singh and Darroch 2000). The most recent, and arguably the most thorough, has been reported by Santelli et al (2007), who calculate, on the basis of using data from a number of longitudinal surveys, that 86% of the decline in the overall pregnancy risk index between 1995 and 2002 for teenage women was due to increased effective use of contraception. The remaining 14% was accounted for by reduced levels of sexual activity (which may not, of course, be directly as a result of abstinence-only education).

Such conceptual and methodological (and moral) issues are not only relevant for purely academic debates, nor just for guiding attempts to reduce levels of teenage pregnancy. They also have a significant global impact. A proportion of the overseas aid finance provided by the previous US Government (PEPFAR) to support efforts to reduce levels of HIV and AIDS in poorer countries was tied to the introduction of abstinence-only programmes in these countries (Murphy et al 2006). This was despite there being no evidence that such programmes are effective in reducing levels of sexual activity; indeed, what evidence there is points in the opposite direction (Kirby 2002, 2008; Ellis and Grey 2004; Santelli et al 2004; Swann et al 2003; Trivedi et al 2007). It is clear that the vulnerability of young people to infection (and death) may be increased by the religious and moral decisions of those who allocate resources for programmatic and intervention efforts.

Measures to improve sexual health: towards some conclusions

We have demonstrated that the understanding of sexual health outcomes—in particular, rates of teenage conceptions—are inexorably related to various indices of deprivation and seemingly deep-seated community norms involving lack of educational or employment aspirations, gender roles and expectations, stigma, and so on.

Programmes to address income and social inequalities are complex and need to be seen as long term. Meanwhile, attempts are required to explore what measures may help to alleviate the vulnerability to negative outcomes. A relatively large number of studies have attempted to develop greater understanding of what might 'work', some based on sound theoretical bases with others driven by pure pragmatism. Space does not permit full coverage of these. However, recent evidence reviews, as well as some reviews of reviews, have helped to focus attention on seemingly successful approaches (Swann et al 2003; Harden et al 2006; Downing et al 2006). It is important to stress that reviews (and reviews of reviews) present patterns of results derived from a number of studies that have been selected as meeting certain very strict scientific standards.

In brief, school-based sex education linked with contraceptive services are found to be effective in reducing teenage conception rates, although the precise characteristics of successful programmes are hard to identify with precision. Community-based programmes are also found to be effective, be these focused on contraceptive provision or wider personal development initiatives aimed at young people. The development of personal and academic skills amongst young people at early ages is found to be protective, as is involving the families of vulnerable young people. Supportive antenatal care for young mothers and intensive emotional and material support after birth can help to alleviate some of the negative sequelae of early motherhood as well as lowering the risks of subsequent unplanned pregnancies.

Some reservations need to be expressed about conclusions drawn on the basis of this approach to reviewing the evidence. By giving priority to studies that reach a certain gold standard of scientific design (usually a randomized control trial) then issues that do not lend themselves to such a design are rendered less important (or are not considered at all) (WHO 2008, p 30). Thus, for example, given the ethical difficulties that would be involved in randomly allocating families to high or low sexual discussion groups, the importance of the family context may be relatively ignored. Further, priority is given to studies that can isolate a specific form of intervention (such as a school-based programme) and produce a specific outcome measure (such as knowledge, attitudes, age at first intercourse, actual conception rates, reported contraceptive use, etc). Such studies may lead to an artificially simplistic view of the world—we have shown above how areas that differ in rates of conception vary on a wide range of factors which probably work together to create vulnerability. Isolation of just one or two of these factors may be missing an important point. On the other hand, countries that have different rates differ on a wide range of contextual features and it would be impossible to transfer these over to a new setting. There is pressure to try to identify the one or more key factors that seem to make a difference; but this may be equally as challenging as, for example, reducing income inequalities in Britain!

The Government's target of reducing the England under-18 conception rate by half by 2010 appears to have been rather too ambitious. At the time of writing, the latest annual conception data (2007) show a decrease of around 11% since the 1998 baseline year of the strategy (from 46.6 to 41.7). Although one might expect an acceleration of progress as services and policies become embedded, it is still highly unlikely that the target will be met. Efforts have been made to ascertain what it is about the more successful of the areas, and these have led to the production of interim guidance reports (DCSF 2006).

However, in the glare of the focus of attention on the teenage conception rates themselves, a different change has also been occurring that has gone relatively unnoticed. Since the baseline year of the strategy in 1998, the overall national abortion proportion has increased steadily from 42% to 51%. What this means is that the actual rate of childbearing amongst women aged under 18 (or at least who conceived whilst the woman was under 18 years old) has reduced from 27.0 to 20.4 per thousand. This is a reduction of around 24%. Given that the key thrust of the initial Social Exclusion Unit report was to reduce the likelihood of the further exclusion of young women who become mothers, then the strategy has clearly been more successful than it may appear from just the conception rates. The increase in the abortion proportions also, as it happens, provides little solace to those who argue a rational economic approach to sexual issues; at a time when the benefits and support for young mothers has probably never been higher, fewer are choosing to continue with their pregnancies than have done so earlier.

Research on sexual health, at least as assessed through teenage pregnancy, draws attention to the relationship between risk and vulnerability. Traditional social psychological models tend to emphasize risk-taking as a trait of certain young people (Abraham and Sheeran 2003; de Visser and Smith 2004) and attempts to identify individual cognitive deficits that are in need of 'correcting' through better education, campaigns, and other devices. Whilst such initiatives are undoubtedly important, it must be recognized that the contexts in which many young people live out their lives make them vulnerable to negative outcomes. In the absence of genuine opportunities to achieve educational and/or material success, then being a good mother may be the best option for a young woman; this is not best regarded as risk-taking, but rather as responding in a rational manner to a particular set of material and social circumstances.

Many young people are vulnerable just because they are young, some because they live in areas that have no tradition of educational achievement or lucrative employment, others because they live within gendered discourses from which it is difficult to escape, and so on. What is important to understand is that, whilst material resources may not readily be forthcoming, much of the vulnerability faced by young people in this domain of health outcomes is created by others. Thus, for example, those individuals and organizations that challenge and restrict the opportunity for good sex and relationships education, that fail to address gender issues and homophobia, that discourage the development of knowledge and skills to control one's sexual activities, and that try to impose their own narrow value systems, are themselves creating the very circumstances that increase vulnerability.

Bibliography

Abraham, C and Sheeran, P (2003) 'Implications of goal theories for the theories of reasoned action and planned behaviour' *Current Psychology: Developmental, Learning, Personality, Social* 22/3: 264–80

Alan Guttmacher Institute (1995) *Issues in brief: teenage pregnancy and the welfare reform debate.* Available at <http://www.guttmacher.org/pubs/ib5.html> (accessed 22 September 2008)

Allen, EJ (2003) 'Aims and associations of reducing teenage pregnancy' *British Journal of Midwifery* 11/6: 36–9

Allen, I and Bourke Bowling, S (1998) *Teenage mothers: decisions and outcomes.* London: Policy Studies Institute

Anderson, E (1991) 'Neighborhood effects on teenage pregnancy' in C Jencks and PE Peterson (eds), *The urban underclass*, pp 375–98. Washington: The Brookings Institution

Arai, L (2003a) 'British policy on teenage pregnancy and childbearing: the limitations of comparisons with other European countries' *Critical Social Policy* 23/1: 89–102

Arai, L (2003b) 'Low expectations, sexual attitudes and knowledge; explaining teenage pregnancy and fertility in English communities. Insights from qualitative research' *The Sociological Review* 51/2 199–217

Arai, L (2007) 'Peer and neighbour influences on teenage pregnancy and fertility: Qualitative findings from research in English communities' *Health and Place* 13: 87–98

AVERT (2008) <http://www.avert.org/> (accessed on 25 October 2008)

Berrington, A, Diamond, I, Ingham, R, and Stevenson, J (2004) *Consequences of teenage parenthood; pathways which minimise the long term negative impacts of teenage childbearing*. Final report to Department of Health. Southampton: Division of Social Statistics, University of Southampton Available at: <http://www.dcsf.gov.uk/research/data/uploadfiles/RW52.pdf> (accessed on 21 September 2008)

Berrington, A, Hernandez, IC, Ingham, R, and Stevenson, J (2005) *Antecedents and outcomes of young fatherhood: longitudinal evidence from the 1970 British birth cohort study. Final Report*. Southampton: Division of Social Statistics, University of Southampton. Available at: <http://eprints.soton.ac.uk/18182/01/s3ri-workingpaper-a05-09.pdf> (accessed on 21 September 2008)

BMJ Health Intelligence (2007) *Interventions to reduce inequalities in child health by promoting antenatal care for women from disadvantaged groups*. London: BMJ Publishing Group Ltd. Available at: <http://healthintelligence.bmj.com/hi/do/public-health/topics/content/inequalities-in-health/evidence/HEA.EVI.001.HEA.html> (accessed 25 October 2008)

Botting, B, Rosato, M, and Wood, R (1998) 'Teenage mothers and the health of their children' *Population Trends* 93 19–23

Bourke, J (1994) *Working class cultures in Britain, 1890–1960: gender, class and ethnicity*. London: Routledge

Brewster, KL, Billy, JOG, and Grady, WR (1993) 'Social context and adolescent behaviour: the impact of community on transition to sexual activity' *Social Forces* 71/3: 713–40

Cater, S, and Coleman, L (2006) *Planned teenage pregnancies: views and experiences of young people from poor and disadvantaged backgrounds*. York: Joseph Rowntree Foundation

CEMACH (2004) *Why mothers die, 2000–2002*. London: Royal College of Obstetricians and Gynaecologists Press

Cheesbrough, S, Ingham, R, and Massey, D (2002) *Reducing the rates of teenage conceptions: a review of the international evidence on preventing and reducing teenage conceptions: the United States, Canada, Australia and New Zealand*. London: Health Development Agency

Clements, S, Stone, N, Diamond, I, and Ingham, R (1998) 'Modelling the spatial distribution of teenage conception rates within Wessex' *British Journal of Family Planning*, 24: 61–71

Crawford, M and Popp, D (2003) 'Sexual double standards: a review and methodological critique of two decades of research' *The Journal of Sex Research* 40/1: 13–26

Darroch, J, Singh, S, Frost, J, the Study Team (2001) 'Differences in teenage pregnancy rates among five developed countries; the roles of sexual activity and contraceptive use' *Family Planning Perspectives* 33/6: 244–50 and 281

Dattani, N (1999) 'Mortality in children aged under 4' *Health Statistics Quarterly 02*. London: Office for National Statistics

DCSF (2006) *Teenage pregnancy: accelerating the strategy to 2010*. London: Department for Children, Schools and Families

DCSF (2007) *Improving access to sexual health services for young people in further education settings*. London: Department for Children, Schools and Families

DCSF/DH/RCM (2008a) *Teenage parents: who cares? A guide to commissioning and delivering maternity services for young parents*. London: Department for Children, Schools and Families

DCSF/DH/RCM (2008b) *Getting maternity services right for pregnancy teenagers and young fathers*. London: Department for Children, Schools and Families

DH (Department of Health) (2001) *The national strategy for sexual health and HIV*. London: Department of Health

Diamond, I, Clements, S, Stone, N, and Ingham, R (1999) 'Spatial variation in teenage conceptions in south and west England' *Journal of the Royal Statistical Society, Series A*, 162/3: 273–89

Dickson, N, Paul, C, Herbison, P, and Silva, P (1998) 'First sexual intercourse: age, coercion, and later regrets reported by a birth cohort' *British Medical Journal* 316: 29–33

Downing, J, Jones, L, Cook, PA, and Bellis, MA (2006). *Prevention of sexually transmitted infections (STIs); a review of reviews into the effectiveness of non-clinical interventions. Evidence briefing update*. Liverpool: Centre for Public Health, Liverpool John Mores University, for NICE

De Visser, RO and Smith, AMA (2004) 'Which intention? Whose intention? Condom use and theories of individual decision-making' *Psychology, Health and Medicine* 9/2: 193–204

Drife, J (2004) 'Teenage pregnancy: a problem or what?' *BJOG: An International Journal of Obstetrics and Gynaecology* 111/8: 763–4

Eberhard-Gran, M, Slinning, K, and Eskild, A (2008) 'Fear during labor: the impact of sexual abuse during adult life' *Journal of Psychosomatic Obstetrics and Gynaecology* 28: 1–4

Ellis, S and Grey, A (2004) *Prevention of sexually transmitted infections (STIs); a review of reviews into the effectiveness of non-clinical interventions.* London: Health Development Agency

Ermisch, J (2003) *Does a 'teen-birth' have longer-term impacts on the mother? Suggestive evidence from the British household panel study.* Working papers of the Institute for Social and Economic Research, paper 2003-32. Colchester: University of Essex

Feinstein, L and Sabates, R (2006) *Does education have an impact on mothers' educational attitudes and behaviours? Brief No: RCB01-06.* London: Department for Education and Skills

Fitzpatrick, M (2003) 'Teen dreams' *Lancet* 362: 1248

Frosh, S, Phoenix, A, and Pattman, R, (2002) *Young masculinities: understanding boys in contemporary society.* Basingstoke: Palgrave Macmillan

Goyder, E, Blank, L, and Peters, J (2003) *Supporting teenage parents: the potential contribution. New Deal for Communities Research Report 8.* Sheffield: School of Health and Related Research, University of Sheffield

Griffiths, C and Kirby, L (2000) 'Geographic variations in conceptions to women aged under-18 in Great Britain during the 1990s' *Population Trends* 102: 13–23

Harden, A, Brunton, G, Fletcher, A, Oakley, A, Burchett, H, and Backhans, M (2006) *Young people, pregnancy and social exclusion; a systematic synthesis of research evidence to identify effective, appropriate and promising approaches to prevention and support.* London: EPPI-Centre, Social Science Research Unit, Institute of Education, University of London

Hendessi, M and Dodwell, C (2002) *Supporting young parents; models of good practice.* London: YWCA

Hendessi, M and Rashid, F (2002) *Poverty: the price of young motherhood in Britain.* London: YWCA

Hobcraft, J and Kiernan, K (2001) 'Childhood poverty, early motherhood and adult social exclusion' *British Journal of Sociology* 52/3, 495–517

Holland, J, Ramazanoglu, C, Sharpe, S, and Thomson, R (1998) *The male in the head: young people, heterosexuality and power.* London: The Tufnell Press

HPA (Health Protection Agency) (2008). *STIs Annual Data, 1997–2006, slide set.* Available at <http://www.hpa.org.uk/webw/HPAwebandPageandHPAwebAutoListDate/Page/1203409656940?p=1203409656940> (accessed 20 September 2008)

Ingham, R (2007) 'Variations across countries—the international perspective' in P Baker, K Guthrie, R Kane, C Hutchinson, and K Wellings (eds), *Teenage pregnancy and reproductive health.* London: Royal College of Obstetricians and Gynaecologists

Ingham, R and van Zessen, G (1997) 'Towards an alternative model of sexual behaviour; from individual properties to interactional processes' in L Van Campenhoudt, M Cohen, G Guizzardi, and D Hausser (eds), *Sexual interactions and HIV risk; new conceptual perspectives in European research*, pp 83–99. London: Taylor and Francis

Jewell, D, Tacchi, J, and Donovan, J (2000) 'Teenage pregnancy: whose problem is it?' *Family Practice* 17: 522–8

Johnson, AM, Wadsworth, J, Wellings, K, and Field, J (1994) *Sexual attitudes and lifestyles.* Oxford: Blackwell Scientific Press

Katz, A and Buchanan, A (1999) *Leading lads.* London: Topman/Young Voice

Kendall-Tackett, KA, Williams, LM, and Finkelhor, D (1993) 'Impact of sexual abuse on children; a review and synthesis of recent empirical studies' *Psychological Bulletin* 113/1: 164–80

Kiernan, K (2002) 'Disadvantage and demography—chicken and egg?' in J Hills, J Le Grand, and D Piachaud (eds), *Understanding social exclusion*, pp 84–96. Oxford: Oxford University Press

Kirby, D (2002) *Do abstinence-only programs delay the initiation of sex among young people and reduce teen pregnancy?* Washington DC: National Campaign to Prevent Teen and Unplanned Pregnancies

Kirby, D (2008) 'The impact of abstinence and comprehensive sex and STD/HIV education programs on adolescent sexual behavior' *Sexuality Research and Social Policy* 5/3: 18–27

Kirkengen, AL (2001) *Inscribed bodies: health impact of childhood sexual abuse.* Boston: Kluwer Academic

Lawlor, DA and Shaw, M (2002). 'What a difference a year makes? Too little too late' Int J Epimediol 31: 552–4

Lee, E, Clements, S, Ingham, R, and Stone, N (2004) *A Matter of Choice? Explaining national variation in teenage abortion and motherhood.* York: Joseph Rowntree Foundation. Available at: <http://www.jrf.org.uk/bookshop/eBooks/1859351824.pdf> (accessed on 21 September 2008)

Lesser, J, Koniak-Griffin, D, and Sanderson, NLR (1999) 'Depressed adolescent mothers' perceptions of their own role' *Issues in Mental Health Nursing* 20 131–49

Liao, TF (2003) *Mental health, teenage motherhood, and age at first birth among British women in the 1990s*. Working Papers of the Institute for Social and Economic Research, paper 2003-33. Colchester: University of Essex

Low, N, Daker-White, G, Barlow, D, and Pozniak, A (1997) 'Gonorrhoea in inner London; results of a cross-sectional study' *British Medical Journal* 314: 1719–23

Mac an Ghaill, M (1994) *The making of men: masculinities, sexualities and schooling*. Buckingham: Open University Press

Machin, S, McNally, S, and Rajagopalan, S (2005) *Tackling the poverty of opportunity*. London: The Prince's Trust

McLeod, A (2001) 'Changing patterns of teenage pregnancy; population based study of small areas' *British Medical Journal* 323: 199–203

Moffitt, T and the E-Risk Study Team (2002) 'Teen-aged mothers in contemporary Britain' *Journal of Child Psychology and Psychiatry* 43/6 727–42

Morgan, R (2000) 'Did primary care advice really fail our pregnant teenagers?' *Primary Care Report* 2/4: 38–41

Murphy, EM, Greene, ME, Mihailovic, A, and Oluput-Olupot, P (2006) Was the 'ABC' approach (Abstinence, Being Faithful, Using Condoms) responsible for Uganda's decline in HIV?' *PLoS Medicine*, 3/9: e379 doi:10.1371/journal.pmed.0030379 (accessed 20 September 2008)

Noble, M, Wright, G, Dibben, C, et al (2004) *The English indices of deprivation*. Report to the Office of the Deputy Prime Minister. London: Neighbourhood Renewal Unit

Pheonix, A, Frosh, S, and Pattman, R (2003) 'Producing contradictory masculine subject positions: narratives of threat, homophobia and bullying in 11–14 year old boys' *Journal of Social Issues* 59/1 179–95

Robertson, E, Grace, S, Wallington, T, and Stewart, D (2004) 'Antenatal risk factors for postpartum depression: a synthesis of recent literature' *General Hospital Psychiatry* 26/4, 289–95

Santelli, JS, Abma, J, Ventura, S, et al (2004) 'Can changes in sexual behaviors among high school students explain the decline in teen pregnancy rates in the 1990s?' *Journal of Adolescent Health* 35: 80–90

Santelli, JS, Lindberg, LD, Finer, LB, and Singh, S (2007) 'Explaining recent declines in adolescent pregnancy in the United States: the contribution of abstinence and improved contraceptive use' *American Journal of Public Health* 97/1: 150–6

Shaw, M, Dorling, D, and Davey Smith, G (2006) 'Poverty, social exclusion and minorities' in M Marmot and RG Wilkinson (eds), *Social determinants of health*, pp 196–223. 2nd edn. Oxford: Oxford University Press

Singh, S and Darroch, J (2000) 'Adolescent pregnancy and childbearing; levels and trends in developed countries' *Family Planning Perspectives* 32/1: 14–23

Singh, S, Darroch, JE, Frost, JJ, and the Study Team (2001) 'Socioeconomic disadvantage and adolescent women's sexual and reproductive behaviour: The case of five developed countries' *Family Planning Perspective* 33/6: 251–258 and 289

Smith, DM (2007) *Affluence, deprivation and young parenthood—an exploration of pregnancy decisions in four Local Authorities in London*. Unpublished PhD thesis. Kingston: Department of Psychology, Kingston University

Smith, DM and Elander, J. (2006) 'Effects of area and family deprivation on risk factors for teenage pregnancy among 13 to 15 year old girls' *Psychology, Health and Medicine* 11/4, 399–410

Smith, T (1993) 'Influence of socio-economic factors on attaining targets for reducing teenage pregnancies' *British Medical Journal* 306: 1232–5

Social Exclusion Unit (SEU) (1999) *Teenage pregnancy*. London: Her Majesty's Stationery Office

Speak, S (1999) 'Young single mothers and access to health and support services: problems and possibilities' in Health Education Authority Expert Working Group (ed), *Promoting the health of teenage and lone mothers; setting a research agenda*, pp 103–8. London: Health Education Authority

Swann, C, Bowe, K, McCormick, G, and Kosmin, M (2003) *Teenage pregnancy and parenthood; a review of reviews, evidence briefing*. London: Health Development Agency

Tabberer, S, Hall, C, Prendergast, S, and Webster, A (2000). *Teenage pregnancy and choice. Abortion or motherhood: influences on the decision*. York: Joseph Rowntree Foundation

Thomson, R (2000) 'Dream on: The logic of sexual practice' *Journal of Youth Studies* 3/4 407–27

TPSE (Teenage Pregnancy Strategy Evaluation) (2004). *Interim Report No 3, February 2004*. London: LSHTM

Trivedi, D, Bunn, F, Graham, M, and Wentz, R (2007) *Update on review of reviews on teenage pregnancy and parenthood; submitted as an addendum to the first evidence briefing 2003*. Hertfordshire: Centre for Research in Primary and Community Care, University of Hertfordshire, on behalf of NICE

UNICEF (2001) 'A league of teenage births in rich nations' *Innocenti Report Card, No 3, July 2001*. Florence: UNICEF Innocenti Research Centre

UNICEF (2007) 'Child poverty in perspective: an overview of child well-being in rich country. *Innocenti Report card, No 7*. Florence: UNICEF Innocenti Research Centre

Uren, Z, Sheers, D, and Dattani, N (2007). 'Teenage conceptions by small area deprivation in England and Wales, 2001–2002' *Health Statistics Quarterly* 33, 34–9

Wellings, K and Kane, R (1999) 'Trends in teenage pregnancy in England and Wales: how can we explain them?' *Journal of Royal Society of Medicine* 92: 277–83

Wellings, K, Nanchahal, K, Macdowall, W, et al (2001) 'Sexual behaviour in Britain: early heterosexual experience' *The Lancet* 358/9296: 1843–50

Whitehead, E (2001) 'Teenage pregnancy: on the road to social death' *International Journal of Nursing Studies* 38, 437-46

Whitehead, SM (2002) *Men and masculinities*.Cambridge: Polity Press

WHO (2006) *Defining sexual health; report of a technical consultation on sexual health, held in January 2002*. Available at <http://www.who.int/reproductive-health/publications/sexualhealth/defining_sh.pdf> (accessed 20 September 2008)

WHO (2008) *Closing the gap on a generation: health equity across action on the social determinants of health; report from the Commission on Social Determinants of Health*. Geneva, Switzerland: The World Health Organization Press

Wiggins, M, Oakley, A, Sawtell, M, Austerberry, H, Clemens, F, and Elbourne, D (2005). *Teenage parenthood and social exclusion: a multi-method study. Summary report of findings*. London: Social Science Research Unit Report, Institute of Education, University of London

Wight, D, Henderson, M, Raab, G, et al (2000) 'Extent of regretted sexual intercourse among young teenagers in Scotland: a cross sectional survey' *British Medical Journal* 320: 1243–4

Willis, P (1977) *Learning to Labour*. Farnborough: Saxon House

Wilson, J (1995) 'Maternity policy. Caroline: a case of a pregnant teenager. *Professional Care of Mother and Child* 5/5: 139–142.

Wilson, WJ (1987) *The truly disadvantaged: the inner city, the underclass and public policy*. Chicago: University of Chicago Press

Chapter 7

Social context and youth health: understanding and mitigating exclusion

M Judith Lynam

Introduction

Much of our knowledge about social determinants of health has been developed from population-based studies that identify trends and conditions or indicators associated with different health profiles. In particular, it has been recognized that in addition to being associated with poverty, health inequalities are gendered and 'raced'. Studies have also demonstrated that the impact of determinants of poor health are cumulative over the life course. Such work shows the need to identify critical points in the life course and to understand the ways social determinants of health exert their effect, so that 'upstream' interventions can be implemented.

This chapter will share insights from a research programme (Lynam 2005, 2007; Lynam and Cowley 2007) that aims to extend our understanding of how social conditions, contributing to health inequalities, are experienced by teenagers, including teenagers at risk because of their social and material circumstances. I first locate the research in broader discourses on inequalities in health and then introduce the theoretical perspective that informed the study. The research is guided by Bourdieu's theoretical perspective and was designed to identify the social processes and practices that contribute to, or mitigate, the impact of marginalization and social exclusion. The implications of these insights for policy and practice are discussed.

Perspectives on inequalities in health: Insights for further exploration

Key concepts contributing to inequalities in health that have been identified in population studies in the UK and elsewhere include the recognition that material circumstances have an inverse relationship with health (Gordon et al 1999; Whitehead 1992). While all societies have inequalities in health, analyses by a number of scholars show that the magnitude and nature of inequalities vary depending upon the extent of the gap between the wealthy and the poor and the nature of a country's investment in its social infrastructure, including the infrastructure for education, health, and social programmes (Farmer 2004; Farmer et al 2006; Wilkinson 1996; Williams and Williams-Morris 2000). Such research illustrates the role of social structures in creating social hierarchies and illustrates their consequences for health. These social arrangements influence access to employment, health, education, and social services that arise out of decisions about how resources are allocated and priorities determined.

It is important to note however, that there are additional processes operating that influence social structuring. For example, it has been clearly documented that *particular groups* within the broader population are more likely to be poor and experience inequalities in health over the life course. In this regard it has been noted that health inequalities are gendered (Beiser and Stewart, 2005; Graham 1993, 2000, 2004), 'raced' (Nazroo 2003; Whitehead 1992; Williams and Williams-Morris 2000), and *cumulative over the life course* (Power et al 1997 and 2002).

Communities as resources for health: Issues for Teenagers There is considerable evidence that communities, the opportunities they provide for capacity building, and the relationships established with others in them, can be resources for health. For example, research has repeatedly shown the health protective function of social support, particularly integrated networks of support (Berkman and Smye 1979; Health Education Authority 1999; Haan et al 1987; Kawachi and Berkman 2000). Research on health inequalities concluded that 'access to social resources, including social networks and support, is mediated by social inclusion and material resources' (Shaw et al 2005).

Such evidence indicates the importance of social context in facilitating access to support and resources, and the need for research that moves beyond traditional views to consider the policies and practices that shape processes of social location and contribute to experiences of inclusion or exclusion. Despite the recognition that communities are resources for youth, health research suggests that many youth, but most particularly immigrant and refugee youth, feel on the margins of their communities and do not have access to support and opportunities for capacity building to meet developmental needs. We must consider these as potential social determinants of poor health and seek to examine how such conditions are created and how they influence teenagers' abilities to access resources and meet developmental needs. This is critical given that the impacts of social and material disadvantage are cumulative over the life course (Hertzman and Power 2003; Power and Fox 1991; Power, Hyppönen and Davey Smith 2005).

Families as resources for teenagers' health Families, particularly parents, have been identified as key resources for teenagers as they cope with marked physical and social change and meet developmental needs (Armstrong et al 2005; Lagarin 2004; Levitt et al 2005; Lipshitz-Ellhawi and Itzhahy 2005; Lynam and Tenn 1989; Parker and Benson, 2004; Young et al 2001; Ungar et al 2004). In particular, parents play important roles in facilitating teenagers' connections with resources and opportunities for capacity building in their community. In addition to providing support, most parents seek to facilitate or enhance teenagers' access to other forums of support with varying degrees of success. The challenges many immigrant parents face in fostering access to support and opportunities for themselves and their teenagers has been identified in several studies (Lynam and Young 2002; Lynam and Cowley 2007; Young et al 2001). Findings indicate that parents' efforts at being a resource for their teenagers are undermined when teenagers viewed their parents as lacking credibility in, or knowledge of, their social worlds. This was further compounded when the other forms of 'capital' (credibility, status) parents had to offer were limited because of the material and social circumstances that accrued from downward mobility and being viewed as less credible by their teenagers because of their marginal status subsequent to migration.

The few studies of immigrant youth that have been undertaken in Canada suggest that poorer mental health profiles are related in part to stresses associated with migration and settlement but also that these stresses are compounded by worries and challenges associated with adolescence, including relationships between parents and teenagers (Lynam and Young 2002; Freire 1993; Young et al 2001) and for some by poverty and concerns about their future. Additionally, research undertaken in the UK and Canada has revealed that resources to deal with such stresses are frequently lacking or not readily accessible to immigrant youth (Freire 1993; Status of Women Canada Policy Research Fund 2002). The pathways perspective, such as that conceptualized by Powers and Hertzman, has helped to make visible the multiple sources of influence on child health and development and to illustrate that these influences accumulate and converge over time. Such insights underscore the importance of attending to social influences and of continuing to work to foster multiple domains of development through adolescence.

Childhood influences on health inequalities Schools are central social contexts for teenagers. As well as providing opportunities for development they can be forums for support and affirmation or exclusion with their attendant positive or negative effects. Lynam and Cowley (2007) observed that for some immigrant teenagers, schools were sites of connection, affirmation and capacity building while for others they were sites of failure and exclusion. In the latter situation the school climate contributed to teenagers' questioning their value and potential. Such findings show the need *to understand the processes that create climates of inclusion or exclusion* because of their influence on the teenagers' views of themselves and their futures. With insights into the conditions and processes that influence connectedness and access to resources we may be better positioned to design and implement 'upstream' (Butterfield 1991; Lynam 2005; Wallerstein 1992) interventions to foster health.

Viewing health inequalities from a critical theoretical perspective

Bourdieu's theory of social relations was used as an analytic frame to understand the complex *influences on social relations*—the 'processes' of influence thereby potentially offering means for acting to effect change was also needed.

One goal of Bourdieu's (Bourdieu 1990a, 2001; Bourdieu et al 1999) theorizing was to make visible the ways broader societal practices structure relationships and shape experiences of those largely outside of formal discourses, such as the poor and immigrants (Lynam 2007; Lynam et al 2007). While Bourdieu does not name power as a central concept in his theoretical work he does examine processes that create privilege and disadvantage and he focuses attention on the social processes that assign value to different forms of 'capital' (Bourdieu 1994, 1990b, 2001; Bourdieu and Wacquant 1992; Bourdieu et al 1999). These processes find their expression in what Bourdieu (2001) terms 'symbolic violence', a concept that extends analyses of structural influences to illustrate how they operate.

> I have always been astonished . . . that the established order, with its relations of domination, its rights and prerogatives, privileges and injustices, ultimately perpetuates itself so easily, apart from a few historical accidents, and that most intolerable conditions of existence can so often be perceived as acceptable and even natural. And I have also seen masculine domination, and the way it is imposed and suffered, as the prime example of this paradoxical submission.

> (Bourdieu 2001, pp 1–2)

Bourdieu observed that social relations remain stable over time and illustrated how forms of symbolic violence become 'institutionalized' and viewed as normal through tacit agreement. Moreover, institutional policies and practices reflect such taken-for-granted notions thereby reinforcing and replicating structural influences which in turn continue to shape social relations. Of particular importance to this present research study is that 'symbolic violence manifests its power essentially in *face-to-face* interactions, it constitutes and reproduces domination in the immediate interactions between people' (Krais 2006, p 121). Symbolic violence is the expression of tacit power relations many of which are sanctioned in policy and through tradition and as such, it takes hold most firmly when both the dominated and the oppressed are complicit. And, as Krais (2006) contends, 'complicity can thus only be achieved when both agents, dominants and dominated, have integrated into their habitus[1] the symbolic order that generates the corresponding actions' (Krais 2006, p 42).

Marginalization and marginalizing practices accrue from unquestioned assumptions, stereotypical images. In our case the population of interest is immigrants, asylum seekers, or refugees. Such (stereotypical) notions of 'others' are reinforced when no countervailing images or representations are visible and when prevailing formal and popular discourses, and the social structures that underpin them, reinforce the messages of marginality (Lynam 2007). As such, marginalization is an appropriate concept for examination using discourse analysis and for identifying ways forward. Bourdieu's contention is that one strategy for effecting change in experiences, and the social structures that contribute to them, is to interrupt prevailing discourses by introducing alternative perspectives that challenge the assumptions of the status quo (Bourdieu 2001).

The research aims and methods

The study that is the focus of this chapter sought to: i) examine community-based conditions and processes that create or mitigate challenges in accessing or mobilizing resources

---

[1] Habitus 'refers to features of the individual, his or her viewpoints, and physical "dispositions" towards navigating the social world' (Lynam et al 2007; p 29).

for youth health and development, ii) make visible the ways local policies and practices shape the ways parents and teens navigate the 'social terrain' of the community to access community based resources for health.

The research was undertaken in two neighbourhoods in the Vancouver region that had an explicit commitment to youth engagement and that include Aboriginal and non-Aboriginal families and a large proportion of immigrant families with migration histories from regions of Asia and Central America as well as the Middle East and eastern Europe.

A premise of the methodology is to make visible the day-to-day interactions that are often 'taken for granted' and people's own accounts of such interactions. Therefore, the processes of data gathering and analysis are characterized by reflection and reflexivity (Bourdieu 2001; Bourdieu et al 1999; Reay 1998). The goal of data gathering is not to achieve consensus, or to recount the prevalence of particular examples but to examine, over the series of interviews, individuals' experiences so the analysis can consider these in relation to the context of the community and, the extralocal conditions that organize or shape them (Bourdieu et al 1999; Lynam 2005).

Approaches to sampling data gathering and analysis

The study employed a *purposive sampling strategy* and included families with 12 to 16-year-old sons or daughters. An acategorical approach to sampling was taken as the focus of the analysis was on the ways people interact to form relationships and the influences on this process. Teenagers and families with a range of experiences were included to capture similarities and differences in their experiences.

Taking direction from Bourdieu the transcripts and field notes were analysed to make visible the individuals' accounts of their experiences and the context using Bourdieu's concepts of *habitus*, field, and capital. Exemplars of social situations are drawn upon to illustrate the ways individuals make sense of their situations (*habitus*), the ways they navigate their social worlds (the fields), and the different forms of resources they draw upon or seek to acquire (forms of capital) to gain entry to, or to participate in, different fields. *A central process* evident in all of the interviews was what we have called the 'convoy' process.

The role of 'convoys' as resources for fostering affirmation and connectedness

Here we report specific findings that define this process, trace the ways it influenced teenagers' experiences, and explicate the conditions that influenced how it was enacted.

> Teenager: I think it was just the way I was raised, like my mum she, she raised me to like just stand up for myself and not do anything I don't want to do, she's raised me to really be assertive so, um, also I think its like my friends they really help and also the community center, um, they really stress like the bad things about drugs and about alcohol and I've seen like my friends get into it and they just kind of drift apart, they completely change, . . .

Researcher (R): So you know that you have people you can count on?

Teenager: Yeah, definitely (12-year-old girl).

In reflecting on why she views herself as comfortable and confident in social situations at school, at home, and in the community this teenager credits her mother, her friends, and community workers at the local community centre who run programmes for teenagers.[2] In this case the messages from each source echo one another, thus reinforcing a message of affirmation while also providing consistent information.

In each of the neighbourhoods where this study was being undertaken, there were key workers whose roles included engagement with, and support of Aboriginal[3] youth. In the quote that follows one key informant (KI) who was a resource person in the high school discusses the ways she tries to ensure that the teenagers get the support needed to feel valued and connected, which she hopes will contribute to school success. She does this in part by ensuring teenagers experience the support of their community and 'see' that their community is proud of them and available to them. Such messages are important, particularly as Aboriginal youth must confront negative and pervasive stereotyping as they navigate the broader community, challenges the KI must also confront. The following narrative and data excerpts describe how she enacted the convoy function while also drawing attention to a number of discourses that shaped the way she enacted the role.

The teenagers were raising funds for an exchange trip which, for most, was an opportunity of a lifetime. The KI observes that while the trip provides an important opportunity, it was equally important for these teenagers to experience the support of their community:

Key Informant (KI): They've really had a lot of help from the Nation and, you know, I'm trying to reaffirm to these children, I said, you know, if you learn something, one thing from this, learn that your community cares about you and they want to see you succeed and do well, they just haven't always had a chance or a place to express that support but that's why they're doing this because a lot of these kids are the ones who, who are bypassed, they're the ones who are overlooked because they struggle in different ways, they're the ones who don't get anything in some ways, you know, what I mean, they, its just complicated, its different . . . Yeah, well *I'm* vouching for those kids, I'm saying they're a good bet, you know. They're worth it, *they are so worth it.*

Somebody tried to tell me the investment isn't paying off. 'Oh their attendance rate hasn't improved since then'. And I'm like 'Yeah, but they're still going to the same school now aren't they? They're still there now, you know one step at a time. I don't expect to suddenly make them go to school everyday but I do hope that it encourages their sense of belonging to communities and self esteem and self worth I mean what's the value of that? It's priceless' (KI-2).

---

[2] Of note, this was the only teenager who called the researcher to ask about participating in the research. All other teens were recruited through their parents or others they knew in the community.

[3] Aboriginal communities in Canada are populations that have faced systematic exclusion from full participation in Canadian society (Royal Commission on Aboriginal Peoples 1996). One of many consequences of this is marked health inequalities. Aboriginal youth are much more likely to not complete school than their non-Aboriginal counterparts.

In this account we see that the KI is enacting the convoy function with a view to encourage, nurture, and invest in teenagers, who are on the extreme social and material margins of society. Her goal is that, like the teenager speaking in the first quote, they too will see they are 'worth it' and engage with school.

A number of assumptions are manifest in these quotes. One is that the inherent value of the first teenager is not in question. By contrast the Aboriginal teenagers must first be convinced that they too are of value. These two assumptions construct different starting points for the teenagers in question. They also signal that one's social location is related to both structural conditions and 'markers' such as colour, language, or ethnicity (Lynam and Cowley 2007) that signal the social value of a person and/or their attributes.

As these quotes suggest, the convoy process is a goal directed strategy or way of acting to mobilize support or resources for teenagers. The social convoy model recognizes the importance of enduring social relationships to child development and provides a way to capture the structure of social networks that continue over time (Kahn and Antonucci 1980). Convoys, as conceptualized from this study data however, characterize it as a form of agency that bridges both social and structural conditions. Convoys in this study were parents, but also key informants, and in some instances teenagers themselves.

The capacity of the convoy to be successful across a range of conditions was influenced in part by the 'authority' the convoy was viewed as holding in the social context. Bourdieu's concept of symbolic violence as introduced above focuses attention on the *social processes that shape interactions*, in effect, the embodiment of social structures. Such embodiment is underpinned by socially sanctioned views of 'authority' or credibility. Authority then, is one form of power that is drawn upon in social interactions. The KI speaking above had authority because of her formal role in the school. She also held a form of authority with the teenagers and their families because she shared, and had experienced the legacy of exclusion. Her authority, however, was not without question as others did not 'get it' and did not appreciate the challenges the teenagers faced. Similarly, the teenager quoted at the outset, valued her mother's input and position. Her mother's views, however, were reinforced and supported by formal and popular discourses the teenager was exposed to.

As Bourdieu explains, however, such forms of authority are socially assigned and are therefore 'arbitrary'. For example, parents are legally and socially accorded particular forms of authority, these two forms can reinforce one another and can be further augmented if a parent also has other forms of capital that accrue from their social status or standing such as their work role or their education. However, if a parent does not 'parent' in ways viewed to be 'appropriate'—that is, if the parent 'dissents' or challenges the tacitly agreed upon norms, these different forms of authority can be undermined and the parents' ability to have their authority recognized is also undermined. Symbolic violence is the way traditional or socially sanctioned forms of authority are maintained.

Adolescence presented developmental challenges some immigrant parents felt ill-equipped to deal with in the Canadian context. As the following quote suggests, some parents successfully enlisted the support of others on their teenager's behalf. The teacher responded to this mother's concern, recognized the teenager's interests, and created avenues for the teenager's interests and talents to be recognized with a positive outcome.

> Mother: Now I think she is very confident. It is a realistic confidence, not a blind confidence (1-5—Mother).

Here, the teacher acted as a resource for both the mother and a 'convoy' for the teenager. Her positioning within the school offered knowledge of the broader social network but what is also critically important here is that this teacher, and others at this school, held the view that supporting a teenager's development was a part of their role.

In the following account a teenager, who has a passion for art as well as sports activities, describes how her interest was extinguished and then rekindled because of the ways art was being taught.

> Teenager: Well it was kind of the opposite because I was always interested in art and then it was school that kind of upset me with art.

> R: Oh because they wanted you to do it this way?

> Teenager: Grade five it would be you measure two inches from the right and two inches from the left then you draw a diagonal point and then we'd all draw the same picture in the end. So I stopped doing a lot of art and then it was kind of, like in the summer when I'm thinking I haven't done art for awhile, so then I just started painting or sewing or clay or something like that. High school art wasn't as tragic as elementary school art, I use the word tragic because everybody's art looked the same, yeah.

> R: Yeah, so high school has been a little bit more freeing in the sense in relation to art?

> Teenager: Yes absolutely.

In this example, the authoritative voice of the teacher regulated the way art was to be undertaken. The teenager saw this as belying her view of art as an expressive form, instead art became 'tragic'. The teenager 'followed the rules' but as a consequence it was her interest in art that was the casualty.

As the following quotes suggest, however, all parents were not successful in gaining the support of others, with devastating consequences for herself and for her son.

> Mother: With my, you know, I'd like an explanation, he doesn't have any problem but this one, he's talking of even killing himself, and it's killing me, killing my parents who are living with me and I just don't know what I have to do, even that I'm a family counselor, my mum always say (name) you are a family counselor, you've been helping so many people for twenty-seven years, can you believe it?

> R: So you're worried, so when you say killing himself, are you worried that he's depressed?

> Mother: He's depressed.

> R: And he's resisting letting you mobilize help for him?

> Mother: Yes.

This too was an immigrant family. The parents were well educated and the family had lived in the community for more than ten years. The parents had, however recently, separated and the son was unhappy about his father's departure. The teenager had been an excellent student and talented athlete but, following his father's departure, his behaviour changed and he started missing school.

Mother: He lost his imagination, his responsibility and everything, started to be with his friends and skipping his school and, oh gosh, when I just remember this I get emotional. But I have to tell you like a few months ago, Christmas time I was really concerned about that he's keeping from school, I went to school. That's the part that makes me really angry about the system, very angry.

R: They didn't call you or anything?

Mother: They just call to say that your son or daughter has been missing one or two or more classes, if you're concerned contact the school. I was concerned. I went to school and I said I know that my son is skipping and I know that he's at home because he's sleeping and he's depressed and these people didn't do anything.

R: They didn't care?

Mother: They didn't care, they just said their concern is that, okay, he's going to be okay, don't worry about it. I'm worried, I'm a counselor I know what's going on with my son please give me some help, some resources even that I know all the resources more than them.

R: Right.

Mother: I wanted to hear it from them maybe they have some different things to tell me.

R: Right, I mean you're trying to be the parent not the counselor.

No support was forthcoming despite the mother's plea. She was also upset that her concerns were dismissed, an affront that was particularly painful because she was educated as a counsellor. Instead, when the teenager continued to miss school, they cut him from the sports team which was, at the time, the only activity that he felt good about. Rather than using this as means for re-engaging with the teenager. The teenager became angry and depressed and continued to miss school with the result that he was excluded. At the time of the interviews the teenager had become a part of a group of other teenagers also excluded from school. He was drinking alcohol and was clinically depressed. His mother was devastated that not only had he been excluded, but the school had not involved her in the decision and no one seemed to see that this teenager's bright future was compromised.

The message this mother received was that it was her problem to deal with. Such comments echo popular discourses and institutional practices that hold parents responsible for their children's 'bad' behaviour, even if, the behaviour is more harmful to the teenager than anyone else. In addition to trying to mobilize supports from teachers and counsellors at school she sought counselling for him and even approached the police in an effort to have them help her to deal with his underage drinking. They too declined to assist saying you're his mother, it's your problem.

Mother: Look at the police, (they said) 'you are his mum, do something for him'. Okay, tell me what should I do? I want to do something for him but I don't know what especially being as a foreigner, as a person who has come from the different country, you know, imagine you as a mum (referring to the researcher) being a Canadian, its quite different, you know, your rights, you know.

. . .

> And still I'm stuck and I still don't have any help for my son after all these, you know, places that I've gone, all these people that I've seen, still cannot see any help for my son, how about the other poor people that they don't have any support, not pulling in, I mean financial, I'm just talking about the ability to speak English, knowledge about the community and everything.

In this case the son is viewed as not playing by the rules by not attending school, even though the teenager's issues were not with the school; the school became a forum in which his anger and sadness played out. While in the earlier quotes, requests for support for teenagers are responded to in positive ways, here the 'system' does not respond to the plea for help, but asserts its authority by making an example of the teenager. As this quote suggests, when one is mobilizing support for a 'problem', particularly a behavioural problem, there is stigma attached. As noted above, Bourdieu directs the analyst to focus attention on the dissenting voice for through such voices one gains insight on the tacit assumptions that structure social relations. As a dissenter the son is not supported. But also, in this case the mother's credibility as a parent was eroded by her son's behaviour, her sense of being a capable parent was undermined because, as an immigrant, she did not know the best way to effectively engage with resources of the community. And, her credibility as a counsellor was undermined by a lack of recognition of her expertise. Moreover, because of the stigma associated with having a child excluded from school for 'bad' behaviour she was isolated from other parents in the community. This mother's capacity to act as a convoy was further eroded by the largely unquestioned authority of the agents of the school.

In what follows an additional example of students missing school is described. But here, although 30% of the students in the school walked out to protest a decision made by the administration, students were not sanctioned. Parents who attended a meeting to discuss the administrative decision were told 'it's too late for dialogue'. When the mother I spoke with noted that parents had not been consulted, administrators responded 'we didn't have to ask for dialogue'. Here parents also experienced the 'authoritative voice' and, as a consequence, supported their teenagers' decision to protest.

> Mother: There is nothing more frustrating than, *growing up in a community where your voice is important, where you're heard, where you're valued and then suddenly somebody comes along and takes a different approach*, . . . It was really *nice to hear how many parents at that school made it really clear that when those children walk out you, respect them.*

Are these examples of symbolic violence achieved and thwarted? Symbolic violence, Goldstein (2005) argues, relies upon the presupposition of the existence of the authority of those who set and enforce policy (p 35). Moreover, to question such authority, one risks the consequences of being named a 'deviant'—which was effectively the fate of one family above. Under certain conditions schools do have the authority to exclude students. But, as the second example shows they also have the mandate to work with students, to engage them, to guide them, to help them to be successful. In one case the school choose to exclude and effectively give up on, a talented and gifted teenager, while in the other the administration was put on warning by the parent and teenager community.

Discussion

Symbolic violence is the use of authority and the structuring or practices that reinforce the voice of authority. By examining the ways parents, and others, were, or were not, able to enact the convoy function, we gain insights into the ways social processes structure interactions and influence connection and the capacity to mobilize resources. Some communities are better at creating a sense of belonging while others foster marginalization or limit access to diverse groups for support. The analytic perspective taken here considers individuals' experiences in context and enables an analysis of the ways broader social conditions shape intergroup relations and contribute to the creation of conditions of privilege or disadvantage.

As Krais (2006) observes 'symbolic violence is the acting out of a worldview and social order anchored deeply in the habitus of both dominants and dominated'. It thus requires harmony between subjective structures—the *habitus*—and objective relations, and incorporation of 'the way things are supposed to be' within each social agent. Symbolic violence then implies, in a certain sense, what may be termed 'complicity' on the part of the dominated, as it 'can only be exerted on a person predisposed (in his habitus) to feel it, whereas others will ignore it' (Bourdieu, 1991: 51). This 'complicity' can thus only be achieved when both agents, dominants and dominated, have integrated into their *habitus* the symbolic order that generates the corresponding actions' (p 122). Those who dissent, those who do not 'go along' and challenge the practices may be the voice of change, but they also risk different consequences. *Habitus* mediates structures and practices. Our predispositions (ways of making sense of situations) guide our interpretations of structural processes and how we act on/towards them. If for example, it has been our experience that 'systems' work in our favour, that the 'rules' work for us, then, we are less likely to question or to challenge them. But in this way we may also overlook the impact of such conditions on others, particularly those with fewer (social and material) resources to draw upon.

As many of the examples offered here suggest, when one stands on the outside it is easier to question the way things 'are'. All of the study participants had not 'integrated the symbolic order' into their way of being. In many cases, they or their observations can be seen as calling the 'symbolic order' into question. Some parents effectively navigated around the social order, taking advantage of situations that were available to them.

This study provides some insights into why new theoretical and analytical perspectives on health inequalities are needed. Population analyses that identify groups at risk are frequently taken to mean that such groups are (or should be) responsible for their poor health. As such, a central focus of many interventions is to change individuals' behaviours through education. While education is always important, attention must also be paid to addressing the social structural conditions that place such groups at risk.

It is clear that people do not engage with institutions or with policy. Rather, they engage with individuals. As such, to be effective, policies of inclusion, or policies of engagement, must be enacted through all levels of society and social organizations so that they can be experienced at the 'face' of the organization. That is, to be effective, policies must be taken up, throughout social organizations. In designing this study I took the position that Bourdieu's analytic perspective offers a means to recognize the ways multiple axes of disadvantage, that can include: gender, class, and 'race', intersect and create challenges for individuals. In health professionals' practice such insights may translate into an awareness of the ways different axes of disadvantage influence individuals' capacities to manage their own health and illness, but it may also prompt a realization of the ways each of our assumptions about such individuals shape our responses to them. Our *habitus* or 'predispositions' as professionals is shaped by the intuitive perception of objective possibilities. We are therefore disinclined to question the logic that underpins our reasoning—that may for example prompt us to conflate ethnicity with—risk; to consider risk as arising from inherent capabilities rather than being mediated by social conditions (Moore 2004).

Without critical reflection on the assumptions that inform how we practice, or how we make sense of our day-to-day interactions, or how we make sense of our data, we become complicit in reproducing and replicating the structures and processes that create privilege for some while disadvantaging others. In being complicit we play a role in the continuing exclusion and marginalization of those whose views are not reflected, or not pervasive in the social organization of society.

The insights from this analysis will not solve the problems of health inequalities but they do introduce new perspectives to the discourses of health inequalities and the conditions that contribute to them. Such research is needed, for as Muhajarine, Vu, and Labonte (2006) suggest, there is a need for more research 'in areas that do not lend themselves to quick fixes, particularly the accumulation of evidence regarding the pervasive impact of social inequity and exclusion on health of children. If healthy families produce healthy children, the societal milieu with its structures, norms and values is the fundamental platform upon which lasting change must occur' (p 216).

Acknowledgements

The research that informs this chapter was funded by a grant from the Canadian Social Sciences and Humanities Research Council (SSHRC).

Bibliography

Armstrong, M, Bernie-Lifcovitch, S, and Ungar, M (2005) 'Social support, mastery, self esteem and individual adjustment among at-risk youth' *Child & Youth Care Forum* 34/5: 329–46

Beiser, M and Stewart, M (2005) 'Reducing health disparities: a priority for Canada' *Canadian Journal of Public Health* 96/2: S4–S5

Berkman, L and Syme, L (1979) 'Social networks, host resistance, and mortality. A nine year follow up of Alameda County residents' *American Journal of Epidemiology* 109/2: 186–204

Bourdieu, P (1990a) *The logic of practice*. Translated by R Nice. Cambridge: Polity Press

Bourdieu, P (1990b) *In other words: essays towards a reflexive sociology*. Cambridge: Polity Press

Bourdieu, P (1991) *Language and symbolic power*. Cambridge: Harvard University Press and Polity Press

Bourdieu, P (1994) 'Structures, habitus, power: Basis for a theory of symbolic power' in NB Dirks, G Eley, and S Ortner (eds), *Culture/power/history: a reader in contemporary theory*, pp 155–99. Princeton: Princeton University Press

Bourdieu, P (2001) *Masculine domination*. Translated by R Nice. Stanford: Stanford University Press

Bourdieu, P and Wacquant, L (1992) *An invitation to reflexive sociology*. Oxford: Polity Press

Bourdieu, P, Accardo, A, Balacs, G, Beaud, S, Bonvin, F, and Bourdieu, E (1999) *The weight of the world: social suffering in contemporary society*. Cambridge: Polity Press

Butterfield, P (1991) 'Thinking upstream: nurturing a conceptual understanding of the social context of health behaviour' in K Saucier (ed), *Perspectives in family and community health*, pp 66–71. Toronto: CV Mobsy

Farmer, P (2004) 'An anthropology of structural violence' *Current Anthropology* 45: 305–26

Farmer, PE, Nizeye, B, Stulac, S, and Keshavjee, S (2006) 'Structural violence and clinical medicine' *PLoS Medicine* 3: 1686–91

Freire, M (1993) 'Mental health, culture, children and youth' in R Masi, L Mensah, and K McLeod (eds), *Health and cultures exploring the relationships. Volume II: Programs, services and care*, p 119. Oakville: Mosaic Press

Goldstein, R (2005) 'Symbolic and institutional violence and critical educational spaces: in the name of education' *Journal of Peace Education* 2/1: 33–52

Gordon, D, Shaw, M, Dorling, D, and Davey Smith, G (1999) *Inequalities in health: the evidence*. Bristol: The Policy Press

Graham, H (1993) *Hardship and health in women's lives*. London: Harvester Wheatsheaf

Graham, H (2000) 'Socio-economic change and inequalities in men and women's health in the U.K.' in E Annandale and K Hunt (eds), *Gender inequalities in health*, pp 90–122. Buckingham: Open University Press

Graham, H (2004) 'Social determinants and their unequal distribution: clarifying policy understandings' *The Milbank Quarterly* 82/1: 101–24

Haan, M, Kaplan, G, and Camacho, T (1987) 'Poverty and health: prospective evidence from the Alameda County Study' *American Journal of Epidemiology* 125/6: 989–98

Health Education Authority (1999) *The influence of social support and social capital on health. A review and analysis of British data*. Report prepared by Cooper, H, Arber, S, Lin, F, and Ginn, J. London: Health Education Authority.

Hertzman, C and Power, C (2003) 'Health and human development: understandings from life- course research' *Developmental Neuropsychology* 24/2–3: 719–45

Kahn, RL and Antonucci, TC (1980) 'Convoys over the life course: attachment, roles and social support' in P Bakes and O Brim (eds), *Life span development and behavior*. Volume 3, pp 253–86. San Diego, CA: Academic Press

Kawachi, I and Berkman, L (2000) 'Social cohesion, social capital, and health' in L Berkman and I Kawachi (eds), *Social epidemiology*, pp 174–90. Oxford: Oxford University Press

Krais, B (2006) 'Gender, sociological theory and Bourdieu's sociology of practice' *Theory, culture & society* 26/6: 119–34

Lagarin, M (2004) 'Protective factors for inner-city adolescents at risk of school drop out: family factors and social support' *Children & Schools* 26/4: 211–20

Levitt, MJ, Levitt, J, Bustos, G, Crooks, N, Santos, J, Telan, P, Hodgetts, J, and Milevsky, A (2005) 'Patterns of social support in the middle childhood and early adolescent transition: implications for adjustment' *Social Development* 14/3: 398–420

Lipshitz-Ellhawi, R and Itzhahy, H (2005) 'Social support, mastery, self esteem and individual adjustment among at-risk youth' *Child & Youth Care Forum* 34/5: 329–46

Lynam, MJ (2005) 'Health as a socially mediated process: theoretical & practice imperatives emerging from research on health inequalities' *Advances in Nursing Science* 28/1: 25–37

Lynam, MJ (2007) 'Does discourse matter? Using critical inquiry to engage in knowledge development for practice' *Primary Health Care Research and Development* 8: 54–67

Lynam, MJ and Tenn, L (1989) 'Communication: a tool for the negotiation of independence in families with adolescents' *Journal of Advanced Nursing* 14: 653–60

Lynam, MJ and Young, R (2002)'Empowerment, praxis, and action theory in health promotion research' in L Valach, R Young, and MJ Lynam (eds), *Action theory: a primer for applied research in the social sciences*, pp 123–38. Westport: Praeger

Lynam, MJ, Browne, A, Reimer, S, and Anderson, J (2007) 'Rethinking the complexities of "culture": what might we learn from Bourdieu?' *Nursing Inquiry* 14/1: 23–34

Lynam, MJ and Cowley, S (2007) 'Understanding marginalization as a social determinant of health' *Critical Public Health* 17: 137–49

Moore, R (2004) 'Cultural capital: objective probability and the cultural arbitrary' *British Journal of Sociology of Education* 25/4: 445–56

Muhajarine, N, Vu, L, and Labonte, R (2006) 'Social contexts and children's health outcomes: researching across the boundaries' *Critical Public Health* 16/3: 205–218

Nazroo, JY (2003) 'The structuring of ethnic inequalities in health: economic position, racial discrimination, and racism' *American Journal of Public Health* 93/2: 277–84

Parker, JS and Benson, M (2004) 'Parent–adolescent relations and adolescent functioning: self-esteem, substance abuse & delinquency' *Adolescence* 39/155: 519–30

Power, C, Manor, O, and Fox, J (1991) *Health and class: the early years.* London: Chapman & Hall

Power, C, Hertzman, C, Matthews, S, and Manor, O (1997) 'Social differences in health: life-cycle effects between ages 23 and 33 in the 1958 British birth cohort' *American Journal of Public Health* 87/9: 1499–503

Power, C, Stansfeld, S, Matthews, S, Manor, O, and Hope, S (2002) 'Childhood and adulthood risk factors for socio-economic differentials in psychological distress: evidence from the 1958 British birth cohort' *Social Science & Medicine* 55: 1989–2004

Power, C, Hyppönen, E, and Davey Smith, G (2005) 'Socioeconomic position in childhood and early adult life and risk of mortality: a prospective study of the mothers of the 1958 British Birth Cohort' *American Journal of Public Health* 95/8: 1396–402

Reay, D (1998) *Class work: mothers' involvement in their children's primary schooling.* London: UCL Press

Royal Commission on Aboriginal Peoples (RCAP) (1996) 'Royal Commission Report on Aboriginal Peoples', Indian and Northern Affairs Canada <http://www.ainc-inac.gc.ca/ch/rcap/sg/sgmm_e.html> (viewed September 30 2004)

Shaw, M, Dorling, D, and Davey Smith, G (2005) 'Poverty, social exclusion, and minorities' in M Marmot and RG Williamson (eds), *Social determinants of health*, pp 211–39. Oxford: Oxford University Press

Status of Women Canada Policy Research Fund (2002) *Mental health promotion among newcomer female youth: post-migration experiences and self-esteem.* Report prepared by N Khanlou, M Beiser, E Cole, M Freire, I Hyman, and KM Kilbride, Ottawa

Ungar, M (2004) 'The importance of parents and other caregivers to the resilience of high-risk adolescents' *Family Process* 43/1: 23–41

Wallerstein, N (1992) 'Powerless, empowerment and health: Implications for health promotion programmes' *International Journal of Health Promotion* 6/3: 197–205

Whitehead, M (1992) *The health divide. With the Black Report, in inequalities in health.* London: Penguin Books

Wilkinson, RG (1996) *Unhealthy societies: the afflictions of inequality.* London: Routledge

Williams, DR and Williams-Morris, R (2000) 'Racism and mental health: the African American experience' *Ethnicity & Health* 5/34: 243–68

Young, RA, Lynam, MJ, Valach, L, Novak, H, Brierton, I, and Christopher, A (2001) 'Joint actions of parents and adolescents in health conversations' *Qualitative Health Research* 11/1: 40–57

Chapter 8

Economic evaluation of public health interventions

Susan Griffin, Nigel Rice, and Mark Sculpher

Introduction

Economic evaluation is an increasingly used tool which aims to provide a formal, explicit and transparent framework for informing decisions about allocating public funds in the health care sector. By utilizing economic evaluation in the field of public health, it is possible to address questions about the efficiency of allocating resources to fund interventions aimed at improving public health. Economic evaluation of medical interventions and programmes within the health care sector typically utilizes a framework which aims to maximize health outcomes subject to the health sector budget constraint (an 'extra welfarist' perspective). This differs from the approaches generally used in some other areas of economic evaluation (eg transport).

In this chapter we discuss whether this extra welfarist normative framework can be extended to the evaluation of public health interventions, which may have objectives other than health maximization and may operate across multiple sectors and budget constraints. The extensions to the framework that would enable intersectoral comparisons and a consideration of equity are considered as well as frameworks used in other areas of policy evaluation (eg cost–benefit analysis based on conventional 'welfarist' normative principles). The chapter considers how the current elements of economic evaluation, such as statistical analysis of individual patient data, systematic review, evidence synthesis, and decision-analytic modelling can be applied to evaluate public health interventions with the view to informing policy. Methods for valuing health outcomes are considered to determine the need to move beyond the quality adjusted life year (QALY) in order to reflect concerns about equity, and the determinants of health and health inequalities. Methods for evaluating the opportunity costs of allocating resources from multiple sectors to a particular intervention are examined, with a view to calculating the net benefits of alternative interventions. The chapter concludes by considering whether methodological standards for the economic evaluation of public health interventions can be established.

Economic evaluation in the health care sector

The recognition within health care systems that the amount of resources required to provide all available health technologies exceeds current capacities has led, in many countries, to institutes being created to take a prominent role in the rationing process and to have power over the allocation of health care resources. Decisions about allocating collective resources need to be made in a justifiable and auditable manner, so any methods need to make explicit the underlying scientific and social value judgements. Economic evaluation tackles the problem of making choices in the presence of scarce resources in an explicit, formal framework by evaluating the resources required to provide health care interventions and comparing the generated outcomes to those that could have been achieved with an alternative use of those resources. The most cost-effective use of available resources is the one that provides the best outcome. Knowing what resources to evaluate and how to measure outcomes depends on the normative framework or collection of principles which underlies the economic evaluation.

Current methods for economic evaluation in health technology appraisal

The methods for health economic evaluation have largely been developed to satisfy the purpose of informing resource allocation decisions in the field of health technology assessment. Within the health care sector, the outcome of interest for economic evaluation has generally been regarded as some measure of health. In order to facilitate comparisons between alternative health care technologies, it is necessary to have a single index measure of health. One such measure is the quality adjusted life year (QALY), which is calculated as a function of length of life and a preference-based measure of quality of life. Quality of life is generally measured in terms of freedom from symptoms of ill health such as pain, with the quality weight determined by estimating the quantity-quality trade-off. In other words, people are asked how much of a reduction in length of life or how much of an increased risk of death they would be willing to accept for an improvement in quality of life. This allows quality of life to be valued on a scale from zero (death) to one (full health) that is exchangeable with quantity of life.

The view that health is the outcome to be maximized (ie the 'maximand') in the decision maker's objective function when choosing between alternative health care technologies, represents a departure from a classical economic approach which would regard the sum of individuals' subjective utilities as the maximand (Brouwer and Koopmanschap 2000). The departure results in part from disagreement with the implicit social value judgements underpinning welfare economics by those institutes with the remit to allocate health care resources. In brief, cost–benefit analysis (CBA) would value health gains (and potentially other sorts of outcomes) using individuals' willingness to pay values, and willingness to pay is dependent on ability to pay. Hence a CBA approach has been perceived as prioritizing health care interventions aimed at the rich over those aimed at the poor, raising ethical concerns (Claxton et al 2007). This is perhaps the main reason why cost-effectiveness analysis (CEA), in which the benefits of health care interventions are measured in terms of health, is the dominant form of economic evaluation in the health care sector.

In determining the cost of providing any health care intervention the resources to be measured depend on the perspective for the analysis and the source of the budget constraint.

In the United Kingdom, for example, the budget for health care is determined by the government, and once defined is regarded as fixed by institutes with the remit to make resource allocation decisions within the National Health Service. The view of the budget constraint, and the objective function, as exogenously determined conforms to the social decision-making framework (Sugden and Williams 1978). Economic evaluations then take the form of a solution to a constrained optimization problem to maximize health gains subject to a given budget constraint. With this in mind, the resources of interest are simply those that fall on the budget constraint, ie resources within the health care sector. The budget is fully allocated, so introducing a new health technology displaces another. The health gains forgone by displacing existing health care technologies represent the opportunity cost of introducing the new technology. If the health gains from the new technology exceed this opportunity cost then it is regarded as cost-effective. An illustration of this decision rule is provided in Box 8.1. In practice in the UK, the technologies that would be displaced are not identified, and the opportunity cost is approximated by a cost-effectiveness threshold value. Thus new health technologies assessed by the National Institute for Health and Clinical Excellence are regarded as cost-effective if the additional cost required to gain an additional QALY relative to a competing technology is less than

Box 8.1 Evaluating the cost-effectiveness of new health care interventions

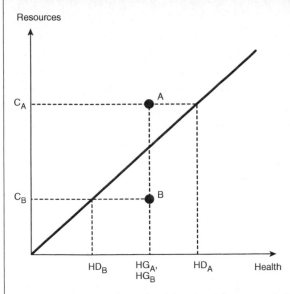

The slope of the diagonal line represents the amount of health that can be generated per unit of resources used to provide existing health care interventions.

Two new interventions are evaluated to determine whether they should be provided within the healthcare system.

Intervention A offers a health gain HG_A at an additional cost of C_A. Reducing provision of existing services to fund A would displace amount of health HD_A, resulting in a loss of health overall as $HG_A - HD_A < 0$.

Intervention B offers a health gain HG_B at an additional cost of C_B. Reducing provision of existing services to fund B would displace amount of health HD_B, resulting in a gain of health overall as $HG_B - HD_B > 0$.

£20,000–£30,000, although factors other than cost-effectiveness are also considered (NICE 2008).

The marginal effect of an intervention is described by the cost per QALY gained ($\Delta C / \Delta Q$), or the incremental cost-effectiveness ratio (ICER). However, it is possible to rearrange a decision rule based on observing an ICER less than the cost-effectiveness threshold to calculate a decision rule based on net health benefits, NHB (or net monetary benefits if desired):

$$(1) \qquad ICER = \Delta C / \Delta Q < threshold; \quad NHB = \Delta Q - \Delta C / threshold > 0.$$

In contrast, if the budget is not viewed as fixed, the introduction of a new health technology does not necessarily displace another, so the benchmark for establishing cost-effectiveness is no longer the amount of health displaced. Instead the health gains must be described in terms of their value to society. Treating health as a socially desirable outcome in addition to the well-being individuals derive from consumption may conform to the principles of Extra Welfarism (Culyer 1991). The resources do not have to be limited to those that fall on the budget constraint, and may for example include personal expenditure by patients. The amount of health care resources that are required to provide all of the health technologies that are deemed cost-effective determines the budget constraint. The process for evaluation remains the same, but the threshold has a different interpretation as the societal willingness to pay for health and the opportunity cost of new technologies are seen in terms of consumption of all other goods and services.

Public health interventions

The analytical frameworks reflected in many of the existing guidelines for economic evaluation were developed with the focus on health care technologies provided within the health care sector. However, it is increasingly recognized that the marginal improvements in population health offered by new pharmaceutical products, medical devices, and surgical techniques may well be outstripped by the improvements achievable with more broad-spectrum interventions that extend beyond health care (Wanless 2004). Public health interventions may be broader than medical interventions in both scope and purpose, with wider aims than the simple improvement of health overall. A significant economic impact on the wider public sector is not unique to public health interventions, but it is certainly more common, particularly when the process of delivering those interventions places demands on sectors outside of health care. The question is how to extend the analytical frameworks to reflect the wider economic impact of public health interventions. This requires consideration of how to measure the benefits of public health interventions, how to assess the opportunity costs of providing those interventions, and how to define the objective function.

As well as discussing the appropriate analytical framework for evaluating public health interventions, it is important to take a more detailed look at the methods that can be applied to conduct those analyses. The processes involved in cost-effectiveness analysis include the identification of evidence on the costs and benefits of interventions and the synthesis of that evidence to provide a unified assessment of cost-effectiveness. For example, in evaluating health technologies it is common to have available data from randomized controlled trials to establish efficacy. This is less common with public health interventions where randomization may be regarded as more problematical and as a result efficacy may need to be established on the basis of non-experimental evidence. It is thus necessary to assess whether the methods for systematic review, evidence synthesis, and decision-analytic modelling that are routinely applied in the evaluation of health care technologies can be applied to evidence characterized by different methods of data collection.

A framework for evaluating public health interventions

Public health policy has traditionally been concerned with improving health equity in addition to improving health. The decision maker's objective function is not simply to maximize health gains, but also to ensure an equitable *distribution* of health. Health equity can be regarded as the fair distribution of health care resources according to some measure of 'need'. If the intervention or programme that is identified as most cost-effective in terms of maximizing health gains is also the intervention that most improves the distribution of health, then it could be regarded as dominant (unequivocally better in terms of the key decision criteria) and should be funded. However, in those cases where one intervention is most cost-effective, but another offers a greater improvement in equity for example, then we require an extension to the standard decision rules in order to identify the alternative which should be provided. In the same way that standard CEA as used in health technology appraisal compares the improvement in health gains with a new intervention to the health gains forgone by diverting resources from (reducing provision of) existing activities to fund the new intervention, it is possible to take an opportunity cost approach to valuing improvements in equity. By evaluating the health gains forgone as a result of selecting the intervention offering the greater improvement in equity rather than the one offering the greater improvement in health, the opportunity cost of improving equity would be expressed in health terms (Epstein et al 2007). It is then necessary to value the improvement in equity to establish whether the opportunity costs exceed the benefits.

Defining equity

Inequity is most often measured in terms of an inequality in either health inputs or health outcomes according to some identifying characteristic within a population. However, it must be noted that inequity and inequality are not interchangeable, as only for particular patient characteristics will inequality in health be considered unfair or inequitable. Williams and Cookson (2006) point to the multitude of health inequalities that could be identified in relation to the characteristics of the population of interest, including inequalities by sex, social class, ethnicity, smoking status and many more. Williams and Cookson also note that each health inequality may be regarded as inequitable to a different degree, with, for example, inequalities by smoking status viewed as less important than inequalities by social class. Some health inequalities may not be regarded as inequitable at all. For example, women are known to have a longer life expectancy than men, but most people would not regard this as unfair and simply a result of differing biological endowments. Taking steps to ensure that the distribution of health is more equal between men and women by prioritizing health care interventions targeted at men could, under these circumstances, actually be regarded as reducing equity (Sen 2002). Thus, the value in making the distribution of health more equal will vary according to the characteristic over which the inequality is assessed.

One way to identify those inequalities that are regarded as inequitable would be to undertake surveys of the general public, and this approach has been used by researchers trying to estimate the components of the social welfare function (Dolan et al 2008). The National Institute for Health and Clinical Excellence takes advice from a Citizens Council that is tasked with representing the public's view in the process of decision making. The Citizens Council has been asked to consider a number of extensions to a simple QALY maximization framework including the role of health inequalities, the rule of rescue, and whether orphan drugs should be assessed on a different basis to other interventions. The reports have demonstrated that it is difficult to achieve unanimity on extensions to the objective function, and that defining additional attributes, such as equity, presents an additional challenge. Alternatively, it is likely that, for a given public health intervention, the targeted inequality will be specified by stakeholders, with the implicit assumption that a more equal distribution would be regarded as more equitable. Once the inequality of interest is defined, the process of measuring the existing level in the population of interest, and valuing any potential improvements, can begin.

Measuring and valuing equity

Routine data on mortality and morbidity, or data collected during health research, can make it possible to identify health inequalities, where groups with different characteristics experience different health outcomes. Concentration indices can then be used to quantify the level of inequality (O'Donnell et al 2008). Figure 8.1(a) compares the distribution of total health in a population to the distribution of total wealth. An equal distribution of health would be represented by the diagonal, with each quintile of the population divided according to wealth sharing 20% of the overall population health. However, it can be seen from the unequal distribution in Figure 8.1(a) that the poorest 20% share only 10% of overall health, and the next poorest 20% also share only 10% of overall health. In contrast, the richest 20% of the population share 40% of overall health. The shaded area between the observed distribution and the line of equality can be measured and used to generate concentration indices to quantify the level of inequality.

The impact of public health interventions on reducing inequalities can be obtained by collecting data on equity-relevant characteristics alongside estimates of costs and effectiveness and performing appropriate subgroup analyses. For example, an intervention targeted at low-income groups could improve the distribution of health if care were taken to ensure that existing programmes displaced to fund the new intervention were not also

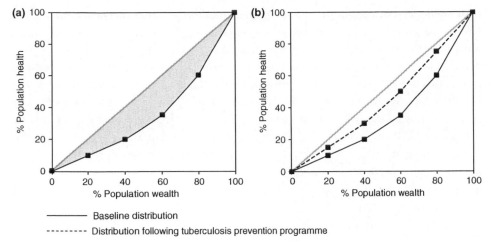

Baseline distribution

-------- Distribution following tuberculosis prevention programme

Fig. 8.1 Measuring the distribution of health and quantifying the level of inequality

targeted at those groups. An intervention targeted at reducing the prevalence of tuberculosis in a population may be expected to improve health outcomes in low income groups but have little effect on health outcomes in high income groups. By ensuring that the programme was funded by displacing existing interventions that were neutral in their impact on the distribution of health (or those that if removed would reduce inequality), a more equal distribution of health could be achieved, as illustrated by the dashed line in Figure 8.1(b). The challenge may be to ensure that health care interventions are more widely routinely assessed for their impact on the distribution of health, to enable fair comparisons between public health interventions and those competing for the same resources within the health care sector.

The decision about whether to fund the tuberculosis prevention programme is not clear if in total the tuberculosis prevention programme offers a smaller health gain than that displaced in order to fund the programme. Under these circumstances the improvement in equity will only have been achieved at the expense of a loss in overall health, and this opportunity cost must be valued. A likely source of such opportunity costs may arise where disadvantaged groups are less likely to seek or receive health care, such that additional resources must be invested in order to achieve the health gains attainable with a given intervention in those groups.

One way to arrive at values for the amount of health decision makers should be willing to forgo to improve health equity is to rely on informal analysis, such as the deliberative process undertaken by the Appraisal Committees for the National Institute for Health and Clinical Excellence. When determining whether to approve an intervention for reimbursement the Appraisal Committee is presented with a range of evidence including a formal CEA and statements from relevant stakeholders that can be used to identify additional considerations not yet incorporated into assessments of cost-effectiveness. Where equity concerns are considered to be important, the Committee may choose to approve an intervention with an ICER higher than the notional threshold of £20,000–£30,000 per QALY gained. The amount by which the ICER exceeds the threshold represents the value of the health gains the Committee considers it is reasonable to forgo in order to address those equity concerns. In this way precedents are set and propagated through later decisions. Trade-offs between equity and efficiency routinely occur within health services when it is determined that patients with the same disease should have access to the same treatments regardless of any other characteristics that could influence the expected costs or benefits from treatment. Many health care systems incorporate this notion of equality of access without quantifying the consequences. Epstein et al (2007) consider the effects of horizontal equity restrictions using a mathematical programming framework. By comparing the health gains achieved by offering all patients the same treatment to those achievable if perfect discrimination were allowed, the opportunity costs in terms of the health lost overall are quantified.

An alternative method to value improvements in equity is to perform a direct valuation task in which respondents are asked to specify how much health they would be willing to forgo to produce a more equal distribution of health across a given characteristic. Williams and Cookson demonstrated such a valuation task that could be used to generate weights to express the benefits of reducing inequalities in health terms (2006). Once values are established, reductions in inequality can be expressed in terms of the equivalent improvement in health, allowing the benefits from all interventions to be expressed on the same scale.

Cross-sector comparisons

In the context of public health, a narrow health care sector perspective would not be fully able to reflect the resource implications of interventions that drew on resources from multiple sectors of the economy. The perspective should, at the minimum, be widened to include the whole public sector. A wider perspective is taken by the National Institute for Health and Clinical Excellence for its public health evaluation activities. The outcomes that could be generated with an alternative use of resources taken from educational, criminal, and transport applications might not be measurable solely in terms of health. This leads us to consider how to reflect the opportunity cost of those resources.

A classical welfarist approach for CBA would value all outcomes in terms of the benefit individuals derive from consumption, placing the outcomes on a monetary scale that could be compared directly with costs across all sectors. Where markets do not exist to provide direct values, this approach requires the use of alternative measures to derive a monetary value for outcomes. Thus, an intervention that affected educational outcomes might be valued directly according to the earning potential associated with those education outcomes in addition to any improvement in public health, whereas for an intervention that affected reoffending rates, an indirect valuation may need to be acquired using a willingness to pay exercise. Given that a CBA approach is generally not used for the evaluation of health care technologies, there may be issues about its suitability for the evaluation of public health interventions. It might be that outcomes in other sectors are considered desirable in addition to the well-being derived from consumption, similar to health, or that the implicit value judgements inherent to the CBA approach are not accepted.

Claxton et al (2007) proposed a means for assessing interventions with multi-sectoral impacts by comparing a series of sector-specific CEAs. Assuming each sector's budget is determined exogenously, the evaluation requires only that each sector has an index measure of outcome. The existence of suitable measures, such as the QALY in the healthcare sector, may depend on whether cost-effectiveness analysis is routinely applied to inform resource allocation decisions within each sector. A public health intervention with impacts across multiple sectors is then assessed on the basis of each sector-specific measure of net benefit. The net benefit within each sector is calculated using the sector specific outcome measure and the costs that fall on that sector's budget constraint. If the intervention is found to have a positive net benefit in all sectors, then it should be reimbursed. However, if the intervention is found to have a positive net benefit in some sectors, but a negative net benefit in others, then it should only be recommended if the sectors in which the intervention is cost-effective could compensate the other sectors such that funding the intervention could provide a positive net benefit (or at least neutrality in net benefit) in every sector. Thus, a compensation test can be defined to establish whether a public health intervention with multi-sectoral impacts represents a potential cost-effective use of resources. An illustration of this decision rule is provided in Box 8.2.

Box 8.2 Evaluating public health interventions with multi-sectoral impacts

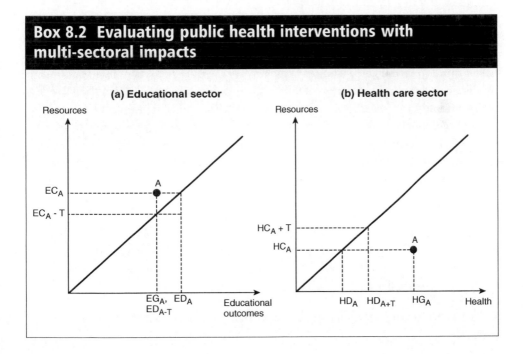

Evaluating public health interventions with multi-sectoral impacts (*continued*)

The slope of the diagonal lines represent the amount of educational outcomes (panel a) or health (panel b) that can be generated per unit of resources used to provide existing programmes. A new public health intervention is evaluated to determine whether it should be provided within the public sector. Intervention A might represent a vaccination programme that is delivered by nurses, aided by teaching staff, in a school setting.

The amount of health care resources required to deliver intervention A is equivalent to HC_A and its provision would result in a gain in health equivalent to HG_A. Reducing provision of existing services to provide A would displace amount of health HD_A, resulting in an overall gain in health as $HG_A - HD_A > 0$.

The amount of educational resources required to deliver intervention A is equivalent to EC_A and its provision would result in a gain in educational outcomes equivalent to EG_A (for example by reducing schooling days lost to illness). Reducing provision of existing services to provide A would displace amount of health ED_A, resulting in an overall loss in educational outcomes as $EG_A - ED_A < 0$.

However, if the health care sector is able to compensate the educational sector by amount T, the amount of educational outcomes displaced by provision of A falls to ED_{A-T}, and intervention A is now cost-effective in the educational sector. The amount of health displaced in the health care sector rises to HD_{A+T}, but intervention A remains cost-effective as $HG_A - HD_{A+T} > 0$.

Methods

In evaluating the cost-effectiveness of medical technologies, randomized controlled trials have proved to be the gold standard in identifying the causal effects of interventions. In public health research, experimental data from randomized controlled trials are less prevalent and the researcher is more often faced with identifying causal relationships from observational or non-experimental sources of data where the assignment of individuals to treatment or control groups is beyond the control of the researcher. This may create substantial challenges to the analyst wanting to estimate the impact of an intervention. Additionally, any cost-effectiveness analysis should incorporate the full range of existing evidence to support the use of the intervention in order that the remaining decision uncertainty be fully characterized. It is therefore advantageous to perform systematic reviews to identify and collate the body of supporting evidence, which will often include more than a single study. Where multiple sources of data are available, these must be synthesized to describe the combined weight of the evidence, using appropriate statistical methods. These challenges are discussed briefly below.

Establishing the effectiveness of public health interventions

For public health research we might be interested in the evaluation of a particular intervention, but we might also be interested in the evaluation of a broader programme, such as a ban on smoking in public places. In the context of a randomized controlled trial, the average treatment effect can be estimated by a simple comparison of the mean of costs and effects in the treatment and control groups. This is justified on the basis that randomization guarantees no systematic differences in the baseline characteristics of individuals within the treated and control groups. However, in the context of non-randomized experimental data, treatment assignment is not randomly allocated and accordingly a simple comparison of the mean costs and outcomes in a treated and control group is likely to yield biased estimates of the underlying treatment effect due to confounding between treatment assignment and characteristics of individuals. This is due to selection bias whereby certain patient characteristics are important in determining both whether a patient would receive an intervention and their post-intervention health gains. An unadjusted comparison of treated and non-treated patients would erroneously attribute some difference in health outcomes caused by disparities in patient characteristics to the intervention under assessment. Instead, it is necessary to conduct analyses that adjust for the effects of selection. Such analyses are common in the field of econometrics, where there exist a range of methods to extract unbiased estimates of the treatment effect from non-randomized data. These include the use of regression analysis, methods of matching and propensity scores, difference-in-differences estimation and instrumental variables (Angrist and Krueger 1999; Meyer 1995). A simplified taxonomy of the methods is provided in Box 8.3. All these methods have potential application in the evaluation of public health interventions where reliance on non-experimental sources of information is likely to be a prominent consideration.

Where selection into treatment (intervention) assignment is thought to be determined by characteristics of individuals observed by the analyst, then regression analysis and the methods of matching, including propensity scores, can be used to recover unbiased estimates of the impact of an intervention. In a regression framework, it might be sufficient to simply condition on the set of confounding characteristics when estimating the relationship between the intervention and outcomes of interest. Assuming the specification of the model conforms to the underlying data-generating process this will lead to an unbiased estimate of the treatment effect. An alternative method that does not rely on the parametric assumptions underpinning the regression approach is the method of matching. The idea of matching is to use outcome data from a set of chosen comparison individuals for whom observed pre-treatment characteristics match those of treated individuals up to some chosen degree of proximity. Where suitably matched individuals can be identified, then the average outcome across these individuals provides the counterfactual for the average outcome for treated individuals. A key assumption of the approach is that, conditional on the set of observed matched characteristics, selection into treatment is independent of the outcome of interest. A number of methods have been proposed for defining a suitably matched group of individuals and a leading method is propensity score matching (Rosenbaum and Rubin 1983). This approach is based on estimating an individual's propensity to receive treatment. Once obtained, matching is based on finding suitable individuals from within the control group to match to treated individuals based on proximity of propensity scores. For all methods of matching it is assumed that there is common support, or overlap, in the distributions of propensity scores across treated and control groups. Enhancements to the method include matching with replacement and multiple matching. Matching with replacement allows an individual within the control group to be matched to more than one individual in the treatment group. Multiple matching allows multiple individuals from within the control group to be matched to a single individual in the treatment group. The contribution of matched individuals to each treated individual is weighted in accordance to the proximity of their respective propensity scores. These extensions are often chosen to enhance the closeness of matched control individuals to treated individuals and to increase the amount of information used in the matching estimator. The closer the respective propensity scores, the closer the matches and the less bias in the matching estimator of the treatment effect.

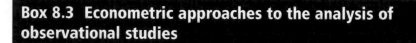

Box 8.3 Econometric approaches to the analysis of observational studies

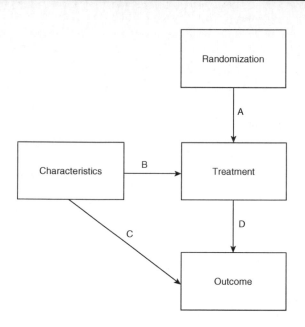

The goal of evaluative research is to identify the effect of treatment on outcomes, D. Randomization ensures that patient characteristics do not influence the likelihood of receiving treatment; every patient has an equal chance of receiving treatment, and consequently the treated and untreated groups should have equal characteristics. A comparison of the outcomes in the treated and untreated groups allows us to estimate D.

$$H_{treated} - H_{untreated} = D$$

In non-randomized studies, patient characteristics influence the likelihood of receiving treatment, through mechanism B. Patients have differing chances of receiving

---

Econometric approaches to the analysis of observational studies *(continued)*

treatments, and consequently treated and untreated groups have unequal characteristics. A comparison of the outcomes in the treated and untreated groups provides an estimate of the combined impact of treatment and patient characteristics on outcomes, D + C.

$$H_{treated} - H_{untreated} = D + C$$

Regression analysis seeks to explain the outcome as a function of observed characteristics, X, and treatment, T, allowing D and C to be identified independently.

$$H = \alpha + D.T + C.X + \varepsilon$$

Matching methods seek to identify treated and untreated groups that have equal characteristics, either by directly identifying groups of patients with equal characteristics $X_{treated} = X_{untreated}$, or by identifying groups with equal likelihood of receiving treatment $B_{treated} = B_{untreated}$.

$$H_{treated} - H_{untreated} = D + C.X_{treated} - C.X_{untreated} = D$$

Where unobserved characteristics, Y, influence the likelihood of receiving treatment, regression methods and matching methods can identify only D + C.($Y_{treated} - Y_{untreated}$). Instrumental variable methods seek to identify a patient characteristic, Z, that acts in the same way as randomization (ie through mechanism A): influencing the likelihood of receiving treatment but having no influence on outcomes. Utilizing independent information in the instrument to determine treatment assignment, the method seeks to infer the underlying treatment effect, D.

Where selection into treatment is based on unobservable, rather than observable, characteristics of individuals the method of instrumental variables (IV) can be used to identify the impact of an intervention (see Grootendorst 2007). The approach consists of locating a set of variables, the instruments, with the properties of being predictive of treatment assignment (instrument relevance) but not correlated with the error term in the outcome regression of interest (instrument validity). Provided these conditions hold and that the instruments are not 'weak' (by ensuring the instruments strongly predict treatment assignment), then the method of instrumental variables can be used to derive a consistent estimate of the treatment effect. The intuition behind the approach is that the instruments provide an exogenous source of variation about treatment assignment, independent of the outcome, that can be used to identify the relationship between the intervention and outcomes. A number of statistics exist to test the underlying assumptions (relevance, validity and non-weak instruments) behind the implementation of instrumental variables. In practice, the choice of instruments should be guided both by a theoretical rationale as to why they can be considered relevant and valid and also by the rigorous application of relevant test statistics. While the method of instrumental variables produces bias in finite samples, the degree of bias can be substantially smaller than that obtained by simple regression techniques, such as ordinary least squares, which fails to account for selection effects due to unobservable characteristics. Test statistics exist to allow the analyst to assess the degree of instrumental variable bias relative to ordinary least squares regression bias.

Where information is available across multiple time periods a commonly used method for evaluating the average treatment effect of a policy intervention is the difference-in-differences approach. The method requires data in both a pre-intervention and post-intervention period on a set of treated and non-treated individuals, and is illustrated in Figure 8.2. In its basic form the method simply compares the mean difference in outcomes before and after treatment for the group of treated individuals to the mean difference for non-treated individuals. A comparison of these differences across the treated and control groups provides an estimate of the impact of the intervention. The validity of the method relies on the assumption that the time trend in the absence of treatment is the same across treated and non-treated groups. A failure of this assumption will confound the estimated treatment effect with a natural time trend producing a biased estimate. A strength of the method is that by comparing outcomes pre- and post-intervention, individuals act as their own controls. The difference-in-differences approach can be formulated within a regression framework and extended to control for time-varying characteristics correlated with outcomes and treatment assignment that would otherwise potentially confound the effect of the intervention. The closer the control and treatment groups in terms of baseline characteristics, the greater the credibility of the difference-in-differences approach. To enhance comparability, the approach can be combined with the method of matching so that control individuals are matched to individuals experiencing the intervention on the basis of pre-treatment characteristics prior to implementing difference-in-differences.

Identifying evidence

The search criteria for systematic reviews of the efficacy of clinical interventions typically include only randomized controlled trials. These can be widened to identify other forms of experimental evidence, such as that obtained from observational studies. As the range of studies expands, the specificity of the search will decline, which may have implications for the time required to conduct the review. The body of evidence relevant to a particular public health intervention may include previously conducted econometric analyses. However, the methods for systematic review are less well developed for identifying these types of econometric analyses and for extracting the relevant data from those identified studies (Ogilvie et al 2008).

Establishing the weight of evidence

In the presence of a homogenous set of trials of similar design, reporting similar outcome measures, a standard meta-analysis is often applied (see for example Whitehead 2002; Egger et al 2003). A well-conducted meta-analysis allows a more systematic and objective appraisal of study results than can be achieved through the more traditional narrative synthesis. By specifying characteristics of individual studies as a set of explanatory variables, and the outcome of interest as the dependent variable, a meta-regression allows the

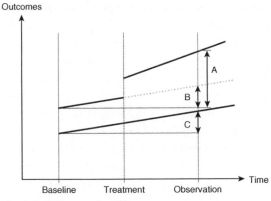

The lower solid line represents the trajectory of outcomes over time for the group of non-treated individuals and the upper solid line the trajectory for treated individuals.

For non-treated individuals a pre- and post-treatment comparison reveals a mean difference of C.

Similarly, the mean difference for treated individuals is given by the distance A. However, this difference ignores the increase in outcomes that would have occurred in the absence of treatment, B. The true impact of the intervention is simply A – B, which is equal to the difference in differences (A – C).

Fig. 8.2 Difference in differences

statistical exploration of the quantitative relevance of differences in study designs on outcomes. The resulting information may help in defining the impact of interventions, but will also help to reveal heterogeneity between studies and inform areas where further research might be usefully undertaken to further explore observed relationships. In this way, a meta-analysis is often thought of as an analysis of analyses. When pooling evidence across independent studies thought to be sufficiently homogenous to be combinable, in general, greater weight should be placed on evidence derived from larger studies where there is greater confidence in the estimated intervention effect. Statistical approaches to combining evidence and weighting according to some indication of the precision of study evidence is often achieved through the use of fixed or random effects meta-regressions. The methods differ in the way they deal with study variation. This is either assumed to be due solely to random variation such that there exists a single population effect (fixed effects) or that each study estimates a different underlying effect and that variability exists both within and across studies (random effects). Careful consideration needs to be given to the selection of studies to contribute to a meta-analysis. Where evidence is thought to be unreliable, due perhaps to poor study design, then either this should be omitted from the analysis or the analysis weighted to reflect study quality. This is likely to be most relevant to analyses of evidence from non-experimental study designs where the quality of sources of data is likely to vary between studies. Recent methods for generalized evidence synthesis, using Bayesian techniques, have been developed to allow the inclusion of non-randomized studies and the synthesis of evidence from a more heterogeneous group of studies than those found in more traditional meta-analysis based on experimental designs.

Summary

Economic evaluation may have a role to play in informing decisions to allocate resources to fund interventions aimed at improving public health. The basic economic principle of establishing the opportunity cost of devoting resources to a particular intervention, ie whether the benefits of devoting resources to a particular intervention exceed the benefits that could have been achieved with an alternative use of those resources, can be used to ensure that public funds are directed to the most valuable interventions. The extra welfarist normative framework that is characteristic of economic evaluations that assess medical interventions should be extended to take account of any additional objectives of public health interventions beyond simple health maximization, and to reflect the impact of those interventions across multiple sectors and budget constraints.

Equity considerations may be one of the key additional considerations when evaluating public health interventions. That is, public health interventions may seek to improve the distribution of health between patients defined by characteristics such as wealth by making the distribution more equal. Methodological work to estimate health inequalities can be used to incorporate equity considerations in a quantitative manner, for example with the use of concentration indices which quantify the level of inequality. The benefits of reducing inequality can be assessed by performing valuation exercises with the general public, or by examining previous decisions that have allocated resources to interventions that would have appeared cost-ineffective without consideration of equity issues. By valuing improvements in equity on the same scale as improvements in overall health, the trade-off between the two objectives can be established. The process of defining health equity and identifying which health inequalities to target is not straightforward, and here the transparent and formal nature of economic evaluation is of benefit. By making explicit the assumptions underlying the analysis, the process is auditable, reproducible, and open to challenge. In contrast, an informal analysis of equity considerations may not make explicit the trade-off between overall health and other objectives, and could result in a series of decisions that each imply different values for those trade-offs.

The process of examining the impact of a health care intervention within the health care sector can be extended to consider the impact of a public health intervention within each relevant public sector. In this manner, a series of sector-specific cost-effectiveness analyses is performed. Compensation tests can be introduced where public health interventions appear cost-effective in only a subset of the relevant sectors, to establish whether those sectors that benefit can offset excess opportunity costs in other sectors. The issue of whether compensation is actually paid, or whether budgets are adjusted over time to account for this compensation, would still need to be established. However, the evaluation of the level of any compensation required represents a more formal approach than a simple cost-consequences analysis which would present the impacts across multiple sectors and rely on informal analysis by decision makers to weigh up the overall benefits. Again, the transparency of the formal approach makes the trade-offs explicit and makes them open to challenge.

The evidence base to support the use of public health interventions may be more likely to include non-randomized trials than is the case for medical interventions. Thus the methods for systematic review, analysis, and evidence synthesis should be able to incorporate these alternative sources of efficacy data. A range of econometric methods of analysis have been developed to try and identify an unbiased estimate of the treatment effect from observational datasets. Methods for assessing the quality of studies included in systematic reviews can be used to indicate the level of bias that may exist relative to a well-conducted randomized trial. Bayesian methods for evidence synthesis can be used to incorporate these quality assessments in meta-analysis by down-weighting evidence from studies considered to be of poorer quality. All of these methods have application in the economic evaluation of medical technologies, but may become more prevalent in the move to consider public health interventions. Establishing a methodological framework for the economic evaluation of public health interventions appears feasible, and once established this framework could equally be applied to medical interventions, allowing both to be assessed on the same basis.

Acknowledgements

Nigel Rice gratefully acknowledges funding from the Economic and Social Research Council (ESRC) under grant reference RES-060-25-0045. The Centre for Health Economics also receives support from the Medical Research Council for a programme of work on the methods of economic evaluation.

Bibliography

Angrist, JD and Krueger, A (1999) 'Empirical strategies in labor economics' in: O Ashenfelter and D Card (eds), *Handbook of Labor Economics*. Amsterdam: Elsevier

Brouwer, WBF and Koopmanschap, MA (2000) 'On the economic foundations of CEA. Ladies and gentlemen, take your positions!' *Journal of Health Economics* 19: 439–59

Claxton, K, Sculpher, MJ, and Culyer, AJ (2007) 'Mark versus Luke? Appropriate methods for the evaluation of public health interventions'. York: Centre for Health Economics

Culyer, AJ (1991) 'The normative economics of health care finance and provision' In: A McGuire, P Fenn, and K Mayhew (eds), *Providing health care: the economics of alternative systems of finance and provision*, pp 65–98. Oxford: Oxford University Press

Dolan, P, Edlin, R, and Tsuchiya, A (2008) *The relative societal value of health gains to different beneficiaries*. Discussion Paper. Sheffield: Health Economics Group, University of Sheffield

Egger, M, Smith, D, and Altman, DG (2003) *Systematic reviews in health care. Meta-analysis in context*. London: BMJ

Epstein, DM, Chalabi, Z, Claxton, K, and Sculpher, M (2007) 'Efficiency, equity and budgetary policies: informing decisions using mathematical programming' *Medical Decision Making* 27: 128–37

Grootendorst, P (2007) *A review of instrumental variables estimation of treatment effects in the applied health sciences. Social and economic dimensions of an aging population*. Canada: McMaster University

Meyer, B (1995) 'Natural and quasi-experiments in economics' *Journal of Business and Economic Statistics* 12: 151–61

National Institute for Health and Clinical Excellence (NICE) (2008) *Guide to the methods of technology appraisal*. London: NICE

O'Donnell, O, van Doorslaer, E, Wagstaff, A, and Lindelow, M (2008) *Analyzing health equity using household survey data. A guide to techniques and their implementation*. Washington DC: World Bank Institute

Ogilvie, D, Fayter, D, Petticrew, M, Sowden, A, Thomas, S, Whitehead, M, et al (2008) 'The harvest plot: a method for synthesising evidence about the differential effects of interventions' *Medical Research Methodology* 8/8:1–7

Rosenbaum, P and Rubin, DB (1983) 'The central role of propensity score in observational studies for causal effects'. *Biometrika* 70: 41–55

Sen, A (2002) 'Why health equity?' *Health Economics* 11: 659–66

Sugden, R and Williams, A (1978) *The principles of practical cost–benefit analysis*. Oxford: Oxford University Press

Wanless, D (2004) *Securing good health for the whole population*. Norwich: HMSO

Whitehead, A (2002) *Meta-analysis of controlled clinical trials. Statistics in practice*. Chicester: John Wiley & Sons

Williams, AH and Cookson, RA (2006) 'Equity-efficiency trade-offs in health technology assessment' *International Journal of Technology Assessment in Health Care* 22/1: 1–9

Chapter 9

Equity and efficiency in public health: the contribution of health economics

Stephen Morris, David Parkin, and Nancy Devlin

Introduction

Health economics has been defined as 'the application of economic theory, models and empirical techniques to the analysis of decision making by individuals, health care providers and governments with respect to health and health care' (Morris et al 2007). It is a branch of economics, but it is not just the application of standard economic theory to health and health care. It has been developed specifically to understand the behaviour both of people, as members of the population, as patients, and as health professionals, and of institutions, such as hospitals and insurance companies, and to facilitate resource allocation decisions in health care. Health economics has evolved into a highly specialized field, drawing on related disciplines including epidemiology, statistics, psychology, sociology, operations research, and mathematics.

In this chapter we investigate the notions of efficiency and equity, which are commonly used in health economics to judge the appropriate use of health care resources, and which are arguably the main contribution of health economics to decision making in health care. We apply these to the provision of public health programmes and investigate the role that NICE plays in this.

Health care as an economic good

Economics studies the behaviour of economic agents—individuals, firms, governments, and other organizations—when confronted with *scarcity of resources*. This arises from the fact that resources, such as labour, capital, and raw materials, are limited while the potential uses of those resources are unbounded. Choices must therefore be made about the production and consumption of *economic goods*, which are defined as goods or services that are scarce relative to our wants for them.

Health care is an economic good, because the resources used to provide it are finite: more of these resources can be devoted to the production and consumption of health care only by diverting them from some other use. By contrast, our *wants* for health care— what we would choose to consume in the absence of constraints on our ability to pay for it as a society or as a consumer—have no known bounds. No health care system, anywhere in the world, has achieved levels of spending sufficient to meet all its citizens' wants for health care.

Choices must therefore be made about how much health care of different kinds to produce, how to produce it, who is to pay for it, and how it is to be distributed amongst the population. Answering these economic questions is unavoidable at two levels. First, the more health care we choose, the more that some other desirable goods and services must be given up. For example, in a predominantly publicly funded health care system, if more money is spent on health care then less is available to be spent on other parts of the public sector, such as education, housing, and national defence. Second, within a health care system with a fixed budget, the more of one type of health care we choose, for example public health interventions, the more of another type of health care must be sacrificed, for example secondary care. Because health care is important to our welfare as human beings, these choices are difficult and contentious ones to make.

The choices that arise because health care is an economic good, and the inevitable trade-offs encountered in making these choices, are captured in an idea that is fundamental in economics: *opportunity cost*. The opportunity cost of committing resources to produce a good or service is the benefits that are foregone by not devoting those same resources to their next best alternative use. Each action taken by patients, by health care providers, or by governments with respect to the use of health care involves the sacrifice of the benefits that would have been enjoyed by other, alternative uses of the resources used to provide that care. This applies as much to public health interventions as to other types of health care. For example, running a health promotion campaign may mean that some other health-promoting activities will not be carried out; but equally a decision to concentrate on curative secondary care will limit the resources available to undertake primary prevention.

When economists refer to cost, we really mean opportunity cost, which is not the same as financial cost, although we may measure opportunity costs in monetary terms. Weighing up the costs and benefits of a decision to provide public health programmes involves assessing the benefits to society from such programmes compared to the benefits that would have been possible using those same resources elsewhere in the health care system. Box 9.1 illustrates the concept of opportunity cost in relation to a 2007

Box 9.1 The opportunity cost of one-to-one interventions to reduce teenage pregnancies

In February 2007 NICE issued guidance on strategies to reduce sexually transmitted infections and teenage conceptions in the UK (NICE 2007). Among other things, the guidance promotes universal provision of one-to-one counselling where appropriate for the prevention of teenage conceptions, recommending that this should be part of the routine care offered in primary care and by contraceptive services.

The NHS would pay around £44 per person to provide practice nurse-led counselling on a one-to-one basis. Counselling was projected to reduce the conception rate by around 2%. Does this represent good value for money? Answering this question

The opportunity cost of one-to-one interventions to reduce teenage pregnancies *(continued)*

requires us explicitly to weigh up this benefit against the opportunity cost. The resources devoted to each person for one-to-one counselling could instead be used to provide:

In the health care sector:

Two and a half years'
supply of statins

One two-hundredth of a
heart bypass operation

One five-hundredth of
a nurse for a year

One and a half vaccinations for
Measles, Mumps, and Rubella

Elsewhere in the public sector:

One hundred-thousandth
of a Challenger 2 military tank

One five-hundredth of a
teacher for a year

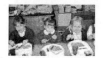

24 school dinners

From a limited budget, the most efficient mix of services to fund will be that which generates the greatest aggregate benefit. But efficiency is not the only criterion: equity is also an important consideration in many health care systems.

Data sources:
Statins: <http://www.bnf.org>
Heart bypass: <http://www.dh.gov.uk/en/index.htm>. Schedule of Reference Costs 2006–07—NHS Trusts and PCTs Combined.
Nurse: <http://www.nhscareers.nhs.uk/details/Default.aspx?Id=766>
Vaccination for MMR: <http://www.dh.gov.uk/en/index.htm>. Schedule of Reference Costs 2006–07—NHS Trusts and PCTs Combined.
Challenger 2 tank: <http://www.armedforces.co.uk/army/listings/l0023.html>
Teacher: <http://www.tda.gov.uk/Recruit/lifeasateacher/payandbenefits.aspx>
School dinner: <http://www.express.co.uk/posts/view/42794/Cost-of-a-school-dinner-hits-2-as-food-prices-soar>

recommendation by NICE that the NHS should promote provision of one to one counselling for the prevention of teenage conceptions (NICE 2007).

Efficiency and equity in health care

In economics, it is conventional to judge the use of resources using the criteria of efficiency and equity. A general definition of efficiency is the allocation of scarce resources that maximizes the achievement of aims (Knapp 1984). The economic problem described above is that there are scarce resources and potentially unbounded uses for them. If our aim is to obtain the 'best' set of uses, defined in whatever way we like, then efficiency is simply the use of resources that maximizes our achievement of that aim. For example, if we want to maximize the health of the population, an efficient allocation of resources is one that produces the greatest health benefit given the budget and resources available. Inefficiency exists if greater health benefit could be gained from the available resources by reallocating them between different uses.

Efficiency is concerned with the relation between resource inputs, sometimes called factors of production, and outputs. In health care, we can think of output in two different ways; as services produced, such as the number of interventions, or as health outcomes measured, for example in terms of gains in quality adjusted life expectancy. Three types of efficiency are commonly used in economics. *Technical* efficiency and *economic* efficiency refer to relationships between resource inputs and outputs. A technically efficient allocation of resources occurs when the maximum output is obtained from a particular combination and quantity of resource inputs. An intervention is technically inefficient if the same or greater output could be produced with less of one type of input. Economic efficiency, which is also known as cost-effectiveness, is similar but refers not to the quantity of resource inputs but their cost. Interventions are inefficiently produced if the same or greater output could be achieved at lower cost. Using the example above of one to one counselling to reduce teenage conceptions, it was found that practice nurse counselling was as effective as GP counselling. Since practice nurse consultations are less costly they are more economically efficient.

In health care, the ideas of technical and economic efficiency are useful when comparing interventions for treating the same condition that have directly comparable outcomes. For example, in the delivery of a population screening programme, the interest may be in issues to do with the correct mix of staff and of facilities. However, these ideas cannot be used to address the impact of reallocating resources at a broader level, for example from secondary care to public health. To do this we use the notion of *allocative* efficiency.

Allocative efficiency, sometimes referred to as Pareto efficiency, accounts not only for the efficiency with which health care resources are used to produce health outcomes, but also the efficiency with which these outcomes are distributed among the population. An allocatively efficient allocation of resources is one such that any alternative allocation would make at least one person worse off. In practice, strict adherence to this criterion is unlikely to be feasible. It would mean, for example, that we would regard as inefficient any health care intervention that resulted in many people becoming much healthier, at the cost of a few relatively rich people having their incomes slightly reduced. Consequently, a common adaptation of the theoretical definition of allocative efficiency is that it is achieved when resources are allocated so as to maximize the health of society. (Drummond 1991; Palmer and Torgerson 1999). The question that is addressed therefore concerns obtaining the best mix of health care programmes: what broad balance of resources across preventive and curative strategies and between specific treatments and interventions within each of these strategies maximizes improvements in health?

Many economic issues in health care are about the efficiency with which scarce resources are used, but an equally important criterion for judging the use of health care resources is *equity*, which is a synonym of fairness. In this context, it means fairness in the distribution of health and health care between people. Equity is also relevant when judging who pays for health care and how they do so, but this issue is beyond the scope of this chapter.

Equity is not a synonym of equality, but it is usually analysed with respect to equality. For example, equity might be defined according to whether or not people who have equal needs for health care have equal access to or equal use of it. Whether a particular distribution of health care can be judged to be fair depends on views about what constitutes fairness, for example equal health outcomes for equal need, or equal access to health care services for equal need. There is far less agreement within economics about what equity means than about efficiency and other disciplines, such as philosophy and law, have views about what constitutes fairness as well. Nonetheless, equity is always an important consideration in economics, and one of the special characteristics of health and health care is that people attach more importance to equity in them than in many other goods and services.

Is there a trade-off between efficiency and equity?

Since we have two criteria, how do we judge the allocation of resources where these are in conflict? What if we have an efficient use of resources that is inequitable or an equitable use of resources that is inefficient? What if there is a trade-off between the two, so that more of one can only be obtained if we have less of the other?

To address this question we first need a working definition of equity. Since 1977 financial resources have been allocated to NHS organizations in England using a funding formula. The initial objective of the formula was '[t]o secure, through resource allocation, that there would eventually be equal opportunity of access to health care for people at equal risk' (Department of Health and Social Security 1976). In 1998 this was revised to be 'to contribute to the reduction in avoidable health inequalities'. Using the latter as our notion of equity, the question of whether or not there is a trade-off between efficiency and equity can be restated to ask whether or not there is a trade-off between cost-effectiveness and reducing health inequality.

The answer to this question in the context of public health interventions depends on whether interventions are designed to affect the whole population or are targeted to specific population groups, and whether they require access to health care services or are community-based. Some cost-effective public health interventions tend to increase socio-economic inequalities in health. One reason for this is that they are designed to achieve overall reductions in risk factors for disease across the population and are not targeted at specific population groups. For example, interventions aimed at reducing smoking, reducing cholesterol, and reducing blood pressure also typically require access to primary care, for detecting risk factors and delivering preventive care. Because there are inequalities in access to primary care (Department of Health 1998), these interventions may widen inequalities in health (Woodward and Kawachi 2000). Hence, in the case of untargeted population interventions that require direct access to health care services there is likely to be an efficiency-equity trade-off.

However, some public health interventions both reduce health inequalities and are cost-effective (Woodward and Kawachi 2000). For instance, fluoridation of the public water supply has been shown in certain studies to be cost-effective (Griffin et al 2001) and to reduce inequalities in dental health across social classes (McDonagh et al 2000). Since fluoridation of the public water supply is a community-based intervention, there is equal access to the health benefits across the socio-economic gradient, but people in lower social classes have higher levels of dental caries and are therefore likely to obtain greater health benefits. This intervention does not require people to access health services and is therefore unaffected by inequalities in access to them.

There are some public health interventions that do require direct access to health care services, but because they are targeted to specific populations groups, they may be cost-effective and also reduce health inequalities. An example is active case finding for tuberculosis among the homeless. A number of studies have demonstrated that tuberculosis is associated with deprivation and that much higher rates of tuberculosis disease are found in street homeless people and hostel dwellers than in the general population. Based on a systematic review of the literature, NICE recommended in its recent tuberculosis guideline (National Collaborating Centre for Chronic Conditions 2006) that active case finding should be carried out among street homeless people, including those using direct access hostels for the homeless, by chest X-ray screening on an opportunistic and/or symptomatic basis. NICE also recommended that in an effort to target this group, incentives for attending testing, such as hot drinks and snacks, should be used. For public health interventions of this type, improvements in both efficiency and equity are possible.

Achieving efficiency and equity in public health

Health economics is concerned with allocating scarce health care resources: *What* health care should be provided? *How* should it be provided? *Who* should receive it? We can judge the answers to these questions with reference to efficiency and equity. But how is an efficient and equitable allocation of scarce health care resources to be achieved?

One option is to allow market forces to allocate scarce resources. This is the way in which decisions are made about the provision and consumption of most economic goods, such as clothes, books, food, games machines, and music concerts. In the absence of government intervention, privately-owned firms decide how much to produce and how to produce it. Consumers decide how much to purchase and from where to purchase it, guided by their own view of what is in their best interests. Through the price system, the market decides which goods and services, and how much of these, should be produced. This is achieved by finding the price at which the wishes of the buyers and sellers coincide. Goods and services are consumed by people who are willing and able to pay the market price for them.

One of the most important results of economic theory is the First Fundamental Theorem of Welfare Economics. This proves that a market operating perfectly will generate an allocation of resources that is allocatively efficient. This idea is the basis for many economists' arguments in favour of free markets and minimal government interference. However, in most countries and for most health care services a reliance on unfettered market forces is rare. Typically, governments intervene in health care markets to a far greater extent than for most other economic goods. In health care governments commonly regulate who may provide services and what they can charge or what profits they may earn, subsidise health care either partially or fully via various types of taxes and directly provide certain types of health care. Public health interventions are one type of health care that are commonly provided directly by governments rather than in a market by private firms. Why are governments so often involved in the provision of public health interventions? What is it that makes these types of service 'different' from other economic goods? In the next section we examine this issue further.

Why are markets not widely used to provide public health programmes?

The theory that markets generate allocative efficiency relies on those markets being perfect. Any breakdown in the operation of the market will lead to allocative inefficiency. The term *market failure* is used to cover all circumstances in which allocative efficiency is not achieved by the market. Of course, in the real world no market is perfect, but that does not mean that there is a feasible alternative that would be better. It is necessary to examine in each particular case the causes of market failure and whether or not government intervention could remedy that. Failure to achieve efficiency is not the only reason why governments might intervene in markets; it may also be that there are equity considerations. The following are the main reasons that explain why public health care interventions are not more widely provided by markets.

Externalities

Externalities, or spillover effects, are the uncompensated effects of an economic activity on other members of society who are not directly involved in that activity. These effects may be positive or negative: if other members of society are affected beneficially there are external benefits; if they are affected adversely there are external costs. Externalities may arise from either the consumption or the production of goods and services. As examples, consumption of tobacco products in public places may impose external costs on others, and maintenance of water drainage systems for agricultural purposes may generate benefits by reducing water-borne diseases for those living nearby. Health care markets will in most cases ignore these externalities, and will therefore not lead to allocative efficiency. If there are external benefits, markets will lead to too little being consumed or provided; if there are external costs there will be too much.

Without government intervention, people left to their own devices will choose to consume levels of public health interventions based on the costs and benefits to themselves (private costs and benefits), which may be different from the costs and benefits to society (social costs and benefits). A good illustration of this is the external benefits that arise from the prevention of infectious diseases. Box 9.2 gives an example related to mass vaccination programmes and herd immunity.

Public goods

Public goods are goods that can only be consumed in a collective way. They are often publicly provided (ie provided by the government) but this is not their defining feature: they are defined by how they are consumed, not how they are produced. Public goods have two characteristics. The first is *non-rivalry*, which means that if one person consumes a good or service, this will not prevent others from consuming it. An example of a non-rival good is television or radio broadcasting as means of delivering public health messages.

Box 9.2 Externalities and public health programmes: herd immunity

Mass public vaccination programmes for communicable diseases can result in herd immunity because when people are vaccinated and become immune to the disease it is more difficult for it to be passed on to others. The greater the number of people who are immune to a communicable disease, the less likely it is that a susceptible person will come into contact with someone who has the disease. Herd immunity is an externality because it is a spillover effect on others—an external benefit—arising from an individual's decision to be vaccinated, which is based on their private costs and benefits.

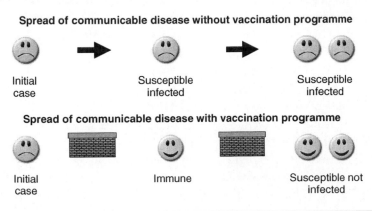

Spread of communicable disease without vaccination programme

Initial case — Susceptible infected — Susceptible infected

Spread of communicable disease with vaccination programme

Initial case — Immune — Susceptible not infected

Externalities and public health programmes: herd immunity *(continued)*

The table below shows the number of usual secondary cases from a single case for a number of communicable diseases, plus the estimated herd immunity thresholds needed to prevent transmission.

Disease	No secondary transmissions per single case	Herd immunity (%)
Diptheria	6–7	85
Measles	12–18	83–94
Mumps	4–7	75–86
Pertussis	12–17	92–94
Polio	5–7	80–86
Rubella	6–7	83–85
Smallpox	5–7	80–85

Data source:<http://www.bt.cdc.gov/agent/smallpox/training/overview/pdf/readicationhistory.pdf>

One way to view this is that if a non-rival good is provided privately, it will have large external benefits. This may make it socially very desirable, even if it was in fact privately unprofitable to provide.

The second characteristic is *non-excludability*, which means that if a good or service is provided at all, it is not possible to exclude anyone from consuming it. In other words, it is not possible to provide a good or service to one person without letting others also consume it. As a result, if a non-excludable good is provided, anyone can obtain the benefits from consuming it without paying for it. No one therefore has an incentive to pay for a non-excludable good if someone else will do so, which is known as the *free-rider* problem. If everyone free-rides, then the good or service will not be provided at all, even if what society as a whole is willing to pay for it is greater than what it costs to provide it. Television or radio broadcasting is excludable because it can be encrypted and provided on a pay-per-view basis. Unencrypted broadcasting is non-excludable.

The concepts of non-rivalry and non-excludability are not the same. The first is the idea that consumption of a good by one person does not prevent another from consuming it. The second is that it is not possible to prevent people from consuming it. Goods that have these two features are unlikely to be provided privately. So, if their benefits to society as a whole exceed their costs, then there is a case for them to be provided by the government, funded by taxation of those who potentially benefit.

Most types of health care, even those that can be classified as public health interventions, are not public goods. In fact, many are purely private goods, because they are both rival and excludable. The receipt of health care by one person will usually prevent another person from consuming that same health care. For example, although mammography screening can be provided to many people, each scan can only be used for one woman. It is also quite possible to exclude a woman from screening, even if it is unethical to do so.

However, some public health programmes are non-rival or non-excludable or both, and therefore do have some public good properties. Box 9.3 gives an example of public health measures aimed at preventing the spread of bird flu.

Information imperfections

Market failure arises in the provision of public health programmes due to information imperfections. Unless members of the population are well informed, they may take actions that are not in their best interests.

To be able to act in their own best interests in a health care market, consumers need to be aware of their health status and of all the options open to them to maintain or improve their health. Although this may be the case for some illnesses, it is not the case for the majority, and the market for health care is characterized by imperfect knowledge. For many types of public health problem there is imperfect knowledge. For example, individuals may indulge in risky health behaviours and they may not access health care services appropriately. Some public health interventions aim to educate the population about

---

Box 9.3 Public goods and public health programmes: preventing a bird flu pandemic

Like humans, birds are susceptible to flu. There are currently 15 known types of bird flu, and the type currently causing concern is strain H5N1, which can be fatal in humans. Bird flu spreads via migratory birds, who can then pass it on to domestic birds, and then on to humans. It was thought only to infect birds until the first human cases were confirmed in Hong Kong in 1997. Humans catch the disease by being in close contact with live infected birds: the birds excrete the virus in their faeces, which then dry and become pulverised, and are then inhaled.

By February 2006, the World Health Organization (WHO) confirmed 169 cases of H5N1 in humans worldwide, which have resulted in 91 deaths. If the virus mutates and gains the ability to pass between humans the experts predict there may be between two and 50 million deaths worldwide.

A variety of public health measures have been taken to try to stop the spread of bird flu. The WHO has devised a rapid-response plan to detect and contain a global flu pandemic (WHO 2005). Millions of farmyard birds have been culled, and millions more have been vaccinated and confined indoors where they are less likely to be contaminated by migratory birds. Regions where the disease has been found have been quarantined and some countries have banned imports of live birds and poultry products.

These measures have public good aspects. By imposing controls the protection provided is non-rival in the sense that if one individual is protected then so others are also protected. It is also non-excludable in that it is not possible to exclude people in a region from being protected, and individuals who did not pay for the protection privately could not be excluded from receiving it.

Box 9.4 Information imperfections and public health programmes: the MMR vaccine

The MMR vaccine provides immunization against measles, mumps, and rubella. It is commonly given to children at around one year of age; a booster dose is usually administered at three to five years of age. The MMR vaccine is widely used around the world, having been administered in over 90 countries since its introduction in the 1970s.

Controversy has arisen surrounding the safety of the MMR vaccine. In February 1998, the authors of a paper published in the journal The Lancet suggested a link between the MMR vaccine and autism (Wakefield et al 1998). As a result, the uptake of the MMR vaccine fell sharply, leading to fears of a measles epidemic.

Due to the controversy and uncertainty surrounding the safety of the MMR and the potential effect on uptake, the Department of Health and others stressed and continue to stress that extensive research in numerous studies shows no link between MMR and autism.

The Lancet paper was further discredited when it emerged there was an undisclosed conflict of interest in the submission of the original Lancet paper. Had this been known the paper would probably not have been published. The result was a partial retraction of the paper by some of its authors.

The Department of Health continues to try and reassure parents about the safety of the MMR vaccine, stating categorically that there is no link between MMR and autism. In a Department of Health press release on 12 January 2001 the Chief Medical Officer, Professor Liam Donaldson, said: 'Scare stories clearly worry parents but giving children separate vaccines unnecessarily exposes them to the risk of life-threatening infection. MMR remains the safest way to protect our children.'

the health risks associated with certain health problems and about ways to reduce the associated health risks. See Box 9.4 for an example of the MMR vaccine.

Merit and demerit goods

Merit goods are goods that from society's viewpoint are better for people than they perceive them to be. Demerit goods are worse for people than they perceive them to be. As a result, if people are free to choose how much to consume of a merit good, it will usually be consumed at a lower level than is optimal from society's viewpoint. Similarly, too much will be consumed of demerit goods. There is therefore a case for government intervention to increase consumption of merit goods and lower consumption of demerit goods.

Some public health programmes are merit goods. For example, interventions designed to reduce the number of car crash fatalities, reduce obesity, reduce smoking, reduce alcohol consumption, and reduce the consumption of illicit drugs all have merit good aspects. Other public health programmes are not merit goods, but are aimed at increasing the consumption of merit goods or decreasing the consumption of demerit goods. For example, health promotion activities are usually concerned with promoting merit goods such as the uptake of influenza jabs in the elderly, or discouraging demerit goods such as smoking.

Inequity

Market provision of public health programmes may lead to inequity, because goods and services are consumed by people who are willing and able to pay the market price for them. As a result, resources are allocated according to ability to pay, which is likely to lead to pro-rich inequality in consumption since rich people are more likely to be willing and able to purchase goods in the market place. This is usually viewed as inequitable in health care, especially if it is the poor that have greater needs for health care, as it is a widespread view that health care should be distributed not according to ability to pay but according to need. Of course, the problem that markets generate *inequalities* may apply to very many goods and services, but it seems to be a special characteristic of health care that people are more likely to view inequalities as inequitable.

Government intervention in public health

It will be obvious from the above that public health programmes are heterogeneous in terms of their economic characteristics, and that different types of public health interventions have different rationales for their public provision. Although some public health programmes produce benefits that are public goods, most do not. Most public health programmes are preventive, and while some have strong positive externalities, for example the control and prevention of infectious diseases, others do not, for example reducing obesity. Some are delivered to populations, for example water fluoridation and health education, but some are similar to other forms of health care in that they are delivered to individuals, for example prostate cancer screening.

Government interventions in the provision of public health programmes therefore take a number of forms. First, the government may be involved directly in the provision of public health programmes, making the public pay for them via taxation. Such programmes might include those targeted at specific population groups with a view to reducing health inequality, for example the identification and treatment of disease in ethic minority groups, or those with public good characteristics, for example controls to reduce the spread of swine flu.

Second, governments may introduce taxes or subsidies to bring about an allocatively efficient level of consumption of public health goods and services. Taxes are imposed on activities where the current level of provision in the market is greater than the allocatively efficient level. Subsidies are given when the current level of provision is lower than the socially efficient level. Taxes and subsidies might be used to alter the level of consumption of merit and demerit goods. For example, the government may subsidise gym membership fees in target population groups such as the elderly, or it may impose taxes on unhealthy activities such as smoking in order to curtail these activities.

Third, governments influence the allocation of resources in the health market by establishing rules and regulations. Regulation in health care can take many different forms, including price-setting, quantity-setting and quality controls. At one extreme the government may prohibit certain activities entirely due to the adverse consequences they have on health, for example the consumption of certain types of recreational drugs. At the other extreme the government might compel individuals to undertake certain activities, judging it is in their best interests to do so, for example the compulsory wearing of seatbelts in cars.

Finally, when market failure in health care arises due to imperfect knowledge then the government may help to correct the problem via the provision of information. An example is the provision of information for the general public on the effect of risky health behaviours such as smoking, lack of exercise or an unhealthy diet, or on the benefits of certain types of public health programmes, for example influenza jabs for the elderly during the winter.

The role of NICE

As discussed, one of the ways in which the government intervenes in health care is via the provision of information to reduce imperfect knowledge and therefore reduce inefficiency and inequity. The introduction of NICE, and in particular, the formation of the Centre for Public Health Excellence (CPHE) at NICE, can be seen as one way in which the British Government has attempted to reduce imperfect knowledge in public health. Although NICE is independent from government, it is a statutory public body and is financed from government funds.

NICE produces guidance in three areas; public health, health technologies, and clinical practice. The guidance on health technologies and clinical practice is primarily for health professionals and patients. The audience for public health guidance is much broader than the NHS, and includes those working in the fields of education, transport, environment, and criminal justice, in both the public and private sectors.

NICE was given its remit for producing public health guidance in April 2005. The aim of this guidance is to help achieve national targets for health improvement and reducing health inequalities. Its initial areas of guidance focused on health behaviours targets set out in the 2004 white paper 'Choosing Health: making healthy choices easier' (Department of Health 2004). In the white paper the government set out a series of principles, centred around the provision of information to improve public health.

> [P]eople told us that they want to take responsibility for their own health. They were clear that many choices they made—such as what to eat or drink, whether to smoke, whether to have sex and what contraception to use—were very personal issues. People do not want Government, or anyone else, to make these decisions for them.

> [W]hat they did expect was that the Government would support them in making these choices. They wanted clear and credible information, and where they wanted to make a change and found it hard to make a healthy choice they expected to be provided with support in doing so—whether directly or through changes in the environment around them—so that it is easier to 'do the right thing'.
>
> Choosing health sets out key principles for that support. Our starting point is informed choice. People cannot be instructed to follow a healthy lifestyle in a democratic society. Health improvement depends upon people's motivation and their willingness to act on it. The Government will provide information and practical support to get people motivated and improve emotional wellbeing and access to services so that healthy choices are easier to make. (Preface)

They acknowledge the existence of market failures in public health and a role for government in overcoming these failures:

> While we respect individuals' rights to make their own choices, we need to respond to public concern that some people's choices can cause a nuisance and have a damaging impact on other people's health. We need to strike the right balance between allowing people to decide their own actions, while not allowing those actions to unduly inconvenience or damage the health of others. (Preface)

The CPHE provides specific guidance to inform choices in the provision of public health programmes. It produces two types of guidance, though other aspects of NICE's work, for example clinical guidelines and technology appraisals, also contain public health aspects. *Public health intervention guidance* makes recommendations on specific interventions to promote healthy lifestyles and reduce the risk of ill health. The types of interventions considered in this type of guidance include giving advice, for example GPs giving advice to encourage exercise; the provision of services, for example needle exchange programmes for injecting drug users; and the provision of support, for example supporting new mothers with breastfeeding. *Public health programme guidance* deals with broader activities for promoting good health and preventing ill health. This guidance may focus on a broad topic, for example smoking; a particular population group, for example young people; or a particular setting, for example the workplace. Examples of the kinds of advice produce by CPHE are described in Box 9.5.

But how does the public health guidance produced by NICE aim to improve efficiency and equity? The CPHE publishes guidance on whether or not particular interventions should be considered worthwhile both by the NHS and by others outside the NHS such as local authorities and employers. An important component of public health guidance is whether or not the interventions are cost-effective; underpinning the guidance is the idea that resources should be allocated to maximize the health of the population subject to the resources available (Rawlins and Culyer 2004). In order to assess cost-effectiveness the CPHE has produced guidance on the methods that should be used to compute cost-effectiveness estimates, specifically designed for public health guidance (NICE 2009). This includes guidance on the critical appraisal of economic studies, and approaches to and principles for modelling cost-effectiveness. NICE uses the quality adjusted life year (QALY) as its principal measure of health outcomes in economic evaluations (NICE 2008). NICE's public health methods guidance endorses the view that QALYs are the

Box 9.5 NICE public health guidance

(As of September 2009)

Completed public health guidance:

- Behaviour change
- Brief interventions and referral for smoking cessation
- Community engagement
- Four commonly used methods to increase physical activity
- Identifying and supporting people most at risk of dying prematurely
- Interventions to reduce substance misuse among vulnerable young people
- Maternal and child nutrition
- Mental well-being and older people
- Needle and syringe programmes
- Physical activity and the environment
- Preventing the uptake of smoking by children and young people
- Prevention of sexually transmitted infections and under-18 conceptions
- Promoting young people's social and emotional well-being in secondary education
- Promoting mental well-being at work
- Promoting physical activity for children and young people
- Promoting physical activity in the workplace
- Reducing differences in the uptake of immunizations
- School-based interventions on alcohol
- Smoking cessation services
- Social and emotional well-being in primary education
- Workplace interventions to promote smoking cessation

Public health guidance in development:

- Alcohol-use disorders (prevention)
- Contraceptive services for socially disadvantaged young people
- Home-based approaches to promoting children's well-being
- Identification and weight management of overweight and obese children in primary care
- Increasing fruit and vegetable provision for deprived communities
- Looked after children
- Personal, social, and health education focusing on sex and relationships and alcohol education

NICE public health guidance *(continued)*

- Pre-school approaches to promoting children's well-being
- Preventing and reducing HIV transmission among African communities
- Preventing and reducing HIV transmission among men who have sex with men
- Preventing children's unintentional injuries outside the home
- Preventing domestic violence
- Preventing obesity: whole system approaches
- Preventing unintentional injuries among under-15s in the home
- Preventing unintentional road injuries among under-15s: road design
- Preventing unintentional road injuries among young people
- Prevention of cardiovascular disease
- Prevention of type 2 diabetes: preventing prediabetes
- Providing public information to prevent skin cancer
- Quitting smoking in pregnancy and following childbirth
- Reducing infant mortality among those living in disadvantaged circumstances
- Resources and environmental changes to prevent skin cancer
- School-based interventions to prevent smoking
- Spatial planning for health
- Strategies to prevent unintentional injuries among under-15s
- Transport policies that prioritize walking and cycling
- Using the media to promote healthy eating
- Weight management following childbirth
- Weight management for overweight and obese children: community interventions
- Weight management in pregnancy

Data source: <http://www.nice.org.uk/Guidance/Type>

preferred outcome measure, but it admits other measures if there are insufficient data to estimate QALYs; if it is important to consider other health measures to capture the multi-dimensional nature of specific public health interventions; or if there are other non-health-related measures that are important to stakeholders outside of the health sector (NICE 2009). In terms of costs, NICE recommends that economic analyses relating to public health guidance should adopt both a public sector and an NHS and personal social services perspective. This differs from the perspective used for technology appraisals and clinical guidelines, which consider only the costs to the NHS and personal social services. In public health guidance it is also permissible to present results from other perspectives where applicable, for example from an employer's perspective to demonstrate the business case for a public health intervention.

NICE also considers equity. The equity goal for public health guidance is to improve health in all population groups while at the same time reducing health inequalities between groups (NICE 2009). Hence, in its public health guidance, NICE does aim to improve efficiency and equity. We reflect on the challenges to achieving these goals in the final section.

Government failure

As noted, government intervention in the provision of public health interventions occurs because of the likelihood of market failure and the likely inequitable outcomes from market provision. However, there are potential pitfalls arising from government intervention, and it is possible that the work carried out by organizations such as NICE may not, ultimately, be desirable. For NICE's involvement in public health to be advantageous, it must improve efficiency and equity; involvement may not be desirable if it fails to achieve these goals. If the problems created by intervention are greater than the problems overcome by it, then there may be *government* failure, which would provide a case for reduced involvement.

Government failure with respect to NICE's intervention in public health might arise for a number of reasons. These centre on whether or not NICE's views as to what constitutes allocative efficiency and equity are wrong, because they do not reflect society's view. One way in which this might occur derives from the way that NICE measures benefits. The preference for QALYs may be problematic for public health interventions if they do not capture outcomes appropriately, for example because there are health benefits not captured appropriately by QALYs, or there are non-health benefits. This is acknowledged by NICE and other outcome measures are admitted, for example life years gained, cases averted, and some other disease-specific outcomes. However, it is not clear whether or how these alternatives relate to allocative efficiency and equity. Is cost-effectiveness measured in terms of these outcomes suitable for measuring allocative efficiency? Are these outcome measures appropriate for assessing equity? These issues are unresolved.

Another way in which NICE's views as to what constitutes efficiency and equity may be wrong is that the cost-effectiveness threshold—the critical value that NICE uses to judge whether or not interventions represent good value for money—may be incorrect. If it is, there will be an inefficient use of resources. In terms of its current threshold, NICE's view is that interventions with an incremental cost-effectiveness ratio of less than £20,000 per QALY are cost-effective, and that there should be stronger reasons for accepting as cost-effective any interventions with an incremental cost-effectiveness ratio of more than £30,000 per QALY (NICE 2008). In the context of public health guidance, there are a number of ways in the threshold may be incorrect. First, the £20,000–£30,000 threshold may not just be incorrect for public health interventions but for technology appraisals and clinical guidelines as well. It has been argued that 'the uncomfortable truth is that NICE's threshold has no basis in either theory or evidence' (Appleby et al 2007).

The cost-effectiveness threshold emerged as a key factor in the House of Commons Health Select Committee recent inquiry into the role of NICE. The Committee received evidence from manufacturers and patient groups that the threshold is too low and from academic researchers that it is too high, crowding out other cost-effective interventions (House of Commons Health Select Committee 2008). Secondly, while it is accepted that for public health interventions it may be important to consider outcome measures other than QALYs to capture adequately the multidimensional nature of public health interventions, the cost-effectiveness thresholds for these alternative measures in the NHS is unknown. Thirdly, public health interventions that impose costs and benefits that fall outside the NHS, for example interventions to improve mental well-being in schools, are also problematic, because cost-effectiveness thresholds do not exist outside the health sector, making it difficult to judge whether or not these interventions represent good value for money. NICE acknowledges that cost-effectiveness thresholds are not available universally (NICE 2009), but it is unclear how this problem is dealt with in the production of public health guidance.

There may also be a lack of comprehensive cost-effectiveness data with which to judge allocative efficiency accurately. This is because the existing health economics literature is rarely comprehensive or conclusive enough to inform fully the production of public health guidance. Additional economic analyses are usually required, but for pragmatic reasons these rarely cover all aspects of the interventions being considered (NICE 2009), and the selection of topics for economic analysis within a specific guidance is usually made on a case-by-case basis. It is unclear how the selective use of additional economic analyses affects the guidance produced, and whether or not it permits an accurate assessment of allocative efficiency.

Finally, NICE's views on equity may be incorrect. It is clear what the equity principles underlying NICE's public health guidance are: the improvement of health in all population groups and the reduction of health inequalities between groups. However, it is unclear what weight is and should be given to each of these principles when one is achieved at the expense of the other, for example in the case of population-based versus targeted interventions discussed above. Whichever of these principles is preferred—which is considered on a case-by-case basis (NICE 2009)—does this reflect society's view?

So, we conclude this chapter on a note of caution. One of the aims of health economics is to improve efficiency and equity in health care. Involvement by organizations such as NICE in the provision of public health should be perceived as a good thing because the aim is to reduce the inefficiencies and inequities of the health care market. But in order to ensure that NICE does not do more harm than good, it is important that the social value judgements concerning efficiency and equity underpinning the guidance that NICE makes are scrutinized and explicitly discussed and accepted, and it is also important to ensure that the processes NICE uses to produce its guidance achieve its stated goals.

Glossary

Allocative efficiency: Also known as Pareto efficiency. A measure of efficiency that accounts not only for the efficiency with which inputs are used to produce outputs, but also the efficiency with which these outputs are distributed among the population. An allocatively efficient allocation of resources is one such that any alternative allocation would make at least one person worse off.

Demerit good: A good that from society's viewpoint is worse for people than they themselves perceive it to be.

Economic efficiency: Also known as cost-effectiveness. An allocation of resources is economically efficient when the maximum output is obtained from a given input cost.

Economic goods: Goods or services that are scarce relative to our wants for them.

Equity: A synonym of fairness commonly used to assess the finance and the distribution of health care.

Externalities: Spillover effects. The uncompensated effects of an economic activity on other members of society who are not directly involved in that activity.

First Fundamental Theorem of Welfare Economics: A theorem proving that a market operating perfectly will generate an allocation of resources that is allocatively efficient.

Free-rider: A person who enjoys the benefits of a good without paying for them. A common problem for non-excludable goods.

Government failure: A situation in which government intervention causes a more inefficient allocation of goods and services than would occur without government intervention.

Market failure: A condition in which the allocation of goods and services produced by the market is not allocatively efficient.

Market forces: The interaction of supply and demand in the market that causes prices to rise and fall.

Merit good: A good that from society's viewpoint is better for people than they themselves perceive it to be.

Non-excludable good: A good that once provided is not possible to exclude anyone from consuming.

Non-rival good: A good that if one person consumes, another person cannot be prevented from consuming.

Opportunity cost: the benefits foregone when choosing one option over another.

Public goods: Goods that are non-rival and non-excludable. They can only be consumed in a collective way.

Technical efficiency: A measure of the effectiveness with which inputs are used to produce outputs. An allocation of resources is technically efficient when the maximum output is obtained from a particular combination and quantity of resource inputs.

Bibliography

Appleby, J, Devlin, NJ, and Parkin, D (2007) 'NICE's cost effectiveness threshold' *British Medical Journal* 335: 358–9

Cairns, J (2007) 'Slow slow, quick quick slow: the health technology guidance tango' *Journal of Health Services Research and Policy* 12: 130–1

Department of Health (1998) *Independent inquiry into inequalities in health—report* (Chairman: Sir Donald Acheson). London: The Stationery Office

Department of Health (2004) *Choosing health: making healthy choices easier*. London: The Stationery Office.

Department of Health and Social Security (1976) *Sharing resources for health in England. Report of the Resource Allocation Working Party*. London: Her Majesty's Stationery Office

Dolan, P, Tsuchiya, A, and Wailoo, A (2003) 'NICE's citizen's council: what do we ask them, and how?' *Lancet* 362: 918–9

Drummond, M (1991) 'Output measurement for resource allocation decisions in health care' in A McGuire, P Fenn, and K Mayhew (ed), *Providing health care. The economics of alternative systems of finance and delivery*. Oxford: Oxford University Press

Griffin, SO, Jones, K, and Tomar, SL (2001) 'An economic evaluation of community water fluoridation' *Journal of Public Health Dentistry* 61: 78–86

House of Commons Health Select Committee (2008) HC 27-I, National Institute for Health and Clinical Excellence, First Report of Session 2007-08, Volume I

Knapp, M (1984) *The economics of social care*. London: Macmillan

Maynard, A, Bloor, K, and Freemantle, N (2004) 'Challenges for the National Institute for Clinical Excellence' *British Medical Journal* 329: 227–9

McDonagh, M, Whiting, P, Bradley, M, et al (2000) *A systematic review of public water fluoridation*. York: NHS Centre for Reviews and Dissemination, University of York

Morris, S, Devlin, NJ, and Parkin, D (2007) *Economic analysis in health care*. London: Wiley

National Collaborating Centre for Chronic Conditions (2006) *Tuberculosis: clinical diagnosis and management of tuberculosis, and measures for its prevention and control*. London: Royal College of Physicians

NICE (2007) *One to one interventions to reduce the transmission of sexually transmitted infections (STIs) including HIV, and to reduce the rate of under 18 conceptions, especially among vulnerable and at risk groups.* London: NICE

NICE (2008) *Guide to the methods of technology appraisal.* London: NICE

NICE (2009) *Methods for development of NICE public health guidance.* London: NICE

NICE Citizens Council (2003) *Report on age.* London: NICE

Palmer, S and Torgerson, DJ (1999) 'Economic notes: definitions of efficiency' *British Medical Journal* 318: 1136

Rawlins, M and Culyer, AJ (2004) 'National Institute for Clinical Excellence and its value judgements' *British Medical Journal* 329: 224–7

Woodward, A and Kawachi, I (2000) 'Why reduce health inequalities?' *Journal of Epidemiology and Community Health* 54: 923–9

Chapter 10

Measuring overall population health: the use and abuse of QALYs

Richard Cookson and Anthony Culyer

Introduction

Evidence-based public health obviously needs to measure population health. To do so, it can draw on a battery of epidemiological, biomedical, behavioural and psycho-social measures of the many different aspects of population health. These include mortality (eg death rates from heart disease and cancer), morbidity (eg rates of obesity, heart attack, heart disease, high blood pressure, self-rated good health), health-related behaviour (eg rates of smoking, poor diet, no physical exercise) and health-related quality of life (eg self-reported levels of pain, mobility, anxiety, energy, ability to care for oneself, ability to undertake work and social activities). Amongst the reasons for wanting such measures is a desire to be able to measure the impact on them of interventions intended to improve them for the better. Another is to measure health inequalities and assess the impact of interventions intended to reduce them. But why also try to measure *overall* population health? That is, why construct a summary measure of population health—such as the Quality Adjusted Life Year (QALY)—which aims to weigh up the most important aspects of health and reach an *overall* assessment of whether population health has got better or worse, and by how much?

One reason for wanting *overall* measures is that health sector policy objectives are often couched in overall terms such as 'the health of the nation', or 'the health of the whole population', or 'the health of all' (Department of Health 1999, Wanless 2003, HM Treasury 2007). Another is that health inequality cuts across *all* of the narrower aspects of public health mentioned above. Yet another is that efficiency or value for money—in the sense of making health sector resources have the largest possible impact on population health—requires an overall measure so that the comparative impacts of interventions of many different kinds in many different settings can be assessed. Public health scholars routinely combine data on mortality with simple binary data on morbidity (eg the presence or absence of one particular disease or disability or health state) to compute summary measures of population health such as healthy life expectancy and disability-free life years (Field and Gold 1998). A further step is to incorporate detailed data on health-related quality of life across multiple diseases and health states, which examines how the presence of disease actually influences people's physical, mental, and social functioning as they go about their daily lives (Mathers 2002; Murray, Salomon, and Mathers 2002).

The QALY can be used to do this, by generating measures of quality-adjusted life expectancy (QALE) among the whole population and by population subgroups.

Where QALYs really come into their own, however, is the evaluation of public health programmes to inform public resource allocation decisions (Dolan 2000). The QALY can be used to measure gains and losses in overall population health to inform decision makers faced with 'hard choices' between alternative programmes. All sensible public health programmes are likely to offer *some* benefit on *some* health outcomes. However, not all can be funded. In choosing between programmes, an important difficulty is the sheer mind-boggling diversity of health outcome measures used in public health. For instance, effectiveness studies of smoking cessation programmes might measure an increase in the 12-month quit rate. Evidence about this short-term behaviour change outcome might then be combined with evidence from clinical and epidemiological studies to model long-term population health outcomes such as mortality rates and prevalence of lung cancer, chronic obstructive pulmonary disease (COPD), and cardiovascular disease. However, in relation to programmes for reducing alcohol use in young people, the outcome measure might be the reduction in the number of teenagers prevented from '30-day heavy use' (defined as consuming five or more drinks in a row in the last 30 days) during a two-year period. Ideally, one would then extrapolate from this behaviour change outcome to model health outcomes such as rates of alcohol-related accidents, mental illness, and liver disease? Yet after all the evidence is in, and all the modelling is done, how can 30-day smoking quit rates and rates of mortality, lung cancer, COPD, and cardiovascular disease be compared with rates of 30-day heavy alcohol use, accidents, mental illness, and liver disease? How can a cash-strapped decision maker (say, a local authority) decide whether to adopt one, both, parts of, or neither of these programmes? How can these programmes be compared with the vast assortment of other possible public health programmes, delivering a vast range of other different kinds of health benefit, all of which are competing for scarce public funds?

Another way of putting the problem of health outcome comparison is in terms of opportunity cost. Few public health programmes are costless, even after purported future cost savings are taken into account. They therefore divert scarce resources away from alternative public health programmes which yield different health outcomes. Decision makers therefore need to weigh up the benefits of any proposed programme (ie one battery of health outcomes) against its opportunity costs (ie a quite different battery of health outcomes). In practice, these comparisons are often not explicitly considered by decision makers. Nevertheless, the inescapable logic of opportunity cost means that these comparisons are implicit in any public health decision with substantial resource implications.

The QALY facilitates these comparisons, and makes the comparison explicit rather than implicit. It also allows comparisons between health outcomes in public health and health outcomes in medicine. However, the QALY does not offer a complete solution for the cash-strapped public health decision maker, since there may also be important non-health outcomes to consider. In the case of alcohol reduction, for example, important non-health outcomes might include reductions in criminal offences, accidents, truancy, and unprotected sex, and increases in future employment and earnings prospects. Furthermore, the opportunity costs may fall on public organizations outside the health sector—such as schools and local authorities—thus diverting scarce resources away from education and other local government services with important non-health outcomes. The QALY does not address this wider problem of comparison between health and non-health outcomes, since it aims only to measure overall population health, not overall social welfare. This is important to appreciate. The QALY, despite the claims that are sometimes made about it, is not a measure of overall welfare, utility, or strength of preference. It is a measure of health or health gain. The critical issue for those who want to use it concerns how good a measure of health it is and the extent to which the nature of its construction should limit its application.

This chapter first explains how the QALY is produced (in section 2), setting out the basic arithmetic of the QALY, and then describing how QALYs incorporate evidence on health-related quality of life from surveys of patients and the general public. We then turn to potential uses and abuses of the QALY (in sections 3 and 4). The final section discusses future research directions, focusing in particular on how one might try to value QALYs *vis-à-vis* the many non-health outcomes that are often important in public health (section 5). The main aim of the chapter is to provide a clear introduction to the QALY with an emphasis on practical application to public health. A secondary aim is to assuage, if not dispel, some of the methodological and ethical concerns that can arise in relation to the QALY (Williams 1996). The QALY is simply a tool. Few tools are fit for all purposes, just as few horses are fit for all courses. The emphasis ought, as always, to be on sensible application and interpretation—based on a full appreciation of the pros and cons.

Anatomy of the QALY

Basic QALY arithmetic

The QALY is a measure of overall health calibrated over one year. It represents one year of life, adjusted for health-related quality of life. It thus incorporates both length of life and health-related quality of life in a single index (Williams 1985). Health-related quality of life focuses on health outcomes specifically, and does not aim to capture non-health outcomes that contribute to overall quality of life or well-being. The quality adjustment to life years is made by assigning a value of one to 'full health', and a value of zero to the state of 'death'. Intermediate values represent intermediate health states. In principle, negative values can be used to represent states worse than death, though in practice negative values are almost never encountered in applied cost per QALY studies in either health care or public health.

To measure the overall health of an individual, QALYs are summed over that individual's lifetime. To measure the overall health of a population, QALYs are summed across all the individuals within that population. Risk and uncertainty about health outcomes are dealt with by computing the *expected* number of QALYs (ie the probability of an outcome times the number of QALYs associated with it). The timing of health gains may be dealt with by *discounting* future QALYs, such that the present value of a future QALY

Box 10.1 QALY arithmetic for measuring individual health

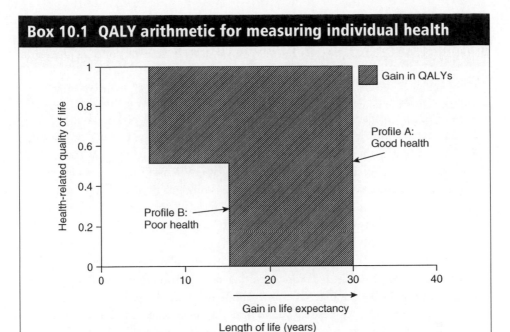

Fig. 10.1 Hypothetical QALY profiles: the value of an individual's health over time

To understand how QALYs are calculated, consider the simple hypothetical example in Figure 10.1. This shows two possible health profiles over time for an individual. In Profile A, the individual lives for another 30 years in full health, then dies instantly. In Profile B, the individual lives for 5 years in full health, with a quality of life score of 1, but then suffers a serious health event (such as a stroke) which severely impairs quality of life down to a score of 0.5 from then on. The individual then dies instantly in year 15. Compared with Profile B, Profile A yields a gain of 30 minus 15 equals 15 years in length of life. However, this does not take into account the improved quality of life in Profile A. The QALY score for each health profile is the time spent alive, adjusted for quality of life at each moment in time. So the QALY score for Profile A is 30 times 1 QALY equals 30 QALYs. Whereas the QALY score for Profile B is 5 years in full health (5 times 1 QALY equals 5 QALYs) plus 10 years in 0.5 health (10 times 0.5 QALY equals 5 QALYS), which adds up to only 10 QALYs in total. Compared with Profile B, Profile A thus yields a QALY gain of 30 minus 10 equals 20 QALYs. This is larger than the 15 year gain in length of life, because it accounts for improved quality of life as well as longer length of life.

To recap the QALY calculation so far:

Profile A: Good health	30 years in full health (30 times 1)	30 QALYs
	Total for Profile A	30 QALYs
Profile B: Poor health	5 years in full health (5 times 1)	5 QALYs
	10 years in 0.5 health (10 times 0.5)	5 QALYs
	Total for Profile B	10 QALYs

Box 10.2 QALY arithmetic for measuring changes in population health

Assume we have a population of 1,000 individuals. Of these, 800 will experience Profile A and 200 will experience Profile B. The population QALY score is thus 800 times 30 QALYs (for the Profile A group) plus 200 times 10 QALYs (for Profile B group) equals 26,000 QALYs. Now imagine that a public health programme costing 20 million pounds can reduce the prevalence of Profile B from 200 to 100 cases, while correspondingly increasing the prevalence of Profile A from 800 to 900. In this new post-programme scenario, the population QALY score is now 900 times 30 QALYs plus 100 times 10 QALYs equals 28,000 QALYs. The gain in QALYs in moving from the baseline scenario to the post-programme scenario is thus 28,000 − 26,000 = 2,000 QALYs.

This health gain can then be compared with the cost of the programme. Of course, the *opportunity cost* of the programme is not simply 20 million pounds but rather the opportunity forgone to use this money in other programmes that would have delivered other benefits. For example, the money might otherwise have been spent on other health-improving programmes that would have delivered other health benefits. If so, the health benefits of the programme need to be compared against those forgone health benefits. To make this comparison, current standard practice at NICE is to assume that the 20 million pounds would otherwise have been spent on other health-improving programmes that cost 20,000 pounds per QALY gained. If so, those alternative programmes would have delivered 1,000 QALYs. So the *net* health gain of a decision to pay 20 million pounds for this programme would then be 2,000 QALYs minus the opportunity cost of 1,000 QALYs equals 1,000 QALYs.

is less than the present value of a current QALY. For example, discounting may account for 'pure' social time preference for earlier rather than later health gains. This can of course make a large difference in relation to public health programmes with long-term health outcomes. The question of whether to discount future health gains, and if so by how much, is a matter of controversy which turns on issues of both factual and value judgement (Claxton et al 2009). However, this controversy reigns irrespective of how long-term health outcomes are measured, and is not specific to the QALY.

Incorporating data on health-related quality of life

The most difficult part of computing QALYs is quantifying the quality adjustment to life years. This requires us to measure an individual's health-related quality of life for a period of time in terms of a quality of life score on a ratio scale with 1 representing full health and 0 representing the state of death. Let us call this a QoL score, for short. A critical issue at this stage is that of 'construct validity'. That is, is the measure we are constructing truly a measure of 'health' or 'health gain'. The answer to this question largely depends upon judgement and introspection. For example, and as we shall see, there are some interventions that one can reasonably expect to have an impact on health that will hardly cause the QALY as currently constructed to change at all (impacts that reduce only fatigue is such an example). So one must judge whether the context is a suitable one for use of the QALY. Introspection comes in if you reflect on what you think are the key attributes of one's quality of life that lead one to consider oneself, or someone else, to be 'in good health' or not.

The QoL score is measured on a ratio scale. The ratio scale implies that a QoL score of 1 represents twice as much health as a QoL score of 0.5. This is required so that QoL scores can be added up over time and between individuals to yield an overall measure of population health. In the past, QoL scores were typically assigned using expert judgement. These days, however, more evidence-based approaches are available, drawing on self-reported individual survey data (Torrance 1986, Brazier et al 2007).

By placing a tick in one box in each group below, please indicate which statements best describe your own health state today.

Mobility

I have no problems in walking about ☐

I have some problems in walking about ☐

I am confined to bed ☐

Self-Care

I have no problems with self-care ☐

I have some problems washing or dressing myself ☐

I am unable to wash or dress myself ☐

Usual Activities (e.g. work, study, housework, family or leisure activities)

I have no problems with performing my usual activities ☐

I have some problems with performing my usual activities ☐

I am unable to perform my usual activities ☐

Pain/Discomfort

I have no pain or discomfort ☐

I have moderate pain or discomfort ☐

I have extreme pain or discomfort ☐

Anxiety/Depression

I am not anxious or depressed ☐

I am moderately anxious or depressed ☐

I am extremely anxious or depressed ☐

Fig. 10.2 EQ-5D Health State Classification System
© EuroQoL Group 1990

The standard survey-based approach has two stages. First, *classification* of individual health states in terms of a suitable generic multi-dimensional health state classification system, such as the five dimensional EQ-5D developed by a European group called 'EuroQol' (see Figure 10.2). This is the stage at which you have to ask about the construct validity of the measure. Second, *scoring* of health state classifications to generate QoL scores, by attaching numerical weights to each dimension and any interactions between dimensions. Both of these stages involve value judgements. In stipulating the dimensions of health, one is effectively saying not only that 'this is what we mean for present purposes by *health*' but also 'these are the elements of personal functioning and feeling in relation to health that it is good to have more of and bad to have less of'. In scoring the states one is effectively saying that 'this element counts for this much more or less than this other element'. That is not a scientific judgement but a judgement about what is good (or bad) for members of society in relation to their health.

It is usually felt that these value judgements ought not to be those of the inventors of QALYs but that they should come from the people affected by the decisions that are being informed by the use of QALYs. So it becomes important to examine data on the dimensions of health that matter most to people, and the values that people actually hold. In the case of the EQ-5D instrument, considerable effort was made to gather data of both kinds during development and validation stages (Euroqol Group 1990; Brookes 1996; Williams 1995).

The classification stage thus requires data on health-related quality of life from a survey of the individuals affected (or likely to be affected) by the public health intervention in question. By contrast, the scoring stage is typically done using off-the-shelf dimensional weights based on data from a national sample survey of the general public (Dolan et al 1996). Not all generic health state classification systems are suitable for the scoring stage. For example, the popular SF-36 instrument had to be shortened into a six dimensional version, the SF-6D, before preference-based QoL scoring could be done (Brazier, Roberts, and Deverill 2002). This is because the SF-36 generates many millions of possible health states with its 35 multi-level dimensions, whereas most respondents can only process five to nine pieces of information at a time. This provides a reminder that construct validity and more sophisticated measures of health can rapidly come up against practical (including financial) constraints. The measure could doubtless be made more perfect than it is, but only at a cost. Another judgement call is required to decide how 'perfect' the QALY should be for it to be useful and how valuable in actual practice further refinements are likely to be. As well as EQ-5D and SF-6D, other QALY-ready classification systems include the US Quality of Well-Being scale (QWB), the Canadian Health Utility Index (Mark 2 for children and Mark 3 for adults), the Finnish 15D descriptive system, and the Australian Assessment of Quality of Life index (AQoL) (Brazier et al 2007).

In the case of EQ-5D, the description stage results in a five digit code which classifies the individual's health-related quality of life state in five dimensions (mobility, self-care, usual activities, pain/discomfort, anxiety/depression). Each dimension has three levels with scores from 1 to 3, in decreasing order of healthiness for that dimension. This gives rise to 3 to the power of five (ie 3 times 3 times 3 times 3 times 3) equals 243 possible health states, plus the states of 'being dead' and 'being unconscious', making 245 states altogether. In the valuation stage, each health state needs then to be given a value, on a scale with 1 representing full health (a code of 1,1,1,1,1) and 0 representing the state of death.

The classification stage can be undertaken by asking a sample of relevant individuals to complete a QALY-ready health state classification questionnaire about their own health state. If direct survey data of this kind are not available, however, there are alternative indirect procedures which map whatever proxy health-related quality of life data are available on to a QALY-ready health state classification system. These indirect mapping procedures are sometimes based on expert judgement. Sometimes, however, a more evidence-based approach is possible, based on correlation analysis of data from a sample of individuals who have completed both the proxy health indicator questionnaire and the QALY-ready health state classification questionnaire.

The scoring stage is typically based on a survey of the general public. The usual justification for this is that public resource allocation decisions should be based upon public values, rather than the values of any particular interest group such as individuals targeted by a particular public health intervention. Even here there are subtle embodied value judgements (for example which 'public'—the taxpaying public or the health care receiving public? Current patients or prospective patients? Those directly affected or those, like informal carers, who are indirectly affected?). Many different survey-based value elicitation methods have been used for the purpose of eliciting health dimension weights, the most popular ones being Visual Analogue Scale (VAS), Time Trade-Off (TTO) and Standard Gamble (SG). The VAS simply asks people to mark how good or bad each state is on a visual scale from 0 to 100 that looks a bit like a thermometer (see Figure 10.3). The TTO asks people to make choices between health profiles under certainty, involving trade-offs between length of life and quality of life—for instance, many years in poor health versus fewer years in good health. Finally, the SG asks people to make choices under uncertainty between scenarios involving different probabilities of health outcomes—for instance, a small chance of death versus certainty of chronic ill-health. Other methods include Person Trade Off (PTO), in which respondents trade off numbers of persons in one health state against numbers of persons in another health state, Discrete Choice Experiments (DCE), in which respondents make pair-wise comparisons between health states, and ranking exercises in which respondents rank health states in order (Brazier et al 2007). Each method has numerous variants, with different questionnaire styles, modes of administration, and 'props' to help people understand the question and make their responses.

For logistical reasons, it is not possible to ask people enough questions to value all possible health states in a health state classification system. Based on piloting work, for example, Dolan (1997) suggests that no one respondent can be expected to compare more than 13 health states using TTO questions. So a selection of questions is asked about a carefully chosen subset of health states, and regression methods are used to estimate the dimensional weights that best fit the pattern of responses. These estimated dimensional weights are then used indirectly to predict QoL scores for the health states that have not been

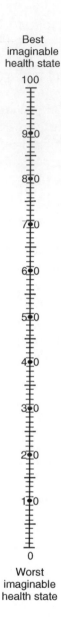

To help people say how good or bad a health state is, we have drawn a scale (rather like a thermometer) on which the best state you can imagine is marked 100 and the worst state you can imagine is marked 0.

We would like you to indicate on this scale how good or bad your own health is today, in your opinion. Please do this by drawing a line from the box below to whichever point on the scale indicates how good or bad your health state is today.

Your own health state today

Fig. 10.3 EQ-5D Visual Analogue Scale
© EuroQoL Group 1990

directly valued. For example, Dolan (1997) uses direct TTO valuations on 42 of the 243 health states in EQ-5D from 2,997 respondents in a UK survey, each of whom valued about 13 different health states each, to estimate dimension weights and thus model QoL values for the remaining health states.

One variant of the TTO question is illustrated in Figure 10.4. The respondent is taken through various 'warm up' exercises which compare different health states. The respondent is then asked to focus on one particular state of ill-health, h. To set a QoL score on

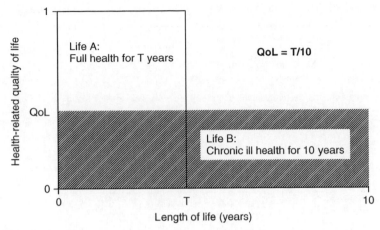

Fig. 10.4 Time trade-off

this state of ill health, the respondent is asked to choose between full health for T years ('Life A') and chronic ill health in state *h* for 10 years ('Life B'). The interviewer than varies T, in terms of years and months, until the respondent cannot choose between Life A and Life B. At this point of indecision, the QALY scores for Life A and Life B must be the same. The QALY score for Life A is T years times 1 equals T QALYs. The QALY score for Life B is 10 years times the QoL score for state *h*. Therefore T equals ten times the QoL score for state *h*, and so the QoL score for state *h* is T divided by ten.

Finally, a variant of the SG question is illustrated in Figure 10.5. Under various assumptions, the stated minimum chance of success, p%, is the value of one year in the chronic ill-health state.

Different value elicitation methods, and different ways of analysing the responses, can yield systematically different sets of QoL scores for the same health states. Hence there remains controversy about the best way of doing it. NICE currently recommends the use of weights based on TTO or SG questions from a large and (historically) representative sample survey of members of the UK population, such as the TTO weights from Dolan (1997) presented in Figure 10.6.

Due to remaining methodological uncertainty, however, NICE is willing to consider QALY data based on alternative sets of weights in sensitivity analysis, especially if good reasons can be given for diverting from the NICE 'reference case' in a particular decision context. This reminds us that the QALY is not a fixed and permanent concept in all respects. It would scarcely be the QALY if it were not a system for weighting life-years, so that is a given. Similarly, the system will be based on dimensions and their weights. But the EQ-5D is but one version and, as we have seen there are many ways of attaching values, even if the EQ-5D is deemed to be the appropriate version to use. One's choice depends partly on the general acceptability of the value judgements and partly on other attributes that are specific to the context in hand. For some the QALY may be too insensitive to small changes, for others there may be omitted aspects of QoL, for yet others the values relating to trade-off between dimensions may be culturally specific. In all these

Imagine you have a chronic illness. In terms of EQ-5D, your health state can be described as:

Mobility: 1 No problems walking about
Self-care: 1 No problem with self-care
Usual activities   2 Some problems performing usual activities
Pain/discomfort   2 Moderate pain or discomfort
Anxiety/depression   3 Extremely anxious or depressed

Your doctor informs you that two different treatments are available. With the first treatment, you will live for ten more years in poor health and then die. With the second treatment, you have a chance of returning to full health for ten years before death. However, there is also a chance that the treatment would kill you immediately.

So, your two options are:

1. Take the first treatment and live for 10 years in chronic ill health, with 100% certainty.

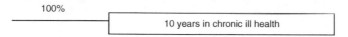

2. Take the second treatment for a p% chance of returning to full health but risk a (100% − p%) chance of immediate death.

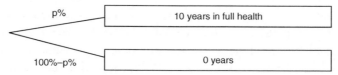

If the second treatment is successful, you will live for ten years in full health. If not, you will die immediately.

Your doctor tells you that the chance the second treatment will succeed is not known.

Please indicate on the scale below **the minimum chance of success—ie p%—** that you would require for you to accept the second treatment.

0%   10%   20%   30%   40%   50%   60%   70%   80%   90%   100%

Fig. 10.5 Stylized standard gamble question (modified for a readership familiar with the EQ-5D and with probability notation)

Item	Penalty
Starting from 1.000 for full health	
Any dimension higher than 1	−0.081
Any dimension at level 3	−0.269
Mobility level 2	−0.069
Mobility level 3	−0.314
Self-care level 2	−0.104
Self-care level 3	−0.214
Usual activities level 2	−0.036
Usual activities level 3	−0.094
Pain or discomfort level 2	−0.123
Pain or discomfort level 3	−0.386
Anxiety or depression level 2	−0.071
Anxiety or depression level 3	−0.236

Example QoL calculation for health state 11223

(Health state code 11223 represents: no problems walking about, no problems with self-care, some problems performing usual activities, moderate pain or discomfort, extremely anxious or depressed)

Start from full health	1.000
Any dimension higher than 1	−0.081
Any dimension at level 3	−0.269
Usual activities level 2	−0.036
Pain or discomfort level 2	−0.123
Anxiety or depression level 3	−0.236
Resulting QoL score	0.255

Fig. 10.6 Example dimensional weights for QoI scoring of EQ-Sd health states
(Based on data from Williams (1995) and Dolan (1997))

respects, good judgement has to be exercised as to the suitability of QALYs, the suitability and availability of alternatives, and the consequences of working with a measure that is not as good as may be wished for the purpose in hand. These consequences can be revealed by a sensitivity analysis which would test whether different assumptions in the QALY would lead to substantially different conclusions about efficiency or equity. The key question to ask is 'is the QALY in the form available good enough for the purposes to hand?'

Potential uses of the QALY

Health impact assessment and health inequality impact assessment

The QALY can be used to facilitate health impact assessment for a particular public health programme. That is, one can compute the total number of QALYs gained by a public health programme, compared with the status quo or an alternative programme. The advantage of using the QALY, rather than a battery of different indicators, is, as we have seen, that it yields a single overall assessment of health impact which accounts for both for changes in length of life and health-related quality of life. The same applies to health inequality impact assessment. The QALY also allows one to assess differential health impacts on different social groups, incorporating differential impacts on quality of life and length of life into a single overall index.

Cost-effectiveness analysis

The most common use of the QALY is in cost-effectiveness analysis (sometimes called 'cost-utility analysis'[1] when QALYs are used). The basic idea is to compute the extra cost per QALY gained of the proposed public health programme, as compared with the status quo or an alternative programme. Different proposals can then be compared on an equivalent footing, in terms of their incremental cost per QALY gained.

With experience, a benchmark or 'threshold'[2] cost per QALY can be established, allowing a judgement to be made about whether a programme is cost-effective or not compared with other uses of public money to improve health in medicine and public health. This 'threshold' may be interpreted as the opportunity cost of diverting resources from alternative medical or public programmes (ie the 'typical' cost per QALY of alternative programmes). More ambitiously, it may be interpreted as a social value judgement by decision makers and/or the general public about how much society is willing to pay for a

---

[1] We think use of the term 'utility' here is somewhat misleading. Although the QALY has many characteristics of utility measurement as understood in economics, the QALY does not have to be based on individual subjective preferences, nor indeed on preferences at all. It could, for example, be simply interpreted as an empirically descriptive and pragmatic indicator of health. Or the values embodied in it could be recognized as such but be the values of a benevolent dictator or (less controversially!) an accountable public official.

[2] It is conventional to talk of a 'threshold' such as £20,000 per QALY above which a technology would be of doubtful cost-effectiveness. However, the door joinery analogy ought really to be 'lintel' since it has the character of an upper rather than a lower limit.

QALY. The threshold implicitly adopted by NICE lies in the range £20,000 to £30,000 per QALY, and this threshold is interpreted by NICE in terms of the opportunity cost of alternative uses of public money in medicine and public health (Culyer et al 2007).

The use of the QALY in cost-effectiveness analysis is perfectly compatible with the use of other health and non-health outcomes in supplementary economic evaluations. The production of multiple cost-effectiveness analyses using different outcome measures is sometimes known as 'cost-consequence analysis'.

Cost–benefit analysis

A drawback with cost-effectiveness and cost-consequence analyses in public health is that they fail to integrate health and non-health outcomes within the same analysis despite the frequency with which effects of both kinds may be present. This makes it hard to take a 'whole systems' approach that allows for different outcomes and the interactions between them. Since both health and non-health outcomes come in a bewildering variety of different shapes and sizes, it also makes it hard to draw an overall conclusion from the analysis about whether a programme is worthwhile[3], or to seek a degree of consistency between decisions in different areas. One potential solution to this is the use of cost–benefit analysis, which converts all health and non-health benefits into the common currency of money. Cost–benefit analysis may potentially be useful when there are important non-health benefits of a public health programme—for instance, improvements in education outcomes, employment outcomes, crime outcomes, environmental outcomes, private consumption outcomes, and so on.

The QALY can be used in cost–benefit analysis by 'simply' attaching a monetary value to the QALY. There are various ways of attaching a monetary value to a QALY, none of which is entirely satisfactory. One obvious option is simply to use the NICE 'threshold'. One way of justifying the use of such 'thresholds' to value sector specific outcomes is in terms of the delegated decision-making responsibility of different public sector agencies (Claxton, Sculpher, and Culyer 2007). Another approach is to conduct surveys of the general public to estimate collective 'willingness to pay'. The traditional approach in economics is to value all health and non-health outcomes as the sum total of *individual* 'willingness to pay' for these outcomes among the population. However, this traditional approach has had limited success in the health sector, having come under criticism both on theoretical grounds—eg that willingness to pay is influenced by ability to pay, misperceptions of the actual effects of changes in QoL, and by misperceptions of risk—and on the practical grounds that 'willingness to pay' surveys are particularly vulnerable to framing effects and can produce 'rubber-money' estimates (Cookson 2003). Different methods give different answers, so sensitivity analysis is likely to be needed in any applied cost–benefit analysis, using a range of different monetary values for a QALY. As ever, the legitimacy of the alternative methods also depends upon the nature of the decision that the analysis is designed to inform.

---

[3] In this section we set aside analyses intended to reduce inequities.

Cost–equity analysis

The QALY can also be used to analyse the trade-offs that arise when the policy goal of improving population health conflicts with equity goals such as reducing socio-economic health inequality (Cookson, Weatherly, and Drummond 2009). This is sometimes referred to as an 'equity-efficiency trade off'. Strictly speaking, however, improving population health is not necessarily the same thing as improving efficiency in the technical economic sense of 'Pareto efficiency': a situation in which no individual can be made better off unless some other individual is made worse off (Culyer 2006). Improving overall population health may not improve Pareto efficiency, if one group of individuals gains a large health benefit at the expense of another group which loses a small health benefit. And improving Pareto efficiency may not improve population health, if some individuals are better off overall but worse off in terms of health specifically. Moreover, improving population health inevitably involves, as we have seen, adding up the QoLs of different individuals and groups, which inherently involves distributional value judgements. To treat them all the same (ie assigning a weight on unity to each QALY gain per person) is no less a social value judgement than to weight them differently.

To analyse equity issues, it is possible to examine how cost per QALY varies by equity-relevant subgroups—for example, by socio-economic status, ethnicity, gender, geographical location. In some cases, cost-per-QALY will be higher for 'hard-to-reach' individuals in lower socio-economic groups, who may be less attentive to public health messages and less able and willing to attend public health clinics. If so, the reduction of health inequality may require diverting additional resources towards targeting 'hard-to-reach' groups. The cost-per-QALY of these additional resources may be relatively high. If so, these resources could deliver larger health gains if used elsewhere—leading to a bigger improvement in population health and increased health inequality at the same time. Hence there may be a trade-off between maximizing population health and reducing socio-economic health inequality, even if the equal weighting of QALY gains is deemed to be equitable. The QALY can be used to explore such trade-offs, by quantifying the opportunity cost of tackling health inequality. For example, it may be possible to compute the number of QALYs forgone among 'easy-to-reach' groups by a policy of devoting additional resources to 'hard-to-reach' groups. Decision makers can then make a more informed judgement about how large a sacrifice in total population health is worth making for the sake of tackling health inequality. More ambitiously, it may be possible to 'equity weight' QALYs in order to deliver more explicit and consistent answers to questions about equity-efficiency trade-offs. However, an evidence-based approach to equity weighting is some way off: although valuation methods have been developed and piloted, there is as yet no evidence from a large and representative sample survey of members of the general public.

Burden of disease

A quite different context in which QALYs could be used is that of estimating the cost of illness or burden of disease. We may be interested to know the overall scale of a health problem compared with other health problems. In this context, a variant of the QALY known as the Disability Adjusted Life Year (DALY) has been extensively used to monitor the burden of disease in developing countries (Murray and Lopez 1996). However, some economists are sceptical of burden of disease calculations, since they only tell us about the size of the problem. There is a considerable step between understanding the size of the problem and the payoff to resources devoted to reducing it, which has not always been perceived by commentators (Williams 1999, Murray and Lopez 2000, Mooney and Wiseman 2000).

International comparisons and performance monitoring

Another context in which QALYs are potentially useful—although hitherto rarely used—is that of international comparisons and national performance monitoring in public health. We may be interested to know how well (or badly) a particular country or jurisdiction is doing *overall* on public health, and on tackling health inequalities, over time and compared with other jurisdictions and countries. It may not be enough to know a country is doing well on some health indicators and badly on others. Public health professionals, politicians, and voters alike may want to know how well their country is doing *overall* on public health. In this context, the most commonly used summary measures of population health are based on mortality and morbidity data, such as health expectancy, disability-free life expectancy and impairment-free life expectancy (Field and Gold 1998). The QALY can improve upon these measures by incorporating data on health-related quality of life—rather than merely morbidity data on disease and disability—to produce estimates of quality adjusted life expectancy (QALE).

Potential abuses of the QALY

Excessive focus on young and healthy rather than elderly and sick populations

One potential abuse of the QALY is that it could be used (wittingly or unwittingly) to focus public health efforts excessively on young and healthy rather than elderly and sick populations. Elderly and sick people tend to have fewer life years left to go than young people, more chronic disease, and lower health-related quality of life (Kind et al 1998). Hence young and healthy people tend to have better overall health than elderly people and more QALYs left to go. So when measuring population health gains with long-lasting benefits for the individuals concerned—such as reducing rates of death and disability—the QALY will register a larger overall health gain in a young and healthy population than an elderly and sick population.

To take an extreme hypothetical case, saving a newborn baby from instant death might yield 100 QALYs, if that baby is expected to live for another 100 years in full health. Whereas saving a frail elderly individual from instant death might only yield 1 QALY, if that individual is otherwise expected to live for another 2 years with a QoL score of 0.5 (ie a gain of $2 \times 0.5 = 1$ QALY). In practice, of course, things are less extreme than this, as public health programmes are preventative rather than curative, and are typically not in the business of saving babies or terminally ill adults from instant death. Furthermore, alongside the lifetime QALY gains there is also the stream of lifetime costs to consider, which may impose opportunity costs and QALY losses on others.[4] And the same point can of course be made about any outcome measure based on life expectancy, or indeed almost any outcome measure that is not a 'life saved'.

In some cases and to some extent, of course, it may be appropriate, and in line with wider social values, to focus public health efforts on children and young people. The danger, however, is that QALY estimates (or other estimates based on life expectancy) could be misused to exaggerate the case against public health efforts among elderly populations and to get the balance wrong.

This example reminds us again that it may often be important not to focus exclusively on the potential for health gain but also to consider carefully the character of those receiving the gain (and, conversely, those likely to bear the opportunity cost). From time to time it is to be entirely expected that public policy will want to emphasize particular client groups—perhaps the old, or the young, or the newly immigrated, or single mothers, . . .). In such cases, while the QALY may provide an adequate account of their expected health gain, it will not express the social significance attaching to it on account of their being members of a targeted group.

It is thus important to understand that the QALY is a measure of health gain and not a measure of overall social value. The QALY merely informs the decision maker which option delivers the largest overall gain in population health or to various population groups, and what the cost might be to those not receiving the resources in question. It does not inform the decision maker which is the 'best' option in terms of overall social value. And it certainly does not tell the decision maker which is the 'right' decision to take.

Capricious decisions about young children and the mentally ill

QALY assessment for young children and the mentally ill is particularly difficult and unreliable. One reason is that young children and the mentally ill are less able to give reliable answers to questionnaires asking them about their health-related quality of life. Another reason is that generic health state valuation instruments were typically developed with 'normal' adult populations in mind, and may not be well adapted to the special circumstances and needs of young children and the mentally ill. QALY estimates in these groups must therefore be interpreted with particular caution, and special consideration given to methodological uncertainty and potential bias.

---

[4] It is sometimes claimed that the use of QALYs in cost-utility analyses is inherently ageist, favouring those with a longer life expectancy. While it is certainly true that some public health interventions may be judged not to be cost-effective in elderly populations, this is not to say that the use of QALYs in CUA is *inherently* ageist. For one thing, it is not the quality adjustment that creates the effect, rather it is the prospective relative life span of the beneficiaries. For another, a judgement about cost-effectiveness depends on both benefit *and cost*. Thus, in the case of ongoing interventions with costs that continue throughout a person's life, the 'ageist' argument goes into reverse: for any given benefit the advantage lies with those having the shorter life expectancy (Claxton and Culyer 2008).

There is nothing intrinsic in the very idea of the QALY that discriminates either in favour of or against young children and the mentally ill. The problem is just that QALY estimates are unreliable in these groups, and so there is a danger of capricious decision making if potential errors and biases are not carefully considered. The QALY is more like a kitchen knife than a thumb screw: it is a useful instrument that can be abused, not an instrument of abuse! And despite its imperfections it may still be better than using life-years unadjusted at all.

Unethical treatment of individuals

The QALY focuses on outcomes. If too much attention is paid to outcomes, there is a risk of downplaying important considerations relating to process rather than outcome—such as the importance of respecting rights and treating individuals with humanity, dignity, and compassion. Of course, if decision makers pay less attention to QALYs they may not pay more attention to rights, humanity, dignity and compassion, and vice versa. As ever, the issue is about paying appropriate attention to QALYs *vis-à-vis* other considerations. It is, however, extremely unlikely that all the relevant matters that need to be taken into account when addressing matters of fair treatment can be encompassed within methods that use only QALYs. So, while to allow excessive attention to QALY effects would indeed be excessive, by the same token so is excessive attention to anything else. Every single one of these concepts and the empirical measures and interpretations that are built upon them need to be understood and critically evaluated case by case. None is ever a substitute for careful thought! One hopes that each can, however, be a useful aid to careful thought.

Excessive focus on health outcomes rather than non-health outcomes

The QALY measures only health outcomes. It does not measure non-health outcomes which are often important in public health, such as education outcomes, employment outcomes, crime outcomes, and so on. If too much time is spent on producing and discussing QALY outcomes, there is a danger that decision makers may pay insufficient attention to important non-health benefits. Again, however, it is not necessarily the case that paying less attention to health outcomes automatically means paying more attention to non-health outcomes. In practice, decision makers may pay little attention to either, preferring to focus instead on anecdotes and opinions and the lobbying of special interest groups. Once again, the 'aid to thought' message needs to be borne in mind and a sensible balance struck—which includes a sensible balance of time in research and any discussion of its implications for policy.

Future research directions

There are at least three important areas in which further methodological research is needed:

1 improving methods of measuring health-related quality of life in order to construct QALYs;

2 developing methods for adjusting QALYs to accommodate equity concerns; and

3 developing methods for bringing together and weighing both QALY and non-QALY outcomes, including private consumption as well as outcomes in other public policy sectors (eg education, employment, crime, and so on).

In all three areas, the nature of future research is likely to be guided by underlying philosophical views about the nature and purpose of economic evaluation. There is general consensus (at least among economists) that the purpose of economic evaluation is to compare alternative public policy decisions in terms of their outcomes for individual well-being. However, there is little consensus on the best theory of individual well-being. We can distinguish three main views in the general economics and philosophy literature:

1 Preference theories (aka desire theories). According to preference theories, individual well-being is defined by the individual's own subjective preferences between states of the world. The relevant preferences may or may not be the same ones that drive the individual's actual behaviour and choices in the marketplace; they may be 'informed' or 'considered' or 'laundered' or otherwise 'improved' preferences (Goodin 1986). This is the standard approach in 'welfare economics' and among some practitioners of cost-effectiveness analysis.

2 Experience theories (aka happiness theories). According to experience theories, individual well-being is defined by the individual's own subjective experiences of actual states of the world from moment to moment (Kruger and Kahneman 2006). Individual well-being over time is (usually) the sum total of momentary experiences; and population well-being is (usually) the sum total of individual well-being.

3 Capability theories (aka objective list theories). According to capability theories, individual well-being is defined by the individual's opportunities to do valuable activities and to achieve valuable states of being (Coast et al 2008, Vizard and Burchardt 2007). Capabilities might include things like the ability to live a long and healthy life, to access adequate education and social services, to undertake productive activity, to enjoy a reasonable standard of living, to engage in family and social life, to participate in and influence public life, to enjoy self-respect, and so on. This approach in broad terms is that embodied in NICE's methods.

It is possible to consider revolutionary change in current valuation methods, if one is willing to sign up wholeheartedly to one of these theories. A 'preference revolution' might involve valuing entire public health intervention programmes in terms of direct 'referendum style' questions. An 'experience revolution' might involve asking people to complete experience sampling questionnaires that ask how you are feeling at different moments in time (eg on a scale of 1 to 10). Finally, a 'capability revolution' might involve constructing a new all-purpose index of well-being with multiple dimensions reflecting both health and non-health-related quality of life—a sort of 'super-QALY'.

Our own personal view, however, is that each theory probably contains an element of the truth. We are not monoethicists. Hence the most sensible direction for future research probably involves evolutionary change, in which existing approaches are gradually refined and improved through pragmatic methodological development guided by elements of all three theories, an evolving public understanding of the issues, and an increasing public ability to articulate the relevant social values. Indeed, in a way, the QALY already has been guided by elements from all three schools of thought. The explicit focus on multiple dimensions of health-related quality of life to classify health states aligns with capability theories. The use of preference-based value elicitation methods to weigh the health dimensions and generate QoL scores aligns with preference theories. And the adding up of QoL scores across moments in time and between persons aligns with experience theories.

Even if there are no methodological developments in this area, however, there is scope for a vast improvement in evidence-based public health policy making by applying existing standard QALY methods more extensively and more rigorously to public health. Almost all primary effectiveness studies in public health should use a standard, well-validated, and QALY-ready health state classification questionnaire, such as EQ-5D, which is relatively cheap and simple to administer. And almost all secondary evaluations of public health programmes should construct QALYs alongside a battery of other outcome measures.

The first of these recommendations has three advantages over current practice. First, it would provide information on the health outcomes that matter—ie quality of life outcomes for people's physical, mental, and social functioning as they carry out their daily lives—rather than merely surrogate behaviour change outcomes. Second, it would allow statisticians to synthesize evidence from different studies in order to estimate the overall size of the population health gain, and not merely to count the number of studies in which there was or was not a significant effect. At present, different studies of similar public health programmes typically use different outcome measures, and so it is often impossible to synthesize evidence from different studies to estimate an overall effect size. So all the decision maker can know for sure is that the programme has some effect, in some studies. Since almost all programmes have some effect in some studies, that is a thoroughly inadequate evidence base for decision making in the face of scarce resources. Third, this would allow more rigorous comparisons of overall population health gain and cost-per-QALY between programmes in different areas of public health and medicine.

More extensive use of standard QALY methods and standard QALY-ready survey instruments for measuring health-related quality of life would thus mark a huge practical leap forward compared with the information on surrogate behavioural outcomes that NICE public health advisory committees all too often currently have to work with when evaluating public health programmes.

Acknowledgements

We would like to thank John Brazier, Amanda Killoran, Chris McCabe, Adam Oliver, and Aki Tsuchiya for extremely helpful and detailed comments on an earlier draft. However, our errors and opinions about QALYs are our own.

Bibliography

Brazier JE, Ratcliffe J, Tsuchiya, A, and Salomon, J (2007) *Measuring and valuing health for economic evaluation.* Oxford: Oxford University Press

Brazier, J, Roberts, J, Deverill, M (2002) 'The estimation a preference-based single index measure for health from the SF-36' *Journal of Health Economics* 21/2: 271–92

Brookes, R (1996) 'EuroQol: the current state of play' *Health Policy* 37/1: 53–72

Claxton, K and Culyer, AJ (2008) 'Not a NICE fallacy: a reply to Dr Quigley' *Journal of Medical Ethics* 34: 598–601

Claxton, K, Sculpher, M, and Culyer, AJ (2007) *Mark versus Luke? Appropriate methods for the evaluation of public health interventions.* CHE Research Paper 31. York: University of York

Claxton, K, Paulden, M, Gravelle, H, Brouwer, W, and Culyer, AJ (2009) *Discounting and decision making in the economic evaluation of health care technologies.* Paper presented to Health Economists Study Group Meeting, Manchester, January 2009

Coast, J, Flynn, TN, Natarajan, L, Sproston, K, Lewis, J, Louviere, JJ, Peters, TJ (2008) 'Valuing the ICECAP capability index for older people' *Social Science and Medicine* 67: 874–82

Cookson, R (2003) 'Willingness to pay methods in health care: a sceptical view' *Health Economics* 12/11: 891–4

Cookson, R, Weatherly, H, and Drummond, M (2009) 'Explicit incorporation of equity considerations into economic evaluation of public health interventions' *Journal of Health Economics*, Policy and Law 4: 231–45

Culyer, A (2006) 'The bogus conflict between efficiency and vertical equity' *Health Economics* 15: 1155–8

Culyer, A, McCabe, C, Briggs, A, Claxton, K, Buxton, M, Akehurst, R, Sculpher, M, and Brazier, J (2007) 'Searching for a threshold, not setting one: the role of the National Institute for Health and Clinical Excellence' *Journal of Health Services Research and Policy* 12/1: 56–8

Department of Health (1999) *Saving lives: our healthier nation.* Cm 4386. London: Her Majesty's Stationary Office. Accessible via <http://www.archive.official-documents.co.uk/document/cm43/4386/4386.htm> (accessed 18 February 2009)

Dolan, P (1997) 'Valuations for EuroQol Health States' *Medical Care* 35/11: 1095–108

Dolan, P (2000) 'The measurement of health-related quality of life for use in resource allocation decisions in health care'. in A Culyer and J Newhouse, *Handbook of health economics.* North Holland: Elsevier. Publicly available via <http://ideas.repec.org/h/eee/heachp/1-32.html> (accessed 19 February 2009)

Dolan, P, Gudex, C, Kind, P, and Williams, A (1996) 'The time trade-off method: results from a general population study' *Health Economics* 5/2: 141–54

EuroQol Group (1990) 'EuroQol—a new facility for the measurement of health-related quality of life' *Health Policy* 16/3: 199–208

Field, MJ and Gold, GM (eds) (1998) *Summarizing population health: directions for the de6elopment and application of population metrics.* Washington, DC: Institute of Medicine, National Academy Press

Goodin, R (1986) 'Laundering preferences' in Jon Elster and Aanund Hylland (eds), *Foundations of Social Choice Theory,* pp 75–101. Cambridge: Cambridge University Press

HM Treasury (2007) *PSA Delivery Agreement 18: Promote better health and wellbeing for all.* Downloadable via <http://www.hm-treasury.gov.uk/d/pbr_csr07_psa18.pdf> (accessed 18 February 2009)

Kind, P, Dolan, P, Gudex, C, and Williams, A (1998) 'Variations in population health status: results from a United Kingdom national questionnaire survey' *British Medical Journal* 316: 736–41

Kruger, A and Kahneman, D (2006) 'Developments in the measurement of subjective well-being' *Journal of Economic Perspectives* 20/1: 3–24

Mooney, G and Wiseman, V (2000) 'Burden of disease and priority setting' *Health Economics* 9: 369–72

Mathers, C (2002) 'Health expectancies: an overview and critical appraisal' Chapter 4.1 in CJL Murray, JA Salomon, CD Mathers, and AD Lopez, *Summary measures of population health: concepts, ethics, measurement and applications.* Geneva: World Health Organization. This WHO book is publicly available via <http://whqlibdoc. who.int/publications/2002/9241545518.pdf> (accessed 19 February 2008)

Murray, CJL, Saloman, JA, and Mathers, C (2002) 'A critical examination of summary measures of population health' Chapter 1.2 in CJL Murray, JA Salomon, CD Mathers, and AD Lopez, *Summary measures of population health: concepts, ethics, measurement and applications.* Geneva: World Health Organization

Murray, CJL and AD Lopez (1996) *The global burden of disease.* Geneva: World Health Organization

Murray, CJL and Lopez, AD (2000) 'Progress and directions in refining the global burden of disease approach: a response to Williams' *Health Economics* 9: 69–82

Torrance, GW (1986) 'Measurement of health state utilities for economic appraisal' *Journal of Health Economics* 5: 1–30

Vizard, P and Burchardt, T (2007) 'Developing a capability list: final recommendations of the Equalities Review Steering Group on Measurement' Available at: <http://archive.cabinetoffice.gov.uk/equalitiesreview/publications. html>

Wanless, D (2003) *Securing good health for the whole population—population health trends*. London: Her Majesty's Stationery Office. Available via <http://www.hm-treasury.gov.uk/consult_wanless03_index.htm> (accessed 18 February 2009)

Williams, A (1985) 'Economics of coronary artery bypass grafting' *British Medical Journal* 291: 326–9

Williams, A (1995) *The measurement and valuation of health: a chronicle*. Centre for Health Economics Discussion Paper 136. York: University of York. Downloadable via <http://www.york.ac.uk/inst/che/pdf/DP136.pdf> (accessed 18 February 2009)

Williams, A (1996) 'QALYs and ethics: a health economist's perspective' *Social Science and Medicine* 43: 1795–804

Williams, A (1999) 'Calculating the global burden of disease: time for a strategic reappraisal?' *Health Economics* 8: 1–8

Chapter 11

Ethics and public health: the ethics of intervention choices

Lord Krebs and Harald Schmidt

Introduction

The Faculty of Public Health of the Royal Colleges of Physicians of the United Kingdom understands public health as: 'The science and art of preventing disease, prolonging life and promoting health through the organized efforts of society' (Griffiths et al 2005). But how should 'society' be understood here, and whose job specifically is it to ensure that we lead a healthy life? Should society be taken to refer to the collective of people that make up the population of a state, and is it entirely up to us as individuals to choose how to lead our lives? Alternatively, does the state also have a role to play? And if so, what kind of intervention would be most appropriate and effective?

In January 2006, the Nuffield Council on Bioethics set up a Working Party to examine the ethical issues surrounding public health. The Council is an independent body that identifies, examines, and reports on ethical questions raised by advances in biological and medical research. It seeks to contribute to policy making and stimulate debate in bioethics, and has published major reports on a range of topics, including genetic screening, healthcare research in developing countries, research involving animals, and the forensic use of DNA.

This article summarizes some of the conclusions and recommendations that were published in the report *Public health: ethical issues* (Nuffield Council on Bioethics 2007) in November 2007. The context to the public health debate is set out in the first section and the 'stewardship model' is presented and the role of evidence is considered. This model outlines the legitimate goals and constraints of liberal states in pursuing public health measures. In the next section we describe the 'intervention ladder', which is a tool that helps use of the stewardship model in practice. It enables an assessment of the acceptability of different interventions in terms of their level of intrusiveness and evidence that is required. In the final section we consider the case of obesity which illustrates the role of both the stewardship model and the intervention ladder in policy and practice.

The discussion emphasizes the need to consider in particular the situation of vulnerable groups such as children and the socio-economically disadvantaged, and underlines that public health issues concern not only tensions between the individual and the state, but also require consideration of the role of third parties, such as industries.

Public health context: the key ethical issues

The role of the state

A question that was fundamental to the Council's inquiry was the relationship between the state's authority and the individual. A spectrum of views exists on this matter, from those who give priority to the individual, to those who believe that the collective interests of the population as a whole are the most important.

At one end of the spectrum we find the Libertarian perspective. Proponents of this view argue that the authority of the state needs to be limited to ensuring that members of the population are able to enjoy the 'natural' rights of man, such as life, liberty, and property, without interference from others. Accordingly, the state has no particular obligations to use funds to promote the welfare of the population through public health measures.

At the other end of the spectrum we find what can be called Collectivist positions. There are several forms, for example Utilitarian and Social Contract approaches. The primary aim of the Utilitarian approach is to maximize utility by focusing on achieving the greatest possible collective benefit. This means that actions or rules are generally measured by the degree to which they reduce pain and suffering, and promote overall happiness and well-being. In principle, they may allow the welfare or interests of some people to be 'sacrificed' if this were to lead to an increase in overall welfare. The Social Contract approach finds that the state's authority is based on the collective will of a community (for example, as expressed in a democratic vote) to live together as an enduring nation state. This position will typically favour measures to promote the welfare of its citizens, including public goods and services of all kinds.

There are, of course, a range of intermediate positions in between these two ends of the spectrum. Essentially they would recognize that the state should uphold certain fundamental individual rights, but also that it has a responsibility to care for the welfare of all citizens. These welfare considerations may include ensuring that all have a fair opportunity to make a decent life for themselves, and that efforts are made to address and reduce unfair inequalities (ie pursue equity). Positions of this kind are generally thought of as liberal.

Mill's harm principle

Most modern Western states are, according to this analysis, liberal. An important question is how far it is proper for the state to introduce programmes that interfere to different degrees in the lives of its population in order to reduce the risks to the health of all or some of them. One way to start thinking about resolving this tension is provided by the 'harm principle', first established by the philosopher John Stuart Mill in his *On liberty* of 1859. According to Mill:

> The object of this Essay is to assert one very simple principle, as entitled to govern absolutely the dealings of society with the individual in the way of compulsion and control, whether the means used be physical force in the form of legal penalties, or the moral coercion of public opinion. That principle is, that the sole end for which mankind are warranted, individually or collectively in interfering with the liberty of action of any of their number, is self-protection. That the only purpose for which power can be rightfully exercised over any member of a civilized community,

against his will, is to prevent harm to others. His own good, either physical or moral, is not a sufficient warrant. He cannot rightfully be compelled to do or forbear because it will be better for him to do so, because it will make him happier, because, in the opinions of others, to do so would be wise, or even right. These are good reasons for remonstrating with him, or reasoning with him, or persuading him, or entreating him, but not for compelling him, or visiting him with any evil, in case he do otherwise. To justify that, the conduct from which it is desired to deter him must be calculated to produce evil to someone else. The only part of the conduct of any one, for which he is amenable to society, is that which concerns others. Over himself, over his own body and mind, the individual is sovereign.

(Mill 1859)

Mill's harm principle is often seen as being closer to the libertarian rather than the collectivist perspective. A minimal state is favoured over one that would seek to actively help people develop certain capabilities or attain certain levels of welfare. However, Mill's discussion is not limited to only preventing harms to others. He also argued that: 'those who are still in a state to require being taken care of by others, must be protected against their own actions as well as against external injury' (Mill 1859). So Mill recognized that the state can rightfully intervene to protect children, and other similarly vulnerable people who require protection, from, for example, damaging their own health.

Mill furthermore makes it clear that his defence of individual liberty is founded on his commitment to advancing 'utility', which can be understood as general welfare. Hence his principle is to be interpreted to allow the state to support 'joint work necessary to the interest of society' (Mill 1859) including, for example, the provision of clean water and regulations that limit working hours (Mill 1859). In the context of public health policy this provision is especially important as such policy is often directed at public goods and services.

Lastly, Mill was also clear about the importance of educating and informing people so that they can make up their own minds about important questions concerning both the public affairs of the state, and their own personal decisions as to how to lead their lives. Hence, although Mill's discussion of the harm principle shows that he would strongly oppose public health programmes which simply aim to coerce people to lead healthy lives, he would be likely to support programmes which seek to 'advise, instruct and persuade' (Mill 1859) them so that they can make informed decisions about, for example, what to eat and how to exercise.

Beyond Mill

A closer reading of Mill therefore shows that he is far more sympathetic to broader public health measures than might be thought initially. Nonetheless, for a more comprehensive framework suited to address public health issues in the 21st century, further values need to be incorporated that have played a role in ethical debates and political theory since Mill. Here, we consider first autonomy and individual consent and then equity.

The core notion underlying the concept of consent that currently features in the bioethical literature and much healthcare law and policy can be traced back to the 1947 Nuremberg Trials of German physicians (US Adjutant General's Department 1949), and it was later incorporated into the Declaration of Helsinki of the World Medical Association (WMA), and other ethical codes and laws. These codes thus established consent as a powerful and indispensable condition: any intervention that may expose someone to significant risk is morally unacceptable unless the person concerned agrees to being exposed to the risks, and, in legal terms, waives the corresponding rights. Within the clinical context, the feasibility of consent, the degree to which it is, or should be, informed, genuine, specific, or explicit, and the general conditions required for it to be ethically acceptable, have continued to be the subject of intense debate (Beyleveld and Brownsword 2007; Manson and O'Neill 2007; Nuffield Council on Bioethics 1995).

The concept of consent is rightly at the centre of the practice of clinical medicine. Consent for public health measures, however, is more complex. Public health interventions may interfere to different degrees with people's choices or liberties. For example, in the case of quarantine and isolation used to control the spread of infectious diseases, the degree of intrusion is considerable, but restricting the movement of people suspected of having a severe infectious disease, whether or not they agree with it, can be justified on the basis of the harm principle. Many other interventions do not concern this degree of intrusion, and it is important to recognize the difference between consent requirements that are relevant in the context of clinical medicine and research, and those for infringements of people's choices or liberties in the non-clinical context of public health. Often, requiring each person to consent individually to nonintrusive public health measures is almost impossible and certainly impractical. More importantly, the possible harms and restriction of liberties that are entailed by a range of public health measures may not be severe. The essential point is that a greater, more explicit justification is needed for the state to interfere in a situation where individual consent would otherwise be required due to the considerable health or other risks involved. In contrast, such justification may not be needed where an interference merely limits certain choices.

Health is not distributed evenly across the population. Further to the 1980 Black report (DHSS 1980) and the Whitehall studies (Marmot et al 1984; Marmot 1991) which paved the way for much research on the social gradient in health, the 2008 report by the WHO Commission on Social Determinants of Health emphasized the importance of the socio-economic environment and provided a wealth of empirical evidence demonstrating its effect. The report showed, for example, that a boy growing up in the deprived Glasgow suburb of Calton will live on average 28 years less than a boy born in nearby affluent Lenzie (54 vs 82 years) (WHO 2008). Often, the causes of poor health or reduced life expectancy can be traced to people jeopardizing their health through risky behaviour. But it is short-sighted to stop the analysis here, for the causes of the causes of poor health also need to be considered. And here a wide range of factors are of relevance, including education, housing, living, and working conditions, and access to health-conducive environments and health services. Often, clear inequalities exist between different socio-economic groups, as described above. But differences in age, gender, racial or ethnic background, disability, and geographical location also need to be addressed.

The UK Government has made an explicit policy commitment to reducing health inequalities. It has set national targets for reducing inequity, measured in terms of life expectancy and infant mortality. It recognizes that achievement of these targets requires that the health status of least well off groups must improve at a faster rate than those who are better off. This has clear ethical implications for policy choices.

Therefore, while Mill's initial framework can go some way towards supporting a public health framework, it still needs to be expanded, in particular to accommodate the value of the community. This value is the basis of efforts aimed at reducing socially determined health inequalities. This may raise the question of whether the Working Party advocates some form of paternalism, usually understood as the 'interference of a state or an individual with another person, against their will, and justified by a claim that the person interfered with will be better off or protected from harm' (Dworkin 2002). We suggest that it does not, principally because democratic societies have a range of different methods in place to provide mandate or authorization for particular public health measures, and because it can be questionable whether public health measures are in fact in contravention of people's individual wills. For example, while some people might prefer to opt out of the NHS, it is far from clear that many, the majority, or everybody would prefer to do so. So, the question is whether respect for the wishes of a particular group (or possibly even one single person) should be sufficient to counter arrangements that benefit a larger group of people, especially where these benefits can only be sustainably achieved through collective efforts.

The stewardship model

The concept of stewardship means that liberal states have responsibilities to look after important needs of people both individually and collectively. Therefore, states are stewards both to individual people, taking account of different needs arising from factors such as age, gender, ethnic background or socio-economic status, and to the population as a whole (WHO 2000; Jochelson 2005). In the Working Party's view, the notion of stewardship gives expression to the obligation on states to seek to provide conditions that allow people to be healthy, focusing attention, in particular, on reducing health inequalities.

Summarized below are the core characteristics that public health programmes carried out by a stewardship-guided state should have.

Concerning goals, public health programmes should:

- aim to reduce the risks of ill health that people might impose on each other;
- aim to reduce causes of ill health by regulations that ensure environmental conditions that sustain good health, such as the provision of clean air and water, safe food, and decent housing;
- pay special attention to the health of children and other vulnerable people;
- promote health not only by providing information and advice, but also with programmes to help people to overcome addictions and other unhealthy behaviours;
- aim to ensure that it is easy for people to lead a healthy life, for example by providing convenient and safe opportunities for exercise;
- ensure that people have appropriate access to medical services; and
- aim to reduce unfair health inequalities.

In terms of constraints, such programmes should:

+ not attempt to coerce adults to lead healthy lives;

+ minimize interventions that are introduced without the individual consent of those affected, or without procedural justice arrangements (such as democratic decision-making procedures) which provide adequate mandate; and

+ seek to minimize interventions that are perceived as unduly intrusive and in conflict with important personal values.

These positive goals and negative constraints are not listed in any hierarchical order, and the implementation of these principles may, of course, lead to conflicting policies. It is furthermore possible that difficulties arise from needing to reconcile multiple tensions. However, in each particular case, it should be possible to resolve these conflicts by applying those policies or strategies that achieve the desired social goals while minimizing significant limitations on individual freedom. The stewardship model therefore does not provide an off-the-shelf solution for public health policy, but it specifies clearly the areas in which justification needs to be provided. While it has a strong proceduralist element, the provisions also have substantive content which helps achieve the above-mentioned goals of public health, centred around 'preventing disease, prolonging life and promoting health through the organised efforts of society.'

Third parties

The stewardship model might be understood to address the relationship between the state and the people only. However, this would be a short-sighted interpretation. For various third parties also have a role in the delivery of public health, and they need to recognize their responsibilities. These third parties may be medical institutions, charities, businesses, or local authorities. They include, in particular, businesses producing, marketing, and selling food, alcohol, and tobacco, and others whose products and services can either contribute to public health problems or help to alleviate them.

Regarding corporate agents, sometimes the view is taken that as long as they act within the law they are behaving ethically. However, in the same way that one would not judge the ethical acceptability of actions of individuals by merely assessing whether or not they have broken the law, it is reasonable to argue that commercial companies have responsibilities beyond merely complying with legal and regulatory requirements. Recent years have seen a significant rise in respective initiatives, and many large companies publish annually the results of their corporate social responsibility activities alongside their financial reports. The extent to which such initiatives are driven by marketing strategies rather than genuine social concern is difficult to assess. The emergence of corporate social responsibility is noteworthy nonetheless: if it is not driven by companies actively reflecting on their social responsibilities it seems more than likely that consumer expectations have played an active role and created a new kind of 'ethical' demand. Corporate social responsibility clearly has a role to play in public health. But, if there is a lack of corporate responsibility, or a 'market failure', it is acceptable for the state to intervene, where the health of the population is significantly at risk.

The role of evidence

Before we consider the way in which the stewardship model can be used to guide state intervention, we need to consider the role of evidence in public health. Broadly, two types of evidence are central: evidence about causes of ill health and about the usefulness of particular interventions. Ideally, evidence should be based on peer-reviewed research, and not on preliminary results or unpublished reports. Selective use of evidence or 'policy-based evidence' (House of Commons Science and Technology Committee 2006) that has been commissioned or interpreted to support existing or planned policies is unhelpful and can lead to confusion. But even peer-reviewed evidence requires careful interpretation, as it is often incomplete, or it may be ambiguous, and usually it will be contested. Moreover, public health interventions often concern people's deeply engrained habits and personal preferences. Changing these behaviours is highly complex (National Institute for Health and Clinical Excellence 2007). Regarding evidence about the efficacy and effectiveness of promising interventions two distinct but related questions hence need to be answered: 'Can it work?' relates to the potential which different paths of action, in principle, have, to promote health or reduce harm. A further question is whether an intervention that can be shown to be efficacious in a research setting will have a similar degree of effectiveness in a particular real-world context. This has been called the 'Does it work?' (Haynes 1996) question, and may often require considerable time.

Although scientific experts may sometimes be tempted or pressured into offering precise answers to policy makers, regarding, for example, whether policy X or Y is the more effective one, the honest answer will often be 'we don't know (yet)' or 'we can only estimate the risk to within certain, sometimes wide, limits'. Claims of absolute safety or certainty should therefore generally be treated with great caution.

The ethics of policy choices in practice

The intervention ladder

Evidence and ethics are equally central in public health policy making. In order to use the stewardship model in practice the Working Party devised what was termed the 'intervention ladder', a tool for evaluating the acceptability and justification of different policy interventions to improve public health. In general, the higher the rung on the ladder at which the policy maker intervenes, the stronger the justification has to be, both in ethical terms, and with regard to the evidence about causes of good and ill health and about the potential of particular interventions to promote the former, and reduce the latter:

- **Do nothing/monitor:** At the bottom of the ladder, the policy option might be to simply 'do nothing', or merely to monitor the situation. While, in some sense, this might be the lowest rung of the ladder, it is important to realize that inaction is also in need of justification and not value-free.
- **Information:** On the next rung up, policy makers might provide information, for example through campaigns that encourage people to walk more or eat five portions of fruit and vegetables per day.

- **Enable choice:** Under this option, cycle lanes might be built, or free fruit might be provided in schools.

- **Changing the default:** while the previous steps at best appeal to people to make use of certain health-promoting activities, a slightly more intrusive option, which nonetheless respects the value of choice, would be to guide behaviour through changing what is the default policy in particular areas. For example, in a restaurant, instead of providing chips as a standard side dish (with healthier options available), menus could be changed to provide a more healthy option as standard (with chips as an option available). In this way, people would be 'nudged' (Thaler et al 2008), but not coerced, to adopt a more healthy behaviour. In another version, salt levels in ready-made food could be regulated to be very low, while enabling customers to add more salt through the provision of salt shakers at the place of purchase.

- **Incentives:** There are different ways in which choices can be guided through incentives. For example, tax breaks might be offered for the purchase of bicycles that are used as a means of travelling to work, or people can secure vouchers for taking part in exercise or weight loss programmes (Jochelson 2007).

- **Disincentives:** Means such as taxes or charges can work as strong disincentives, for example the use of cars in inner cities can be discouraged through charging schemes or limitations of parking spaces.

- **Restrict choice:** For example, banning so-called junk food from schools, while not preventing children from consuming such food outside of schools, or imposing similar limitations on food provided in work canteens.

- **Eliminate choice:** On this option, laws and regulations might be put in place that lead to the removal of what are judged to be unhealthy food ingredients, such as transfats.

The intervention ladder is a useful tool for deciding which of several policy options to prefer in a given context, and for designing policy and interventions in the first place. We have noted above that the general rule is that the higher up one moves on the ladder, the stronger the need for sound evidence. But we also noted above that evidence can sometimes be incomplete or ambiguous, and that practical constraints may mean that decisions need to be made in situations where there is lack of certainty as to which intervention the best evidence favours. Policy makers generally have limited time and resources, and issues that pose severe and urgent threats to the health of many people are rightly prioritized over those that are only 'possible threats', affect health in a relatively minor way or involve fewer people. The need for a public health intervention may be dictated by urgency, most obviously with the emergence of an epidemic of a serious infectious disease. In such situations, evidence may be patchy, albeit the need for action is strong, illustrating that tensions between ethical justification and the weight of the evidence can arise, and that the former needs to be the stronger, the weaker the latter is. Tensions may also arise between public health policies and those of other government departments, and different interventions may have different effects on particular socio-economic groups, particularly information campaigns. We explore some of these tensions next by illustrating in more detail how the Working Party applied the stewardship model and the intervention ladder for particular obesity related policies.

The public health challenge of obesity

Being overweight or obese is a risk factor for several health conditions, including diabetes, stroke, some cancers, and lung and liver problems. The number of people who are obese has increased substantially over the past few decades in the UK and in many other countries. In 2008, the UK had the highest rate of obesity in Europe, and if trends continue at a similar pace it is expected that by 2050, 60 per cent of adult men, 50 per cent of adult women and about 25 per cent of all children under 16 could be obese (Foresight 2007). The causes of obesity (and especially the causes of the causes) are complex. There are no simple solutions, or 'magic bullets', as the Government's Foresight Report on Obesity, which was published shortly before the Working Party's Report, clearly illustrated, drawing on a vast amount of evidence that had been reviewed (Foresight 2007).

Information and the corporate sector

There is a strong case for clear labelling of food so that people know what they are choosing. Readily understandable food labelling might also exert consumer pressure on manufacturers and shops to produce and stock foods or 'varieties' that are less unhealthy. At the time of writing, as at the time when the Working Party's report was published, there was no agreement by the food industry in the UK on appropriate, 'at a glance' front-of-pack labelling for the nutritional composition of food sold in shops. Two different strategies were introduced in 2005–6, focusing on Guideline Daily Amounts (GDAs) and the so-called 'traffic light' system, respectively. However, the evidence to date remains inconclusive about which scheme is likely to be more effective, although the Food Standards Agency (FSA) commissioned a formal evaluation of both models. Agreed standards on any requirements of an equivalent kind for catered food are also lacking, although the FSA recently proposed a system whereby consumers at catering outlets would be provided with nutritional information, such as calorie levels. The proposal is based on recent consumer research, which indicated that consumers would like simple and consistent information on the nutritional qualities of the food purchased at the point of sale (BBC News 2009; Food Standards Agency 2009).

The stewardship model emphasizes providing conditions that make it easy for people to lead healthy lives, paying special attention to vulnerable people and reducing causes of ill health through appropriate regulations. The Working Party therefore concluded that businesses, including the food industry, have an ethical duty to help individuals to make healthier choices, and that the composition of manufactured products, and the way they are marketed and sold needs to be reviewed. Where the market fails to uphold its responsibility, for instance in failing to provide universal, readily understandable front-of-pack nutrition labelling or in the marketing of food more generally, regulation by the government is ethically justifiable.

Information campaigns rank relatively low on the intervention ladder, and are attractive to policy makers for this reason. In considering their potential to achieve public health goals, it is particularly important to assess their implications for different socio-economic groups. There is some evidence that information strategies may actually increase social inequalities as more advantaged groups in society are more likely to avail themselves of health promotion advice (Acheson 1998; Gepkins and Gunning-Schepers 1996; National Institute of Clinical Excellence 2008; Association of Directors of Public Health 2008). In such a case, there would be a tension between two competing goals of the stewardship model (reducing inequalities and seeking to minimize intrusion). Given the clear social gradient in health regarding obesity, and given the potential for different socio-economic groups to benefit to differing degrees from front-of-package information, it is crucial to monitor the effect of any introduced schemes particularly on health inequalities between different socio-economic groups.

The Working Party was equally clear that the power of information in a different sense needed to be addressed, namely, in relation to food advertising to children, an especially vulnerable group. The group considered the protracted debates around 'watersheds' for television advertising of food and drink products high in fat, salt, and sugar (HFSS), and concluded that a proportionate level of action cannot be determined in a formulaic way. Whether to intervene is a complex decision, not least because the evidence base on where to set the watershed is incomplete. However, evidence does demonstrate clearly that children's early diet affects their health later in life, and that obesity in childhood is strongly associated with obesity in adulthood (Deckelbaum and Williams 2001). It is also clear that that children are especially vulnerable because they are more susceptible to external influences, including marketing by industry, and that they have limited control and ability to make genuine choices (American Academy of Pediatrics 2006). Moreover, HFSS products may be advertised not only on television, but also on the internet, which is typically far more difficult to regulate. In May 2007, the European Commission published a White Paper entitled *A Strategy for Europe on Nutrition, Overweight and Obesity-related Health Issues*, (European Commission 2007) which included details of a best practice model for self-regulation of food advertising for children, and the Working Party recommended that following the planned review of the EU Strategy in 2010, the European Commission should consider whether there are cases in which self-regulation of food advertising for children has proved unsatisfactory and whether more binding regulation across the EU is required.

Environmental factors

The previous examples have focused on the responsibilities of producers, marketers, and sellers of foods. Energy intake is an important part of the equation, and producing more healthy food is as important as ensuring that it is available to people of all socio-economic groups with equal ease—however, research has shown that so-called 'food deserts' exist in certain disadvantaged areas (Acheson 1998). Such areas may suffer from a dearth of outlets offering healthy food, the result being that simply living in some areas can prevent access to healthy food, and contribute to the 'mechanism by which poverty and social inequality' can cause poor health (Cummins and Macintyre 2002). In addition to optimizing energy intake, options for energy expenditure must also be given due consideration. Here, the environment established by infrastructures in towns, living and work environments play an important role. The Working Party was clear that planning decisions by central and local government should include the objective of encouraging people to be physically active. While this may entail some restrictions of people's freedoms, for instance to drive anywhere they wish to, and may therefore be seen to be ranking relatively high on the intervention ladder, these restrictions would be justified in terms of public health benefits. Furthermore, the training of architects and town planners should include measures for increasing people's physical activity through the design of buildings and public spaces. This can be viewed as analogous to the recent incorporation of the study of energy efficiency and sustainability of buildings.

Vulnerable groups

We noted above the particularly vulnerable position of children, which was also recognized in a recommendation aimed at the UK Government departments responsible for food, health, and education to develop long-term strategies for schools with the aim of preventing obesity, and changing food and exercise culture, accompanied by monitoring and follow up. However, such interventions may themselves result in harm. Data on the prevalence of obesity are a crucial part of understanding trends and the impact of interventions. Weighing and measuring young children is ethically justifiable, provided the data are anonymized and collected in a sensitive way. In particular, it is important to manage the collection of childhood obesity data in a way that minimizes the risks of stigmatization, for instance by encompassing it within a broader programme of health checks, and the Working Party recommended that the UK health departments should give consideration to how this could be best realized in practice.

One of the most difficult issues in preventing childhood obesity and responding to the weak position of children arises from cases where parents overfeed their children, and do not encourage them to exercise. If parents were to severely harm the health of their children, for example by underfeeding them, action would be taken by social services and they could be charged with neglect. In recent years there have been cases in the UK where issues of neglect were raised in relation to a child who became severely obese (BBC News 2007). In general, direct regulation of food provided to children in the home would be disproportionate, as any health benefits achieved would be outweighed by the value of private and family life. However, where severe obesity is caused by overfeeding by parents or guardians, child protection issues would be raised if the child was at risk of significant harm to health. The Working Party recognized that such scenarios present 'no-win' situations, as, either way, a non-ideal outcome would be achieved. However, this is no excuse for lack of clear policy, and the welfare of the children must not be neglected. The Working Party therefore recommended that the relevant government bodies should develop criteria for deciding when interventions, such as removing a child from their home, would be appropriate.

A similarly controversial issue relates to whether obese people should be entitled to NHS treatment in the same way as healthy people, if, the argument might go, they could have avoided becoming obese in the first place by eating less and exercising more. Due to the complexity of causes that lead to obesity, the Working Party was not persuaded by such arguments. Moreover, there is a significant risk of stigmatization and unfair 'victim-blaming', where already-disadvantaged people are held unduly responsible for their poor health state. The group therefore concluded that it would not generally be appropriate for NHS treatment of health problems associated with obesity to be denied to people simply on the basis of their obesity. However, appeals to change behaviour before or subsequent to an intervention could be justified, provided that the change would enhance the effectiveness of the medical intervention, and people were offered help to do this. On the whole, the Working Party was clear that although the case of obesity raises some valid considerations about making the most efficient use of resources at the point of providing treatment, and although difficult decisions have to be made in allocating necessarily limited resources, in terms of public health policy the focus of efforts should be on avoiding the need for treatment in the first place. This is a fairer approach, and also seems likely to be more promising in economic terms.

Conclusions

Improving public health touches on some of the most personal decisions people make about their own lives, and the lives of others. Two typical, and contradictory, attitudes people sometimes hold simultaneously are 'We don't want the nanny state interfering with our lives' and 'The Government should do more to make people healthy'. We have tried to show here, first, that such views are problematic because population health is not merely a matter of individual and government action, but is also affected significantly by third parties, such as the food and drink industry. Secondly, we sought to argue that the apparently value-free option of not interfering is in fact not what might be seen as the neutral default, but rather also a choice that requires justification. In view of the established evidence on the social gradient in health, and current and predicted future trends for obesity, not intervening is an option that simply cannot be justified by a stewardship guided state.

While the evidence on the factors influencing obesity is relatively clear, the evidence regarding what successful interventions are is far more patchy. A number of interventions have been initiated under the Department of Health's 'Healthy weight, healthy lives' strategy, a £372 million cross-government approach to tackling the causes of obesity (Department of Health and Department of Children, Schools and Families 2008). The strategy addresses many of the Council's recommendations on food labelling, advertising to children, and the promotion of physical activity. As outlined above, it is likely to be some time before any impact of these measures can be measured, but monitoring is crucial not only to determine the most successful interventions, but also to ensure that policy can be redesigned if it should emerge that, for example, labelling strategies exacerbate, rather than close the gap in health inequalities.

Bibliography

Association of Directors of Public Health (2008) *Memorandum by the Association of Directors of Public Health.* Available at: <http://www.publications.parliament.uk/pa/cm200708/cmselect/cmhealth/422/422we221.htm> (accessed 09 December 2008)

Acheson, D (1998) *Independent inquiry into inequalities in health: report.* London: The Stationery Office

American Academy of Pediatrics Committee on Communications (2006) 'Children, adolescents, and advertising' *Pediatrics* 118: 2563–9

BBC News (2007) *Child obesity 'a form of neglect',* 14 June. Available at: <http://news.bbc.co.uk/1/hi/health/6749037.stm>

BBC News (2009) *Calorie information on menus call,* 15 January. Available at: <http://news.bbc.co.uk/1/hi/health/7830343.stm>

Beyleveld, D and Brownsword, R (2007) *Consent in the law.* Oxford: Hart

Commission on Social Determinants of Health (2008) *Closing the gap in a generation: health equity through action on the social determinants of health.* Geneva: WHO

Clegg, S and Lawless, S (2008) *Comprehension and use of UK nutrition signpost labelling schemes. Interim report on qualitative phase prepared for the Food Standards Agency.* Available at: <http://www.food.gov.uk/multimedia/pdfs/quantannexa.pdf> (accessed 08 December 2008)

Cross-Government Obesity Unit, Department of Health and Department of Children, Schools and Families (2008) *Healthy weight, healthy lives: a cross-government strategy for England,* p xv. London: COI. Available at: <http://www.dh.gov.uk/en/Publicationsandstatistics/Publications/PublicationsPolicyAndGuidance/DH_082378?IdcService=GET_FILE&dID=163391&Rendition=Web> (accessed 08 December 2008)

Cummins, S and Macintyre, S (2002) '"Food deserts"—evidence and assumption in health policy making' *British Medical Jurnal* 325: 436–8

Deckelbaum, RJ and Williams, CL (2001) 'Childhood obesity: the health issue' *Obesity Research* 9: S239–43

DHSS (1980) *Inequalities in health.* London: DHSS

Dworkin, G (2002) 'Paternalism' in *Stanford encyclopedia of philosophy.* Available at: <http://plato.stanford.edu/entries/paternalism/> (accessed on 08 December 2008)

European Commission (2007) *A strategy for Europe on nutrition, overweight and obesity-related health issues.* Available at:.<http://ec.europa.eu/health/ph_determinants/life_style/nutrition/documents/nutrition_wp_en.pdf> (accessed on 08 December 2008)

Food Standards Agency (2009) *First steps in providing nutrition information for consumers eating out,* 15 January. Available at: <http://www.food.gov.uk/news/newsarchive/2009/jan/eatoutinfo>

Foresight (2007) *Tackling obesities: future choices.* London: Department of Innovation Universities and Skills. Available at: <http://www.foresight.gov.uk/Obesity/17.pdf> (accessed 08 December 2008)

Gepkens, A and Gunning-Schepers, LJ (1996) 'Interventions to reduce socioeconomic health differences: a review of the international literature' *European Journal of Public Health* 6/3: 218–26

Griffiths, S, Jewell, T, and Donnelly, P (2005) 'Public health in practice: the three domains of public health' *Public Health* 119: 907–13

Haynes, B (1999) 'Can it work? Does it work? Is it worth it?' *British Medical Journal* 319: 652–3

House of Commons Science and Technology Committee (2006) *Scientific advice, risk and evidence based policy making.* Available at: <http://www.publications.parliament.uk/pa/cm200506/cmselect/cmsctech/900/900-i.pdf> (accessed 09 December 2008)

Jochelson, K (2005) *Nanny or steward? The role of government in public health.* London: King's Fund

Jochelson, K (2007) *Paying the patient—improving health using financial incentives.* London: The King's Fund

Manson, N and O'Neill, O (2007) *Rethinking informed consent in bioethics.* Cambridge: Cambridge University Press

Marmot, M, Shipley, MJ, and Rose, G (1984) 'Inequalities in death-specific explanations of a general pattern' *The Lancet* 5: 1003–6

Marmot, MG, Davey Smith, G, Stanfield S, et al (1991) 'Health inequalities among British civil servants: the Whitehall II study' *The Lancet* 337: 1387–93

Mill, JS (1859) 'On liberty' in *On liberty and other essays* (1989) Collini S (ed), p13. Cambridge: Cambridge University Press

National Institute for Health and Clinical Excellence (2007) *Behaviour change at population, community and individual levels—NICE public health guidance 6.* London: National Institute for Health and Clinical Excellence. Available at: <http://www.nice.org.uk/nicemedia/pdf/PH006guidance.pdf> (accessed 08 December 2008)

National Institute for Health and Clinical Excellence (2008) *Select Committee on Health Written Evidence—Memorandum by the National Institute for Health and Clinical Excellence.* Available at: <http://www.publications.parliament.uk/pa/cm200708/cmselect/cmhealth/422/422we137.htm> (accessed 09 December 2008)

Nuffield Council on Bioethics (1995) *Human tissue: ethical and legal issues.* London: Nuffield Council on Bioethics

Nuffield Council on Bioethics (2007) *Public health: ethical issues.* London: Nuffield Council on Bioethics. Available at: <http://www.nuffieldbioethics.org/go/ourwork/publichealth/introduction> (accessed 08 December 2008)

Royal Colleges of Physicians of the United Kingdom (2008) *What is public health.* Available at: <http://www.fphm.org.uk/about_faculty/what_public_health/default.asp> (accessed 08 December 2008)

Thaler, RH and Sunstein, CR (2008) *Nudge: improving decisions about health, wealth, and happiness.* New Haven: Yale University Press

US Adjutant General's Department (1949) 'Directives for human experimentation' in *Nuremberg Code Trials of War Criminals before the Nuremberg Military Tribunals under Control Council Law No. 10.* Volume 2, pp 181–2. Washington, DC: US Government Printing Office. Available at: <http://ohsr.od.nih.gov/guidelines/nuremberg.html> (accessed 08 December 2008)

World Health Organization (2000) *World health report 2000.* Geneva: WHO

Part 3

Generating evidence

Chapter 12

Developing and evaluating complex interventions: an introduction to the new Medical Research Council guidance

Peter Craig, Paul Dieppe, Sally Macintyre, Susan Michie, Irwin Nazareth, and Mark Petticrew

Introduction

Complex interventions are widely used in the health service, in public health practice, and in areas of social policy that have important consequences for population health, such as education, transport, and housing. They present a number of problems for evaluators, in addition to the practical and methodological difficulties that any successful evaluation must overcome. In 2008, the Medical Research Council (MRC) published revised and updated guidance (Craig et al 2008) to help researchers and research funders to recognize and adopt appropriate methods. The full guidance, with detailed case studies of successful approaches, is available online (<http://www.mrc.ac.uk/complexinterventions guidance>). This chapter summarizes key messages for the evaluation of public health interventions, and discusses some of the issues that have been raised since the guidance was published.

What makes an intervention complex?

Complex interventions are usually described as interventions that contain several interacting components, but this is only one dimension of complexity (Box 12.1). There is no sharp boundary between simple and complex interventions. Few interventions are truly simple, although they are often treated as though they were (Francis et al 2008), but there is a wide range of complexity.

How complexity is dealt with will depend on the aims of the evaluation. A key question in evaluating complex interventions is whether they are effective in everyday practice (Haynes 1999). It is therefore important to understand the whole range of effects, and how they vary, for example among recipients or between sites. A second key question in evaluating complex interventions is *how* the intervention works: what are the active ingredients within the intervention, and how are they exerting their effect? Answers to

Box 12.1 What makes an intervention complex?

- Number of interacting components within the experimental and control interventions
- Number and difficulty of behaviours required by those delivering or receiving the intervention
- Number of groups or organizational levels targeted by the intervention
- Number and variability of outcomes
- Degree of flexibility or tailoring of the intervention permitted

Implications for development and evaluation

- A good theoretical understanding is needed of how the intervention causes change, so that weak links in the causal chain can be identified and strengthened
- Lack of impact may reflect implementation failure (or teething problems) rather than genuine ineffectiveness; a thorough process evaluation is needed to identify implementation problems.
- Variability in individual level outcomes may reflect higher level processes; sample sizes may need to be larger to take account of the extra variability, and cluster rather than individually-randomized designs considered.
- Identifying a single primary outcome may not make best use of the data; a range of measures will be needed, and unintended consequences picked up where possible.
- Ensuring strict fidelity may be inappropriate; the intervention may work better if a specified degree of adaptation to local setting is allowed for in the protocol.

this kind of question are needed to design more effective interventions and apply them appropriately across groups and settings in future (Michie and Abraham 2004).

The development-evaluation-implementation process

It is useful to think of the process of development through to implementation of a complex intervention in terms of stages, though these may not follow a linear or even a cyclical sequence (Figure 12.1)(Campbell et al 2007).

Best practice is to develop interventions systematically, using the best available evidence and appropriate theory, then to test them using a carefully phased approach, starting with a series of pilot studies targeted at each of the key uncertainties in the design, and moving on to an exploratory and then a definitive evaluation. The results should be disseminated as widely and persuasively as possible, with further research to assist and monitor the process of implementation.

In practice, evaluation takes place in a wide range of settings that constrain researchers' choice of interventions to evaluate and their choice of evaluation methods. Ideas for complex interventions emerge from various sources, which may have a significant impact on

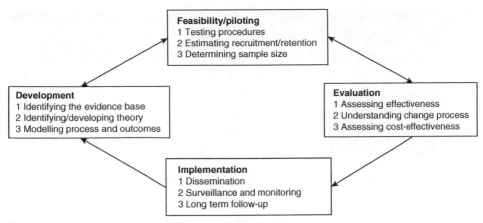

Fig. 12.1 Key elements of the development and evaluation process

how much leeway the researcher has to modify the intervention, to influence the way it is implemented, or to adopt an ideal evaluation design. Evaluation may take place alongside or after large-scale implementation, rather than starting beforehand. Strong evidence may be ignored or weak evidence taken up, depending on its political acceptability or fit with other ideas about what works. The design of Sure Start Local Programmes in England, for example, reflected a mixture of evidence about the effectiveness of early years interventions, and value judgements about the desirability of community-led approaches, which created huge problems for the evaluation (see Box 12.2). The emphasis on 'joined-up' approaches to tackling common problems such as obesity (Butland et al 2007) means that evaluators are often working in settings where traditional biomedical hierarchies of evidence are not generally accepted, and methods that are well established in other areas of health research may still be viewed with suspicion.

Researchers need to consider carefully the trade-off between the importance of the intervention, and the value of the evidence that can be gathered given these constraints. In an evaluation of the health impact of a social intervention, such as a programme of housing improvement, the researcher may have no say in what the intervention consists of, and little influence over how or when the programme is implemented, limiting the scope to undertake development work or to determine allocation. Experimental and quasi-experimental methods are slowly becoming accepted as methods of policy evaluation (Creegan and Hedges 2007; Purdon et al 2001). Even so, as Sure Start and many other recent examples show (House of Commons Health Committee 2009), there may still be political or ethical objections to using them to assess health impact, especially where the intervention provides significant non-health benefits (Thomson et al 2004). Given the cost of such interventions, evaluation should still be considered: 'best available' methods, even if they are not theoretically optimum, may yield useful results (Ogilvie et al 2006; Petticrew et al 2005).

If such methods are used, researchers should be aware of their limitations, and interpret and present the findings with due caution. Wherever possible, evidence should be

Box 12.2 Sure Start: evaluating highly complex social interventions

The evaluation of Sure Start is one of the largest ever attempted in the UK: a £20 million study of an intervention costing £1.8 billion per year by 2008. It has yielded positive evidence of effectiveness, though the early results also showed some negative effects. The design has been praised as the best possible in the circumstances, but also criticized as a second-best solution. It is an informative case study of the problems facing the evaluation of large-scale social interventions.

Sure Start Local Programmes (SSLPs) are area-based interventions to improve services for young children and their families in deprived communities in England. The programme as a whole was informed by the success of early years interventions in other countries, but the approach adopted in England differed markedly from those that worked elsewhere (for a more detailed account, see chapter 13). The first SSLPs were established in 1999. Initially the range of services was not specified; instead providers were expected to work with their local communities to determine how best to improve existing services. From 2004 onwards, the model of service delivery changed to one in which services were more tightly prescribed, with a closer focus on improving children's well-being in the most vulnerable families, and the local programmes were renamed Sure Start Children's Centres (SSCCs).

An extensive programme of evaluation research was commissioned when Sure Start was set up, and two rounds of results on the effectiveness of the scheme have been published to date. The first compared mothers and children in 150 Sure Start areas and 50 areas chosen to receive the programme, but where services had not yet been delivered. Small beneficial effects were found among the less deprived families exposed to Sure Start, but there were adverse effects on teenage mothers, lone parents, and families in workless households (Belsky et al 2006). The second round, which took place after the reorientation of SSLPs, was based on comparisons between families in 93 Sure Start areas and 72 matched non-Sure Start areas corresponding to sampling points in the Millennium Cohort Study. This time, there was no evidence of adverse effects, or of differential subgroup effects, and positive outcomes on five of the 14 measures used (Melhuish et al 2008).

The authors attribute the positive outcomes to the adoption of a more focused and prescribed model of service improvement, following the first wave of results. This claim is consistent with other evidence that such interventions tend to be more effective, but is hard to judge as the two Sure Start variants were not directly compared, and the two studies use somewhat different methods. Commentary on the evaluation, while acknowledging the thoroughness with which the researchers tried to overcome the limitations of the design, has been highly critical of the decision by the sponsoring government departments to rule out a randomized trial, to implement such a loosely specified intervention on such a large scale, and to make changes before the evaluation was complete (Academy of Medical Sciences 2007; House of Commons Science and Technology Committee 2006a; Kane 2008; Rutter 2006).

> **Sure Start: evaluating highly complex social interventions** *(continued)*
>
> Given the need to phase introduction of Sure Start over a number of years, an experimental design may have been possible, without delaying implementation. Given the uncertainty, then and now, over the effectiveness of the programmes, there was in any case no ethical imperative for rapid implementation, and the speed with which the programme was rolled out dismayed some of those involved in its development (House of Commons Science and Technology Committee 2006b). Would a randomized controlled trial have provided more definitive answers? A trial (Hutchings et al 2007) of a parenting intervention in Sure Start areas in Wales, which found consistently positive effects on both parents and children, suggests the answer is yes.

combined from a variety of sources that do not share the same weaknesses (Academy of Medical Sciences 2007). Researchers should also be prepared to explain to decision makers the need for adequate development work, the pros and cons of experimental and non-experimental approaches, and the trade-offs involved in settling for weaker methods. They should be prepared to challenge decision makers when interventions of uncertain effectiveness are being implemented in a way that would make strengthening the evidence through a rigorous evaluation difficult, or when a modification of the implementation strategy would open up the possibility of a much more informative evaluation.

Developing a complex intervention

Identifying existing evidence Before a substantial evaluation is undertaken, the intervention must be developed to the point where it can reasonably be expected to have a worthwhile effect. The first step is to identify the relevant evidence base. Unless there is a recent, high quality systematic review that covers the planned intervention, a review should be conducted, and kept up to date as the evaluation proceeds.

Identifying/developing theory The rationale for a complex intervention, the changes that are expected, and how change is to be achieved, may not be clear at the outset. A key early task is to develop a theoretical understanding of the likely process of change by drawing on existing evidence and theory, supplemented if necessary by new primary research (Michie et al 2005). This should be done whether the researcher is developing the intervention, or evaluating one that has already been developed.

Modelling process and outcomes Modelling a complex intervention prior to a full scale evaluation can provide important information about the design of both the intervention and the evaluation (Hardeman et al 2005). One useful approach is to undertake a pre-trial economic evaluation (Torgerson and Byford 2002). This may identify weaknesses and lead to refinements, or show that a full-scale evaluation is unwarranted (Eldridge et al 2005).

It is important to begin thinking about implementation at an early stage and to ask the question 'would it be possible to use this?' before embarking on a lengthy and expensive process of evaluation (Tunis et al 2002; Glasgow et al 2003).

Assessing feasibility

Evaluations are often undermined by problems of acceptability, compliance, delivery of the intervention, recruitment, and retention, and smaller-than-expected effect sizes that could be anticipated by thorough piloting (Eldridge et al 2004). A pilot study need not be a scale model of the planned mainstage evaluation, but should address the key uncertainties that have been identified in the development work. Pilot study results should be interpreted cautiously when making assumptions about the numbers required when the evaluation is scaled up. Effects may be smaller or more variable and response rates lower when the intervention is rolled out across a wider range of settings. A series of studies may be required to progressively refine the design, before embarking on a full-scale evaluation.

Evaluating a complex intervention

There are many study designs to choose from, and different designs suit different questions and different circumstances. Researchers should beware of blanket statements about what designs are suitable for what kind of intervention and make their choice on the basis of specific characteristics of the study, such as expected effect size and likelihood of selection or allocation bias. Awareness of the whole range of experimental and non-experimental approaches should lead to more appropriate methodological choices.

Assessing effectiveness Randomization is the most robust method of preventing the selection bias that occurs whenever those who receive the intervention differ systematically from those who do not, in ways likely to affect outcomes. The key advantage of randomization is that it can deal with unknown or unmeasured confounders, so the possibility of using a randomized approach should always be considered. If a conventional parallel group randomized trial is not appropriate, there are a number of other experimental designs that should be considered (Box 12.3).

If an experimental approach is not feasible, because the intervention is irreversible, necessarily applies to the whole population, or because large scale implementation is already under way, a quasi-experimental or an observational design may be considered. In some circumstances, a non-randomized design may be preferred, but the conditions under which observational methods can yield reliable estimates of effect are very limited (Box 12.4) (MacMahon and Collins 2001). Successful examples, such as the evaluation of legislation to restrict access to means of suicide (Gunnell et al 2007), reduce air pollution (Clancy et al 2002), or ban smoking in public places (Haw and Gruer 2007), tend to involve interventions with rapid, large impacts.

Measuring outcomes Researchers need to decide which outcomes are most important, and which are secondary, and how they will deal with multiple outcomes in the analysis. A single primary outcome, and a small number of secondary outcomes, is the most straightforward for statistical analysis, but may not represent the best use of the data, and may not provide an adequate assessment of the success or otherwise of an intervention which has effects across a range of domains. It is important also to consider which sources of variation in outcomes matter, and to plan appropriate subgroup analyses, or use methods that take into account the hierarchical structure of the data.

Box 12.3 Experimental designs for evaluating complex interventions

Individually randomized trials: Individuals are randomly allocated to receive either an experimental intervention, or an alternative such as standard treatment, a placebo, or remaining on a waiting list. Such trials are sometimes dismissed as inapplicable to complex interventions, but there are many variants of the basic method, and often solutions can be found to the technical and ethical problems associated with randomization.

Cluster randomized trials: Contamination of the control group, leading to biased estimates of effect size, is often cited as a drawback of randomized trials of population level interventions (Ukoumunne et al 1999), but cluster randomization, widely used in health services research, is one solution. Here, groups such as patients in a GP practice or tenants in a housing scheme are randomly allocated to the experimental or a control intervention.

Stepped wedge designs (Brown and Lilford 2006; Hall et al 1987; Stone et al 2007): The randomized stepped wedge design may be used to overcome practical or ethical objections to experimentally evaluating an intervention for which there is some evidence of effectiveness, or which cannot be made available to the whole population at once. It allows a randomized controlled trial to be conducted without delaying roll-out of the intervention. Eventually, the whole population receives the intervention, but with randomization built into the phasing of implementation

Preference trials (King et al 2005; McPherson and Chalmers 1998; Torgerson and Sibbald 1998) *and randomized consent designs* (Altman et al 1995; Torgerson and Roland 1998): Practical or ethical obstacles to randomization can sometimes be overcome by the use of non-standard designs. Where patients have very strong preferences among treatments, basing treatment allocation on patients' preferences, or randomizing patients before seeking consent, may be appropriate.

N-of-1 designs (Brookes et al 2007; Guyatt et al 1990; Guyatt et al 1988; Zucker et al 1997): Conventional trials aim to estimate the average effect of an intervention in a population, and provide little information about within or between person variability in response to interventions, or about the mechanisms by which effective interventions achieve change. N-of-1 trials, in which individuals undergo interventions with the order or scheduling decided at random, can be used to assess between and within person change, and to investigate theoretically predicted mediators of that change.

Understanding processes Process evaluation can provide valuable insight into why an intervention fails unexpectedly or has unanticipated consequences, or why a successful intervention works and how it can be optimized. A process evaluation nested inside a trial can be used to assess fidelity and quality of implementation, clarify causal mechanisms, and identify contextual factors associated with variation in outcomes (Oakley et al 2006). However, it is not a substitute for an outcome evaluation, and interpreting the results is crucially dependent on knowledge of outcomes.

Box 12.4 Choosing between randomized and non-randomized designs

Size and timing of effects: randomization may be unnecessary if the effects of the intervention are so large or immediate that confounding or underlying trends are unlikely to explain differences in outcomes before and after exposure (Black 1996; Glasziou et al 2007). It may be inappropriate if the changes are very small, or take a very long time to appear. In these circumstances a non-randomized design may be the only feasible option, in which case firm conclusions about the impact of the intervention may be unattainable.

Likelihood of selection bias: randomization is needed if exposure to the intervention is likely to be associated with other factors that influence outcomes. Post-hoc adjustment is a second-best solution, its effectiveness limited by errors in the measurement of the confounding variables (Deeks et al 2003; MacLehose et al 2003) and the difficulty of dealing with unknown or unmeasured confounders.

Feasibility and acceptability of experimentation: randomization may be impractical if the intervention is already in widespread use, or if key decisions about how it will be implemented have already been taken, as is often the case with policy changes and interventions whose impact on health is secondary to their main purpose.

Cost: if an experimental study is feasible, and would provide more reliable information than an observational study, but would also cost more, the additional cost should be weighed against the value of having better information.

Assessing cost-effectiveness An economic evaluation should be conducted, as this will make the results more useful for decision makers. Ideally, economic considerations should be taken fully into account in the design of the evaluation, to ensure that the cost of the study is justified by the potential benefit of the evidence it will generate, appropriate outcomes are measured, and the study has enough power to detect economically important differences (Torgerson and Byford 2002; Torgerson and Campbell 2000). The main purpose of an economic evaluation is estimation rather than hypothesis testing (Briggs 2000), so it is worth including one even if the study cannot identify clear cost or effect differences, so long as the uncertainty is handled appropriately (Briggs 1999).

Implementation and beyond

Getting evidence into practice Publication in peer-reviewed journals is essential, and should follow established guidelines, but it is only part of an effective implementation strategy. Asking relevant questions at the outset is critical, as is an active and systematic approach to encouraging uptake of results (NHS Centre for Reviews and Dissemination, 1999). Successful implementation depends on changing the behaviour of people in the implementing organizations. It requires a scientific understanding of the behaviours that need to change, the factors maintaining current behaviour, the barriers and facilitators of change, and the expertise to develop strategies to achieve change based on this under-standing (Michie et al 2005). Implementation research teams should therefore include a behavioural scientist. The evidence base for effective implementation remains limited, but some promising approaches have been identified (Box 12.5).

Surveillance, monitoring and long term outcomes A single study is unlikely to provide a comprehensive, generalizable account of the effectiveness of an intervention. Few trials are powered to detect rare adverse events (Collins and MacMahon 2001; MacMahon and Collins 2001), and even pragmatic studies with wide inclusion criteria are likely to take place in a population and range of settings that are to some extent self-selected. Effects may be smaller and more variable once the intervention is implemented more widely, and unanticipated consequences may emerge. Long-term follow-up may be needed to deter-mine whether outcomes predicted by interim or surrogate measures do occur, or that short term changes persist. Although long-term follow-up of complex interventions is uncommon, such studies can be highly informative (Wortman, 1995). Researchers should consider how to measure rare or long-term impacts, for example through routine data sources and record linkage, or by recontacting study participants. Plans for the collection of appropriate outcome data, and obtaining appropriate consents, should be built into the study design at the outset.

Further questions

There are many other important questions that arise in the development and evaluation of complex questions (Box 12.6).

Unresolved issues

The guidance is intended to help researchers, research funders, and other decision makers to make appropriate methodological and practical choices. We have primarily aimed our

---

Box 12.5 Promising approaches to implementation

- Involve stakeholders in the choice of question and design of the research to ensure relevance (Glasgow et al 2003; Tunis et al 2002).

- Provide evidence in an integrated and graded way: reviews not individual studies, and variable length summaries that allow for rapid scanning (Lavis et al 2005).

- Take account of context, and identify the elements relevant to decision making, such as benefits, harms, and costs (Lavis et al 2005).

- Make recommendations as specific as possible (Michie and Johnston 2004).

- Use a multifaceted approach involving a mixture of interactive rather than didactic educational meetings, audit, feedback, reminders, and local consensus processes (Bero et al 1998).

Box 12.6 Further questions for evaluators

1 *Have you conducted a systematic review?* Systematic reviews of complex interventions can be problematic because of the wide scope for variation in the way interventions are delivered (Herbert and Bo 2005). To make sense of variability in outcomes, you will need to classify variants of a complex intervention in terms of components, mode of delivery, or intensity, and this will require a theoretically informed understanding of the mechanisms of change underlying the intervention.

2 *Who is the intervention aimed at?* If your intervention is seeking to achieve change at more than one level, eg by influencing a practice-level outcome, such as prescribing behaviour, as well as patient outcomes, then you will need to measure processes and outcomes at each level. Changes in practice, such as the adoption of guidelines or implementation of service frameworks, are not necessarily mirrored by improvements in patient outcomes (Moher et al 2001).

3 *Can you describe the intervention fully?* A complex intervention should strive to be reproducible. This means that you need a full description of the intervention, and an understanding of its components, so that it can be delivered faithfully during the evaluation, allowing for any planned variation (see Question 4 below), and so that others can implement it outside your study (Abraham and Michie 2008).

4 *How variable is the intervention: between sites, over time, etc?* 'Fidelity' is not straightforward in relation to complex interventions (Bellg et al 2004; Leventhal and Friedman 2004). In some evaluations, eg those seeking to identify active ingredients within a complex intervention, strict standardization may be required and controls put in place to limit unplanned variation (Farmer et al 2007). But some interventions are deliberately designed to be adapted to local circumstances (Patton et al 2003; Patton et al 2006). You need to be clear about how much change or adaptation would be permissible (Hawe et al 2004a; Hawe et al 2004b), and record any variation in the intervention so that fidelity can be assessed in relation to the degree of standardization required by the study protocol.

5 *Can you describe the context and environment in which the evaluation is being undertaken?* What works in one setting may not be as effective, or may even be harmful, elsewhere (Campbell et al 2007). The impact of a new intervention will depend on what provision already exists and interventions may have to be explicitly designed to fit different contexts (National Institute for Health and Clinical Excellence 2007). You should develop a good understanding of the context in which the study is being carried out, and monitor and document any significant changes.

Further questions for evaluators *(continued)*

6 *How are you going to involve users in the study?* Appropriate 'users' should be involved at all stages of the development, process, and outcome analysis of a complex intervention, as this is likely to result in better, more relevant science and a higher chance of producing implementable data. Qualitative research, as well as providing important insights into processes of change, can be a good way to involve users (Yardley et al 2006).

7 *Is your study ethical?* Ethical problems of evaluating complex interventions need careful consideration. You need to think about the ethics of the design in terms of the autonomy of participants and informed consent, and think through the possible effects of their trial in terms of effects on communities, possible adverse events, etc, in as robust a way as possible before seeking ethical approval.

8 *What arrangements will you put in place to monitor and oversee the evaluation?* Any complex intervention study should have appropriate data monitoring and steering committees (Prescott et al 1999) and comply with the relevant ethical and research governance frameworks. Appropriate in this context means proportionate to the various risks involved, such as risks to participants, financial risks, etc. Whatever framework you adopt, it is important to incorporate an element of independent oversight, as difficult decisions may need to be taken about the direction and even continuation of the study.

9 *Have you reported your evaluation appropriately?* Where possible, evaluations should be reported according to established guidelines, as this will help to ensure that the key information is available for replication studies, systematic reviews, and guideline development. A common failing in the reporting of complex intervention studies is an inadequate description of the intervention (Michie and Abraham 2004; Glasziou et al 2008), but work is under way to improve this, for example through the WIDER recommendations (see <http://interventiondesign.co.uk/>). A range of reporting guidelines (<http://www.equator-network.org>), is now available, covering non-drug trials (Boutron et al 2008), pragmatic trials (Zwarenstein et al 2008), and non-randomized studies (DesJarlais and Lyles 2004), which should lead to improvement.

key messages at researchers. Perhaps the key message for research funders is the need to invest in developmental studies prior to large-scale evaluations, and in implementation research. Both forms of investment will help to ensure a better return on investment in evaluation studies. The key message for policy makers and other public health decision makers is the need to incorporate evaluation considerations in the implementation of new initiatives, and wherever possible to allow for an experimental or a high quality non-experimental approach to the evaluation of significant initiatives where there is uncertainty about their effectiveness.

We recognize that many of the issues that we have covered are still debated, that methods will continue to develop, and that further experience will accumulate. Responses to publication of the new guidance have raised a number of important issues, which we briefly address below, in the form of a dialogue.

1 Your definition of complex interventions is too broad. It scarcely leaves anything out—what use is that?

Although, as we say in the guidance, few interventions are truly simple, what often happens in practice is that much of the complexity is ignored for the sake of generating clear-cut answers to relatively simple questions—for example, to satisfy regulatory authorities that a new drug is safe and effective, or to answer questions about efficacy. In an efficacy trial, many components of a complex intervention might be balanced between the trial arms, so that differences in outcome are clearly attributable to a particular component of interest. But this approach will fail to capture sources of variation, within and between patients, practitioners, sites, etc, that are important for considering whether and how to implement on a larger scale. The dangers of too narrow a definition may therefore be greater than those of a broader one, and much of our guidance is aimed at encouraging researchers to think carefully about which aspects of complexity, or which sources of variation, they need to address.

2 Your definition of complex interventions is too narrow. You've neglected 'complexity science' and the valuable insights it can bring to understanding the interaction between complex interventions and complex systems (Kernick 2008).

Many of the claimed insights, such as sensitive dependence on local context and unanticipated consequences, while important, are not dependent on the theory. Others, such as phase transitions and non-linear effects, seem to rely on metaphorical parallels between the kind of complexity that some mathematicians and physicists are interested in, and the kind that health researchers are faced with. Complexity science has enjoyed a minor vogue in the health sciences for some years, and there is no shortage of advocacy or theoretical justification for the approach (Kernick 2006; Shiell et al 2008). What is lacking is an account of how to engineer the theory into the nuts and bolts of a practical research strategy, let alone any empirical underpinning in the form of successful evaluations using these methods (even the advocates admit these are lacking at present) (Anderson 2008). It will be interesting to see whether such examples begin to emerge over the next few years, but there are good reasons to doubt that an approach focused on unexpected and unpredictable changes, rather than on those whose uncertainty can be quantified, will turn out to be practically useful.

3 You haven't addressed the problem of inter-individual variability in the evaluation of complex interventions. Understanding who benefits (and who is harmed) is what matters, not just the average effect.

That's true, though this is primarily an issue for individual-level treatments rather than public health interventions directed at whole populations. The corollary for population interventions (see (1) above) is the need to take into account variation between places or sites of intervention. It is not a problem specific to complex interventions, but one that affects all trials, as authors such as Senn have stressed. A trial in which 70% of patients benefit from a new treatment will not usually distinguish between 70% of recipients benefiting all the time and all benefiting 70% of the time (Senn 2004). There is therefore a danger that evidence of benefit for a new treatment will lead to the replacement of existing treatments that are more effective, or less harmful, for some people. Skilful application of evidence-based practice, rather than rote following of guidance is one solution (Kendrick et al 2008). Others are carefully planned subgroup analyses, crossover and n-of-1 trials to provide a better understanding of within and between subject variability.

4 Population health strategies nowadays are trying to tackle problems such as obesity, which affect a large fraction of the population. We can't rely on individual level interventions, so the top priority is for methods that can address large-scale environmental interventions in a rigorous way.

We agree, though this is not a new problem. At the peak of the tobacco epidemic, smoking was more common than obesity is now. The problems of evaluating large-scale interventions are primarily political and practical, rather than methodological. The challenge is to ensure that such interventions are developed and tested on an appropriate scale, prior to large-scale roll-out, and that if real uncertainty remains about their effectiveness (or about possible harms), implementation is planned in a way that allows for further testing, and adaptation on the basis of emerging evidence. In this respect, the recent record of large scale public health interventions in the UK is patchy at best (House of Commons Health Committee 2009). There are some good examples, such as the evaluation of the legislation to ban smoking in public places in Scotland, but there are others, such as Sure Start, where huge resources have been invested in interventions that are extremely difficult to evaluate in a rigorous way—as those involved in developing and evaluating the programme acknowledge (see Box 12.2). There are signs too that the lessons of recent experiences are not being learnt. The health trainers' initiative, announced in the 2004 *Choosing Health* White Paper, has been rolled out in phases since 2006, suggesting opportunities for evaluation to be built in, possibly using a stepped wedge design, but an evaluation contract was only awarded in 2008 (Department of Health 2008b). Likewise the Healthy Towns initiative, announced in 2008, is being implemented in a way that makes for good publicity but also makes evaluation difficult, by focusing resources on a small number of highly selected, heterogeneous intervention sites in which a diverse array of co-interventions are taking place (Department of Health 2008a).

5 If you tried to follow the guidance faithfully, evaluation would be impossibly time-consuming and costly. There is a risk that the best will be the enemy of the good.

That would be worrying if people were reluctant to intervene in the absence of perfect evidence, or unwilling to use anything but the most ideal trial designs. But the chief risk, we suggest, is in the other direction: that costly new interventions lacking a good evidence base will continue to be rolled out in ways that preclude an evaluation rigorous enough to make either a worthwhile reduction in the uncertainty around decisions to continue with the programme, or a useful contribution to refining the design or delivery of the intervention.

We acknowledge that it costs more and takes longer to develop and evaluate interventions thoroughly, and we don't imagine that all of our recommendations can be applied in all cases. But the guidance has to be as complete as we can make it. We urge evaluators, policy makers, etc, to use it judiciously and implement the best possible evaluation designs given time and cost constraints, but also to recognize that where there is real uncertainty about the effectiveness or safety of expensive interventions, they should be implemented in ways that allow good evaluation. Given the range of evaluation designs, this is not as hard as some people think, and it is very encouraging that the recent Health Select Committee Report on Health Inequalities made this one of its main recommendations (House of Commons Health Committee 2009). The choice is not between doing nothing until the evidence is ready, or going for broke and hoping that observational data will show that the programme works; the challenge is to phase implementation so that useful comparisons can be made. Evaluations using approaches such as the stepped wedge design, are surprisingly rare, and much greater use should be made of them.

There is great interest in the development and evaluation of complex interventions, and a healthy debate. We hope this will continue, that progress will be made, and that we can incorporate good examples of successful evaluations using high quality, innovative approaches in future revisions of the guidance.

Acknowledgements

Preparation of the guidance on which this chapter is based was supported by the MRC Health Services and Public Health Research Board and the MRC Population Health Sciences Research Network. The original MRC framework, published in 2000 (Campbell et al 2000) has been highly influential, but much valuable experience has accumulated since it was published. The chapter authors formed a writing group convened following a PHSRN-funded workshop in London on 15–16 May 2006 which concluded that it was timely to revise and update the guidance. Workshop participants (see <http://www.populationhealthsciences.org>) and others with an interest in the evaluation of complex interventions (for a full list see <http://www.mrc.ac.uk/complexinterventionsguidance>) were invited to comment on a draft of the revised guidance, which was also reviewed by members of the MRC Health Services and Public Health Research Board. We are grateful to all of the above for their help, and also to participants in a seminar at the UK Society for Behavioural Medicine Annual Conference, 6–7 January 2009, who raised many of the issues we discuss in the final section of the chapter.

Bibliography

Abraham, C, and Michie, S (2008) 'A taxonomy of behaviour change techniques used in interventions' *Health Psychology* 27: 379–87

Academy of Medical Sciences (2007) *Identifying the environmental causes of disease: how should we decide what to believe and when to take action.* London: Academy of Medical Sciences

Altman, D, Whitehead, J, Parmar, M, Stenning, S, Fayers, P, and Machin, D (1995) 'Randomised consent designs in cancer clinical trials' *European Journal of Cancer* 31A/12: 1934–44

Anderson, R (2008) 'New MRC guidance on evaluating complex interventions' *British Medical Journal* 337: a1937

Bellg, AJ, Borrelli, B, Resnick, B, Hecht, J, Sharp Minicuchi, D, Ory, M, et al (2004) 'Enhancing treatment fidelity in health behaviour change studies: best practices and recommendations from the NIH Behaviour Change Consortium' *Health Psychology* 23/5: 543–51

Belsky, J, Melhuish, E,Barnes, J, Leyland, AH, Romaniuk, H, and National Evaluation of Sure Start Research Team (2006) 'Effects of Sure Start local programmes on children and families: early findings from a quasi-experimental, cross sectional study' *British Medical Journal* 332: 1476–81

Bero, LA,Grilli, R,Grimshaw, J, Harvey, E, Oxman, AD, and Thomson, MA (1998) 'Closing the gap between research and practice: an overview of systematic reviews of interventions to promote the implementation of research findings' *British Medical Journal* 317: 465–8

Black, N (1996) 'Why we need observational studies to evaluate the effectiveness of health care' *British Medical Journal* 312: 1215–18

Boutron, I, Moher, D, Altman, D, Scultz, K, and Ravaud, P (2008) 'Extending the CONSORT statement to randomized trials of non-pharmacologic treatment: explanation and elaboration' *Annals of Internal Medicine* 148: 295–309

Briggs, A (1999) 'Handling uncertainty in economic evaluation' *British Medical Journal* 319: 120

Briggs, A (2000) 'Economic evaluation and clinical trials: size matters' *British Medical Journal* 321: 1362–3

Brookes, ST, Biddle, L, Paterson, C, Woolhead, G, and Dieppe, P (2007) '"Me's me and you's you": exploring patients' perspectives of single patient (n-of-1) trials in the UK' *Trials* 8: 10–18

Brown, CA and Lilford, RJ (2006) 'The stepped wedge trial design: a systematic review' *BMC Medical Research Methodology* 6: 54–63

Butland, B, Jebb, S, Kopelman, P, McPherson, K, Thomas, S, Mardell, J, et al (2007) *Tackling obesities: future choices—project report.* London: Government Office for Science

Campbell, M, Fitzpatrick, R, Haines, A, Kinmonth, AL, Sandercock, P, Spiegelhalter, D, et al (2000) 'Framework for the design and evaluation of complex interventions to improve health' *British Medical Journal* 321: 694–6

Campbell, NC, Murray, E, Darbyshire, J, Emery, J, Farmer, A, Griffiths, F, et al (2007) 'Designing and evaluating complex interventions to improve health care' *British Medical Journal* 334: 455–9

Clancy, L, Goodman, P, Sinclair, H, and Dockery, DW (2002) 'Effect of air pollution control on death rates in Dublin, Ireland: an intervention study' *Lancet* 360: 1210–14

Collins, R and MacMahon, S (2001) 'Reliable assessment of the effects of treatment on mortality and major morbidity' *Lancet* 357: 373–80

Craig, P, Dieppe, P, Macintyre, S, Michie, S, Nazareth, I, and Petticrew, M (2008) *Developing and evaluating complex interventions: new guidance.* London: Medical Research Council

Creegan, C and Hedges, A (2007) *Towards a policy evaluation service: developing infrastructure to support the use of experimental and quasi-experimental methods.* Ministry of Justice Research Series. London: Ministry of Justice

Deeks, J, Dinnes, J, D'Amico, R, Sowden, A, Sakarovich, C, Song, F, et al (2003) 'Evaluating non-randomised intervention studies' *Health Technology Assessment* 7/27

Department of Health (2008a) '£30 million "Healthy Towns" kickstart Change4life' London: COI News Distribution Service

Department of Health (2008b) *Health trainers—review to date—July 2008.* London: Department of Health

DesJarlais, DC, and Lyles, C (2004) 'Improving the reporting quality of nonrandomized evaluations of behavioural and public health interventions: the TREND statement' *American Journal of Public Health* 94/3: 361–6

Eldridge, S, Ashby, D, Feder, G, Rudnicka, AR, and Ukoumunne, OC (2004) 'Lessons for cluster randomized trials in the twenty-first century: a systematic review of trials in primary care' *Clinical Trials* 1: 80–90

Eldridge, S, Spencer, A, Cryer, C, Pearsons, S, Underwood, M, and Feder, G (2005) 'Why modelling a complex intervention is an important precursor to trial design: lessons from studying an intervention to reduce falls-related injuries in elderly people' *Journal of Health Services Research and Policy* 10/3: 133–42

Farmer, A, Wade, A, Goyder, E, Yudkin, P, French, D, Craven, A, et al (2007) 'Impact of self-monitoring of blood glucose in the management of patients with non-insulin treated diabetes: open parallel group randomised trial' *British Medical Journal* 335: 132–9

Francis, JJ, Johnston, M, Burr, J, Avenell, A, Ramsay, C, Campbell, MK, et al (2008) 'Importance of behaviour in interventions' Letter. *British Medical Journal* 337: a2472

Glasgow, RE, Lichtenstein, E, and Marcus, AC (2003) 'Why don't we see more translation of health promotion research into practice? Rethinking the efficacy-to-effectiveness transition' *American Journal of Public Health* 93/8: 1261–7

Glasziou, P, Chalmers, I, Rawlins, M, and McCulloch, P (2007) 'When are randomised trials unnecessary? Picking signal from noise' *British Medical Journal* 334: 349–51

Glasziou, P, Meats, E, Heneghan, C, and Shepperd, S (2008) 'What is missing from descriptions of treatments in trials and reviews?' *British Medical Journal* 336: 1472–4

Gunnell, D, Fernando, R, Hewagama, M, Priyangika, W, Konradsen, F, and Eddleston, M (2007) 'The impact of pesticide regulations on suicide in Sri Lanka' *International Journal of Epidemiology* 36: 1235–42

Guyatt, G, Sackett, D, Adachi, J, Roberts, R, Chong, J, Rosenbloom, D, et al (1988) 'A clinician's guide for conducting randomised trials in individual patients' *Canadian Medical Association Journal* 139/6: 497–503

Guyatt, G, Heyting, A, Jaeschke, R, Keller, J, Adachi, J, and Roberts, R (1990) 'N-of-1 randomised trials for investigating new drugs' *Controlled Clinical Trials* 11: 88–100

Hall, A, Inskip, H, Loik, F, Day, N, and The_Gambia_Hepatitis_Study_Group (1987) 'The Gambia Hepatitis Intervention Study' *Cancer Research* 47: 5782–7

Hardeman, W, Sutton, S, Griffin, S, Johnston, M, White, A, Wareham, NJ, et al (2005) 'A causal modelling approach to the development of theory-based behaviour change programmes for trial evaluation' *Health Education Research* 20/6: 676–87

Haw, SJ and Gruer, L (2007) 'Changes in exposure of adult non-smokers to secondhand smoke after implementation of smoke-free legislation in Scotland: national cross sectional survey' *British Medical Journal* 335: 549–52

Hawe, P, Shiell, A, and Riley, T (2004a) 'Complex interventions: how "out of control" can a randomised trial be?' *British Medical Journal* 328: 1561–3

Hawe, P, Shiell, A, Riley, T, and Gold, L (2004b) 'Methods for exploring intervention variation and local context within a cluster randomised community intervention trial' *Journal of Epidemiology and Community Health* 58: 788–93

Haynes, B (1999) 'Can it work? Does it work? Is it worth it? The testing of healthcare interventions is evolving' *British Medical Journal* 319: 652–3

Herbert, RD and Bo, K (2005) 'Analysis of quality of interventions in systematic reviews' *British Medical Journal* 331: 507–509

House of Commons Health Committee (2009) *Health inequalities. Third report of session 2008–09*. London: The Stationery Office

House of Commons Science and Technology Committee (2006a) *Scientific advice, risk and evidence-based policy making. Seventh report of session 2006*. Volume 1 Report together with formal minutes. London: House of Commons

House of Commons Science and Technology Committee (2006b) *Minutes of evidence taken before the Science and Technology Committee enquiry on scientific evidence, risk and evidence: how the government handles them*. Uncorrected transcript of oral evidence, 24 May 2006, Norman Glass. London: House of Commons

Hutchings, J, Gardner, F, Bywater, T, Daley, D, Whitaker, C, Jones, K, et al (2007) 'Parenting intervention in Sure Start services for children at risk of developing conduct disorder: pragmatic randomised controlled trial' *British Medical Journal* 334: 678–82

Kane, P (2008) 'Sure Start local programmes in England' *The Lancet* 372: 1610–11

Kendrick, T, Hegarty, K, and Glasziou, P (2008) 'Interpreting research findings to guide treatment in practice' *British Medical Journal* 337: a1499

Kernick, D (2006) 'Wanted: new methodologies for health services research. Is complexity theory the answer?' *Family Practice* 3: 385–90

Kernick, D (2008) 'Guidelines perpetuate inappropriate methods' Letter. *British Medical Journal* 337: 1128

King, M, Nazareth, I, Lampe, F, Bower, P, Chandler, M, Morou, M, et al (2005) 'Impact of participant and physician intervention preferences on randomised trials' *Journal of the American Medical Association* 293/9: 1089–99

Lavis, J, Davies, H, Oxman, A, Denis, J-L, Golden-Biddle, K, and Ferlie, E (2005) 'Towards systematic reviews that inform healthcare management and policy-making' *Journal of Health Services Research and Policy* 10/Suppl 1: 35–48

Leventhal, H and Friedman, MA (2004) 'Does establishing fidelity of treatment help in understanding treatment efficacy? Comment on Bellg et al (2004)' *Health Psychology* 23/5: 452–6

MacLehose, R, Reeves, B, Harvey, I, Sheldon, T, Russell, I, and Black, A (2003) 'A systematic review of comparisons of effect sizes derived from randomised and non-randomised studies' *Health Technology Assessment* 4/34

MacMahon, S and Collins, R (2001) 'Reliable assessment of the effects of treatment on mortality and major morbidity, II: observational studies' *The Lancet* 357: 455–62

McPherson, K, and Chalmers, I (1998) 'Incorporating patient preferences into clinical trials—information about patients' preference must be obtained first' *British Medical Journal* 317: 78

Melhuish, E, Belsky, J, Leyland, AH, Barnes, J, and National Evaluation of Sure Start Research Team (2008) 'Effects of fully established Sure Start Local Programmes on 3 year old children and their families living in England: a quasi-experimental observational study' *The Lancet* 372: 1641–7

Michie, S and Abraham, C (2004) 'Interventions to change health behaviours: evidence-based or evidence-inspired?' *Psychology and Health* 19/1: 29–49

Michie, S and Johnston, M (2004) 'Changing clinical behaviour by making guidelines specific' *British Medical Journal* 328: 343–5

Michie, S, Johnston, M, Abraham, C, Lawton, R, Parker, D, and Walker, A (2005) 'Making psychological theory useful for implementing evidence-based practice: a consensus approach' *Quality and Safety in Healthcare* 14: 26–33

Moher, M, Yudkin, P, Wright, L, Turner, R, Fuller, A, Schofield, T, et al (2001) 'Cluster-randomised controlled trial to compare three methods of promoting secondary prevention of coronary heart disease in primary care' *British Medical Journal* 322: 1–7

National Institute for Health and Clinical Excellence (2007) '*Behaviour change at population, community and individual levels. NICE Public Health Guidance*. London: NICE

NHS Centre for Reviews and Dissemination (1999) 'Getting evidence into practice' *Effective Healthcare* 5/1

Oakley, A, Strange, V, Bonell, C, Allen, E, Stephenson, J, and Ripple Study Team (2006) 'Process evaluation in randomised controlled trials of complex interventions' *British Medical Journal* 332: 413–16

Ogilvie, D, Mitchell, R, Mutrie, N, Petticrew, M, and Platt, S (2006) 'Evaluating health effects of transport interventions: methodologic case study' *American Journal of Preventive Medicine* 31/2: 118–26

Patton, G, Bond, L, Butler, H, and Glover, S (2003) 'Changing schools, changing health? Design and implementation of the Gatehouse Project' *Journal of Adolescent Health* 33: 231–9

Patton, GC, Bond, L, Carlin, JB, Thomas, L, Butler, H, Glover, S, et al (2006) 'Promoting social inclusion on schools: a group-randomized trial of effects on student health risk behaviour and well-being' *American Journal of Public Health* 96/9: 1582–7

Petticrew, M, Cummins, S, Ferrell, C, Findlay, A, Higgins, C, Hoy, C, et al (2005) 'Natural experiments: an underused tool for public health' *Public Health* 119: 751–7

Prescott, R, Counsell, C, Gillespie, W, Grant, A, Russell, I, Kiauka, S, et al (1999) 'Factors that limit the quality, number and progress of randomised controlled trials' *Health Technology Assessment* 3/20

Purdon, S, Lessof, C, Woodfield, K, and Bryson, C (2001) *Research methods for policy evaluation*. Department for Work and Pensions Research Working Papers. London: Department for Work and Pensions

Rutter, M (2006) 'Is Sure Start an effective preventive intervention?' *Child and Adolescent Mental Health* 11/6: 135–41

Senn, S (2004) 'Individual response to treatment: is it a valid assumption?' *British Medical Journal* 329: 966–8

Shiell, A, Hawe, P, and Gold, L (2008) 'Complex interventions or complex systems? Implications for health economic evaluation' *British Medical Journal* 336: 1281–3

Stone, S, Slade, R, Fuller, C, Charlett, A, Cookson, B, Teare, L, et al (2007) 'Early communication: does a national campaign to improve hand hygiene in the NHS work? Initial English and Welsh experience from the NOSEC study (National Observational Study to Evaluate the CleanYourHands Campaign)' *Journal of Hospital Infection* 66/3: 293–6

Thomson, H, Hoskins, R, Petticrew, M, Ogilvie, D, Craig, N, Quinn, T, et al (2004) 'Evaluating the health effects of social interventions' *British Medical Journal* 328: 282–5

Torgerson, D and Roland, M (1998) 'Understanding controlled trials: what is Zelen's design?' *British Medical Journal* 316: 606

Torgerson, D and Sibbald, B (1998) 'Understanding controlled trials: what is a patient preference trial?' *British Medical Journal* 316: 360

Torgerson, D and Campbell, M (2000) 'Cost effectiveness calculations and sample size' *British Journal of General Practice* 321: 627

Torgerson, D and Byford, S (2002) 'Economic modelling before clinical trials' *British Medical Journal* 325: 98

Tunis, SR, Stryer, DB, and Clancy, CM (2002) 'Practical clinical trials: increasing the value of research for decision-making in clinical and health policy' *Journal of the American Medical Association* 290/12: 1624–32

Ukoumunne, OC, Gulliford, MC, Chinn, S, Sterne, JAC, Burney, PGJ, and Donner, A (1999) 'Methods in health service research: evaluation of health interventions at area and organisation level' *British Medical Journal* 319: 376–9

Wortman, PM (1995) 'An exemplary evaluation of a program that worked: the High/Scope Perry Preschool Project' *American Journal of Evaluation* 16/3: 257–65

Yardley, L, Donovan-Hall, M, Francis, K, and Todd, C (2006) 'Older people's views of advice about falls prevention: a qualitative study' *Health Educ. Res.* 21/4L: 508–17

Zucker, D, Schmid, C, McIntosh, M, D'Agostino, R, Selker, H, and Lau, J (1997) 'Combining single patient (n-of-1) trials to estimate population treatment effects and to evaluate individual patient responses to treatment' *Journal of Clinical Epidemiology* 50/4: 401–10

Zwarenstein, M, Treweek, S, Gagnier, JJ, Altman, D, Tunis, SR, Haynes, B, et al (2008) 'Improving the reporting of randomised trials: an extension of the CONSORT statement' *British Medical Journal* 337: a2390

Chapter 13

Child health and well-being in the early years: the National Evaluation of Sure Start

Edward Melhuish, Jay Belsky, and Jacqueline Barnes

Introduction

The Labour election victory of May 1997 provided an opportunity to change policy. The intention was to place the improvement of people's lives at the centre of government strategy. The Government wanted to break the cycle whereby disadvantaged children repeated their parents' experiences of poor education, physical and mental ill-health, and poverty.

At this time the notion of 'joined-up' services was in vogue, and Prime Minister Tony Blair commented in the Foreword to the first Comprehensive Spending Review of his tenure (Blair 1998) that 'We have looked at key problems across government. The old departmental boundaries often do not work. Provision for young children—health, childcare, support—will be co-ordinated across departments so that when children start school they are ready to learn.'

Here we describe the development of the Sure Start Programme for children and report the findings of the national evaluation. This has been a key component of the Government's policy to breaking the cycle of deprivation.

Cross-cutting review of services for children: the evidence base

A cross-cutting review was established to deal with services for young children. It was to consider all available evidence and produce policy recommendations for counteracting the cycle of disadvantage. Research evidence from American early intervention programmes that were rigorously evaluated by means of randomised controlled trials proved especially influential in this review, which concluded that model early intervention programmes involving high quality childcare provision, whether started in infancy (Abecedarian Project, Ramey and Campbell 1991) or at three years of age (Perry Pre-school Project, Schweinhart et al 1993), enhanced the development of disadvantaged children. Also of developmental benefit were high-quality home visiting programmes designed to deliver parent education and family support (Olds et al 1999). Moreover, where quasi-experimental studies had rigorous methodology, they produced similar results. Small-scale tightly controlled interventions had produced larger effects than the more extensive large-scale interventions, such as the Chicago Child-Parent Centers (Reynolds et al 2001) and Head Start (Karoly et al 1998). Nevertheless, the impact of large-scale interventions was still substantial, producing worthwhile benefits for children, families, and communities.

The cross-cutting review contained a wide-ranging analysis of the state of services and made a number of recommendations and conclusions including the following (Treasury 1998): (1) The earliest years in life were the most important for child development, and very early development was much more vulnerable to adverse environmental influences than had previously been realized. (2) Multiple disadvantage for young children was a severe and growing problem, with such disadvantage greatly enhancing the chances of social exclusion later in life. (3) The quality of service provision for young children and their families varied enormously across localities and districts, with uncoordinated and patchy services being the norm in many areas. Services were particularly dislocated for the under-fours—an age group that tended to get missed by other government programmes. (4) The provision of a comprehensive community-based programme of early intervention and family support which built on existing services could have positive and persistent effects, not only on child and family development but also in helping break the intergenerational cycle of social exclusion, possibly leading to significant long-term gain to the Exchequer.

When it came to making recommendations, the review argued that while there was no single blueprint for the ideal early interventions, they should be: (1) two-generational, involving parents as well as children; (2) non-stigmatizing, avoiding labelling 'problem families'; (3) multifaceted, targeting a number of factors, not just, for example, education or health or parenting; (4) persistent, lasting long enough to make a real difference; (5) locally driven, based on consultation with and involvement of parents and local communities; and (6) culturally appropriate and sensitive to the needs of children and parents.

It was argued also that a range of services should ideally be integrated to support the complex and varied physical, developmental, and emotional needs of young children and families. Such services should be easily accessible and backed up by outreach to offer support in the home. In essence, a programme was to be *area-based*, with *all* children under four and their families living in a prescribed area being clients of the local programme, with the right to a say in the services provided.

Creating Sure Start (Local Programmes)

The findings of the Cross-Departmental review were incorporated into the 1998 Comprehensive Spending Review that delineated future government expenditure. On 14 July 1998, the Chancellor of the Exchequer introduced the plan for what would be known as Sure Start (to become Sure Start Local Programmes and later Sure Start Children's Centres), aiming to bring together quality services for children under four and their parents—nursery, childcare, and playgroup provision, and pre-natal and other health services. A total of £542 million became available to be spent over three years, with £452 million designated for England so that there would be 250 programmes by 2001–02, supporting about 187,000 children, or 18% of all poor children under four. This commitment and investment transformed early years services in the UK, while representing a relatively small contribution from the perspective of Treasury—just 0.05% of public expenditure.

The Sure Start Unit (SSU) responsible for administering the new initiative was cross-departmental, involving many ministries, though the principal departments involved were Health and Education. Guidance for local programmes (SSU 1998) laid out how Sure Start Local Programmes (SSLPs) were to be a completely new way of working, were meant to bring 'joined-up' services of health, childcare and play, early education, and parental support to families with a child under four years of age. SSLPs were to coordinate, streamline, and add value to existing services in the local-programme area, including signposting to existing services; involve parents; avoid stigma; ensure lasting support by linking with services for older children; be culturally appropriate and sensitive to particular needs; be designed to achieve specific objectives relating to Sure Start's overall objectives; and promote accessibility for all local families, later changed to 'promote the participation of all local families in the design and working of the programme'.

The first SSU guidance also outlined the core services that all SSLPs were to provide: (1) outreach and home visiting; (2) support for families and parents; (3) support for good quality play, learning and childcare experiences for children; (4) primary and community health care and advice about child health and development and family health; and (5) support for people with special needs, including help getting access to specialized services. Programmes were directed to provide outreach for hard-to-reach families and could add extra services to suit local needs, such as debt counselling, employment, and benefits' advice.

Community control was to be exercised through local partnerships. Initially, service providers in a deprived area were invited to submit a bid for SSLP funding. A partnership of local stakeholders had to be constituted and this partnership needed to draw up a plan for a local programme, nominating a lead agency. These partnerships were to be at the heart of the initiative and bring together everyone concerned with children in the local community, including health, social services, education, the private sector, the voluntary sector, and parents. Thus, partnerships were to provide community input in the design of SSLPs and, as a consequence, even though core services were required, no specification was provided of how they would be delivered, only what they should aim to achieve. Funding was to flow from the SSU directly to programmes, that could act largely independently of local government, although local government departments including education and social services would typically be part of the partnership.

The speed of SSLP funding was to some extent overwhelming for staff unused to such resources, and services were slow to reach operational status. Despite this slower-than-expected start, and without any evidence of success, the Treasury, in its 2000 Spending Review, expanded the programme—doubling the planned number of local programmes from 250 by 2002 to over 500 by 2004, thereby more than doubling expenditure to almost £500 million by 2003–04! The expanded SSLP initiative was to reach one third of poor children under four years of age.

Thus it was that SSLPs became a cornerstone of the UK Government's campaign to reduce child poverty and social exclusion. SSLPs were to serve *all* children under four and their families in a prescribed area. This area-based strategy allowed the relatively efficient delivery of services to those living in deprived areas without stigmatizing those receiving services: disadvantaged areas were targeted, but within the area the service was universal.

As a consequence of the local autonomy central to the community control of SSLPs, they did not have a prescribed 'protocol' of services to promote adherence to a prescribed model even though they had a set of core services to deliver. Thus, each SSLP had freedom to improve and create services as they saw fit, with general goals and some specified targets (eg reduce incidence of low birth weight, improve language development of young children), but without specification of exactly how services were to be delivered. This contrasted markedly with interventions with clear models of provision and demonstrable effectiveness that formed the basis of the research evidence justifying the creation of Sure Start. Even though research evidence was critical to winning the argument for increased Early Years' expenditure, it was largely overlooked in the detailed planning for and actual operation of programmes, despite entreaties to local programmes that their services be 'evidence based'.

National Evaluation of Sure Start

The Treasury's involvement with Sure Start was central to the creation of the programme and the changes to it that have occurred and they required a rigorous evaluation. Following competitive tender, the National Evaluation of Sure Start (NESS) was commissioned in early 2001 to undertake a multifaceted evaluation of SSLPs, addressing (1) the nature of the communities in which SSLPs were situated; (2) the ways in which SSLPs were implemented; (3) the impact of SSLPs on children, families, and communities; and (4) the cost-effectiveness of SSLPs. In addition, NESS was charged with (5) providing technical support to local programmes so that each could undertake its own local evaluation to inform service development.

The great diversity amongst SSLPs posed particular challenges for evaluation in that there were not several hundred programmes delivering one well-defined intervention, but several hundred unique and multifaceted interventions operating in different places. In the evaluation, NESS used a variety of strategies to study the first 260 SSLPs that were rolled out, in particular studying children and families in 150 of these with great intensity. These included the gathering of administrative data already available on the small geographic areas that defined SSLP communities (eg census data, police records, work and pension records); developing geographical information systems that allowed the collating of information in non-standard geographic units (SSLP areas); conducting surveys of SSLPs dealing with many aspects of SSLPs; carrying out face-to-face and telephone interviews with programme managers, programme employees, and parents about the operation of their local programme; and conducting a large-scale survey of child and family functioning in thousands of households in SSLP areas, and in SSLP-to-be areas.

The Evaluation up to 2006

While NESS had many components, most attention focused on the evaluation of impact upon children and families. In the evaluation tender the Government ruled out the possibility of a randomized controlled trial. It appeared that politicians were unwilling to give up control of which areas would receive the initiative. Hence NESS adopted a quasi-experimental design, involving multi-level modelling, in its impact evaluation. The first phase of impact evaluation compared the functioning of thousands of 9- and 36-month-old children and their families living in 150 SSLP communities across England with counterparts living in 50 communities destined to eventually become SSLP areas but that had not yet done so. Results proved somewhat disappointing to the Government, as evidence of both small positive and negative effects emerged (NESS 2005a; Belsky et al 2006). Whereas the relatively less disadvantaged of the predominantly disadvantaged families living in SSLP areas benefited somewhat from the programme, adverse effects emerged for the most disadvantaged families. Specifically, non-teen mothers (86% of sample) engaged in less negative parenting when living in SSLP areas rather than the comparison communities and, apparently as a result, their three-year-old children exhibited fewer behaviour problems and greater social competence (ie, SSLP→Parenting→Child). Children in SSLP areas living in workless households (39%) or in lone-parent families (36%) or born to teenage mothers (14%), however, scored lower than their counterparts in comparison communities on verbal ability, with those born to teenage mothers also manifesting more behaviour problems and less social competence. Consideration of these findings along with other NESS reports on implementation (eg Tunstill and Alnock 2007) raised the possibility that in many SSLP areas those families most in need and also hardest to reach were receiving fewer services than they would have, had they been in areas without SSLPs. Although this possibility was never confirmed definitively, it did lead to changes in programme emphasis (see below).

While there was limited early impact of programmes overall, the impact evaluation revealed that programmes differed widely in their effectiveness for child and family outcomes. Therefore, further work investigated variation amongst programmes.

Programme variability

One of the strengths of the NESS research design was that it afforded the opportunity to illuminate the conditions that might have made some SSLPs more effective than others. Detailed information across a number of years on each programme (Anning and Ball 2007; Meadows 2007; Tunstill and Allnock 2007) was subjected to systematic quantitative analysis (NESS 2005b; Melhuish et al 2007). Programmes could be differentiated on many dimensions including the range and balance of services, providing quality training for staff, exercising effective leadership and management, and having effective strategies for identifying families in the community, to name just several of 18 distinct dimensions of implementation subject to quantitative scoring. Programmes that tended to be rated as high on realizing one of these dimensions tended to score high on the others, so that there were essentially better and more poorly implemented programmes. When NESS looked at how these implementation differences related to outcomes it emerged that better implemented programmes yielded somewhat greater benefits for children and families. While the evidence was by no means overwhelming, it was consistent with theory about the conditions under which programmes should prove most effective and provided guidance as to what it takes to generate the kinds of benefits that SSLPs were intended to achieve. In addition there was some evidence that programmes led by health agencies had some advantages, possibly reflecting their better access to birth records and health visitors providing a ready-made home-visiting service that was generally accepted by disadvantaged families.

Community-level change

SSLPs varied not only in the manner in which services were provided but also at a more fundamental level, by the nature of the geographical area being served. A defining feature of the Sure Start initiative was that it was area-based, founded on the premise that communities, not just children and/or families, should be the target of intervention. Ultimately, the view was that children and families could be affected by the programme both directly, via services encountered, and indirectly, via community changes that derived from the programme (eg reductions in crime, feelings of cohesion, and changed 'local norms' about parenting). Reflecting this focus on community change, NESS documented the status of communities served by SSLPs over time, created a typology to represent their variability (Barnes et al 2005), and examined the relationship between any changes and programme operations. A large number of community characteristics were tracked over five years, drawing on a wide variety of administrative data sources (Barnes 2007a; 2007b). It was possible to link these data with the very particular areas that were defined by local Sure Start partnership boards using geographic information systems strategies (Frost and Harper 2007). Community changes were chronicled from 2000/01 to 2004/05 and compared with changes taking place in England over the same period of time (Barnes 2007b; Barnes et al 2007). It would have been preferable to compare change in SSLP areas to data from similarly disadvantaged neighbourhoods without Sure Start, but annual information on most of the indicators in question was not available in a sufficiently detailed format. However, the statistical comparison with change in England has proved instructive.

Over the five-year period (2001 to 2005) covered by the NESS analysis of the local contexts in which SSLPs operated, some improvements in SSLP areas were detected, though many simply mirrored trends in England and few could be linked in a straightforward way to factors such as the length of time that the SSLP had been in operation or other programme characteristics. For instance, changes were generally not related to the amount spent per child. However, some changes could be associated with other aspects of the local area, either other local services in terms of the number of other 'area-based initiatives', to the extent of deprivation relative to other SSLP areas, to the proportion of the population that were from minority ethnic groups, or to the variability within the area in housing or deprivation. Overall, the SSLP areas became home to more young children over time while the proportion living in households totally dependent on benefits, or in receipt of benefits indicating a job seeker or someone on a low wage, decreased markedly. For instance, the average proportion of children under four living in 'workless' households in SSLP areas dipped just below 40%, having started out at 45% in 2000/01. On average one third were living in a household in receipt of Income Support, down from 39%. These average levels were still much higher than the England rates (22% and 18%), but revealed important improvements though there was vast variability between the SSLP areas in these factors.

Some aspects of crime and disorder in SSLP areas also changed for the better, notably burglary and exclusions of both primary age and secondary age children from school, as well as unauthorized absences from schools. Moreover, children from 11 upwards demonstrated improved academic achievement, particularly when there are other area-based initiatives operating locally. There was not an identifiable improvement in the achievement of younger children, but examination of change over time was complicated by alterations in the manner by which national tests were administered during the five years, changing from group testing to teacher ratings.

While infant health did not improve over the period of study, reductions in emergency hospitalizations of young children (aged 0 to 3) for severe injury and for lower respiratory infection provided some potential indication that more families in SSLP areas may be accessing routine health care, at GP surgeries or child health clinics, supported by possibly more 'joined-up' working between health and social services. In addition, a decrease in the rate of low birth weight infants was identified in areas typified by proportionately more families from the Indian subcontinent, though their rate was still high in comparison to other SSLP neighbourhoods. Increases in the health screening of young children apparently occurred in SSLP areas over time, as the percentage of children identified with special educational needs or eligible for benefits related to disability increased across the five-year study period.

Ongoing policy developments in Sure Start

The policy-making process did not stand still while the evaluation was being carried out (Melhuish and Hall 2007). In fact the early NESS results contributed to a fundamental change in the structure of SSLPs. Also influential were the results of another Government-sponsored research project, the Effective Provision of Pre-school Education (EPPE) (Sylva, Melhuish, Sammons, Siraj-Blatchford and Taggart 2004), showing that a particular type of early-years' provision, integrated Children's Centres, was particularly beneficial to children's development. Evidence from both NESS and EPPE thus proved central in changing SSLPs into Children's Centres. This was announced in 2005 alongside a move to transfer the new Sure Start Children's Centres into Local Authority control. This transfer of control from central to local government was politically inspired to ensure that Sure Start Children's Centres became embedded within the welfare state by government statute and would thus be difficult to eradicate by any future government.

Also, concern about child protection that had been mounting in the 1990s reached a crisis with the horrific case of Victoria Climbié, who, despite being supposedly monitored by several agencies (health, social services, police, etc), was tortured and murdered in 2000. This triggered a major governmental review, which emphasized the importance of high quality work and research by all relevant professionals, so interagency collaboration and training was once again stressed. This resulted in a series of government reports, including 'Every Child Matters' (HM Government 2003; 2004a, b) which set out plans to reform and improve children's services. These plans were incorporated into the Children Act (HM Government 2004c), which set out a new framework for children's services, ensuring accountability and partnership at local level.

Within a similar time-frame, various reports on children's health care criticized the long-term neglect of children's services and led to a National Service Framework (Department of Health and Department for Education and Skills 2004). It was probably the most comprehensive exposition of child health policy anywhere, reflecting a very broad view of what is meant by health. It endorsed previous policy developments in the fields of early detection, child mental health, and child protection, reinforcing guidance on inter-disciplinary collaboration. The concepts underpinning Sure Start were strongly supported for future policy.

These changes meant that from April 2006, local authorities became the accountable body for the whole Children's Centre programme, and health agencies were legally obliged to cooperate in the provision of services within Children's Centres. The spend on Children's Centres and the associated programmes was £1.3 billion in 2005–06. For 2006–07 £1.7 billion was provided to local authorities for Children's Centres. For 2007–08, £1.8 billion was set aside. This represented four times the amount spent on equivalent services in 2001–02. Sure Start thus became a significant part of the Welfare State. As then Prime Minister Blair (2006) stated:

> Sure Start is one of the government's greatest achievements. It is a programme that gives antenatal advice, and early-years help for children who need it. It is a vital source of learning to parents who often find work on the back of it; and a community facility that becomes a focal point for local health, childcare and educational networks. It has become a new frontier of a changing welfare state.

Latest NESS results

The longitudinal phase of the impact evaluation compared thousands of children first seen at age nine months and again at age three living in SSLP areas with those involved in a large UK cohort study, the Millennium Cohort Study (MCS), who were not living in SSLP areas. This second phase took place nearly three years after the first phase. By this time the three-year-olds and families living in SSLP areas had not only been exposed to more mature SSLP programmes and for longer periods of their lives than those included in the first phase, but probably to programmes that had learned a lot from prior experience, including from the first set of national evaluation findings. Also, ongoing policy changes (see above) had altered the nature of programmes that were now Sure Start Children's Centres.

In order to compare children and families from non-SSLP areas as similar as possible to those in the SSLP areas studied, areas containing MCS children but not having SSLPs

were selected by propensity score matching (Rubin 1997) for having similar area characteristics to SSLPs based on 85 variables from the Indices of Multiple Deprivation (IMD)
and the 2001 Census. For initial comparisons, the SSLP sample was restricted to those
children/families residing in areas most like the non-SSLP areas; this involved excluding
the most disadvantaged SSLP areas due to the absence of comparably deprived areas in
the MCS sample. Thus, the samples included 5,883 children/families in 93 (of the original
150) SSLP areas and 1,879 children/families in 72 non-SSLP areas. In secondary analyses
children/families from SSLP areas excluded from the initial analyses were compared with
those in the 93 SSLP areas in the initial analyses. The results of this second phase of evaluation showed that families in SSLP areas benefited from SSLPs. Parents in SSLP areas
relative to those in non-SSLP areas reported using more services, engaging in more devel-
opmentally facilitative parenting and having children who are socially more competent.
Also, children were more likely to have received all recommended immunizations and to
be less likely to have accidental injuries. However, these latter two benefits associated with
SSLPs may have resulted from time of measurement effects, hence they cannot be accepted
as SSLP effects (NESS 2008; Melhuish, Belsky, Leyland, Barnes, and NESS research team,
2008). In addition, contrary to the earlier NESS (2005) results, all effects associated with
SSLPs were beneficial, and these beneficial effects appeared to apply in all sub-populations
and all SSLP areas.

The latest results of the NESS impact evaluation differed markedly from those found
earlier (Belsky et al 2006; Belsky and Melhuish 2007; NESS 2005). Whereas the earlier
findings indicated that the most disadvantaged three-year-old children and their families
(ie, teen parents, lone parents, workless households) were doing less well in Sure Start
areas, while somewhat less disadvantaged children and families benefited (ie, non-teen
parents, dual parent families, working households), the current phase of the impact
evaluation provided almost no evidence of adverse effects of Sure Start programmes.
Indeed, the Sure Start effects appeared generalizable across population subgroups
(eg workless households, teen mothers) for two reasons: (1) In general, there were almost
no consistent differences in effects of Sure Start programmes for particular subgroups
and, (2) there was almost no consistent evidence that children and families in the
most disadvantaged Sure Start areas, which had more of the most disadvantaged families,
functioned more poorly than children and families in somewhat less disadvantaged Sure
Start areas.

Various explanations can be offered for the dramatic difference in results between the
earlier 2005 findings and the current results. Differences could have occurred because of
methodological differences. Nevertheless, although there is no way to determine whether
methodological variations account for the differences in findings across the two phases of
the NESS impact evaluation, it seems eminently possible that the contrasting results accurately reflect the contrasting experiences of SSLP children and families in the two phases.
Whereas those three-year-olds enrolled in the first phase were exposed to relatively
immature programmes—and probably not for their entire lives—the three-year-old children and their families participating in the second phase were exposed to more mature
and better developed programmes throughout the entire lives of the children. Also, these

latter children and families were exposed to programmes that had the opportunity to learn from the results of the earlier study, especially with respect to the need for greater effort to be made to reach the most vulnerable households. In sum, differences in the amount of exposure to these programmes and the quality of Sure Start programmes may well account for both why the first phase of impact evaluation revealed some adverse effects of the programme for the most disadvantaged children and families and why the second phase of evaluation revealed beneficial effects for almost all children and families living in Sure Start areas.

Conclusions

Sure Start has been undergoing evolutionary change since its inception in 1999. To some extent evaluation results have influenced this process. The early results indicated that lack of specification of how goals are to be achieved in service delivery leads to great diversity with many ineffective programmes. Later developments have tightened up guidelines and the nature of service delivery considerably and also staff themselves have developed and become better trained and more proficient. However, there is scope for extensive further development. The contrast between the latest and earlier findings suggests that children and families may be having increased exposure to Sure Start programmes (Children's Centres) that have become more effective, and indicates that early interventions may improve the life chances of young children in deprived areas. Hence the developments in Sure Start seem to have borne some fruit in that the latest impact results are encouraging, and indicate the beneficial effects of SSLPs are spreading. Nonetheless, it is clear that further developments are desirable. In the meantime it will be some time before the longer term goals of the programme can be realized, and hence the final verdict on Sure Start awaits further evaluation.

Bibliography

Anning, A and Ball, M (2007) 'Living with Sure Start: human experience of an early intervention programme' in J Belsky, J Barnes, and E Melhuish (eds), *The National Evaluation of Sure Start: does area-based early intervention work?*, pp 97–112. Bristol, UK: The Policy Press

Barnes, J (2007a) 'Targeting deprived areas: the nature of the Sure Start Local Programme neighbourhoods' in J Belsky, J Barnes, and E Melhuish (eds), *The National Evaluation of Sure Start: does area-based early intervention work?*, pp 25–44. Bristol, UK: The Policy Press

Barnes, J (2007b) 'How Sure Start Local Programme areas changed' in J Belsky, J Barnes, and E Melhuish (eds), *The National Evaluation of Sure Start: does area-based early intervention work?*, pp 173–94. Bristol, UK: The Policy Press

Barnes, J, Belsky, J, Broomfield, KA, Dave, S, Frost, M, Melhuish, E, and the NESS Research Team (2005) 'Disadvantaged but different: variation among disadvantaged communities in relation to child and family well-being' *Journal of Child Psychology and Psychiatry* 46: 952–62

Barnes, J, Cheng, H, Frost, M, Harper, G, Howden, B, Lattin-Rawstrone, R, Sack, C, and the NESS Team (2007) *Changes in the Characteristics of Sure Start Local Programme Areas in Rounds 1 to 4 between 2000/2001 and 2004/2005*. London: DCSF

Belsky, J, Barnes, J, and Melhuish, E (eds) (2007) *The National Evaluation of Sure Start: does area-based early intervention work?* Bristol, UK: The Policy Press

Belsky, J and Melhuish, E (2007) 'Impact on Sure Start Local Programmes on children and families' in J Belsky, J Barnes, and E Melhuish, E (eds), *The National Evaluation of Sure Start: does area-based early intervention work?*, pp 133–54. Bristol, UK: The Policy Press

Belsky, J, Melhuish, E, Barnes, J, Leyland, AH, Romaniuk, H, and the NESS Research Team (2006) 'Effects of Sure Start Local Programmes on children and families: early findings from a quasi-experimental, cross-sectional study' *British Medical Journal* 33: 1476–578

Blair, T (1998) 'Foreword' in HM Treasury, *Modern public services for Britain: investing in reform. Comprehensive spending review: new public spending plans 1999–2002*. London: HM Treasury. Available at: <http://www.archive. official-documents.co.uk/document/cm40/4011/foreword.htm>(accessed 15 January 2007)

Blair, T (2006) 'A failed test of leadership' *The Guardian*, 5 October. London: The Guardian

Department of Health and Department for Education and Skills (2004) *National service framework for children, young people and maternity services*. London: Department of Health. Available at: <http://www.dh.gov.uk/ PolicyAndGuidance/HealthAndSocialCareTopics/ChildrenServices/ChildrenServicesInformation/fs/en> (accessed 08 July 2008)

Frost, M and Harper, G (2007) 'The challenge of profiling communities' in J Belsky, J Barnes, and E Melhuish (eds), *The National Evaluation of Sure Start: does area-based early intervention work?*, pp 45–62. Bristol, UK: The Policy Press

HM Government (2003) *Every child matters. Green paper*. Nottingham: Department for Education and Skills

HM Government (2004a) *Every child matters: change for children programme*. Nottingham: Department for Education and Skills

HM Government (2004b) *Every child matters: next steps*. Nottingham: Department for Education and Skills

HM Government (2004c) *Children Act 2004*. London: HMSO

Karoly, L, Greenwood, PW, Everingham, SS, et al (1998) *Investing in our children: what we know and don't know about the costs and benefits of early childhood interventions*. Santa Monica, CA: RAND

Meadows, P (2007) 'The costs and benefits of Sure Start Local Programmes' in J Belsky, J Barnes, and E Melhuish (eds), *The National Evaluation of Sure Start: does area-based early intervention work?*, pp 113–30. Bristol, UK: The Policy Press

Melhuish, E and Hall, D (2007) 'The policy background to Sure Start' in J Belsky, J Barnes, and E Melhuish (eds), *The National Evaluation of Sure Start: does area-based early intervention work?*, pp 3–21. Bristol, UK: The Policy Press

Melhuish, EC, Belsky, J, Anning, A, Ball, M, Barnes, J, Romaniuk, H, Leyland, A, and NESS Research Team (2007) 'Variation in Sure Start Local Programme implementation and its consequences for children and families' *Journal of Child Psychology and Psychiatry* 48: 543–51

Melhuish, E, Belsky, J, Leyland, A, Barnes, J, and the NESS Research Team (2008) 'Effects of fully-established Sure Start Local Programmes on 3-year-old children and their families living in England: a quasi-experimental observational study' *Lancet* 372: 1641–7

NESS Research Team (2005a) *Early impacts of Sure Start Local Programmes on children and families. Surestart Report 13*. London: DfES. Available at: <http://www.ness.bbk.ac.uk/documents/activities/impact/1183.pdf> (accessed 08 July 2008)

NESS Research Team (2005b) *Variation in Sure Start Local Programmes effectiveness: early preliminary findings. Surestart Report 14*. London: DfES. Available at: <http://www.ness.bbk.ac.uk/documents/activities/impact/1184. pdf> (accessed 08 July 2008)

NESS Research Team (2008) *The impact of Sure Start Local Programmes on three year olds and their families. Surestart Report 27*. London: DCSF. Available at: <http://www.ness.bbk.ac.uk/documents/activities/impact/41.pdf> (accessed 08 September 2008)

Olds, DL, Henderson, CR, Kitzman, H, Eckenrode, JJ, Cole, RE, and Tatelbaum, RC (1999) 'Prenatal and infancy home visitation by nurses: recent findings' *Future of Children* 9: 44–66

Ramey, CT and Campbell, FA (1991) 'Poverty, early childhood education, and academic competence: the abecedarian experiment' in AC Huston (ed), *Children in poverty: child development and public policy*, pp 190–221. Cambridge, MA: Cambridge University Press

Reynolds, AJ, Temple, JA, Robertson, DL, and Mann, EA (2001) 'Long-term effects of an early childhood intervention on educational achievement and juvenile arrest: a 15-year follow-up of low-income children in public schools' *Journal of American Medical Association* 285: 2339–46

Rubin, DB (1997) 'Estimating causal effects from large datasets using propensity scores' *Annals of Internal Medicine* 127: 757–63

Schweinhart, LJ, Barnes, H, and Weikhart, D (eds) (1993) *Significant benefits: the High/Scope Perry Pre-school Study through age 27*. Ypsilanti, Michigan: High/Scope Press

Sure Start Unit (1998) *Sure Start: guide for trailblazer programmes*. London: Department for Education and Employment

Sylva, K, Melhuish, E, Sammons, P, Siraj-Blatchford, I, and Taggart, B (2004) *Effective pre-school provision*. London: Institute of Education

Treasury, HM (1998) *Comprehensive spending review: cross departmental review of provision for young children*. London: HM Stationery Office. Available at: <http://www.archive.official-documents.co.uk/document/cm40/4011/401122.htm> (accessed on 08 July 2008)

Tunstill, J and Alnock, D (2007) 'Sure Start Local Programmes: an overview of the implementation task' in J Belsky, J Barnes, and E Melhuish (eds), *The National Evaluation of Sure Start: does area-based early intervention work?*, pp 79–96. Bristol, UK: The Policy Press

Chapter 14

Smoking cessation interventions

Robert West and Lion Shahab

Aims of this chapter

This chapter aims 1) to describe all the main interventions that are believed to promote smoking cessation, 2) to show why statements about effectiveness will always require semi-quantitative judgements that go beyond the current 'hard' evidence, and 3) to give estimates of effectiveness based on that evidence. It includes population level interventions such as tax increases and clinical interventions such as use of nicotine replacement therapy. The chapter also presents a model describing how smoking cessation interventions work. It begins with examination of why developing and implementing smoking cessation interventions is such a major public health priority.

The need for interventions to promote smoking cessation

Cigarette smoking is estimated to kill approximately 5 million people worldwide each year (World Health Organization 2002); on current projections this will rise to 10 million by 2020 (World Health Organization 2002). It is the leading preventable cause of premature death worldwide. Half of all smokers who do not stop are killed by their smoking, each one losing an average of approximately 20 years of life (Doll et al 2004). Smokers, whether or not they die prematurely, spend more of their lives with disability and diseases of old age. Table 14.1 lists the fatal and non-fatal diseases to which smoking contributes.

Smoking prevalence varies widely between different countries (Mackay and Eriksen 2006) and between different sociodemographic groups within countries, particularly across gender with smoking prevalence being very low in women in some countries (Mackay and Eriksen 2006). A full statistical analysis of factors that account for variation in smoking prevalence in different countries has not been carried out. However, price and availability of cigarettes, taboos against smoking, level of promotional activity of tobacco companies, level of understanding and salience of the health risks from smoking, presence of measures to restrict situations in which people can smoke, and availability of effective interventions to help with cessation would all be expected to play a role.

There are four main potential targets for reducing tobacco-related harm: 1) Preventing initiation of tobacco use, 2) increasing permanent cessation of use, 3) reducing the harm from continued tobacco use (eg through switching to less harmful products), and 4) reducing exposure to tobacco toxins in non-users. Cessation is extremely effective at mitigating the harm caused by smoking. It almost halts the rising risk of lung cancer,

Table 14.1 Fatal and serious non-fatal disorders for which tobacco use is a known or probable cause or exacerbating factor (from West 2006a)

Smoking	Vascular dementia
Cancer of the lung	Macular degeneration
Cancer of the larynx	Cataract
Cancer of the oesophagus	Hearing loss
Cancer of the oropharynx	Infertility
Cancer of the kidney	Spontaneous abortion
Cancer of the cervix	Stillbirth
Cancer of the pancreas	Low birth weight
Cancer of the stomach	SIDS[1]
Cancer of the bladder	Low back pain
Leukemia	Osteoporosis
COPD[2]	Tuberculosis
Pneumonia	Type II diabetes
Asthma attacks	Peptic ulcer disease
Coronary heart disease	Surgical complications
Aortic aneurism	
Cerebrovascular disease	**Smokeless tobacco use**
Peripheral vascular disease	Cancer of the oropharynx

Sources: All (US Department of Health and Human Services 2004) except vascular dementia (Roman 2005), macular degeneration (Seddon et al 2006), low back pain (Power et al 2001), tuberculosis (Watkins and Plant 2006), diabetes (Meisinger et al 2006), and smokeless tobacco (Critchley and Unal 2003).
[1]Sudden Infant Death Syndrome,
[2]Chronic obstructive pulmonary disease

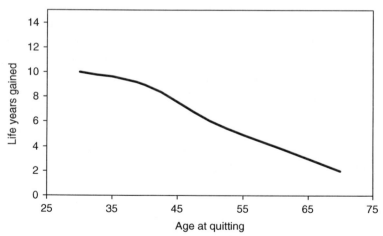

Fig. 14.1 Average years of life saved by stopping smoking at different ages. Data from Doll et al (2004).

radically slows progression of chronic obstructive pulmonary disease, and reduces the risk of cardiovascular disease (USDHHS 1990). From Doll and Peto's large study of British doctors (Doll et al 2004) we can estimate that each year of smoking that is prevented after the age of 40 adds approximately 3 months of life expectancy (Figure 14.1). People who stop smoking before the age of 40 have a life expectancy that is near normal because it appears to take about two decades of smoking to build up a substantial health risk. Interventions are clearly needed to get as many smokers as possible to stop as early as possible.

How interventions that promote smoking cessation work

Any deliberate change in behaviour pattern involves making a personal rule that one will behave differently and then adhering to that rule. Thus there are two parts of the process: making the 'change rule' and then 'implementing it'. Smoking cessation involves initiating a 'quit attempt' and then maintaining abstinence. Initiation and maintenance are influenced by different factors and interventions may act differentially on each of them (West in press-b).

'Initiating a quit attempt' means making a rule not to smoke from that point in time onwards. A simple model of deliberate human behaviour is that people decide to do things when the desire[1] to do them at that moment exceeds the desire to do something else or not to do them (West in press-b). This means that the rate of quit attempts in a population over a period of time will be related to the strength and frequency of feelings of desire to stop smoking and that *interventions will promote quit attempts to the extent that they raise the strength and/or frequency of smokers' desire to stop smoking*. There are potentially many ways of achieving this including creating feelings of concern over health effects and cost, making it inconvenient to smoke, giving direct advice to smokers to stop, increasing feelings that stopping is achievable, and incentivizing cessation (see later). Preventing tobacco companies from putting forward positive messages about smoking could also play a role.

Once the 'no smoking' rule is in place, desire to obey the rule (what one might call 'resolve') opposes the desire to smoke (West in press-b). If the latter is too strong on any given occasion, the rule will be suspended and the smoker 'lapses'. Either immediately or, more commonly, after repeated lapses, the rule is abandoned and the smoker is said to have 'relapsed'. Evidence indicates that risk of relapse to smoking is extremely high in the first week of a quit attempt and then reduces. Thus the risk of relapse in an unaided quit attempt goes from 75% in the first week to less than 1% by the 26th week (Hughes et al 2004).

After the quit attempt has been initiated, it appears that the strength of prior desire to quit has a negligible bearing on the chances of relapse (West et al 2001). Likelihood of relapse seems to be mainly determined by: 1) strength and frequency of 'urges' (immediate feelings of need) to smoke which arise largely out of dependence on nicotine and events in the social and physical environment that trigger these urges and 2) current strength of countervailing motivation. Thus, *interventions will reduce the rate of relapse to the extent that they reduce the strength and frequency of urges to smoke, and increase the resolve not to smoke and the capacity to implement that resolve*. This can be achieved in a

---

[1] 'Desire' here refers to feelings of 'wanting' or 'needing' something which can vary in strength from weak to extremely strong (West R 2006b).

number of ways but usually focuses on medication and 'behavioural support'. Medication primarily targets 'nicotine dependence' to reduce the need to smoke. Behavioural support is more wide ranging in its goals. It has four objectives: 1) to help smokers to find ways of minimizing the need to smoke, 2) to maximise their desire not to smoke, 3) to maximize their capacity to resist the need to smoke, and 4) to help them optimize their use of other forms of assistance such as medication (West in press-b).

Figure 14.2 shows a two-pronged approach to increasing the rate of smoking cessation. Increasing the rate of quit attempts involves targeting the desire to stop by raising concerns about smoking, giving direct advice etc; increasing the success of quit attempts involves reducing the strength and frequency of urges to smoke and bolstering the resolve not to smoke.

Figure 14.3 shows a 'route to quit' model using data from England giving the percentages of smokers trying to quit and using different approaches that would be expected to affect their chances of success. This model can be used to predict the likely effects of focusing on different quitting parameters. For example, a 20% increase in the percentage of smokers trying to quit in a given year would have a greater effect than a 20% increase in the use of behavioural support which in turn would have a greater effect than a 20% increase in the effectiveness of behavioural support. This is because the numbers of people affected in each case are very different. This does not mean, however, that resources should be put exclusively into generating quit attempts as it fails to consider the needs of the more nicotine dependent smokers who cannot quit without help. A comprehensive strategy to promote smoking cessation must address all aspects of the problem.

Types of intervention to promote smoking cessation

There are many different ways of classifying behaviour change interventions. Table 14.2 shows one that is based on the simple model of behaviour change used in this chapter.

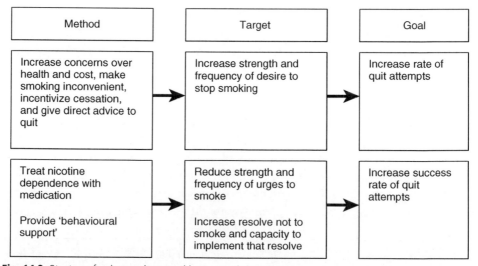

Fig. 14.2 Strategy for increasing smoking cessation rates

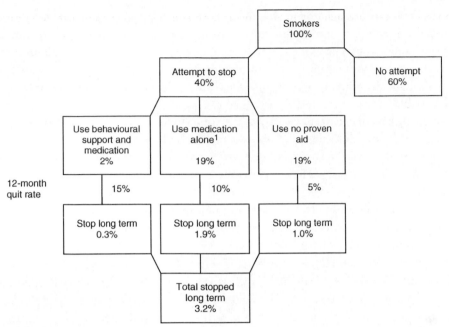

Fig. 14.3 'Route to quit' model with data on quit attempts and use of aids to cessation from England in 2008 (<http://www.smokinginengland.info>). Figures for quit rates are estimated from data from clinical trials.
[1]NRT bought over the counter in most cases.

Table 14.2 The EPICURE classification of behaviour change techniques (West 2006a)

Intervention type	Description	Mechanism of action
Education	Improve knowledge and understanding of the benefits of change or how to change	Increase desire to change or facilitate implementation of the change rule; focus on knowledge and beliefs
Persuasion	Propose the idea of change and make it attractive and salient	Increase desire to change; focus on attitudes
Inducement	Offer extrinsic rewards for making or sustaining the change	Increase desire to change or bolster adherence to the change rule; focus on extrinsic reward
Coercion	Make the old behaviour more aversive or difficult	Increase the desire to change; focus on extrinsic punishment
Upskilling	Train in skills to establish or facilitate the new behaviour	Facilitate implementation of the change rule; focus on capacity
Regulation	Reduce access to the old behaviour	Increase desire to change or facilitate implementation of the change rule; focus on opportunity
Empowerment	Reduce barriers to the new behaviour	Facilitate implementation of the change rule; focus on capacity

Different types of intervention focus differentially on getting people to decide to make the change and getting them to adhere to the 'change rule'. They do this either by bringing about changes in people in the target group (the way they think and feel about things or their capacity to do things), or in the environment (providing extrinsic rewards and punishments or reducing opportunities for the old behaviour or barriers to the new behaviour).

Choosing a set of behaviour change interventions to form part of an overall strategy for a population involves a number of considerations (Table 14.3).

Choice of intervention strategy often involves sacrificing efficacy for reach, or efficacy and reach for acceptability. Thus, coercive measures such as making something unlawful or making it very expensive can be very powerful but if acceptability is low, they can be difficult and costly to implement resulting in high levels of disobedience. This often means that coercive measures have to be preceded by and continue to be accompanied by extensive education and persuasion interventions to maximize acceptability.

A number of different approaches have been tried to get more people to stop smoking permanently. Table 14.4 lists these and their target mechanisms. They vary in terms of the six characteristics described above; thus, paid advertising has the potential for high reach and low unit cost but efficacy is generally likely to be lower than, say, that of smokers clinics.

The list in Table 14.4 is restricted to those that are widely used and have some evidence for effectiveness. There are many others that have been evaluated to some degree but have insufficient evidence to support their use. Systematic reviews of many of these can be found in the Cochrane Library (<http://www.cochrane.org/>). The next section examines how efficacy is determined in the case of smoking cessation interventions.

Methods of establishing the efficacy of smoking cessation interventions

It is common to talk in terms such as 'Intervention X has effect Y' but in the case of public health interventions such as those to promote smoking cessation this involves three simplifications (Table 14.5).

Table 14.3 Important considerations when designing behaviour change interventions

Consideration	Description
Efficacy	What is the effect size on the specified outcome in ideal circumstances?
Reach	How many people are likely to be affected by the intervention?
Cost	What is the overall cost including training and other indirect costs at a given level of implementation?
Barriers	To what extent, and in what way, might the ideal intervention be compromised by practical considerations?
Acceptability	How far will the intervention prove acceptable to the target group and the population at large?
Side-effects	Will there be unwanted consequences of the intervention and if so how extensive and severe will they be?

Table 14.4 Smoking cessation interventions

Intervention type	Description	Possible target mechanisms
Target population: all smokers		
Tax increases	Raise tobacco duty	Increase concern over cost
Controlling smuggling	Increase expenditure on, and/or effectiveness of anti-smuggling activities	Increase concern over cost
Smoking restrictions	Ban smoking in indoor public areas	Make it inconvenient to smoke
Paid advertising	TV, radio, press, or billboard advertising	Increase health concern, direct advice to quit, promote use of effective forms of assistance
Warning labels	Text or pictorial warnings on packets or advertising	Increase health concern (possibly with direct advice to quit and promotion of use of effective forms of assistance)
No Smoking Day	An annual event that uses, PR and paid advertising to promote quitting around a given day	Direct advice to quit, promote use of effective forms of assistance
Quit-and-win competitions, payments, and vouchers to promote quitting	Set up prize draws or direct rewards contingent upon abstinence for a given period	Incentivize cessation
Brief advice from health professionals	Brief advice to quit from GPs etc during routine consultations	Increase health concern, direct advice to quit, promote use of effective forms of assistance
Target population: smokers making an attempt to stop smoking		
'Take home' materials	Books, leaflets, DVD, CDs, and similar materials	Increase health concern, direct advice to quit, promote use of effective forms of assistance, provide behavioural support
Internet-based behavioural support	Web-delivered advice and support, which may be interactive and tailored and involve eg chat rooms	Help find ways of minimizing the need to smoke, maximize desire not to smoke and capacity to resist the need to smoke, and help optimize use of other forms of assistance
Pro-active telephone support	Scheduled telephone sessions with a smoking cessation specialist to help with a quit attempt	Help find ways of minimizing the need to smoke, maximize desire not to smoke and capacity to resist the need to smoke, and help optimize use of other forms of assistance
Group-based behavioural support	Scheduled face-to-face sessions in groups led by a smoking cessation specialist	Help find ways of minimizing the need to smoke, maximize desire not to smoke and capacity to resist the need to smoke, and help optimize use of other forms of assistance

Table 14.4 (continued) Smoking cessation interventions

Intervention type	Description	Possible target mechanisms
Individual face-to-face behavioural support	Scheduled face-to-face sessions with a smoking cessation specialist to help with a quit attempt	Help find ways of minimizing the need to smoke, maximize desire not to smoke and capacity to resist the need to smoke, and help optimize use of other forms of assistance
NRT	One of the many forms of NRT (gum, transdermal patch, inhaler, lozenge, nasal spray) for 8–12 weeks from the quit date	Reduce urges to smoke and rewarding effects of nicotine
Bupropion	300mg/day (after lead-in) of this mild stimulant for 8 weeks from the quit date	Reduce urges to smoke and rewarding effects of nicotine
Varenicline	2mg/day (after lead-in) of this nicotinic partial agonist for 12 weeks from the quit date	Reduce urges to smoke and rewarding effects of nicotine
Nortriptyline	75-100mg/day (after lead-in) of this tricyclic antidepressant for 8 weeks from the quit date	Reduce urges to smoke and rewarding effects of nicotine

Table 14.5 Simplifications needed when making effect size estimates

Homogeneity within intervention category	Treating members of intervention categories as though they were the same
Context generalizability	Assuming that the findings of studies can be generalized to contexts in which they will be applied
Target population generalizability	Assuming that the findings with target populations studied can be generalized to those to which they will be applied

The first is that 'intervention X' is the same across all instances. Thus we talk about 'mass media interventions' or 'providing nicotine gum on prescription'. It is obvious on reflection that this is never the case. Mass media campaigns clearly vary in source, content, and delivery, and it is implausible to imagine that all 'mass media' interventions would have the same effect. 'Providing nicotine gum' may involve different formulations of gum provided for different periods of time in different amounts with different methods of delivery etc. It would not be difficult to construct a scenario in which such an intervention was ineffective: for example, if it were so inconvenient to get hold of enough gum that usage was very low. When testing the 'effectiveness of interventions', therefore, we are always testing the effectiveness of specific instances of a type of intervention and seeking to generalise from those to other instances. Such generalisation will be plausible in some cases and less plausible in others, but they will always require assumptions and therefore conclusions of the kind 'intervention X has effect Y' will always involve a judgement.

The second simplification concerns the context in which the intervention is delivered. This context will very often have an important effect on the effectiveness of the intervention. Context here refers to the state of the world at the time the intervention is delivered. For example, a mass media campaign to encourage people to use stop smoking support services may well have a different effect in the context of other tobacco control interventions such as price rises being implemented than when there are no additional pressures to quit. Brief advice to stop from a physician may have a different effect when given in the middle of a consultation than when given at the beginning or the end of it. A new smoking cessation drug may have a different effect in the context of positive news stories about it than when it is being pilloried by the press. A drug such as varenicline with somewhat unpleasant side effects (nausea) may be less effective when prescribed without any kind of support or explanation because the users would quickly stop taking it but may be highly effective when given with support which could reassure the user and prepare him or her for the experience. It is not possible to obtain data on the effects of interventions in all the contexts in which they are likely to be applied and so, as with the simplification about categories of intervention, a judgement has to be made concerning the likely effect of an intervention in the context of interest based on data that have been collected in other contexts.

The third simplification involves the target of the intervention. Both individual smokers and populations of smokers vary in important ways that affect intervention effectiveness. A smoker who has recently attended a stop smoking service and had a bad experience would be expected to react differently to a recommendation to use the service than one who has never tried to stop before. Nicotine replacement therapy could well be less effective in populations with long experience of this type of treatment because those that remain as smokers may be self-selected as 'treatment resistant'. Tax increases may have different effects on poor than rich smokers. Action-focused mass media campaigns aimed at triggering quit attempts could be less effective in populations that have low levels of concern about smoking than in populations that are already worried about its health effects. As with the other two simplifications, a judgement is inescapable when it comes to estimating the likely effect of interventions in populations or individuals who have not specifically been the target of studies.

The above analysis makes it clear that when we talk about 'hard versus soft evidence' or 'strong versus weak evidence', the way that the evidence was collected and the amount of evidence collected are only two factors to consider. In reality there is no such thing as 'hard evidence' that does not require judgements to be made. This is important because it means that the conventional practice of gathering 'hard evidence' together in systematic reviews to estimate effect sizes with 95% confidence intervals must only be a part of a process which ultimately will lead to a judgement about the likely effect of interventions within a given category, delivered in a range of contexts to a range of target populations. The potential threats to accuracy of such estimates arising from the judgements concerned are at least as great as threats arising from limitations in the studies on which they are based.

This has important implications for the way in which we use evidence to make recommendations about public health interventions. It requires us to pay at least as much attention to factors that limit the generalizability of studies as to the 'quality' of the data available. It also means that our estimates of effect size should be adjusted using judgements about this generalizability and so should the range within which we believe the true figure lies.

With this in mind we can now turn to the nature of the evidence used to make judgements about the effectiveness of smoking cessation interventions. When it is practicable, and doing it does not compromise generalizability, the ideal study is the placebo-controlled, double blind randomized trial. In this design, individuals are randomly assigned to one or more experimental conditions in which they receive different interventions and neither they, nor anyone who has any dealings with them, knows what intervention they have been assigned to (West in press-a). They are then followed up and observations are made to observe what happens to them. There are more than 100 such studies on the effectiveness of nicotine replacement therapy (Stead et al 2008b).

A problem is that the conditions that make RCTs practicable and generalizable are rare in public health interventions. Often it is practicable to undertake an RCT but it is not worthwhile because in striving to achieve it one loses too much by way of generalizability. For example, when trying to evaluate the effectiveness of group-based smoking cessation support versus individual support, it is tempting to propose an RCT comparing the two. But, many smokers will have a strong preference for one kind of support versus the other and one would not be allowed to reason with them that one form was better than another to persuade them to engage with it. So one could only conduct the study on those that were willing to be randomized in the absence of information about which was better. Furthermore, there are many different ways in which a group may be run and some may be counterproductive while others may be very beneficial. The variation within the category of intervention could be at least as great as between it. Worse still, the skill of the 'stop smoking' specialist may have a major role in determining the success of group or individual support. In practice, it may be that while a highly skilled specialist can get better results with a group than with individual support, those that are less skilled have the opposite pattern of results. In that case an RCT with highly skilled staff may give a result that was the opposite of what would be observed were the policy of promoting group support to be implemented.

Thus there are many conditions, probably a majority, in which the RCT is not the appropriate design to evaluate the likely effect of a smoking cessation intervention. Arguably, very large sums of money continue to be spent in the vain hope that an RCT will provide an answer that is simply not there to be had. Recently, new guidance has been provided on the evaluation of 'complex interventions' which include most interventions to promote smoking cessation (Craig et al 2008; Craig et al 2009 this volume). This introduces alternative experimental designs to the traditional RCT, including 'cluster randomised trials', 'preference designs', 'randomised consent' designs, 'stepped wedge' designs and 'N-of-1' studies. These designs have not been widely used in evaluating smoking cessation interventions to date but this may change. Table 14.6 gives brief details of these designs.

Non-experimental designs have to be used when practical or ethical considerations prevent deliberate application of different experimental conditions. Such designs cannot

Table 14.6 Experimental designs that may be used in evaluating intervention efficacy

Type of design	Description	Comments
Double-blind RCT	Individual random allocation of participants to intervention and comparison conditions with researchers and participants unaware which condition has been assigned	Offers strongest evidence for efficacy, but often not practicable, ethical or generalizable
Unblinded RCT	Individual random allocation of participants to intervention and comparison conditions with researchers and participants aware which condition has been assigned	Necessary when blinding is not possible, but cannot rule out bias caused by knowledge of which condition participants have been assigned to
Cluster randomized trial	Randomization of groups of participants to intervention and comparison conditions	Necessary when intervention can only be applied to groups for practical reasons or when there would be high risk of interaction between individual participants that would undermine the integrity of the experimental conditions, but there is loss of statistical power to detect an effect
Preference design	Participants asked to nominate an experimental condition that they prefer. Those that have a strong preference are assigned to that condition and those that do not are randomly allocated to conditions. Statistical analyses compare effect of receiving different interventions and whether preference affects this	Necessary when participants may have strong preferences that would lead to drop-out if they were assigned to a non-preferred condition or limiting study to a small group of people who do not have strong preferences, but if preferences are extreme may not be able to disentangle preference from intervention effects
Informed-consent design	Participants consent to be followed up. They are then randomized to experimental conditions and asked to consent to that condition without being aware of other conditions	Necessary when awareness of the presence of other conditions would be likely to bias the results (for example by participants seeking out elements of other interventions that they had been made aware of)
Stepped wedge design	Roll-out of an intervention is staggered over a number of target groups and measures are taken of the outcome variable before and after implementation for each group	Necessary when an intervention is already planned to be implemented but its effect still needs to be evaluated. Ideally the order in which target groups receive the intervention is randomized
N of 1 design	Outcome measures are taken over a series of time points for individual participants, the intervention is applied once a stable baseline has been achieved and then further measures are taken, then the intervention is terminated and further measures are taken, the cycle being repeated with different interventions	Necessary when individual differences make average across people problematic but can only be used when stable baselines can be achieved and effects of interventions are immediate and reversible

definitely establish a causal link between interventions and outcomes but in many cases such a presumption is reasonable.

The most powerful of the non-experimental designs for evaluating interventions involves some form of time series analysis. A series of measures are taken on an outcome variable and values are linked statistically to implementation of interventions. It is necessary in such analyses to be able to adjust for other factors that might contribute to changes in the outcome measure such as seasonal trends. If one can compare temporal trends in one population with those in another population that has not been subject to a particular intervention, this provides greater confidence in the cause-effect association.

Another potentially useful non-experimental design involves comparisons between different populations that have been subjected to different interventions. A weaker form of evaluation is to assess the rate of self-claimed quitting in response to an intervention. This is clearly subject to significant bias and error but may provide a very broad indication of effectiveness in situations where the extent of bias may be presumed to be low. Evaluations in which opinions are sought about intervention effectiveness are generally not useful because of the potential for bias and error.

In the field of smoking cessation, the choice of outcome measure is of critical importance. Ultimately the outcome of interest is usually abstinence lasting indefinitely, or at least for a sufficient period to result in a significant health gain. In practice, six months of abstinence has become conventional because permanent quit rates can be reliably estimated as about 50% of that figure (West 2007). Quit attempts are of interest as well if it can be assumed that increasing the rate of quit attempts does not at the same time reduce their likelihood of success. In general, changes in attitude to smoking or intentions to quit are too weakly associated with actual quitting to be of any value, though they may provide preliminary information to guide further investigation. Where smokers may feel under social pressure to report abstinence, self-report cannot be taken at face value and normally requires verification using a biochemical marker of smoking such as expired air carbon monoxide concentration or salivary cotinine (West et al 2005). However, even when there is pressure to deny smoking, in the case of many intervention evaluations biochemical verification is not practicable (eg when participants are distributed over a wide geographic area and not in face-to-face contact with researchers). In those circumstances it is important to minimize the differential bias in different intervention conditions. It is also important to minimize bias due to loss to follow up. In clinical intervention studies loss to follow up usually implies a resumption of smoking so the recommendation is to regard those concerned as treatment failures (West et al 2005). However, there may be studies in which participants may be lost to follow up for other reasons so this approach cannot be used. There is no perfect solution and the most important thing is to do everything possible to minimize loss to follow up.

Effectiveness of interventions that promote smoking cessation

Smoking cessation is unique in the field of behaviour change in having a large number of high quality studies showing clear evidence of effectiveness and cost-effectiveness in preventing premature mortality. Interventions can be divided into two main types: those that are applied to the population of smokers to promote and assist quit attempts and those that can be used by individual smokers to help their quit attempt succeed.

Interventions directed at populations such as paid advertising have the weakest evidence to support them but potentially the highest reach while interventions directed at individuals making quit attempts have the strongest evidence but more limited reach. Table 14.7 provides statements relating to effectiveness for each of the interventions listed previously. Bearing in mind the caveats identified earlier in this chapter the statements of effectiveness have to be expressed as 'judgements' and in many cases those judgements are necessarily ambiguous or vague. It is important to recognize that this does not signify a lack of scientific rigour but an application of a rigorous evaluation process to a 'real world' inference. To attempt greater precision would be misleading.

Table 14.7 Effectiveness of smoking cessation interventions

Intervention type	Effectiveness	Nature of the evidence
Target population: all smokers		
Tax increases	1% price increase could have increased long-term cessation by up to 0.4%	Time series analyses of cigarette consumption plus assumption that changes mostly reflect cessation (Colman et al 2003; Jha and Chaloupka 1999; Levy et al 2005; Meng 2004; Observatoire Français des Drogues et des Toxicomanies 2006; Ranson et al 2002; Wilson and Thomson 2005)
Controlling smuggling	Could have had an effect commensurate with price increase caused by increase in tax	No studies directly examining the effects of smuggling countermeasures on cessation (but see Chief Medical Officer 2005)
Smoking restrictions	Could have caused a temporary increase in quit attempts and increase success rates of quit attempts	Time series analyses of quit attempts and success rates (Heloma et al 2001; but see Jha and Chaloupka 1999)
Paid advertising	Could have had an effect whose size varied with content, delivery, and context	Time series analyses of quit attempts and smoking prevalence and comparisons of areas subjected to campaigns with control areas (Bala et al 2008; Jha and Chaloupka 1999; Levy et al 2005)
Warning labels on cigarette packets	Pictorial labels could have had an effect in generating quit attempts	Survey data from Canada found that a substantial proportion of ex-smokers reported that graphic warning labels had been a stimulus to quitting (Hammond et al 2004)
No Smoking Day	Could lead a significant number of smokers to stop	Survey data from England on self-reported quitting in response to No Smoking Day (Owen and Youdan 2006)

Table 14.7 (continued) Effectiveness of smoking cessation interventions

Intervention type	Effectiveness	Nature of the evidence
Quit-and-win competitions, payments, and vouchers to promote quitting	Could have generated quit attempts but uncertain effect on long-term abstinence	A systematic review of RCTs (Cahill and Perera 2008)
Brief advice to quit from health professionals	Has been found to increase long-term[1] abstinence rates by 42%–94%[2]	A systematic review of RCTs involving physicians; no comparable data available from other health professionals (Stead et al 2008a)

Target population: smokers making an attempt to stop smoking

Intervention type	Effectiveness	Nature of the evidence
'Take home' materials	Has been found to increase long-term abstinence rates by 20% on average but depends on the materials	A systematic review of RCTs (Lancaster and Stead 2005b)
Internet-based behavioural support	Has been found to increase the odds of long-term abstinence by 30%–120% on average compared with written materials but depends on the programme	A systematic review of RCTs (Shahab and McEwen In Press)
Proactive telephone support	Has been found to increase the odds of long-term abstinence by 27%–57% on average but depends on the specific programme	A systematic review of RCTs (Stead et al 2006)
Group-based behavioural support	Has been found to increase long-term abstinence rates by 60%–146% compared with brief minimal support	A systematic review of RCTs supported by data from a national sample in England (Stead and Lancaster 2005)
Individual face-to-face behavioural support	Has been found to increase long-term abstinence rates by 24%–57% compared with minimal support	A systematic review of RCTs supported by data from a national sample in England (Lancaster and Stead 2005a)
NRT	Has been found to Increase long-term abstinence rates by 50–70%[3]	A systematic review of RCTs supported by prospective surveys of users vs non-users in national samples (Stead et al 2008b)
Bupropion	Has been found to Increase the odds of long-term abstinence by 72%–119%[3]	A systematic review of RCTs supported by data from NHS smokers clinics (Hughes et al 2007)
Varenicline	Has been found to Increase long-term abstinence rates by 95%–180%[3]	A systematic review of RCTs supported by data from a national sample in England and NHS smokers clinics (Cahill et al 2007)
Nortriptyline	Has been found to increase the odds of long-term abstinence by 61%–241%[3]	A systematic review of RCTs (Hughes et al 2007)

[1]At least six months of abstinence;
[2]Compared with usual care which typically involved not giving advice;
[3]Compared with placebo.

Cost-effectiveness of interventions to promote smoking cessation

The primary reason for stopping smoking is to reduce the loss of healthy life years. Cost-effectiveness is therefore usually stated in terms of the cost per 'quality-adjusted life year' (QALY) gained by an intervention compared with some comparison condition (eg no action) (National Institute for Clinical Excellence 2002; National Institute for Health and Clinical Excellence 2006a, b).

Applying findings of effectiveness to generate cost-effectiveness estimates requires additional information and assumptions. Effectiveness is denoted in different ways in different studies. For example, in RCTs it is typically denoted as an odds ratio or a risk ratio (or 'rate'). The odds ratio is the ratio of the odds of success to those of failure. If an intervention leads 10% of those receiving it to succeed compared with 5% in a comparison group this doubles the success rate but the odds of success are 2.11. Odds and risk ratios have to be converted into the number of long-term ex-smokers generated over and above those who would have arisen without the intervention to be of use. This requires knowledge of what the number of ex-smokers would be in those circumstances which will vary with context and the population. Table 14.8 shows figures that may be used for countries such as the UK and US.

One also has to take into account the fact that ex-smokers continue to relapse for several years. Research shows that the 6-month continuous abstinence rate is about 50% of the permanent cessation rate (West 2007). Thus the permanent effect of an intervention will typically be half that of the 6-month effect.

As shown in Figure 14.1, the number of life years saved by stopping smoking varies with age. At 40 years about 9 years can be saved while at 60 years it is about 3 years. Thus to calculate the cost-effectiveness of a smoking cessation intervention one needs to know the demographic profile of the people using that intervention.

Three further issues need to be considered. One is the rate at which smokers will continue to stop smoking in the years after the intervention: the background cessation rate. This has to be subtracted for the effect of the intervention. Secondly, smoking cessation prevents significant morbidity as well as mortality and so the 'quality-adjusted' life years

Table 14.8 Long-term (6+ months) smoking cessation rates

Population	Cessation rate	Intervention effectiveness	
		50% increase in odds	100% increase in odds
Smokers in the population	2%	3%	4%
Smokers making an unaided quit attempt	5%	7.5%	10%
Smokers quitting with the aid of behavioural support alone	10%	15%	20%
Smokers quitting with the aid of medication alone	10%	15%	20%

saved will be greater than the simple life years saved. There is a tariff for different types of morbidity that can be applied but clearly this involves a degree of judgement. Thirdly, the life years saved will be at some time in the future, perhaps decades after the intervention. It is conventional to 'discount' these life years at a rate of about 3% per year to take account of the preference that we have for immediate versus distant gains. It is not possible here to explain how all these factors go into the final calculation of 'quality adjusted life years' gained by a smoking cessation intervention but in general, in populations such as the UK and US the figure usually works out at about 4 times the 6-month effect size expressed as a percentage when applied to the age distribution of the smoking population. Thus, an intervention that helped 5% of smokers to stop for at least 6 months could be expected to generate approximately 20 QALYs.

The cost-effectiveness is then simply the cost of the intervention, including indirect costs and opportunity costs divided by the number of QALYs achieved. It has been estimated that an intervention that produces a 1 percentage point increase in continuous abstinence rate (eg from 2% to 3%) at a cost of £100 per person receiving the intervention would have a cost per QALY of around £3000 which is more than 5 times better than the average life-saving medical intervention (West 2007).

Summary and conclusions

Smoking kills many millions of people worldwide. Prevalence varies but is above 20% in almost every country in the world. After the age of about 40 years every year of smoking prevented saves an average of 3 months of healthy life. Developing and implementing effective smoking cessation interventions therefore remains one of the most important public health goals globally. These interventions may increase the rate of quit attempts and/or the rate at which those attempts succeed. Different processes are involved in these two objectives. Interventions to promote quit attempts include tax increases, measures to control smuggling, media campaigns, smoking restrictions, and warning labels on packets. These have potentially wide reach but evidence supporting them is mostly indirect or observational. Interventions to aid quit attempts involve use of medications such as nicotine replacement therapies and 'behavioural support'. These have strong evidence for efficacy but are currently used by only a minority of smokers. All these interventions have extremely good cost-effectiveness as ways of preventing premature death. The major challenges now are to find improved ways of implementing these interventions and getting them more widely adopted worldwide.

Acknowledgements

The authors are supported by a grant from Cancer Research UK. We are extremely grateful to Susan Michie and Jenny Fidler for comments on the manuscript.

Conflicts of interest

The author undertakes research and consultancy and has received hospitality and travel funds from companies that develop and manufacture aids to smoking cessation including

Pfizer, GSK, Novartis and Sanofi-Aventis. He also has a share in a patent for a novel nicotine delivery device.

Bibliography

Bala, M, Strzeszynski, L, and Cahill, K (2008) 'Mass media interventions for smoking cessation in adults' *Cochrane Database Syst Rev* 1: CD004704

Cahill, K and Perera, R (2008) 'Quit and Win Contests for Smoking Cessation' *Cochrane Database Syst Rev* 1: CD004986

Cahill, K, Stead, LF, and Lancaster, T (2007) 'Nicotine receptor partial agonists for smoking cessation' *Cochrane Database Syst Rev* 1: CD006103

Chief Medical Officer (2005) *Annual report of the Chief Medical Officer on the state of public health*. London: Department of Health

Colman, G, Grossman, M, and Joyce, T (2003) 'The effect of cigarette excise taxes on smoking before, during and after pregnancy' J Health Econ 22/6: 1053–1072

Craig, P, Dieppe, P, Macintyre, S, Michie, S, Nazareth, I, and Petticrew, M (2008) 'Developing and evaluating complex interventions: the new Medical Research Council guidance' *British Medical Journal* 337: a1655

Critchley, JA and Unal, B (2003) 'Health effects associated with smokeless tobacco: a systematic review' *Thorax* 58/5: 435–443

Doll, R, Peto, R, Boreham, J, and Sutherland, I (2004) 'Mortality in relation to smoking: 50 years' observations on male British doctors' *British Medical Journal* 328(7455): 1519

Hammond, D, McDonald, PW, Fong, GT, Brown, KS, and Cameron, R (2004) 'The impact of cigarette warning labels and smoke-free bylaws on smoking cessation: evidence from former smokers' *Can J Public Health* 95/3: 201–4

Heloma, A, Jaakkola, MS, Kahkonen, E, and Reijula, K (2001) 'The short-term impact of national smoke-free workplace legislation on passive smoking and tobacco use' *American Journal of Public Health* 91/9: 1416–18

Hughes, JR, Keely, J, and Naud, S (2004) 'Shape of the relapse curve and long-term abstinence among untreated smokers' *Addiction* 99/1: 29–38

Hughes, JR, Stead, LF, and Lancaster, T (2007) 'Antidepressants for smoking cessation' *Cochrane Database Syst Rev* 1: CD000031

Jha, P and Chaloupka, FJ (1999) *Curbing the epidemic: governments and the economics of tobacco control*. Washington, DC: World Bank

Lancaster, T and Stead, LF (2005a) 'Individual behavioural counselling for smoking cessation' *Cochrane Database Syst Rev* 2: CD001292

Lancaster, T and Stead, LF (2005b) 'Self-help interventions for smoking cessation' *Cochrane Database Syst Rev* 3: CD001118

Levy, DT, Nikolayev, L, and Mumford, E (2005) 'Recent trends in smoking and the role of public policies: results from the SimSmoke tobacco control policy simulation model' *Addiction* 100/10: 1526–36

Mackay, J and Eriksen, MP (2006) *The Tobacco Atlas*. Geneva: World Health Organization

Meisinger, C, Doring, A, Thorand, B, and Lowel, H (2006) 'Association of cigarette smoking and tar and nicotine intake with development of type 2 diabetes mellitus in men and women from the general population: the MONICA/KORA Augsburg Cohort Study' *Diabetologia* 49/8: 1770–6

Meng, Q (2004) *The effect of cigarette prices on smoking decision and intensity in China*. <http://www.ecu.edu/econ/ecer/kevinpaper.pdf>

National Institute for Clinical Excellence (2002) *National Institute for Clinical Excellence technology appraisal guidance No 38 Nicotine replacement therapy (NRT) and bupropion for smoking cessation*. London: NICE

National Institute for Health and Clinical Excellence (2006a) *An assessment of brief interventions and referral for smoking cessation in primary care and other settings, with particular reference to pregnant smokers and disadvantaged groups with consideration of the tailoring and targeting of interventions*. London: NICE

National Institute for Health and Clinical Excellence (2006b) *Brief interventions and referral for smoking cessation in primary care and other settings PHI001*. London: NICE

Observatoire Français des Drogues et des Toxicomanies (2006) *Tableau de bord mensuel Tabac*. <http://www.ofdt.fr/ofdtdev/live/donneesnat/tabtabac.html>

Owen, L and Youdan, B (2006) '22 years on: the impact and relevance of the UK No Smoking Day' *Tobacco Control* 15/1: 19–25

Power, C, Frank, J, Hertzman, C, Schierhout, G, and Li, L (2001) 'Predictors of low back pain onset in a prospective British study' *American Journal of Public Health* 91/10: 1671–8

Ranson, MK, Jha, P, Chaloupka, FJ, and Nguyen, SN (2002) 'Global and regional estimates of the effectiveness and cost-effectiveness of price increases and other tobacco control policies' *Nicotine Tob Res* 4/3: 311–19

Roman, GC (2005) 'Vascular dementia prevention: a risk factor analysis' *Cerebrovasc Dis* 20(Suppl 2): 91–100

Seddon, JM, George, S, and Rosner, B (2006) 'Cigarette smoking, fish consumption, omega-3 fatty acid intake, and associations with age-related macular degeneration: the US Twin Study of Age-Related Macular Degeneration' *Arch Ophthalmol* 124/7: 995–1001

Shahab, L and McEwen, A (In Press) 'Online support for smoking cessation: a systematic review of the literature' *Addiction*

Stead, LF, Bergson, G, and Lancaster, T (2008a) 'Physician advice for smoking cessation' *Cochrane Database Syst Rev* 2: CD000165

Stead, LF and Lancaster, T (2005) 'Group behaviour therapy programmes for smoking cessation' *Cochrane Database Syst Rev* 2: CD001007

Stead, LF, Perera, R, Bullen, C, Mant, D, and Lancaster, T (2008b) 'Nicotine replacement therapy for smoking cessation' *Cochrane Database Syst Rev* 1: CD000146

Stead, LF, Perera, R, and Lancaster, T (2006) 'Telephone counselling for smoking cessation' *Cochrane Database Syst Rev* 3: CD002850

US Department of Health and Human Services (1990) *The health benefits of smoking cessation: a report of the Surgeon General*. Rockville, MD: USDHHS

US Department of Health and Human Services (2004) *Surgeon General's report. The health consequences of smoking*. Washington: Office on Smoking and Health

Watkins, RE and Plant, AJ (2006) 'Does smoking explain sex differences in the global tuberculosis epidemic?' *Epidemiol Infect* 134/2: 333–9

West, R (In Press-a) 'Experiment design issues in addiction research' in P Miller, J Strang., and P Miller (eds), *Addiction Research Methods*. Oxford: Wiley-Blackwell

West, R (In Press-b) 'The multiple facets of cigarette addiction and what they mean for encouraging and helping smokers to stop'. COPD

West, R (2006a) 'Tobacco control: present and future' *British Medical Bulletin* 77–8: 123–36

West, R (2006b) *Theory of addiction*. Oxford: Blackwells

West, R (2007) 'The clinical significance of "small" effects of smoking cessation treatments' *Addiction* 102/4: 506–9

West, R, Hajek, P, Stead, L, and Stapleton, J (2005) 'Outcome criteria in smoking cessation trials: proposal for a common standard' *Addiction* 100/3: 299–303

West, R, McEwen, A, Bolling, K, and Owen, L (2001) 'Smoking cessation and smoking patterns in the general population: a 1-year follow-up' *Addiction* 96/6: 891–902

Wilson, N and Thomson, G (2005) 'Tobacco tax as a health protecting policy: a brief review of the New Zealand evidence' *NZ Med J* 118/1213: U1403

World Health Organization (2002) *World health report 2002*. Geneva: World Health Organization

Chapter 15

The development of a diabetes prevention programme for a South Asian population: translating evidence and theory into practice

Kamlesh Khunti, Thomas Yates, Jacqui Troughton, Margaret Stone, and Melanie Davies

The aim of this chapter is to provide a transferable framework for developing a structured education programme aimed at preventing type 2 diabetes in people of South Asian ethnic origin. This is timely because governments and health care providers are placing an increasing emphasis on preventing chronic disease. For example, the United Kingdom's Department of Health recently announced plans to systematically screen all individuals between 40 and 75 years of age for vascular disease risk and to treat 'at-risk' individuals with both pharmaceutical products and lifestyle advice. However, as this chapter will highlight, there is a lack of evidence surrounding lifestyle modification programmes that are both effective and suitable for implementation in a primary health care setting. In addition, there has been little attempt to address the specific needs of people from ethnic minority backgrounds, who tend to have an increased risk of many chronic diseases compared to white Europeans and form a large proportion of the population in many urban areas. This chapter will describe a method of addressing this need and provide the health care community with a systematic and reproducible approach to designing and developing a lifestyle modification programme.

Background

Type 2 diabetes mellitus is a chronic and debilitating disease characterized by an inability to adequately regulate blood glucose levels. The symptoms of type 2 diabetes are associated with a reduced quality of life in the short term, whilst in the longer term the disease may lead to serious complications such as cardiovascular disease, blindness, renal failure, and amputation (Massi-Benedetti 2002). The life expectancy of individuals with type 2 diabetes may be shortened by as much as 15 years, with up to 75% dying of cardiovascular disease (Davies et al 2004).

The global prevalence of type 2 diabetes is currently estimated to be 5.1% and is expected to rise to 6.3% by 2025. Type 2 diabetes is commonly referred to as an epidemic (Colagiuri et al 2005; Wareham, Forouhi 2005) and is estimated to be the fifth leading cause of mortality globally (Roglic et al 2005). In the United Kingdom (UK), over two million individuals have been diagnosed with type 2 diabetes and an additional 600,000 cases are estimated to be undiagnosed. Approximately 5% of all National Health Service (NHS) resources and up to 10% of hospital inpatient resources are devoted to the care and treatment of individuals with type 2 diabetes (Department of Health 2001); these figures are set to rise in the future and will represent a serious clinical and financial challenge to the UK's health system (Bagust et al 2002).

Type 2 diabetes is at one end of a continuous glucose control spectrum, with normal glucose control at the other end. In between, there exists a condition called prediabetes or intermediate hyperglycaemia, defined as impaired glucose tolerance (IGT) and/or impaired fasting glucose (IFG) (World Health Organization 2006; American Diabetes Association 2003), where blood glucose levels are elevated above the normal range but do not satisfy the criteria for type 2 diabetes. In most countries around 15% of adults have prediabetes based on WHO criteria (World Health Organization 2006; Santaguida et al 2005), of which an estimated 5 to 12 % develop type 2 diabetes annually (World Health Organization Diabetes 2006; Santaguida et al 2005). Glucose tolerance may start to decline up to twelve years before clinical recognition of T2DM and markedly increases the risk of cardiovascular mortality compared to people with normal glucose tolerance (Balkau et al 1998; Harris et al 1992; Unwin et al 2002). This provides a potential window of opportunity to identify elevated blood glucose levels early, when patients will have been exposed to less hyperglycaemia and fewer coexisting abnormalities. Given these factors, individuals with prediabetes are an important population in the prevention of type 2 diabetes.

Prevention

To date, a coherent nationwide strategy for identifying and treating those at risk of developing type 2 diabetes has been lacking in the UK. However, the Department of Health recently announced plans to introduce a systematic framework for identifying and treating vascular disease risk (including diabetes) using a combination of risk assessment and blood tests (Department of Health 2008). To inform this policy, evidence-based strategies for identifying and treating those at risk of developing type 2 diabetes are urgently required in ethnically diverse settings. There is now clear evidence that lifestyle modification can substantially reduce the risk of type 2 diabetes in those with prediabetes (Gillies et al 2007). For example, data from large diabetes prevention studies in America (Diabetes Prevention Programme) and Finland (Finnish Diabetes Prevention Study) have shown that lifestyle modification programmes, aimed at achieving weight loss through the promotion of physical activity and healthy diet, reduce the risk of type 2 diabetes by 58% (Knowler et al 2002; Tuomilehto et al 2001). Indeed, per protocol analyses of these studies revealed that the risk of type 2 diabetes is reduced by 90% or more when individuals achieve their prescribed lifestyle change goals (Tuomilehto et al 2001; Hamman et al 2006). Successful diabetes prevention programmes have also been carried out in India (Ramachandran et al 2006), China (Pan et al 1997), and Japan (Kosaka et al 2005).

However, in spite of unequivocal evidence that lifestyle modification is effective in pre-venting type 2 diabetes, there are important limitations when it comes to translating this evidence into practice. Previous diabetes prevention programmes have involved multiple and intensive one-to-one counselling appointments with each participant, an approach that is unlikely to be feasible in a real world health care setting (Yates et al 2007). Furthermore, there is a lack of data from diabetes prevention programmes in a UK setting (Davies et al 2004). Although screening and one-to-one counselling programmes for prediabetes may be cost-effective in the longer term (Gillies et al 2008), these initiatives are likely to place a significant strain on health care resources in the shorter term. For this reason a recent review of the evidence commissioned by the NHS in the UK concluded that screening for type 2 diabetes and prediabetes meets most the of National Screening Committees key criteria, although it fails on several, including a lack of adequate staffing and facilities (Waugh et al 2007).

Ethnic-specific risk

Migrant ethnic groups comprise a substantial minority in many countries worldwide. In the UK, individuals of South Asian origin (people of Indian, Pakistani, and Bangladeshi descent) are the largest ethnic minority and now comprise the majority ethnic group in several urban locations. The prevalence of diabetes and prediabetes has consistently been shown to be higher in South Asians compared to white Europeans (Simmons et al 1991, Bhopal et al 1999, Misra and Ganda 2007, Oldroyd et al 2007), indeed the prevalence of known type 2 diabetes is around four times higher in this minority ethnic group (Mather and Keen 1985). Furthermore, in Leicester, progression from prediabetes to diabetes has been observed to be three times greater over a given time period in South Asians com-pared to white Europeans (Srinivasan et al 2007). A further consistent finding is that the incidence and prevalence of premature coronary heart disease, a common co-morbidity of type 2 diabetes, is greater in some migrant communities compared to the indigenous population. For example, in the UK, mortality from coronary heart disease is currently 46% higher for men and 51% higher for women in South Asians compared to the general population (Petersen et al 2004).

A popular hypothesis to explain the increased risk in immigrant South Asian popula-tions is that it reflects adverse gene-environment interactions which are transformed into more potent risk factors by westernization and changes in lifestyle (Williams 1995). A recent study of migrants concluded that increased fat intake and obesity related to migration is likely to largely explain the disproportionate combination of established and emerging cardiovascular disease risk factors prevalent in South Asians in the UK (Patel et al 2006). Furthermore it has consistently been shown that individuals of South Asian descent living in the UK and other industrialized countries are less physically active and less likely to meet the minimum physical activity recommendations than white Europeans (Fischbacher et al 2004, Yates et al 2008a). It is known that for any given BMI or indeed waist circumference, South Asians are more insulin resistant compared to their European counterparts (McKeigue et al 1991).

Although ethnicity in itself is not sufficient to define risk status, it should form part of any risk score or screening strategy developed in a multi-ethnic population. Therefore any at-risk group identified in this way will include a higher proportion of people from ethnic minority backgrounds compared to the underlying population. Given this, it is vital that lifestyle modification programmes are developed which are suitable for implementation in multi-ethnic settings and can respond to the needs of each ethnic community. However, although a large proportion of participants in the American Diabetes Prevention Program came from ethnic minority groups, there has been little attempt to systematically tailor diabetes prevention programmes to the cultural and linguistic needs of people from these groups using well described and reproducible methods. This is also mirrored in diabetes treatment programmes; for example, a recent systematic review identified only five randomized controlled trials investigating diabetes treatment programmes for South Asians living in industrialized countries (Khunti et al 2008). These studies were generally characterized by methodological limitations and a lack of detail regarding the development of the tested interventions. This is an important limitation because interventions designed and evaluated in mono-lingual and/or mono-cultural populations are not necessarily generalizable to other settings; therefore, systematic and reproducible methods of developing lifestyle interventions for people from ethnic minority backgrounds are needed. Whilst we recognize that, by necessity, the broad content and structure of lifestyle interventions should be evidence-based and driven by the needs and resources of national health care providers, it is important that such interventions have some flexibility in terms of adaptation to meet the needs of local communities.

Structured education

It is essential that diabetes prevention programmes recognise the specific needs of local communities and are appropriate for local primary health care services and infrastructure (Yates et al 2007). Until these factors are considered at the development phase, there will continue to be a gap between research and evidence-based practice. Structured education has been widely advocated in the UK as a method of promoting self-management strategies for individuals with type 2 diabetes mellitus (Department of Health 2005). The National Institute for Health and Clinical Excellence (NICE) advises that structured education should be available to all individuals with type 2 diabetes mellitus at the time of diagnosis (National Institute for Health and Clinical Excellence 2008). Structured education refers to group-based, patient-centred educational programmes that: have a clear philosophy; have a written curriculum that is underpinned by appropriate learning and health behaviour theories; are evidence based; and are delivered by trained, quality assessed, educators (Department of Health 2005). The DESMOND programme for individuals with type 2 diabetes has recently demonstrated that a structured education programme, along with educator training and quality assurance protocols, can be delivered within the NHS at a national level (Davies et al 2008). However, evidence for the efficacy of structured education at preventing, rather than treating, chronic disease is lacking from randomized controlled trials.

The development of a structured education programme in a multi-ethnic setting

Given these limitations in the current evidence, we developed a structured education programme aimed at preventing type 2 diabetes in a multi-ethnic population with pre-diabetes. This was achieved by following the Medical Research Council's internationally recognized framework for developing and evaluating complex interventions to improve health (Medical Research Council 2000, Craig et al 2008, Craig et al 2009 this volume). This framework describes how evidence, theory, modelling, and exploratory trials should be used iteratively to develop complex interventions. Importantly this framework also states that complex interventions sometimes need to be adapted to local circumstances rather than being completely standardized.

The following section will describe how each of the developmental phases of the framework for complex interventions was used to inform the development of this structured education programme. In particular this section will describe the processes that were used to modify the programme for the local South Asian population in Leicester.

Theory

There is a growing recognition that using psychological theories to identify determinants of action in promoting behaviour change is essential for the development of behaviour modification programmes. However, this approach has not typically been adequately utilized or described in the past (Michie et al 2005, Brug et al 2005, Rothman 2004). This limitation includes previously evaluated diabetes prevention programmes. However, given that there are more than 20 contending health behaviour theories to choose from (Michie et al 2005), deciding on an appropriate theory to underpin an intervention is not easy. The difficulty is compounded by a lack of empirical evidence for the efficacy of many health behaviour theories in terms of effecting behaviour change, which means that there is often no sound basis for choosing one particular health behaviour theory over another (Michie et al 2005, Brug et al 2005, Rothman 2004). A good example of this is the popular transtheoretical model (TTM). Despite being widely advocated and used, there is little evidence that TTM is successful at effecting or predicting physical activity behaviour change (Brug et al 2005, van Sluijs et al 2004, Sutton 2000). It has also been pointed out that, given its complexity, TTM may be inappropriate for use by practitioners and health promoters (Adams and White 2005).

In order to overcome these difficulties and arrive at an appropriate theoretical framework on which to base the structured education programme, we used the core processes proposed by Bartholomew's intervention mapping (Bartholomew et al 2001). Intervention mapping is an ecological and systematic approach to developing health education programmes that provides a useful and coherent method for identifying which theoretical determinants are likely to be important in the development of an intervention (Bartholomew et al 2001). This approach ensures that empirical evidence is used to confirm or reject a broad range of potentially useful theoretical domains that are not necessarily confined to a particular theory or theories, thus ensuring identification of a comprehensive set of domains that are likely to be important in the promotion of a given health behaviour. Figure 15.1 shows the core steps proposed by intervention mapping and how this approach was adapted for use in the current programme. The key finding from this process was that successful physical activity and multi-factor intervention programmes in individuals with prediabetes and diabetes, regardless of their theoretical underpinning, have consistently utilized methods that are central to Bandura's social cognitive theory (Bandura 1986), such as self-efficacy and self-regulation. As highlighted in Figure 15.1, Gollwitzer's implementation intentions (Gollwitzer 1999) were also identified as an important framework for developing successful strategies around self-regulation and Leventhal's common sense model was thought to be relevant and instructive for targeting risk perceptions (Leventhal et al 1980). These theories were integrated into a single theoretical model of behaviour change.

Leventhal's common sense model was thought to be particularly important because it highlights an area that has typically not been fully utilized in previous diabetes prevention programmes. It suggests that individuals conceptualize a health threat in terms of the causes, consequences, identity, control/treatment, and timeline of the threat and that these domains will influence subsequent coping behaviour (Leventhal et al 1980). The common sense model has been demonstrated across a variety of patient groups, including type 2 diabetes (Hagger and Orbell 2003; Hampson et al 2000; Stenstrom et al 1998; Watkins et al 2000; Hampson et al 2000; Paschalides et al 2004). Importantly it has been suggested that individuals conceptualize any identified health threat in terms of the domains of the common sense model (Leventhal et al 1980). Therefore it is likely that, if the information participants receive about an identified health threat does not include all of the domains identified by the common sense model, individuals are likely to acquire the missing information from elsewhere. They would then be at risk of forming a false set of illness beliefs, which could negatively affect subsequent coping behaviour. This means that if an intervention aimed at promoting health behaviour in individuals with prediabetes fails to target all the domains of the common sense model, it is likely that the intervention could be undermined by participants forming spurious health beliefs. For example, if an individual believes that their prediabetes status is attributable exclusively to their genetic profile, they may be more resistant to increasing their physical activity levels than if they believed that a sedentary lifestyle was a contributing factor. This has particular resonance in South Asian communities, where individuals with type 2 diabetes have been shown to accept their diagnosis with resignation due to a family history of type 2 diabetes (Stone et al 2005).

In addition to establishing theoretical determinants of behaviour change, it is also important for education programmes to establish a relevant philosophy that informs how the identified psychological theories are targeted. The Department of Health puts

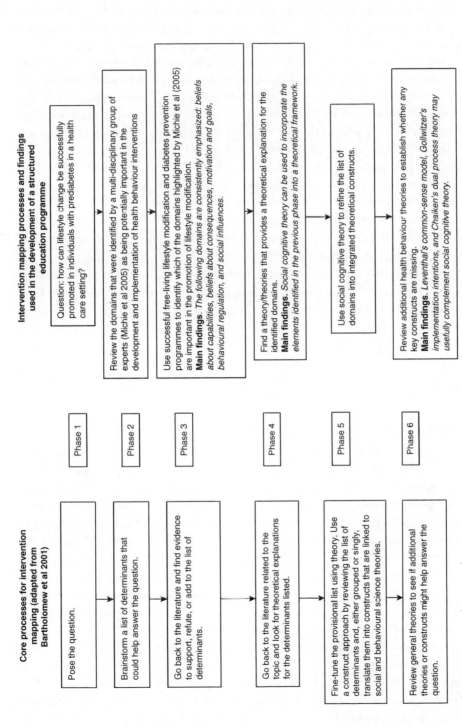

Fig. 15.1 Intervention mapping

particular emphasis on the importance of adopting a patient-centred approach to group education (Department of Health 2005). In the past, most patient education initiatives relied on imparting knowledge through heuristic processing (Skinner et al 2003). In this style of learning, the health professional is placed as the expert who imparts their knowledge to their patients verbally; the patient is therefore a passive entity, who absorbs the information imparted by an expert. The disadvantages of this approach are that individuals can easily rationalize information provided to them in this manner as being irrelevant to their personal circumstances and that, even where attitudes do change, they are vulnerable to further influence from other sources of information perceived as 'expert', and are thus unstable over time (Skinner et al 2003). Chaiken's dual process theory (1987) provides an alternative to the traditional heuristic learning model and makes a distinction between heuristic and systematic processing. In heuristic processing, the patient takes a passive role, whereas systematic processing occurs when an individual takes an active role in their learning experience by looking for evidence, examples, reasoning, and logic within the information they are being provided with. The use of a systematic processing approach in patient education encourages individuals to scrutinize information, ask questions, and work things out for themselves. Systematic processing requires greater cognitive effort from the patient but results in patients making a stronger link between theoretical concepts and their personal situation. It has been reported that individuals who attended a structured education programme based on systematic processing were able to give detailed descriptions of the programme a year later (Skinner et al 2003), in stark contrast to more traditional forms of patient consultation (Parkin and Skinner 2002).

Modelling and piloting

Having established an underlying theoretical model, we then carried out qualitative research in South Asian and white European individuals with prediabetes, to explore how they felt about their condition and what advice and help they would like to receive from health care professionals (Troughton et al 2008). This research found that patients expressed uncertainty about their diagnosis of prediabetes, its physical consequences, and subsequent management. In line with Leventhal's common sense model (Leventhal 1980), patients often articulated spurious beliefs about their prediabetes status because of flawed appraisals made in the absence of sound information. Many had no prior understanding of prediabetes, felt confused or anxious by the diagnosis and wanted clarification of what was meant by being at 'high risk'. All wanted to know why they had developed prediabetes. Many recognized that lifestyle could delay progression to type 2 diabetes but a high proportion also felt that they did not know what to change and lacked confidence in their ability to modify their behaviour. Respondents consistently expressed the need for support and education at diagnosis. Written support alone was not valued but healthcare professional time was. In view of the anticipated increase in the prevalence of prediabetes a group educational approach was considered acceptable to those questioned. The findings of this study are consistent with another qualitative study in the UK where individuals with prediabetes were found to want clear explanations of illness processes and physiology that were in line with Leventhal's common sense model (Evans et al 2007).

We used the underlying theoretical model and the outcomes of the qualitative research to develop a group-based structured education programme, called the Prediabetes Risk Education and Physical Activity Recommendation and Encouragement (PREPARE) programme (Yates et al 2008). This programme was designed to promote walking activity in individuals with prediabetes by targeting perceptions and knowledge of impaired glucose tolerance, self-efficacy beliefs about walking, barriers to walking activity, and self-regulatory strategies based around the use of a pedometer. This programme was aimed at promoting physical activity in the first instance because of the fundamental importance of physical inactivity in the development of metabolic dysfunction and because previous diabetes prevention programmes have failed to demonstrate clinically significant increases in physical activity (Yates et al 2007). This is consistent with the Medical Research Council's framework for complex interventions, which suggests that there is sometimes a need to test key active components within an intervention separately (Medical Research Council 2000; Craig et al 2008).

The PREPARE programme was informed by several small pilot studies before being tested in a proof of concept randomized controlled trial. This trial has been described in detail elsewhere (Yates et al 2008b). Results from this trial found that when the PREPARE programme enabled individuals to set personalized and realistic steps-per-day goals and self-monitor their activity levels with a pedometer it was successful at promoting significant increases in physical activity and decreases in both two-hour post-challenge glucose and fasting glucose compared to control conditions after 12 months (Yates et al 2009). Furthermore the programme positively influenced key risk perceptions, perceived knowledge of prediabetes, and efficacy beliefs.

On the basis of these findings, PREPARE was expanded into a multi-factor programme called Let's Prevent, aimed at reducing the risk of type 2 diabetes by promoting physical activity, diet, and weight loss (see Table 15.1 for a summary of the programme's content). In order to meet national criteria for structured education programmes, a written curriculum and educator training and quality assurance protocols were also developed. The programme is six hours long and is delivered by two educators over one full day or two half days. This is consistent with the DESMOND programme for individuals with newly diagnosed type 2 diabetes (Davies et al 2008), which has been successfully implemented nationally in a primary health care setting.

Initial pilot data from the Let's Prevent programme again demonstrated that the programme was successful at promoting health enhancing behaviours and key underlying psychological determinants.

The South Asian programme

For logistic reasons, the development of the PREPARE programme was informed by and aimed at individuals who spoke and read English. Given the high proportion of

Table 15.1 Content of the Let's Prevent programme

Module	Theory	Sample activity	Time weighting
Session 1			
Introduction			2%
Patient story	Common sense model	Participants asked to tell their story about how they discovered they had prediabetes and their current knowledge of prediabetes	10%
Professional story	Common sense model and dual process theory	Uses participants' stories to support them in learning how the body regulates glucose	15%
Taking control 1 Weight management	Common sense model, social cognitive theory, and dual process theory	Uses participants' stories to support them in discovering how weight/waist affect prediabetes. Provides knowledge and skills for food choices to control weight	10%
Physical activity	Common sense model, social cognitive theory, and dual process theory	Uses participants' stories to support them in discovering how physical activity affects prediabetes. Provides knowledge and skills for activity choices to manage prediabetes	15%
How am I doing?	Social cognitive theory	Participants reflect on what issues have come up in the programme so far	2%
Session 2			
Reflections	Social cognitive theory	Participants reflect issues that have arisen in the programme so far	5%
Professional story	Common sense model and dual process theory	Uses participants' stories to support them in discovering how other risk factors (eg blood pressure and cholesterol) affect prediabetes and the development of complications	13%
Taking control 2 Food choices: focus on fats	Social cognitive theory and dual process theory	Provides knowledge and skills for food choices to reduce risk factors	13%
Self-management plan	Social cognitive theory, implementation intentions	Participants supported in developing their self-management plans	10%
Questions	Common sense model	Checks that all questions raised by participants throughout the programme have been answered and understood	3%
What happens next?		Follow-up care outlines	2%

South Asians within Leicestershire, many of whom do not speak English, we adopted a more inclusive strategy in developing the Let's Prevent programme. Using our experience of modifying the DESMOND module for people newly diagnosed with type 2 diabetes for use in South Asian communities (Stone et al 2008), we were able to concurrently develop standard and modified versions of the programme and educator training protocols, recognizing the needs of the local South Asian population. It was acknowledged that a one-size-fits-all approach in patient education may not necessarily meet the diverse needs of the UK South Asian population, which is not a homogeneous group, for example, in terms of language, place of origin and religion. However, as the majority of South Asians in the Leicester area originate from the Gujarat region of India, our work was predominately aimed at this sub-group.

The South Asian Diabetes Prevention programme was developed to be consistent with the underlying theoretical structure and content of the Let's Prevent programme but was designed to be facilitated by two trained healthcare professionals and two trained interpreters. Previous research in those with type 2 diabetes had identified a need for substantially increased delivery time when interpreters are used (Stone et al 2008); the format of Let's Prevent was therefore amended to be delivered in four three hour sessions.

The core educational messages for the South Asian programme remained the same as for the standard version of Let's Prevent, but changes were made to ensure that food and physical activity messages were culturally appropriate. This included identifying and developing additional or alternative learning resources, including a series of pictures, to ensure that that the programme was not dependent on the written word. Educational resources were developed specifically to take into account the language, literacy, and cultural needs of South Asian people with prediabetes.

Educator and interpreter training protocols building on the Let's Prevent programme were also developed. This was supported with a manual, curriculum, and other resources provided for trainers to retain, read, and reinforce their learning.

An approach including features of action research was used, involving an iterative process and stakeholder involvement. This was broadly based on the model developed for individuals with type 2 diabetes (Stone et al 2008). Both qualitative and quantitative research methods were used to refine the development of the curriculum, resources, and training programme. The aim was to ensure that the programme was effective at initiating behaviour change as well as meeting the language, literacy, and cultural needs of South Asians with prediabetes. This methodology used an iterative and pragmatic approach similar to an audit 'cycle' (see Figure 15.2); this is consistent with the Medical Research Council's framework for complex interventions which highlights the importance of using cyclical process of piloting, evaluating, and developing complex interventions.

This process was carried out in two cycles (see Figure 15.2). During each cycle quantitative data including baseline and follow-up pedometer counts, self-reported physical activity, dietary status, and psychological variables were collected and analysed. In addition, qualitative methods were used to gather and consider the implications of feedback from key stakeholders including health care users (patients attending education sessions)

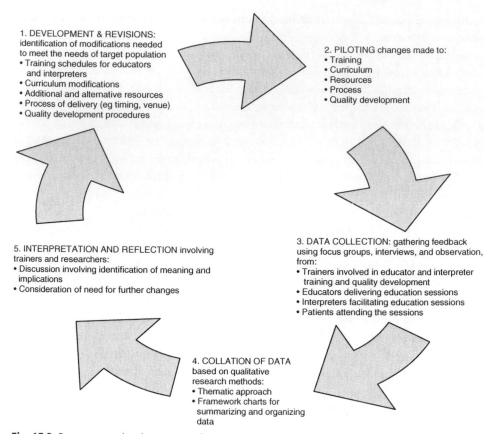

Fig. 15.2 Programme development cycle

and providers and facilitators (trainers, educators, and interpreters). In order to inform and facilitate the qualitative data collection process, trainers and qualitative researchers developed flexible topic guides. Data collection involved one-to-one interviews and focus groups, which were audio recorded. Observations were also recorded, using written notes. Transcriptions were reviewed to achieve familiarization, followed by identification of key themes from the content. Further analysis of the data involved the use of framework charts to summarize and organize the information collected, followed by interpretation and reflection, to inform the next phase of piloting (Richie and Spencer 1994).

First pilot cycle

Twenty-nine South Asian individuals were invited to attend the first pilot phase. Twenty-one individuals indicated that they wished to participate, of whom 14 were able to attend on the allocated pilot dates. Quantitative data collected indicated significant reductions in feelings of depression and anxiety that were attributed to a diagnosis of prediabetes, which in turn may have important implications in terms of the way in which individuals self-manage their risk status in the future. However, no significant changes to health behaviour were observed.

Qualitative feedback showed that participants found the visual resources and the use of interpreters helpful. However, some individuals indicated that interpretation was not required by all South Asian participants as younger people generally possessed good English language skills, although such individuals thought they would still benefit from a culturally adapted education programme. Comments received from all patients suggested that they were more confident about their understanding and knowledge of prediabetes than before the course and that they felt empowered and motivated to do something about it. However, participants indicated that more food models relevant to Asian diets should be included in the food games to support the messages being given. Several participants also expressed confusion over the physical activity messages or had not appreciated the importance of goal setting and action planning.

Qualitative feedback from focus groups with interpreters and educators highlighted areas that needed to be improved to enable educators and interpreters to work together effectively. Educators also expressed a concern about the complexity of the physical activity section. In the light of findings derived from both the quantitative and qualitative data relating to this pilot session, the physical activity section of the curriculum was revised and simplified and the dietary section was modified to include additional models representing foods that are typically consumed by South Asians. Some revisions were also made to the action planning session.

Second pilot cycle

The main purpose of this second pilot phase was to evaluate the changes made to the curriculum, resources, and format of delivery following the first pilot cycle. We delivered the second pilot in two formats depending on the preferences of the individuals attending. In each format, the culturally adapted curriculum and food models were used, but one programme was delivered in English and the other through interpreters. Quantitative analysis demonstrated significant increases in physical activity that were comparable to those demonstrated in the PREPARE study, along with significant changes to key dietary variables and self-efficacy beliefs. Qualitative analysis found that patients were very positive about the food resources, confirming the appropriateness of the changes made. The additional format of delivery in English without interpretation, but using the modified curriculum and resources, was very well received by those who attended. Furthermore, educators and interpreters were happy with the strategies that had been put in place to enable them to work effectively together and with the content of the programme.

Following the implementation of the second cycle of qualitative feedback, it was felt that the methods used had produced a model that was suitable for individuals with prediabetes from a South Asian population.

Randomized controlled trial

Having developed a comprehensive structured education programme aimed at the prevention of type 2 diabetes in a multi-ethnic population and an accompanying educator training and quality assurance protocol, the next key step is to conduct a definitive randomized controlled trial carried out in a primary health care setting with progression to type 2 diabetes as the main outcome measure. This will be carried through a programme grant funded by the National Institute for Health Research in 816 individuals with screening-detected impaired glucose tolerance, of whom we anticipate that around 250 (30%) will be south Asian. Participants will be recruited from 50 GP practices within the Leicestershire and Northampton area. The study will be carried out over three years and will include cost-effectiveness analysis. If successful, this trial will provide the evidence that is required to enable policy makers and primary health care trusts to invest in and promote a successful and feasible strategy for preventing type 2 diabetes.

Conclusion

The prevention of type 2 diabetes is a public health priority. Whilst several lifestyle intervention programmes have proved highly effective at reducing the progression to type 2 diabetes in individuals with prediabetes, important issues remain surrounding the applicability of such interventions to a primary health care setting. In particular, people from black and minority ethnic backgrounds have a substantially increased risk of developing type 2 diabetes compared to white Europeans in the UK and other industrialized countries, but limited research activity and resources have been targeted at preventing type 2 diabetes in this group. We have described the process by which we have attempted to address this need by systematically developing a structured education programme aimed at preventing type 2 diabetes in individuals with prediabetes and tailoring it to the needs of local people of South Asian origin. Future results from several community based randomized controlled trials will establish the efficacy of this programme at promoting behaviour change and improving metabolic health.

Bibliography

Adams, J and White, M (2005) 'Why don't stage-based activity promotion interventions work?' *Health Education Research* 20: 237–43

American Diabetes Association, Alexandria, Virginia, USA and Expert Committee on the Diagnosis and Classification of Diabetes Mellitus (2003) 'Report of the expert committee on the diagnosis and classification of diabetes mellitus' *Diabetes Care* 26/1: S5–20

Bagust, A, Hopkinson, PK, Maslove, L, and Currie, CJ (2002) 'The projected health care burden of Type 2 diabetes in the UK from 2000 to 2060' *Diabetic Medicine* 19/4: 1–5

Balkau, B, Shipley, M, Jarrett, RJ, Pyorala, K, Pyorala, M, and Forhan, A (1998) 'High blood glucose concentration is a risk factor for mortality in middle-aged nondiabetic men: 20-year follow-up in the Whitehall Study, the Paris Prospective Study, and the Helsinki Policemen Study' *Diabetes Care* 21: 360–7

Bandura, A (1986) *Social foundations of thought and action: a social cognitive theory*. Englewood Cliffs, NJ: Prentice-Hall

Bartholomew, L, Parcel, G, Kok, G, and Gottlieb, N (2001) *Intervention mapping: designing theory and evidence-based health promotion programs*. New York: McGraw-Hill

Bhopal, R, Unwin, N, White, M, Yallop, J, Walker, L, Alberti, KG, Harland, J, Patel, S, Ahmad, N, Turner, C, Watson, B, Kaur, D, Kulkarni, A, Laker, M, and Tavridou, A (1999) 'Heterogeneity of coronary heart disease risk factors in Indian, Pakistani, Bangladeshi, and European origin populations: cross sectional study' *British Medical Journal* 319: 215–20

Brug, J, Oenema, A, and Ferreira, I (2005) 'Theory, evidence and Intervention Mapping to improve behavior nutrition and physical activity interventions' *International Journal of Behavioral Nutrition and Physical Activity* 2: 2

Chaiken, S (1987) 'The heuristic model of persuasion' in MP Zanna, JM Olson, and CP Herman (eds), *Social influence: The Ontaio symposium*, pp 3–39. 5th edn. Hillsdale, NJ: Erlbaum

Colagiuri, S, Borch-Johnsen, K, Glümer, C, and Vistisen, D (2005) 'There really is an epidemic of type 2 diabetes' *Diabetologia* 48: 1459–63

Craig, P, Dieppe, P, Macintyre, S, Michie, S, Nazareth, I, Petticrew, M, and Medical Research Council Guidance (2008) 'Developing and evaluating complex interventions: the new Medical Research Council guidance' *British Medical Journal* 337: a1655

Davies, MJ, Heller, S, Campbell, MJ, Carey, ME, Dallosso, HM, Daly, H, Eaton, S, Fox, C, Rantell, K, Rayman, G, Skinner, TC, and Khunti, K (2008) 'Effectiveness of a structured education programme on individuals newly diagnosed with Type 2 diabetes: a cluster randomised controlled trial of the DESMOND programme' *British Medical Journal* 336: 491–5

Davies, MJ, Tringham, JR, Troughton, J, and Khunti, KK (2004) 'Prevention of Type 2 diabetes mellitus. A review of the evidence and its application in a UK setting' *Diabetic Medicine* 21: 403–14

Department of Health (2008) *Putting prevention first. Vascular checks: risk assessment and management*. London: Department of Health

Department of Health (2001) *National service framework for diabetes: standards*. London: Department of Health

Department of Health and Diabetes UK (2005) *Structured patient education in diabetes: Report from the Patient Education Working Group*. London: Department of Health

Evans, P, Greaves, C, Winder, R, Fearn-Smith, J, Campbell, J (2007) 'Development of an educational "toolkit" for health professionals and their patients with prediabetes: the WAKEUP study' *Diabetes Medicine* 24: 770–7

Fischbacher, CM, Hunt, S, and Alexander, L (2004) 'How physically active are South Asians in the United Kingdom? A literature review' *Journal of Public Health* 26: 250–8

Gillies, CL, Abrams, KR, Lambert, PC, Cooper, NJ, Sutton, AJ, Hsu, RT, and Khunti, K (2007) 'Pharmacological and lifestyle interventions to prevent or delay type 2 diabetes in people with impaired glucose tolerance: systematic review and meta-analysis' *British Medical Journal* 334: 299

Gillies, CL, Lambert, PC, Abrams, KR, Sutton, A, Cooper, N, Hsu, R, Davies, M, and Khunti, K (2008) 'Different strategies for screening and prevention of type 2 diabetes in adults: cost effectiveness analysis' *British Medical Journal* 336: 1180–5

Gollwitzer, PM (1999) 'Implementation Intentions: Strong Effects of Simple Plans: How can good intentions become effective behavior change strategies?' *American Psychologist* 54: 493–503

Hagger, MS and Orbell, S (2003) 'A Meta-Analytic Review of the Common-Sense Model of Illness Representations' *Psychology and Health* 18: 141–84

Hamman, RF, Wing, RR, Edelstein, SL, Lachin, JM, Bray, GA, Delahanty, L, Hoskin, M, Kriska, AM, Mayer-Davis, EJ, Pi-Sunyer, X, Regensteiner, J, Venditti, B, and Wylie-Rosett, J (2006) 'Effect of weight loss with lifestyle intervention on risk of diabetes' *Diabetes Care* 29: 2102–7

Hampson, S, Glasgow, R, and Strycker, L (2000) 'Beliefs versus feelings: A comparison of personal models and depression for predicting multiple outcomes in diabetes' *British Journal of Health Psychology* 5: 27–40

Harris, MI, Klein, R, Welborn, TA, Knuiman, MW (1992) 'Onset of NIDDM occurs at least 4–7 years before clinical diagnosis' *Diabetes Care* 15: 815–19

Khunti, K, Camosso-Stefinovic, J, Carey, M, Davies, MJ, and Stone, MA (2008) 'Educational interventions for migrant South Asians with Type 2 diabetes: a systematic review' *Diabetic Medicine* 25: 985–992

Knowler, WC, Barrett-Connor, E, Fowler, SE, Hamman, RF, Lachin, JM, Walker, EA, Nathan, DM, and Diabetes Prevention Program Research Group (2002) 'Reduction in the incidence of type 2 diabetes with lifestyle intervention or metformin' *The New England Journal of Medicine* 346: 393–403

Kosaka, K, Noda, M, and Kuzuya, T (2005) 'Prevention of type 2 diabetes by lifestyle intervention: a Japanese trial in IGT males' *Diabetes Research and Clinical Practice* 67: 152–62

Leventhal, H, Meyer, D, and Nerenz, D (1980) 'The common-sense representation of illness danger' in S Rachman (ed), *Contributions to Medical Psychology*, pp 7–30. 2nd edn. New York: Pergamon

Massi-Benedetti, M and CODE-2 Advisory Board (2002) 'The cost of diabetes Type II in Europe: the CODE-2 Study' *Diabetologia* 45: S1–4

Medical Research Council Health Services and Public Health Research Board (2000) *Framework for Development and Evaluation of RCTs for Complex Intervention to Improve Health*. Available at: <http://www.mrc.ac.uk/prn/pdf-mrc_cpr.pdf> (last accessed 10 July 2005)

McKeigue, PM, Shah, B, and Marmot, MG, (1991) 'Relation of central obesity and insulin resistance with high diabetes prevalence and cardiovascular risk in South Asians' *Lancet* 337: 382–6

Mathers, H and Keen, H (1985) 'Southall Diabetes Survey: prevalence of known diabetes' *British Medical Journal* 291: 1081–4

Michie, S, Johnston, M, Abraham, C, Lawton, R, Parker, D, Walker, A, and 'Psychological Theory' Group (2005) 'Making psychological theory useful for implementing evidence based practice: a consensus approach' *Quality & Safety in Health Care* 14: 26–33

Misra, A and Ganda, OP (2007) 'Migration and its impact on adiposity and type 2 diabetes' *Nutrition (Burbank, Los Angeles County, Calif)* 23: 696–708

National Institute for Health and Clinical Excellence (2008) *Type 2 diabetes: National clinical guideline for management in primary and secondary care (update).* London: Royal College of Physicians

Oldroyd, J, Yallop, J, Fischbacher, C, Bhopal, R, Chamley, J, Ayis, S, Alberti, K, and Unwin, N (2007) 'Transient and persistent impaired glucose tolerance and progression to diabetes in South Asians and Europeans: new, large studies are a priority' *Diabetes Medicine* 24: 98–103

Pan, XR, Li, GW, Hu, YH, Wang, JX, Yang, WY, An, ZX, Hu, ZX, Lin, J, Xiao, JZ, Cao, HB, Liu, PA, Jiang, XG, Jiang, YY, Wang, JP, Zheng, H, Zhang, H, Bennett, PH, and Howard, BV (1997) 'Effects of diet and exercise in preventing NIDDM in people with impaired glucose tolerance. The Da Qing IGT and Diabetes Study' *Diabetes Care* 20: 537–44

Parkin, T and Skinner, T (2002) 'Does patient perception of consultation concord with professional perception of consultation' (Abstract) *Diabetes Medicine* 19: A14

Paschalides, C, Wearden, AJ, Dunkerley, R, Bundy, C, Davies, R, and Dickens, CM (2004) 'The associations of anxiety, depression and personal illness representations with glycaemic control and health-related quality of life in patients with type 2 diabetes mellitus' *Journal of Psychosomatic Research* 57: 557–64

Patel, JV, Vyas, A, Cruickshank, JK, Prabhakaran, D, Hughes, E, Reddy, KS, et al (2006) 'Impact of migration on coronary heart disease risk factors: comparison of Gujaratis in Britain and their contemporaries in villages of origin in India' *Atherosclerosis* 185: 297–306

Petersen, S, Peto, V, and Rayner, M (2004) *Coronary heart disease statistics.* London: BHF

Ramachandran, A, Snehalatha, C, Mary, S, Mukesh, B, Bhaskar, AD, Vijay, V, and Indian Diabetes Prevention Programme (IDPP) (2006) 'The Indian Diabetes Prevention Programme shows that lifestyle modification and metformin prevent type 2 diabetes in Asian Indian subjects with impaired glucose tolerance (IDPP-1)' *Diabetologia* 49: 289–97

Ritchie, J and Spencer, L (1994) 'Qualitative data analysis for applied policy research' in A Bryman and R Burgess (eds), *Analysing Qualitative Data.* London: Routledge

Roglic, G, Unwin, N, Bennett, PH, Mathers, C, Tuomilehto, J, Nag, S, Connolly, V, and King, H (2005) 'The burden of mortality attributable to diabetes: realistic estimates for the year 2000' *Diabetes Care* 28, 2130–5

Rothman, A (2004) '"Is there nothing more practical than a good theory?": Why innovations and advances in health behavior change will arise if interventions are used to test and refine theory' *International Journal of Behavioral Nutrition and Physical Activity* 1: 11

Santaguida, PL, Balion, C, Hunt, D, Morrison, K, Gerstein, H, Raina, P, Booker, L, and Yazdi, H (2005) *Diagnosis, Prognosis, and Treatment of Impaired Glucose Tolerance and Impaired Fasting Glucose.* Evidence Report/ Technology Assessment No. 128. Rockville, MD: Agency for Healthcare Research and Quality

Simmons, D, Williams, DR, and Powell, MJ (1991) 'The Coventry Diabetes Study: prevalence of diabetes and impaired glucose tolerance in Europids and Asians' *The Quarterly Journal of Medicine* 81: 1021–30

Skinner TC, Cradock S, Arundel F and Graham W (2003) 'Lifestyle and Behavior: Four Theories and a Philosophy: Self-Management Education for Individuals Newly Diagnosed With Type 2 Diabetes' *Diabetes Spectrum* 16: 75–80

Srinivasan BT, Davies MJ, Webb D, Healey E, Farooqi A, Hiles S, Mandalia P, Khunti K (2007) 'Baseline characteristics and risk of progression from pre-diabetes to T2DM in a multi-ethnic population based screening' *Diabetes Medicine* 24 S1: P73

Stenstrom U, Wikby A, Andersson P and Ryden O (1998) 'Relationship between locus of control beliefs and metabolic control in insulin-dependent diabetes mellitus' *British Journal of Health Psychology* 3: 15

Stone M, Patel N, Daly H, Martin-Stacey L, Sayjal A, Marian M, Khunti K and Davies M (2008) 'Using qualitative research methods to inform the development of a modified version of a patient education module for non-English speakers with type 2 diabetes: experiences from an action research project on two south Asian populations in the UK' *Diversity in Health and Social Care* 3: 199–206

Stone M, Pound E, Pancholi A, Farooqi A and Khunti K (2005) 'Empowering patients with diabetes: qualitative primary care study focusing on south Asians in Leicester, UK' *Family Practice* 22: 647–52

Sutton, S (2000) 'Interpreting Cross-Sectional Data on Stages of Change' *Psychology Health* 15: 163

Troughton J, Jarvis J, Skinner C, Robertson N, Khunti K and Davies M (2008) 'Waiting for diabetes: Perceptions of people with pre-diabetes: A qualitative study' *Patient Education and Counseling* 72: 88–95

Tuomilehto J, Lindström J, Eriksson JG, Valle TT, Hämäläinen H, Ilanne-Parikka P, Keinänen-Kiukaanniemi S, Laakso M, Louheranta A, Rastas M, Salminen V, Uusitupa M and Finnish Diabetes Prevention Study Group (2001) 'Prevention of type 2 diabetes mellitus by changes in lifestyle among subjects with impaired glucose tolerance' *The New England Journal of Medicine* 344: 1343–50

Unwin N, Shaw J, Zimmet P and Alberti KG (2002) 'Impaired glucose tolerance and impaired fasting glycaemia: the current status on definition and intervention' *Diabetic Medicine* 19: 708–23

van Sluijs EM, van Poppel MN and van Mechelen W (2004) 'Stage-based lifestyle interventions in primary care: are they effective?' *American Journal of Preventive Medicine* 26: 330–43

Wareham NJ and Forouhi NG (2005) 'Is there really an epidemic of diabetes?' *Diabetologia* 48: 1454–5

Waugh N, Scotland G, McNamee P, GilletM, Brennan A, Goyder E, Williams R, John A (2007) 'Executive summary: Screening for type 2 diabetes: literature review and economic modelling' *Health Technology Assessment* 11/17

Watkins KW, Connell CM, Fitzgerald JT, Klem L, Hickey T and Ingersoll-Dayton B (2000) 'Effect of adults' self-regulation of diabetes on quality-of-life outcomes' *Diabetes Care* 23: 1511–15

Williams, B (1995) 'Westernised Asians and cardiovascular disease: nature or nurture?' *Lancet* 345: 401–2

World Health Organization Diabetes Guideline Development Committee (2006) *Definition and diagnoses of diabetes mellitus and intermediate hyperglycemia.* WHO: Geneva

Yates T, Khunti K and Davies MJ (2007) 'Prevention of diabetes: A reality in primary care?' *Primary Care Diabetes* 1: 119–21

Yates T, Khunti K, Bull F, Gorely T and Davies MJ (2007) 'The role of physical activity in the management of impaired glucose tolerance: a systematic review' *Diabetologia* 50: 1116–126

Yates T, Davies M, Brady E, Webb D, Gorely T, Bull F, Talbot D, Sattar N and Kamlesh K (2008a) 'Walking and Inflammatory Markers in Individuals Screened for Type 2 Diabetes' *Preventive Medicine* 47: 417–21

Yates T, Davies M, Gorely T, Bull F and Khuni K (2008b) 'Rationale, design and baseline data from the PREPARE (Pre-diabetes Risk Education and Physical Activity Recommendation and Encouragement) programme study: a randomized controlled trial' *Patient Education and Counseling* 73: 264–71

Yates T, Davies M, Gorely T, Bull F and Khunti K (2009) 'Effectiveness of a pragmatic education programme aimed at promoting walking activity in individuals with impaired glucose tolerance: a randomized controlled trial' *Diabetes Care* 32: 1404–10

Chapter 16

The Gatehouse Project: a multi-level integrated approach to promoting well-being in schools

Lyndal Bond and Helen Butler

Introduction

Over recent decades, there has been a sea change in the conceptualizing of health promotion in educational settings. During this time we have begun to broaden our concept of health promotion in schools from health education focused on changing students' behaviour to creating health promoting contexts (Bond et al 2001; Butler et al 2001; Bonell et al 2007). This change has been built on recognition of the possible inadequacy of traditional health education strategies used in schools to address specific problems such as tobacco and substance use, sexual health or cardiovascular risk factors. Packages and training focused on single issues abound but by themselves may be, in the long term, neither effective nor, given problems of a crowded curriculum, sustainable. The health promoting schools framework (WHO 1995) has been influential in emphasizing the need to address school ethos and environment, community partnerships as well as curriculum and learning but has still often been applied in relation to single health and behavioural issues.

The Gatehouse Project in Australia made a key contribution to this repositioning of emotional and behavioural well-being from a welfare and health education concern to a whole school concern fundamentally integrated into core school programmes, practices and structures. The main objectives of the intervention were to increase levels of emotional well-being and reduce rates of substance use. The project design and intervention strategies were grounded in an understanding of both risk and protective factors common to a range of health and behavioural problems. Implementation was based on an understanding of school change and school improvement processes. As the results of the trial have been disseminated there has been growing interest in the design and implementation of the project and we have had time to reflect on, further investigate, and theorize what was achieved. This chapter presents a detailed description of the Gatehouse Project intervention and presents the results from the cluster-randomized, controlled-trial evaluation. Implications for how we develop, implement, and evaluate complex school-based interventions are discussed.

Approaches to health promotion in schools

It has become increasingly clear over the last decade that school based health promotion programmes which include environment-focused components are more effective than those that use curriculum components alone (Weare 2000; Wells et al 2003). Curriculum programmes to change individuals' social or emotional coping skills, as with similar strategies for drug use and other health risk behaviours, have not been shown to be effective in the long term (Spence and Shortt 2007; White and Pitts 1998). Further, curriculum addressing specific issues fails to take advantage of the fact that the same array of processes is known to be common to many problems (Resnick 2000; Resnick et al 1993; Catalano et al 2004; Hawkins et al 1992) and, as stated above, given problems of a crowded curriculum, creating curricula for every health or social issue is not sustainable. Perhaps, most importantly, a solely curriculum or programme-based approach does not recognize and therefore cannot adequately address the influence of the school social context on both the health and learning outcomes for young people (Bond et al 2007; Fletcher et al 2007).

Whole school approaches aimed at changing the school culture and practices are not simple to implement or evaluate, however. Although often difficult to squeeze into a tight timetable, a programme or curriculum package is a tangible product which can be adopted by individuals or groups of teachers. Whole school approaches require much more coordinated and far-reaching change (Weare 2000).

Taking an ecological approach (Green and Kreuter 1999), and thereby addressing environment or social contexts as well as individual skills, involves developing multilevel interventions that focus on changing risk and protective factors that are common to many problems. Such an approach fits with both the principles of Health Promoting Schools (IUHPE 2009; Lynagh et al 1997; Nutbeam 1992), WHO priorities for adolescent health (Resnick et al 1993), and from the perspective of intervention research, fits with a call to focus more on setting-level contextual factors to enhance adoption, reach, implementation, and maintenance of effective interventions (Glasgow et al 2003).

Community-based health promotion and research in educational reform have both identified a need to understand how to create and sustain change in complex environments. A central concept for both disciplines is the building of local capacity to identify problems and undertake interventions which are then embedded or incorporated within community structures (Fullan 2006; Hargreaves and Fink 2006; Israel et al 2006; Weare 2000; West-Burnham et al 2007). The potential for health promotion to both operate within, and change, the whole-school environment has shifted the perspective from schools as supportive settings for health promotion, to schools as an eco-system that should respond and change with the implementation of an intervention (Hawe et al 2004).

The Gatehouse Project

Drawing on health and health promotion literature and that of school improvement to effect whole school change, the Gatehouse Project was developed to address some of the limitations in earlier school health promotion work. In line with the Health Promoting Schools framework (WHO 1995), the Gatehouse Project was a primary prevention programme, which included both institutional and individual focused components to promote the emotional and behavioural well-being of young people in secondary schools. Specifically, it aimed to increase levels of emotional well-being and reduce rates of substance use, known to be related to emotional well-being (Patton et al 1998; Patton et al 1996; McGee et al 2000; Rey et al 2002; Bovasso 2001).

The intervention was designed to make changes in the social and learning environments of the school and at the individual level by providing schools with strategies to enhance students' sense of connectedness to school and increase individuals' skills and knowledge for dealing with the everyday life challenges. The intervention included strong conceptual and operational frameworks to enhance schools' understanding of adolescent mental health needs and an evidence-based process for planning, implementing, and evaluating a practical intervention, including both individual-focused and environment-focused approaches.

Reflecting on the Project, we believe the key components for the success of the Gatehouse Project were the (1) conceptual and operational frameworks that spoke to and made sense to teachers as well as health researchers; (2) the active combination of health promotion/population health approach with education reform; (3) an educator working closely with schools as facilitator or critical friend; (4) establishment of a broad-based school implementation team to implement the evidence-based process; (5) use of local data to inform direction and strategies and prioritize actions; and (6) integration of the curriculum component with classroom and whole school context.

Conceptual and operational frameworks

The conceptual framework was developed from an understanding of risk processes for adolescents and translated early work on attachment and social support theories into a model relevant for promoting emotional well-being and engagement with learning (Patton et al 2003). It emphasized the importance of healthy attachments and in particular in the school setting a sense of positive connection with teachers and peers. It focused on three areas of action:

+ building a sense of *security* and trust;
+ enhancing *communication* and social connectedness; and
+ building a sense of *positive regard* through valued participation in aspects of school life.

The whole school change component emphasized the development and implementation of strategies that addressed these three areas of action at multiple levels of the school community. These three foci provided schools with 'lenses' to view and critique what they were currently doing and what they might do to promote these.

The operational framework, drawing on the Health Promoting Schools framework (WHO 1995), made it explicit that there was a need to address the three areas of action

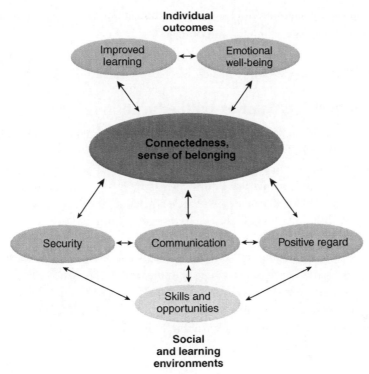

Fig. 16.1 The Gatehouse Project conceptual framework
© The Conceptual Framework of the Gatehouse Project, Centre for Adolescent Health 1997

at all levels of school operations. The comprehensive whole school strategy, therefore sought to:

- introduce relevant and important skills through the curriculum;
- make changes in the schools' social and learning environments; and
- strengthen links between the school and its community.

The Gatehouse Project provided a five-step evidence-based process, through which schools worked to build on existing policies, programmes and practices and develop new policies, programmes and practices that promote connectedness to school. This involved:

- establishing an Adolescent Health Team to coordinate the planning, implementation and evaluation of strategies;
- reviewing policies, programmes, and practices to identify priorities for action, including use of data from their students' perceptions of relationships in the school;
- planning strategies to address areas identified in the review;
- training and implementation, developing a programme of professional development and training for members of the school community to equip them to implement the chosen strategies; and

- monitoring and evaluation of the process of implementation, with a view to informing future cycles of review, planning, and change.

In recognition that promoting emotional well-being in schools required continuous review, planning, and action, the work with schools was based on an action research model.

Combined health promotion with education reform

This project was not driven by health researchers and merely advised by, or implemented by educators. While drawing on health promotion, attachment theory, positive youth development and a risk and protective factor framework, what the intervention looked like and how it was implemented was informed essentially by the, then, current education literature on school change (Fullan 1993; Stoll and Fink 1996; Hargreaves et al 1996). Thus the multi-disciplinary research team with backgrounds in health and education worked together to shape the intervention and its implementation. In this approach robust discussion, challenging each discipline with what could be done or not done in schools, led to a unique development where both the whole school and individual focused approaches were dynamic and were allowed to take advantage of each school's local context. We deliberately and explicitly linked the intervention to education goals and priorities as well as health goals. We talked about well-being not mental illness and related the goals of increasing connectedness to school not just to better health outcomes but to better educational outcomes, the core business for schools (Hargreaves et al 1996; Resnick et al 1993).

The intervention was shaped to account for schools' capacity to take on the intervention in terms of resources and pressures of competing priorities. Our work with the schools involved paying attention to the social and policy environment, facilitating ownership of problems and solutions. Schools' responses to the intervention were therefore allowed to be different from each other, to suit each context. Mediated by the project facilitators, and during professional learning days focused on learning new skills and knowledge and sharing achievements and strategies, schools were encouraged to learn from each other.

Educators facilitating implementation and change

Facilitators were experienced educators and, as described above, were intimately involved in the development of the intervention and its implementation, working intensively with two to four intervention schools each over the life of the project (1997–2001). It is important to note that the facilitators' role encompassed more than the traditional project officer role of providing administrative and technical assistance and professional development (Glover and Butler 2004).They played the role of critical friend to the schools: a role which had both formal and informal dimensions (Butler et al 2001). The formal dimension was one of providing feedback of the data, helping make sense of the data and supporting the planning and implementation of changes, including the provision of resources and professional training. However, the informal dimension was equally important in the process. This involved discussing concerns, building trust, raising questions, reflecting on actions and supporting and encouraging efforts and momentum. School participants often noted the importance of this aspect of the role, one acknowledging for example:

> [facilitator's] magnificent listening skills and intervention at just the right moments and to give individuals encouragement at just the right moments when they needed it. (KII[1] 2000)

> (Butler et al 2007)

Much of this informal work happened outside the scheduled professional learning activities, in lunchtime conversation in staff rooms or debriefing chats with staff. The importance of just being there in places where teachers spent time out of class was important for gaining an understanding of the school culture and practice, building relationships and trust, and hearing individual teachers' hopes and concerns. This 'strategic lurking', as one facilitator called it, enabled facilitators to notice points of synergy and dissonance between the Project's work, the schools' everyday business and involvement with other initiatives and helped schools make meaning and coherence out of all of this. The facilitators' understanding of school life was very helpful here, as acknowledged by a school leader:

> On the whole I would say . . . it wouldn't be possible from someone who doesn't have a teaching background. I think someone who has an understanding of the life of schools is certainly . . . in a more insightful position I think because of the demands that are taking place, the parental demands, the student demands, the staff demands, the curriculum demands, the Board of Study demands, the community demands, so many things impacting upon life in schools. And life in schools is becoming more complicated (AP KII[2] 2000)

> (Butler et al 2007)

Moreover, this time spent building credibility in the schools was fundamentally important to enable work with staff because as one school leader put it:

> Some school staff are suspicious unfortunately of people who come in from outside and it's reality . . . they would be finding a little bit of a battle perhaps to be accepted in some ways . . . (KII 2000)

> (unpublished)

The facilitator also operated as a 'go-between', enabling two-way feedback from the schools to the research team. This enabled dialogue around principles and processes, sometimes challenging assumptions and orthodoxies on both sides. It resulted in some modifications to the planned implementation process and schools appreciated this:

> the model . . . of having that critical friend is vital . . . I understand that there will be tensions between the researchers and the education backed people, teachers, and I know the Project has changed internally over a period of time because of the interaction of the critical friends back into the Centre for Adolescent Health and the fact that there has been that flexibility here to alter has been wonderful. Because people outside of schools don't understand how schools function and

---

[1] Key Informant Interview

[2] Assistant Principal Key Informant Interview

people inside schools don't realise that there are people outside who don't. They think it's obvious, everyone knows how schools function. (KII 2000)

(Butler et al 2007)

This process certainly influenced the evolution of the Gatehouse Project model and future iterations of it.

Establishment of a broad-based school implementation team to implement evidence-based process

The use of project teams or action teams is now a well-established component of many school-based health promotion initiatives. Traditionally, these teams have often mainly comprised staff working in health-related areas such as health teachers, school nurses, student welfare co-ordinators. In the Gatehouse Project, schools were asked to establish teams that not only included health and welfare staff but representatives from school leadership, curriculum and year-level teams, and if possible parents and the wider community. This was important to enable the whole school strategies to span all areas of school operations. Where these teams worked effectively, they:

+ had a formal place in the school's organizational structure (sometimes being an adaptation of an existing team such as a leadership team, faculty team, pastoral care, or student welfare team);
+ were acknowledged and supported by the school leadership; and
+ provided a focus for linkage, priority setting and coordination both within the school and with the school's local community. (Butler et al 2001)

In some cases, it seemed surprising that the staff involved had rarely worked together on whole school planning before, especially on activities spanning curriculum, organizational structures, and services affecting health and well-being. The value of this broad based representation was acknowledged:

Because [the adolescent health team] touches all bases, all aspects to the movement of the school because [one team member] works with heads of learning directly and the welfare dimension of the school works with linking the community and with management and I have a foot in both camps. (KII5-98)

(Bond et al 2001)

The facilitator played an important role in establishing and encouraging these teams, supporting and motivating investigations and discussions, and helping to keep a focus on the themes of the project.

Using local data as a catalyst for local action

Informed by programmes focused on reducing bullying in schools (Olweus 1993) and community prevention programmes such as Communities that Care (Hawkins and Catalano 1993; Hawkins and Catalano 1992), late in the first year of the intervention and each year subsequently we fed back to schools students' perceptions of their relationships with teachers, with peers, and with learning, collected as part of the impact/outcome evaluation. These data included each school's students' data and the aggregated data from the comparison schools. Importantly, we did not feed back data on student health outcomes or health risk behaviours as we wanted schools to focus on aspects of their environment that they had some control over rather than focusing on depression or drug use.

Nor did we use the data diagnostically but rather to create opportunities for discussion of what these data might mean. We asked questions to encourage reflection on how the data profile compared with other data the school had and what the school might want to do about it, for example:

- What general questions are raised for you by this profile?
- How does this information fit with your observations of your students and their experiences of school?
- What might your students mean by their responses?
- What is pleasing about these data and can you celebrate and reinforce this? What are the areas of concern and what resources are available for support in this area?
- What are you already doing to address issues raised and what else needs to be done?
- What circumstances at the time of the survey might have impacted on responses, both positively and negatively?
- Are there any areas of policy, programmes, or practices for which these data have particular implications?

Other questions may arise as teams considered their school's data from this report in conjunction with other data and their school's action plans.

School staff expressed appreciation of this inquiry-based approach and the co-construction of meaning and consequences for action:

> the work that [the facilitator] has done with our staff… has been invaluable and it hasn't been a coming in and saying 'here's the data now do that'. But it's been a listening to what was happening, a giving of advice, a very willingness to be here to address staff, so coming to a staff meeting and talking about it, interpreting the data.
>
> (Butler et al 2007)

Further discussion focused on addressing these risk and protective factors identified in the school environment by choosing strategies to change teacher practice and school culture rather than just implementing further programmes to address student or parent attitudes and behaviours. The opportunity to consider how students perceived their experiences of school, including relationships with each other, their teachers, and with learning was often challenging at first but often yielded rich discussion and powerful motivation for change:

> I think the data provided for teachers an opportunity to look at students from a different perspective. A couple of the key findings in our data related to how students perceived their teachers saw them and where, as their sort of responses to that. And I think for some staff that was a revelation

that they had perhaps not been aware that student[s] felt that way about particular aspects of modes of operation. So I think the data helped to raise awareness for staff about how the student perspective was and so perhaps to revisit some of the ways in which the classroom runs here, that sort of thing, I think for some was also fairly helpful. School leader. (KII 2000)

(unpublished)

So I think the data that provided us that, the particulars of our cohort, informed practice and provided reflection and an opportunity to reflect on our data. (AP KII 2000)

(unpublished)

I mean even with our data when we had it explained to us, as the management team and then we took the pathway of wanting to share it with the staff and you know there was good support then in the school liaison person being prepared to actually come out which is a fairly difficult task to come and have information shared with you that some staff may not be very willing to accept. (AP KII 2000)

(unpublished)

Integration of the curriculum component with classroom and whole school context

The teaching and learning materials were based on principles of cognitive behaviour therapy (CBT), aimed to assist students to explore ways of dealing with difficult feelings that commonly arise in adverse situations. Specifically, the programme was designed to explore and reinforce the key message that:

 • everyone's life has ups and downs;

 • we will experience a range of feelings in response to these; and

 • what we think will influence what we feel.

Sometimes we can change the situation and sometimes we can't but there are always more helpful and less helpful ways of thinking about it. The way we feel and act will depend on how we think about the situation (Glover et al 2002).

The activities were also shaped by a critical literacy approach which encouraged teachers and students to consider the influence of context as well as individual skills and knowledge and to explore situations from multiple perspectives (Lankshear and McLaren 1993).

A CBT approach is common in curriculum-based interventions addressing student mental health (eg Spence et al 2003), however, the approach we used in implementing the curriculum was innovative in a number of ways. Firstly, unlike prescriptive, manualized approaches to health education, we encouraged teachers to understand the key principles underpinning the programme, to incorporate these in their lessons and approaches to teaching and we actively encouraged them to adapt these to best suit the contexts of their students and schools. The manuals the teachers worked with were in draft form and we invited input from them in the further development of these teaching resources.

Secondly, we encouraged the teaching of the key concepts through the study of texts— literature, poetry, song, film, and visual materials. The materials were therefore suited to being taught in the study of English, or other subject areas as determined by the schools. Most Gatehouse Project schools taught these concepts in English, Health/Physical Education, or Pastoral Care/Personal Learning Classes.

Thirdly, teachers were asked to think about their role as more than delivering content. They were asked to think about three strategies for working with the content (see Figure 16.2):

- foster relationships and classroom climate that promote security, communication and positive regard;
- explicit teaching and learning activities which help students develop skills and knowledge for managing the challenges of everyday life; and
- teachers' interactions with students to reinforce strategies 1 and 2 (Glover et al 2002).

While we provided examples of teaching and learning strategies we encouraged staff to look for opportunities in activities they already undertook with students or to create new ones in line with the principles of the teaching and learning approach. We therefore encouraged staff to integrate and extend their learnings from these materials beyond set lesson times and into the teaching context.

Fourthly, the materials did not address mental illness, mental health, or drugs. As described above, the focus was on assisting students to understand the challenges and stresses they may experience, to explore the range of emotional reactions to them and to apply strategies for dealing with them in an everyday context (Glover et al 2002). Themes of the programme included belonging and connectedness, negotiating life's ups and downs, trust and relationships, expectations of self and others, and dealing with anxiety. Strategies explored included recognizing and normalizing feelings, 'self-talk' in dealing

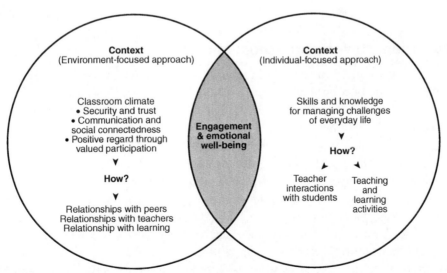

Fig. 16.2 Teaching and learning Venn diagram
© Centre for Adolescent Health 2001

with feelings, seeing common challenging situations from different viewpoints, understanding links between thinking, feeling, and acting (Glover et al 2002).

Overall, what were we asking schools to do that was different from other school-based interventions? We were asking them to implement an evidence-based process to change the social and learning environment to promote well-being. The whole school intervention provided them with a process to do this. Thus, while schools did different things in response to their local data and contexts, and were encouraged to do so within the framework of the trial, they underwent the same processes: establishing or identifying a broadly representative adolescent health team; using local data; examining current policies and practices against the Gatehouse foci of security, communication, and positive regard and choosing and implementing strategies that addressed these; reflecting on the impact of these actions and then refining or choosing new ways to address these key issues for keeping students connected to school. Schools were encouraged to consider and implement multiple changes at multiple levels, to consider simple changes (Principal ensuring he/she greets the students by name) to major structural changes (teaching and learning in small groups; staff teams spanning faculties).

The integration of the curriculum component with classroom and whole school context, and the encouragement of teachers to adapt and extend their use of the processes and materials was aimed at embedding the work beyond the project. The transience of many school-based projects was noted by participants:

> we get you know lots of programs that come and go, and I think they come and go because it may be a good idea but not seeing how it fits within a school setting. And I think a lot of merit of this Project has been in the way in which it has understood the school setting and has set up structures that have worked within a school setting. . . . so it's a big understanding, that, setting it up, understanding administrative, teachers, students, parents and how schools work on a daily basis I think is just fundamental, and this project I think understood that really well. (KII 2000)

(unpublished)

Evaluation: student and school outcomes

The Gatehouse Project was evaluated using a cluster randomized controlled trial in 26 (12 intervention, 14 control) government-funded, Catholic and independent secondary schools in metropolitan and regional Victoria, Australia. Thirty-two schools had been sampled with six declining to participate. No schools dropped out during the trial period (1997–2001).

To assess the effect of the intervention on students' mental health and health risk behaviours a cohort of students in the intervention and control schools were surveyed regularly. Examples of some of these measures are presented in Box 16.1 and a complete list and description can be found in Bond et al (2004a). As well as outcome measures, the questionnaire also included questions assessing students' perceptions of their school climate, and the quality of their relationships with friends and peers.

Figure 16.3 illustrates the timeline for the intervention and when the waves of student data collection were gathered for the intervention and comparisons schools. Supervised

Box 16.1 Examples of self-report impact and outcome measures

School climate	Relationships with peers (eg I like the other students in my classes), relationships with teachers (eg Teachers are fair in dealing with students), relationship to learning (eg Doing well in school is important to me)
Social connectedness	Having someone to trust, depend on, who knows you well
Interpersonal conflict	Having arguments with others recently; being bullied
Mental health status: anxiety/depression	Computerized version of the Clinical Interview Schedule[1]
Substance use	Drinker, regular drinker (≥3 days/week); Smoker, regular smoker (≥6days/week); Used marijuana (in last 6 months)

[1](Lewis et al 1992; Wilkinson and Markus 1989)

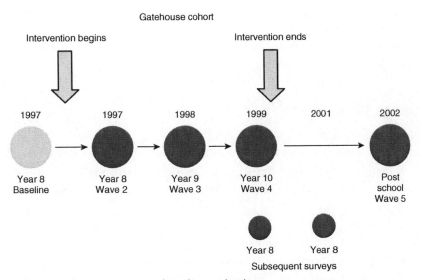

Fig. 16.3 Timeline for intervention and student evaluation

by the research team, students completed a questionnaire at school using laptop computers four times: two waves of data were collected in 1997 at the beginning and end of the participants' second year of secondary school (Year 8, age 13–14) and the third and fourth waves of data were collected at the end of Year 9 (1998) and Year 10 (1999) respectively.

Student participation in the surveys was voluntary and written parental consent was required. About 74% (2,678) of Year 8 students participated in the baseline survey. Absent students were surveyed at school at a later date or by telephone and telephone interviews were completed with students who had left the project schools for the subsequent waves of data collection. Of all the students who participated in the baseline survey 97% completed wave 2 (end of year 8 survey), 92% completed wave 3 (Year 9 survey), and 90% completed the fourth survey. There was no differential response rate between intervention and control groups at the subsequent waves (98% vs 96%; 92% vs 92% and 90% vs 89% for the respective waves).

To determine if changes that had occurred in schools had an effect on students other than those in the Gatehouse cohort, we undertook two repeat cross-sectional surveys of subsequent year 8 students in 1999, and one year after the facilitators had withdrawn from the schools (2001). About 71% of eligible students participated.

We assessed the implementation of the intervention through facilitators' notes and journals; regular team meeting discussions; surveying teachers about their use of the curriculum materials; and annual interviews with key informant in the intervention schools. School socio-demographic information and data about school policies and health promotion programme activities were collected annually from all intervention and control schools. These data have been used to variously describe the implementation of the curriculum components, the factilators' role and to reflect on the content and process of the intervention as experienced by the school staff (Bond et al 2001; Bond et al 2004a; Butler et al 2001; Glover et al 2004).

Outcomes for students

At baseline, the prevalence of depressive symptoms, drug use, and anti-social behaviour was similar for students in intervention and comparison schools. Over the next two years we found that the prevalence of any drinking, smoking, marijuana use, and peers' drug use was between 3% and 5% lower for students in the intervention schools compared to those in the comparison schools. In terms of individuals' risk, there was a 25%–40% risk reduction (ie Odds Ratios between 0.75 and 0.60) in substance use in the cohort of students in the intervention schools followed up longitudinally two and three years after the intervention began. Adjusting for clustering, and baseline measures, these differences remained marginally significant (Bond et al 2004a; Bond et al 2004b). These effects are as strong or stronger than many reported in the drug education literature (Tobler and Stratton 1997; Botvin et al 1995; Botvin et al 1990; Peterson et al 2000).

Importantly, subsequent Year 8 students in the intervention schools surveyed in the third year of the trial and one year after work with schools was finished also reported lower rates of substance use and other health risk behaviours compared with control schools (Patton et al 2006).

As expected from the literature, strong associations were found between depressive symptoms and participants' social relationships and school connectedness but no differences were found in the prevalence of depressive symptoms at any time during the trial. These findings are consistent with other studies of preventive interventions that have failed to demonstrate an effect on depression and related problems (Lister-Sharp et al 1999, Spence and Shortt 2007).

We also found no change in students' reporting of increased connectedness to school, our theoretical explanatory mechanism for change in students' behaviours! Thus, while the findings of this trial appear consistent with a true intervention effect, achieved through a multi-level intervention with a focus not on drugs nor on refusal skills, but on changing social processes underlying these activities, questions remain about these mechanisms.

Over the years, we have pondered on whether we have not measured the right things or whether our measures of school connectedness were sensitive enough to change. We cannot, of course, exclude the possibility that our findings have arisen by chance but it seems unlikely, given (1) the consistency of the reductions across the measures of substance use and (2) across three 'generations' of Year 8 students.

One possible explanation comes from an examination of differential effects of the intervention for those with good school connectedness and those with low school connectedness. While, as with most studies, we have limited capacity to analyse the effect of the intervention on subgroups, adjusting for school connectedness at Year 8, we have found students in the intervention schools who reported good school connectedness in Year 10, were half as likely to smoke and a third less likely to smoke regularly (9.5%, 3.4%) than students in the control schools (20.1%, 12.6%). This was not the case for those who had low school connectedness (Bond et al 2007). Thus, we may have some evidence that the intervention is more effective for those students who are already connected to school. While treating these findings with caution (we found no similar interactions for other outcomes), it makes sense that a school-based intervention may struggle to engage students already disengaging from school.

Should we therefore give up doing things in schools? We would argue no. We need to take into account the amount of time it takes to change organizational structures and cultures. Changing whole school structures, policies, programmes and culture and curriculum is also challenging. It is likely that the extent of change in the lifetime of the Project was probably not sufficient to impact on students already disengaged or disengaging. Perhaps more importantly though, this finding indicates that we need to develop more explicit strategies to engage the disengaging and disengaged students. Some of our more recent research, working with disadvantaged schools, has provided us with some examples of how this might be done successfully. For example, we worked with clusters of primary and secondary schools in disadvantaged areas focused particularly on improving transition from primary to secondary school and involving schools, families, and the communities (Doing it Differently Project Report forthcoming).

Outcomes for schools

Intervention schools reported a strong sense of partnership *with* the research team. They felt respected and valued and appreciated that we worked with them rather than asking them to do things for our research. Schools' perceptions of the student data collection shifted from being a burden and irrelevant to their work, to being a valuable resource, with some schools seeking other opportunities to collect these or similar data either by continuing to use the Gatehouse Student Survey, being involved in other research projects which collected these data, or assessing how they might use the data they routinely collected for the Department of Education (Victoria, Australia) for their own purposes. The use of these data and the process of critical reflection encouraged in the Project therefore enhanced schools' capacity for evidence-based change.

Schools also reported that the conceptual framework and the whole-school process provided a useful framework for change. Involvement in the project provided them with an opportunity to take risks within a safe environment (often what they seek to set up for their students). The three foci—security, communication, and positive regard gave them 'a lens to review activities and practices': how might whatever they do or are asked to do by the education systems, community, or parent body enhance or detract from these for their students and their staff. This project was not just about students, but everyone.

Overall, schools reported a shift in perception that promoting well-being is 'core business'. And ultimately, what became clear for all of us, was that the Gatehouse Project was about changing relationships between students and students, students and learning, and most importantly, between students and staff.

> Gatehouse's greatest contribution was that it forced teachers to accept the fact that we had to change because we hadn't really been properly understanding the circumstances of our clientele . . . certainly the initial stage of Gatehouse forced people to confront the fact that we did have a lot of kids at risk who weren't being connected with. And staff started to take that on board and we then started to see things flow on into our teaching programs that I think before Gatehouse would have been rejected by the staff because I think there was very much an attitude of 'well, I'm the teacher and it all focuses around me'. And I think Gatehouse really caused a change in that teacher-centred view of education and we started to look at the needs of the kids better than we had in the past. (Teacher).

(Drew et al 2008)

Challenges of evaluating school-based interventions

Much of this chapter describes the challenges of implementing whole school interventions and what we have learnt about embedding such interventions within the usual school activities and agendas. Evaluating them is also challenging for researchers and for schools. For the researchers a balance is needed between resourcing the intervention and the evaluation. Importantly, the evaluation of a complex intervention requires sufficient resources to collect not just outcome data but also process or implementation data. In our experience this produces a large quantity of data with little budgeted capacity to fully analyse and utilize it.

For schools the evaluation activities can swamp or may even be seen to *be* the research; these activities can be more apparent than the intervention. For example, for students to participate in the evaluation surveys required active parent consent. This required staff to coordinate parent consent forms, remind students to return forms, liaise with the research survey team about appropriate 'survey dates' and cope with disrupted teaching schedules during these days. Of course, for the comparison schools collecting these data *is* the research so a further challenge is maintaining their interest and cooperation. The carrot of being offered the intervention in due course is again something that is difficult to do in great depth given the research budgets.

In response to these challenges, in the Gatehouse Project, the facilitators and schools annually discussed and agreed upon the type of data we wanted to collect and the time-frame. In our subsequent work with schools we have established written memoranda of understanding including agreements about this. We have also tried, where possible, to ensure that the data has multiple uses—useful for schools to drive change and reflect on activities and practice, and useful for the evaluation. From our feedback from schools, as described in the previous section, this appears to have been a successful strategy.

A further challenge for research where the intervention is theorized as a process of change is to consider what is the unit of interest: the school, the staff and/or the students; and how to measure change processes. This thinking also means that questions of fidelity of implementation and adaptation are different from interventions of products or programmes. Here we want fidelity to process not product and adaptation to context is required.

One aspect of research that in our experience has not been a difficulty is randomization. For the Gatehouse Project we had few refusals to participate and no schools dropping out of the study, but we probably cannot generalize from that. However, for a subsequent national study that we were involved in 150 Victorian schools expressed interest in participating in a randomized trial. We needed 16.

Conclusion

This chapter has described in detail the Gatehouse Project intervention. This intervention had many similarities to other school-based health promotion projects: taking a participatory approach, using local data (Olweus 1993; Hawkins and Catalano 1992), using a CBT framework to build students' skills and capacity to manage everyday ups and downs of life (Spence et al 2003; Spence and Shortt 2007), having a school-based team leading, driving and doing the intervention and using a facilitator or critical friend (Earl et al 2003; MacBeath 1996). So what did Gatehouse do that was different? We would argue several things. The Gatehouse Project:

1 had a theoretical framework that made sense to schools and a simple focus of promoting security, communication and positive regard through valued participation;

2 focused on changing the risk and protective factors in the school environment, that schools had capacity to change, rather than addressing (single) health behaviours or education outcomes;

3 employed all the strategies described above in an integrated approach to change teacher practice and school culture;

4 facilitated this process of change by using critical friends who understood both the demands of education systems and health promotion, were present in the schools and developed the schools' trust and respect;

5 built the capacity of schools to use their local data: not a diagnostic tool interpreted by the researchers. Schools could explore 'what does this mean' in our school and so become critical users of evidence and research;

6 allowed each school to respond to their data and to the Project in their own way, to differ in what they did in response to their data and the Project itself, and to be able to take into account both the strengths and challenges in their school communities;

7 encouraged teachers to understand the principles of the curriculum resources, to embed these in their teaching practice, to be modelled beyond the classroom;

8 encouraged schools to think beyond curriculum-based and knowledge-based solutions to address issues;

9 provided a clear and supported process for reflective practice/action research; and

10 provided support, being there, working with the schools for more than a year, knowing the context and responding to the context.

It is tempting, with complex or multi-level, multi-component interventions, to ask which component really worked. Which bits are necessary and which are ice-breakers, strategies to engage schools and to get them ready and keep them going. Certainly we cannot tell from the evaluation design of the Gatehouse Project, whether it was the curriculum component or the whole school component that was the effective component. But from our experience we would argue that this is not a sensible question. We believe it was the combination of what schools did, the interaction between their contexts and the ingredients/aspects of the Gatehouse Project, which contributed to the success of the Gatehouse Project. For many of the schools, we helped change how they thought about health, health education, and health promotion for their students, themselves, and their communities.

From the work we have been doing over the last ten years in schools, we believe there needs to be a fundamental shift in conceptualizing what mental health promotion in schools might look like and how, therefore, to implement and evaluate it. Rather than developing interventions as products or multiple products delivered at different levels in the school organization we have conceptualized our work in schools as facilitating an overall process of organizational change to enable ongoing promotion of mental health and well-being of young people. Four key components of this process are:

♦ conceptualizing the intervention as an ongoing process of change, not a product to be 'done';

♦ facilitating the change process (not just training and technical assistance);

♦ bringing an in-depth understanding of the educational context and adolescent health and well-being; and

♦ assisting schools to integrate this work within their core business.

Importantly, to be sustainable, this work needs to be supported by, indeed embedded in, educational systems, teacher education programmes, and community support networks.

Acknowledgments

The Gatehouse Project and our subsequent school-based work, has received funding and valued support from the Queen's Trust for Young Australians, the Victorian Health Promotion Foundation, the Department of Human Services, Victoria, Australia, the Sidney Myer Fund, the Catholic Education Office, Melbourne, the National Health and Medical Research Council, Murdoch Childrens Research Institute, and the Baker Foundation. The authors would like to acknowledge the valuable contribution made by the school communities participating in the Gatehouse Project and the project members of Gatehouse Project and the Adolescent Health and Social Environments Programme at the Centre for Adolescent Health.

Bibliography

Bond, L., Butler, H., Thomas, L., Carlin, J. B., Glover, S., Bowes, G., et al (2007) 'Social and school connectedness in early secondary school as predictors of late teenage substance use, mental health and academic outcomes' *Journal of Adolescent Health* 40: 357e9–357e18

Bond, L., Glover, S., Godfrey, C., Butler, H. and Patton, G. (2001) 'Building capacity for system-level change in schools: Lessons from the Gatehouse Project' *Health Education Behavior* 28: 368–83

Bond, L., Patton, G. C., Glover, S., Carlin, J. B., Butler, H., Thomas, L., et al (2004a) 'The Gatehouse Project: can a multi-level school intervention affect emotional well-being and health risk behaviours?' *Journal of Epidemiology and Community Health* 58: 997–1003

Bond, L., Thomas, L., Coffey, C., Glover, S., Butler, H., Carlin, J. B., et al (2004b) 'Long-term impact of the Gatehouse Project on the incidence of cannabis use in 16 year olds: a school-based cluster randomised trial' *Journal of School Health* 74: 23–9

Bonell, C., Fletcher, A. and McCambridge, J. (2007) 'Improving school ethos may reduce substance misuse and teenage pregnancy' *British Medical Journal* 334: 614–16

Botvin, G. J., Baker, E., Dusenbury, L., Botvin, E. M. and Diaz, T. (1995) 'Long-term follow-up results of a randomised drug abuse prevention trial in a white middle-class population' *Journal of the American Medical Association* 273: 1106–12

Botvin, G. J., Baker, E., Dusenbury, L., Tortu, S. and Botvin, E. M. (1990) 'Preventing adolescent drug abuse through a multimodal cognitive-behavioural approach: results of a 3-year study' *Journal of Consulting and Clinical Psychology* 58: 437–46

Bovasso, G. B. (2001) 'Cannabis abuse as a risk factor for depressive symptoms' *American Journal of Psychiatry* 158: 2033–7

Butler, H., Bond, L., Glover, S., Patton, G., Rowling, L., Martin, G., et al (2001) 'The Gatehouse Project: Mental health promotion incorporating school organisational change and health education' in L. Rowling, G. Martin, and L. Walker (eds), *Mental Health Promotion and Young People: Concepts and practice*. Roseville: McGraw Hill

Butler, H., Seal, I., Trafford, L., Drew, S., Hargreaves, J., Martinac, K., et al (2007) *Informed interactions: facilitating evidence-based school change to promote student engagement and wellbeing*. Paper presented at the 6th Australian and New Zealand Youth Health Conference, Christchurch, 23–26 September

Catalano, R. F., Haggerty, K. P., Oesterle, S., Fleming, C. B. and Hawkins, J. D. (2004) 'The importance of bonding to school for healthy development: Findings from the Social Development Research Group' *Journal of School Health* 74: 252–61

Drew, S., Hargreaves, J., Butler, H. and Bond, L. (2008) Horses for Courses: Teachers' perspectives on implementing and sustaining a complex student health and wellbeing intervention (Poster) *5th World Conference on the Promotion of Mental Health and the Prevention of Mental Health Disorders* Melbourne

Earl, L., Torrance, N., Sutherland, S., Fullan, M. and Ali, A. S. (2003) *Manitoba school improvement program: final evaluation report*. Toronto: Ontario The Ontario Institute for Studies in Education of the University of Toronto

Fletcher, A., Bonell, C. and Hargreaves, J. (2007) 'Systematic reviews of intervention and observational studies examining school-level effects on young people's drug use' *Journal of Adolescent Health* 42: 209–20

Fullan, M. (1993) *Change forces: Probing the depths of educational reform*. London: The Falmer Press

Fullan, M. (2006) *Turnaround Leadership*. San Francisco: Jossey-Bass

Glasgow, R. E., Lichtenstein, E. and Marcus, A. C. (2003) 'Why don't we see more translation of health promotion research into practice? Rethinking the efficacy-to-effectiveness transition' *American Journal of Public Health* 93: 1261–7

Glover, S. and Butler, H. (2004) 'Facilitating health promotion within school communities' in R. Moodie and A. Hulme (eds), *Hands-on health promotion*. Melbourne: IP Communications

Glover, S., Patton, G., Butler, H., Di Pietro, G., Begg, B., Ollis, D., et al (2002) *Teaching resources for emotional well-being*. Melbourne: Centre for Adolescent Health

Green, L. W. and Kreuter, M. W. (1999) *Health promotion planning: an educational and ecological approach*. Mountain View, California: Mayfield Publishing Company

Hargreaves, A., Earl, L. and Ryan, J. (1996) *Schooling for change: Reinventing schools for early adolescents*. London: Falmer Press

Hargreaves, A. and Fink, D. (2006) *Sustainable Leadership*. San Francisco: Jossey-Bass

Hawe, P., Shiell, A. and Riley, T. (2004) 'Complex interventions: how "out of control" can a randomised controlled trial be?' *British Medical Journal* 328: 1561–3

Hawkins, J. D, Catalano, R. F. and Associates (1992) *Communities that care: action for drug abuse prevention*. 1st edn. San Francisco: Jossey-Bass Publishers

Hawkins, J. D. and Catalano, R. F. (1993) 'Communities that care: risk and protective factor-focused prevention using the social development strategy' Developmental Research and Programs Inc. Seattle, Washington

Hawkins, J. D., Catalano, R. F. and Miller, J. Y. (1992) 'Risk and protective factors for alcohol and other drug problems in adolescence and early adulthood: implications for substance abuse prevention' *Psychological Bulletin* 112: 64–105

International Union for Health Promotion and Education (IUHPE) (2009) *Achieving Health Promoting Schools: Guidelines to Promote Health in Schools*. Available at International Union for Health Promotion and Education website: <http://www.iuhpe.org/index.html?page=516&lang=en&highlight=schools#sh_guidelines> (accessed 27 July 2009)

Israel B. A., Eng E., Schulz A. J., Parker E. A. (2006) 'Introduction to methods in community-based participatory research for health' in: B.A. Israel, E. Eng, A.J. Schulz, and E.A. Parker (eds), *Methods in community-based participatory research for health*, pp 3–26. California: John Wiley & Sons

Lankshear, C. and McLaren, P. (1993) *Critical Literacy: Politics, Praxis, and the Postmodern*. New York: State University of New York Press

Lewis, G., Pelosi, A., Araya, R. and Dunn, G. (1992) 'Measuring psychiatric disorder in the community: a standardized assessment for use by lay interviewers' *Psychological Medicine*. 22: 465–86

Lister-Sharp, D., Chapman, S., Stewart-Brown, S. and Sowden, A. (1999) 'Health promoting schools and health promotion in schools: two systematic reviews' *Health Technology Assessment* 3/22: 1–207

Lynagh, M., Schofield, M. J. and Sanson-Fisher, R. W. (1997) 'School health promotion programs over the past decade: a review of the smoking, alcohol and solar protection literature' *Health Promotion International* 12: 43–60

MacBeath, J (1996) '"I didn't know he was ill": The role and value of the critical friend' in L. Stoll, and D. Fink (eds), *Changing our Schools: Linking school effectiveness and school improvement*. Buckingham: Open University Press

McGee, R., Williams, S., Poulton, R. and Moffitt, T. (2000) 'A longitudinal study of cannabis use and mental health from adolescence to early adulthood' *Addiction* 95: 491–503

Nutbeam, D. (1992) 'The health promoting school: closing the gap between theory and practice' *Health Promotion International* 7: 151–3

Olweus, D. (1993) *Bullying in school: what we know and what we can do*. Oxford: Blackwell

Patton, G., Bond, L., Butler, H. and Glover, S. (2003) 'Changing schools, changing health?: The design and implementation of the Gatehouse Project' *Journal of Adolescent Health* 33: 231–9

Patton, G., Carlin, J. B., Coffey, C., Wolfe, R. and Bowes, G. (1998) 'Depression, anxiety and the initiation of smoking: a prospective study over three years' *American Journal of Public Health* 88: 1518–22

Patton, G. C., Bond, L., Carlin, J. B., Thomas, L., Butler, H., Glover, S., et al (2006) 'Promoting Social Inclusion in Secondary Schools: A Group-Randomized Trial of Effects on Student Health Risk Behaviour and Well-Being' *American Journal of Public Health* 96: 1582–7

Patton, G. C., Hibbert, M., Rosier, M., Carlin, J. B., Caust, J. and Bowes, G. (1996) 'Is smoking associated with depression and anxiety in teenagers?' *American Journal of Public Health* 86: 225–300

Peterson, A. V., Kealey, K. A., Mann, S. L. and Marek, P. M. (2000) 'Hutchinson smoking prevention project: long-term randomised trial in school-based tobacco use prevention—results on smoking' *Journal of the National Cancer Institute* 92: 1979–91

Resnick, M. D. (2000) 'Protective factors, resiliency, and healthy youth development' *Adolescent Medicine* 11: 157–64

Resnick, M. D., Harris, L. J. and Blum, R. W. (1993) 'The impact of caring and connectedness on adolescent health and well-being' *Journal of Paediatrics and Child Health* 29: s3–s9

Rey, J. M., Sawyer, M. G., Raphael, B., Patton, G. C. and Lynskey, M. (2002) 'Mental health of teenagers who use cannabis' *British Journal of Psychiatry* 180: 216–21

Spence, S. H., Sheffield, J. K. and Donovan, C. L. (2003) 'Preventing adolescent depression: An evaluation of the problem solving for life program' *Journal of Consulting and Clinical Psychology* 71: 3–13

Spence, S. H. and Shortt, A. L. (2007) 'Research Review: Can we justify the widespread dissemination of universal, school-based interventions for the prevention of depression among children and adolescents?' *Journal of Child Psychology and Psychiatry* 48: 526–42

Stoll, L. and Fink, D. (1996) 'Changing our schools: Linking school effectiveness and school improvement' in Hargreaves, A. and Goodson, I. (eds), *Changing our schools: Linking school effectiveness and school improvement*. Buckingham Philadelphia: Open University Press

Tobler, N. S. and Stratton, H. H. (1997) 'Effectiveness of school-based drug prevention programs: a meta-analysis of the research' *The Journal of Primary Prevention* 18: 71–128

Weare, K. (2000) *Promoting Mental, Emotional and Social Health A Whole School Approach*. New York: Routledge

Wells, J., Barlow, J. and Stewart-Brown, S. (2003) 'A systematic review of universal approaches to mental health promotion in schools' *Health Education* 103: 197–220

West-Burnham, J., Farrar, M. and Otero, G. (2007) *Schools and Communities: Working Together to Transform Children's Lives*. London: Network Continuum Education

White, D. and Pitts, M. (1998) 'Educating young people about drugs: a systematic review' *Addiction* 93: 1457–87

Wilkinson, G. and Markus, A. C. (1989) 'PROQSY: a computerised technique for psychiatric case identification in general practice' *British Journal of Psychiatry* 154: 378–82

Chapter 17

Workplace and mental well-being: the Whitehall II study

Mika Kivimäki, Jane E Ferrie, and Michael Marmot

Introduction

The aim of this chapter is to provide policy makers, researchers, organizations and individuals working in the public health sphere with an understanding of the evidence on how factors at work might influence mental well-being. We have used the Whitehall II study, one of the leading cohort studies in the field, as an illustrative example. The chapter provides an overview of major theories, describes the assessment methods used to measure mental well-being in the Whitehall II study, and reviews the main research findings. Finally, we discuss next steps for research, including suggestions for evidence-based interventions to minimize adverse effects on mental health and promote well-being at work.

What is the Whitehall II study?

The first Whitehall study, a prospective occupational cohort of middle-aged men employed in the British Civil Service (Reid et al 1974), showed lower occupational class to be associated with a higher risk of death. Conventional risk factors, such as smoking, hypertension, dyslipidaemia and diabetes, only partially explained this association (Marmot et al 1984; Kivimäki et al 2008).

The Whitehall II study, the focus of this chapter, is modelled on the first Whitehall study and was set up to investigate socioeconomic differences in physical and mental illness among British civil servants (Marmot et al 1991). Importantly, Whitehall II extended the research to include women as well as men and conducted repeated clinical screenings subsequent to baseline. This has enabled the study to track changes in social and economic circumstances, psychological states, health behaviours, and disease outcomes. A leading hypothesis in Whitehall II has been that psychosocial factors at work affect employees' well-being, health, and risk of illness.

Rationale for repeated measurements

Randomized controlled trials are the gold standard for obtaining information about causality in epidemiology. However, participants cannot be randomly allocated to exposures such as socio-economic circumstances or long-term stress at work; and interventions are very costly and difficult to implement in practice. An alternative approach is first to address these questions in observational data and then use this information to develop evidence-based interventions. Through an examination of dose-response relationships, direction of the association, confounding, and other aspects important in terms of establishing causality (Hill 1965), Whitehall II has built up convincing observational evidence of associations between occupational exposures, well-being and disease occurrence. Repeat measures of aspects of the work environment and mental health outcomes have enabled the Whitehall II study to establish temporal order, time sequence and dose-response relationships. At the same time, the inclusion of measures of health behaviours and pre-existing disease has helped us to take into account the role of these factors in the association between work environment and mental health.

One of the strengths of the Whitehall II study is a high participation rate even after 21 years of follow-up. Of the 6,895 men and 3,413 women who participated in the first screening in 1985–88, a total of 7180 (70% of baseline respondents) also participated in 2006.

How mental well-being was measured?

Several generic indicators that measure aspects of mental health and well-being have been used. To date, the 30-item General Health Questionnaire (GHQ) (Goldberg 1972; Goldberg and Williams 1988), a screening instrument that measures common mental disorders, has been included in all nine study phases with the exception of phase 4. Bradburn's Affect Balance Scale (Bradburn 1969), a ten-item scale considered as a measure of well-being, has been elicited twice at baseline and first follow-up. The resulting Affect Balance score is comprised of the five Negative Affect items subtracted from the five Positive Affect items. The 36-item Short Form Medical Outcomes Survey (SF-36, Ware and Sherbourne 1992; McHorney et al 1993, 1994) that measures social, physical, and mental health functioning has been administered five times since 1991 (phase 3) and the Center for Epidemiologic Studies-Depression Scale (CES-D, Radloff 1977) has been administered at phases 5 and 9. Sickness absence records from Civil Service registers are available for the period when the vast majority of the cohort was still in paid employment. These records include causes for absences enabling monitoring of sick leaves from work due to psychiatric reasons. Finally, self-reported information on psychotropic medication has been collected at every phase.

General Health Questionnaire

The GHQ measures common mental disorders. These are the most prevalent conditions classified as depressive episodes, neurotic disorders, stress-related disorders, and somatoform disorders according to the WHO classification of mental and behavioural disorders (Goldberg 1972; Prince et al 2007). Measuring common mental disorders is particularly relevant in community-based samples, such as Whitehall II, as mental disorders in the community are frequently characterized by co-morbidity between the disorders and by shifting patterns of symptoms that resist precise clinical classification (Prince et al 2007).

In Whitehall II, the GHQ questionnaire was validated against the Clinical Interview Schedule (sensitivity 73%, specificity 78%, Stansfeld and Marmot 1992), which gave a cut-off point of 4/5 for dividing 'non-cases' from 'cases'.The GHQ has been shown to have high reliability and has been widely used in large population-based surveys and trials (Pevalin 2000; Blumenthal et al 2005). It also demonstrates high predictive validity such that people classified as being a 'case' have elevated mortality rates relative to others (Huppert and Whittington 1995).

Subscales of the 30-item GHQ measuring symptoms of depression and anxiety have been created through the selection of items that are also present in the scaled 28-item GHQ. The items are as follows: (Depression) 'Have you recently been thinking of yourself as a worthless person,—felt that life is entirely hopeless,—found at times you couldn't do anything because your nerves were too bad?' (Anxiety) 'Have you recently—lost sleep over worry—felt constantly under strain—been getting scared or panicky for no good reason—found everything getting on top of you—been feeling nervous and strung-up all the time?' (Stansfeld et al 1998).

The Short Form Medical Outcomes Survey (SF-36)

The SF-36 is a short-form health survey with 36 questions including physical and mental health summary measures (sample items: 'How much of the time, during the past 4 weeks have you been a happy person?; . . . been a very nervous person?; . . . felt calm and peaceful?', Ware and Sherbourne 1992; McHorney et al 1993, 1994). It is probably the most widely evaluated health outcome measure among the 'quality of life' measures (Garratt et al 2002). The ability of the SF-36 to detect change in health in a general population has been demonstrated in the Whitehall II study (Hemingway, Nicholson et al 1997). As expected, the greatest declines were seen among employees who had physical disease at baseline that limited functioning or were GHQ cases, with the effects of physical disease and common mental disorder being additive. As a given level of objectively assessed morbidity may differently affect individuals' social, physical, and mental health functioning, the SF-36 complements traditional measures of mortality and morbidity by taking account of the functional impact.

Psychiatric sickness absences

Sickness absence is another measure of functioning. In the Whitehall II study, computerized sickness absence records were obtained from Civil Service pay centres. Sickness absence diagnoses coded by the Civil Service were converted to disease categories using the modified morbidity coding system of the Royal College of General Practitioners (RCGP) which is comparable with ICD-8. Disease categories related to mental well-being included: Psychoses (category 5); Headache and migraine (39); Neurosis (40); and Neurosis ill-defined (41).

The validity of the reasons for absence provided by the Civil Service was assessed by obtaining information from the participants' general practitioners (doctors) for all spells > 21 days taken between 1985 and 1990. There was agreement on disease category between the Civil Service and the general practitioner for 64% of absences in the validation study (Feeney, et al 1998). As an indication of the predictive validity of sickness absence as a measure of health, overall certified sickness absence and absences with psychiatric diagnoses have been shown to be associated with mortality in the Whitehall II study (Kivimäki, Head, et al 2003; Head et al 2008).

Main findings

Work-related factors that have received particular attention in the Whitehall II study include occupational class, job insecurity, and work stressors. A review of the main findings is provided below.

The occupational class gradient in mental well-being

A socio-economic gradient in mental health outcomes (lower occupational class–poorer well-being) has been evidenced at several phases of the Whitehall II study (Ferrie et al 2002; Hemingway, Stafford, et al 1997; Stansfeld et al 2003). An early longitudinal analysis documented a nearly twofold excess risk of being in the most rapid quartile of decline in mental health functioning for men in the lower employment grades (Martikainen et al 1999). More recent work has taken advantage of the multiple, repeat measures of the mental health functioning component of the SF-36 now available (Chandola et al 2007).

In contrast to physical health, mental health functioning improved with age from 35 to 74 for all occupational groups. However, this improvement was slower for lower occupational grades, resulting in widening health inequalities in early old age (Figure 17.1, Chandola et al 2007). The widening gap was not a result of differing trajectories by sex or retirement status. Rather it was explained by the better mental health attained by the higher occupational grades after retirement.

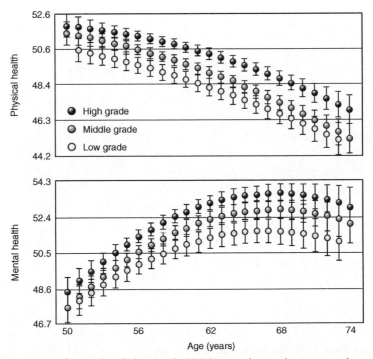

Fig. 17.1 Trajectories of age related changes in SF-36 scores by employment grade
Source: Reproduced from BMJ, Chandola T et al (2007 334, 990–993) with permission from BMJ Publishing group

Further investigation in the Whitehall II study examined how social mobility might contribute to observed occupational grade gradients in symptoms of depression and anxiety. Between baseline and phase 3, 25% of the participants (20% of the women and 27% of the men) were upwardly mobile, moving up at least one grade on the six-level categorization of occupational class. There was good evidence that mental well-being in men was greater and depressive symptom scores lower already at baseline among those who subsequently moved upwards between phases 1 and 3, and in both sexes depression scores at phase 3 were lower among participants who had been upwardly mobile (Stansfeld et al 1998).

Job insecurity and major organizational changes

Several studies have documented adverse effects of self-reported job insecurity on measures of mental well-being (Dooley et al 1987; Roskies et al 1990; Kinnunen et al 1994; Platt et al 1998; Bugard et al 2008; Ferrie et al 2008), and have provided evidence of a dose-response relationship, that is, the higher the level of job insecurity, the greater the increase in mental ill-health (Ferrie et al 2008). While necessary if causality is to be established, a dose-response relationship would be observed whether job insecurity increased mental ill-health or ill-health increased the likelihood of reporting job insecurity. Further evidence of causality is generated if a change in the exposure is matched by a change in the outcome.

As self-reported job insecurity has been assessed repeatedly in Whitehall II, the study was able to examine effects on mental health measures of a change in security. Compared to employees whose jobs were secure at baseline and follow-up (2½ years later), there was an increase in common mental disorders, including depressive symptoms among those who lost job security. Interestingly, those whose jobs were insecure at baseline but secure at follow-up still showed residual adverse effects on mental health; their new-found job security had not completely reversed the adverse effects of their previous insecurity. However, those exposed to chronic job insecurity experienced the worst mental health outcomes (Figure 17.2).

More evidence of the adverse effects of job insecurity has been provided by a study of the effects of major organizational change in the Whitehall II study. In the Civil Service major organizational changes have resulted from reforms introduced in the late 1980s and early 1990s which aimed to transfer the executive functions of government to agencies (Cabinet Office 1997). Executive agencies are run on private sector lines and periodic threats to staffing levels tend to generate job insecurity. Both the prospect of becoming an executive agency and having had one's work transferred to an agency were associated with an excess risk of common mental disorders in men, although no effects were seen in women (Ferrie et al 1998a).

Further Whitehall II analyses took advantage of a series of circumstances that provided the conditions for a 'natural experiment'. Subsequent to the baseline data collection, one of the 20 departments in the Whitehall II study was sold to the private sector, a transfer of business in which most of the workforce lost their jobs. Employees in the department facing privatization were deemed to be subject to job insecurity, ie job insecurity was

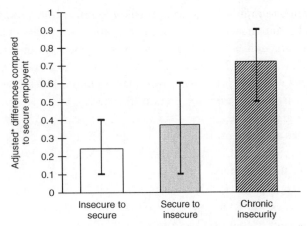

Fig. 17.2 Self-reported job insecurity and depressive symptoms in men
Source: Adapted by permission from BMJ Publishing Group Limited. *J Epidemiol Community Health*, Ferrie JE et al (2002 56, 450–454)

attributed rather than self-reported. The health of study participants in the department facing privatization were compared with those working in departments where jobs were secure, taking account of the health of both groups at baseline. At the group level no effects on common mental disorders were seen in either sex either during the rumour phase, two years prior, or in the immediate three-month run up to the sale (Ferrie et al 1995, 1998b).

An additional follow-up of employees from the privatized department was carried out 18 months after the sale. Health outcomes for the unemployed, those who had left the labour market and those who had found insecure re-employment were compared with participants who had found a secure job. Both unemployment and re-employment in a job that the participant felt was insecure were associated with adverse effects on common mental disorders (Ferrie et al 2001).

A possible explanation of these seemingly contradictory findings has emerged from a similar study that took advantage of a 'natural experiment' within the Maastricht Cohort Study on 'Fatigue at Work'. One of the government agencies included in the study was threatened with closure after the baseline survey. Mental distress among employees in this agency was compared to that in agencies unaffected by closure, adjusting for distress at baseline. Over the 13 months following the closure announcement the incidence of mental distress in the closure group was significantly higher than in the non-closure group. However, the increase in distress among participants in the agency targeted, but who did not perceive themselves to be at risk, was not statistically significant. Thus, self-reported job insecurity and not attributed job insecurity may be driving the association (Swaen et al 2004).

Psychosocial work stressors

As for job insecurity, there may be considerable variation in factors causing stress between individuals. Work stress models aim to describe factors that are likely to elicit harmful stress at work in a large proportion of employees. These factors are conceptualized at a level of generalization that facilitates their identification in a wide range of occupations.

The stress model most often cited and most widely tested is the two-dimensional job strain model (Karasek and Theorell 1990). It proposes that employees who simultaneously have high job demands (eg heavy workload, tight deadlines, conflicting demands) and low control over work are in a job strain situation which, if prolonged, increases the risk of stress-related diseases. An expanded version of the job strain model adds social support as a third component (Johnson et al 1989). The highest risk of illness is assumed to relate to isolated strain or iso-strain jobs, characterized by high demands, low job control, and low social support.

More recent developments in the conceptualization of work stress broadened the view from proximal work characteristics to cover aspects of the person and the labour market context. A promising example is the effort–reward imbalance model (Siegrist 1996). This model maintains that when the employee experiences an imbalance between effort expended at work and reward received the resulting imbalance is particularly stressful. Not only high demands and challenges at work, but also overcommitment and heavy obligations in private life (eg heavy debts) may contribute to a high expenditure of effort. Low rewards can be related to insufficient financial compensation from work, lack of help or acceptance by supervisors and colleagues, and poor career opportunities.

While effort–reward imbalance defines disproportionate costs for an employee in terms of gains received, ie a lack of distributive justice, the latest research on work stress has focused on the two remaining aspects of justice (Elovainio et al 2002; Kivimäki, Elovainio et al 2003, 2005). Procedural justice indicates whether decision-making procedures include input from affected parties, are consistently applied, suppress bias, are accurate, are correctable, and are ethical (Moorman 1991). Relational justice refers to treating individuals with fairness, politeness, and consideration by supervisors (Moorman 1991). Enduring problems in procedural and relational justice have been hypothesized to form an important source of stress at work, the organizational injustice model.

Whitehall II has provided an excellent opportunity to test these general work-stress models in relation to mental well-being. Cross-sectional analyses of the baseline data examined associations between work characteristics (control, work pace, conflicting demands, and social support at work) and mental health outcomes (common mental disorders, well-being measured by the Affect Balance Scale, and symptoms of depression and anxiety). Consistent associations were observed between self-reports of high levels of conflicting demands, low levels of control and low levels of social support, and poorer mental health outcomes in both sexes, with the exception of work pace which associated only with common mental disorders and symptoms of anxiety (Stansfeld, et al 1995). Longitudinal analyses confirmed that high work demands, low control, low social support and also effort-reward imbalance predicted poorer mental health outcomes (Stansfeld, Fuhrer, et al 1997; Stansfeld, et al 1999). Although women have higher rates of common mental disorders than men, an inverse association between social support at baseline and mental disorders (lower support, higher risk) at follow-up has been demonstrated in both sexes. This association remained after taking account of common mental disorders at baseline and social support outside of work (Fuhrer, et al 1999). Conversely, support from colleagues and supervisors has been shown to protect against short spells of psychiatric sickness absence (Stansfeld, Rael et al 1997).

Prospective analyses that examined associations between effort-reward imbalance and subsequent health outcomes have shown a high ratio of efforts in relation to rewards predicts poor mental health functioning (Kuper et al 2002). An association between effort-reward imbalance at work and alcohol dependence among men in the Whitehall II study was found to be partly mediated by via poor mental health (Head et al 2006).

As in the case of job insecurity, analyses of change in work stressors add to evidence in favour of causal associations. In the Whitehall II study recorded sickness absence for psychiatric reasons accounted for just under 10% of all medically-certified, long spells of sickness absence of more than seven days (Head et al 2008). A rigorous study of the effects of changes in demands, control and support at work on long spells of sickness absence showed that an increase in demands, and a decrease in control were associated with a higher risk of sickness absence, whereas an increase in social support at work was associated with a lower risk (Head et al 2006).

More recent work in Whitehall II has examined effort-reward imbalance and organizational justice as predictors of sickness absence. These investigations have demonstrated the existence of a dose-response relationship between both effort-reward imbalance and organizational injustice and sickness absence (Head et al 2007). Other work that focused on a general perception of unfair treatment, which includes unfair treatment at work, has provided strong evidence of a prospective association with poor mental health functioning (De Vogli et al 2007). Analyses of organizational injustice have shown that women and men exposed to low organizational justice at baseline were at increased risk of common mental disorders at follow-up. Supporting reversibility, favourable change in organizational justice between phase 1 and phase 2 was associated with reduced immediate risk of common mental disorder (phase 2) and an adverse change predicted increased immediate (phase 2) and long-term risk (phase 3) (Figure 17.3, Ferrie et al 2006).

In addition to self-reports, external measures for some work stressors were available in Whitehall II. These included personnel managers' assessment of employees' jobs in terms of job control, work pace, and conflicting demands. In cross-sectional and prospective analyses, none of these measures were associated with common mental disorders (Stansfeld et al 1995, 1999).

Interpretation of the evidence

The exact determinants of the development of mental health and well-being are still unknown. It is widely assumed that the aetiology of mental health is multi-factorial involving genetic, biological, and psychosocial factors and this is also likely to apply to well-being. In working populations, psychosocial factors at work, such as job insecurity and work stress, seem plausible correlates of well-being as people spend most of their waking time in workplaces. Moreover, work is the principal source of continuous income for most employees, and related to learning possibilities, opportunities for social contact, meaningful activity, and self esteem (Jahoda et al 1972).

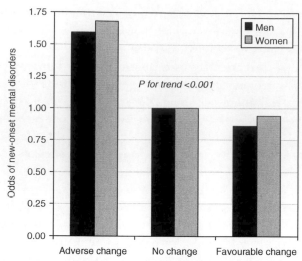

Fig. 17.3 Change in organizational justice between phases 1 and 2 and new-onset common mental disorders at phase 2
Source: Adapted by permission from BMJ Publishing Group Limited. *Occup Environ Med*, Ferrie JE et al (2006 63, 443–450)

The Whitehall II study provides well-characterized observational data on the associations between various workplace factors and mental health and well-being. However, it is important to consider the extent to which (1) selection bias, (2) information bias, and (3) confounding may have contributed to imprecise or incorrect estimations.

Selection bias

The healthy worker effect is a common source of selection bias and occurs when healthier workers are selected into work and those with health problems drop out. As low occupational class, job insecurity and work stressors are related to worse mental health (which in turn can lead to selection out of the workforce), the healthy worker effect may cause some attenuation of associations between these characteristics and mental well-being. To minimize this bias, follow-up screenings in the Whitehall II study target all baseline participants irrespective of their labour market status. However, some attenuation may still be caused by selective non-response if those with more mental health problems are less likely to participate than those with high mental well-being.

Information bias

With the exception of the proxy measure of job insecurity (privatization) and manager-assessed measures of some components of the job strain model, workplace exposures were determined from self-reported data in Whitehall II. As the onset of mental health problems can be insidious, self-reports of job insecurity and work stressors are susceptible to information bias arising from the influence of depressive symptoms below the threshold for detection. Personality and other individual differences may also contribute to information bias. In both these cases, bias is likely artificially to inflate cross-sectional associations between job insecurity, work stressors, and mental well-being.

Three procedures were taken to reduce this possibility: (1) in longitudinal analyses adjustment for mental health problems at baseline (or exclusion of employees with such problems) served to minimize the bias generated by existing problems; (2) analyses explicitly controlled for factors that could lead to exposure misclassification, such as personality traits; and (3) multiple indicators of exposure, including objective proxy measures or supervisory evaluation of the participants work stressors were used.

Associations between work stressors and mental health and well-being were generally robust to the two first procedures, but not the third procedure. When privatization was used as a proxy measure for job insecurity the association observed between self-reported job insecurity and poor mental health was not replicated. Similarly, there were no associations between the manager-assessed measures of job control, work pace, or conflicting demands and employee mental health and well-being. These findings cast doubt on whether variation in self-reports measure true differences in psychosocial work environments or reflect mainly individual differences in perception. On the other hand, null findings might also result if imprecision in the objective proxies and manager-assessed measures led to a failure to detect true associations.

Information bias can affect measurement of the outcome as well as measurement of the exposure; common methods variance. A Whitehall II validation study that used a clinical interview schedule to validate the GHQ found that people in lower occupational classes tend to under-report common mental disorders on the questionnaire relative to those in higher occupational grades (Stansfeld et al 1992). This may have contributed to the changes in the association between occupational class and mental disorders observed over phases 1, 3, and 5 of the Whitehall II study (Head et al 2008), and may also have affected associations with exposures that correlate with occupational class. However, recent work that has specifically examined the potential for common method variance bias between self-reported work characteristics and self-reported health outcomes in the Whitehall II study has concluded that associations are not wholly due to common methods variance (Griffin et al 2007).

Confounding

In observational studies with non-randomly distributed exposures, confounding or residual confounding remains a potential explanation of observed associations. This explanation may also apply to findings on workplace factors and mental well-being, as some relevant confounding factors may remain unaccounted for or may not have been measured with sufficient precision.

Regarding the findings reviewed above, confounding is likely to have affected the occupational class—mental health association, because occupational class acts as a proxy measure for a wide range of work and non-work risk factors, including exposures from before the employment phase of the life-course. Confounding may even affect associations between work stressors and mental well-being despite adjustments for health behaviours and physical disease. For example, adverse childhood socio-economic conditions may be hypothesized directly or indirectly to influence selection into healthy or hazardous working conditions, as well as affect mental well-being in adulthood (Harper et al 2002; Melchior et al 2007). Indeed, evidence from the USA suggests that the first onset of mental disorders is often at a relative early age, well before entry into work life (Kessler et al 2005).

The advantage of Whitehall II is extensive data on potential confounding factors that have facilitated attempts to control confounding by adjustment. In addition, analyses have confirmed that both levels of work stressors and changes in exposure to work stressors are associated with future mental health and well-being in the expected way, providing evidence against confounding.

Complementary evidence from other cohorts

Replication of findings in other populations and settings is essential if the validity of findings is to be established. Studies from various settings confirm the association of low occupational class and other indicators of socio-economic position with reduced mental well-being and increased risk of mental disorders (Qin et al 2003; Everson et al 2002). However, the extent to which occupational class reflects influences from exposures specific to the workplace remains unknown.

Systematic reviews with meta-analyses may provide a useful summary of existing evidence. A meta-analysis of the association between self-reported job insecurity and mental health outcomes in 37 study samples estimated a medium-sized effect (Sverke, et al 2002) and a meta-analysis of temporary work, a proxy measure of job insecurity, also found an association with worse mental well-being (Virtanen, Kivimäki, Joensuu et al 2005). However, it is difficult to determine the extent to which these associations reflect the consequences of job insecurity, on one hand, and selection into insecure jobs, on the other hand. For example, there is evidence that psychological problems already evident at primary school age predict future unemployment and employment in temporary jobs in middle age (Virtanen, Kivimäki, Elovainio et al 2005; Kokko and Pulkkinen 2000), and alcohol-related mortality has been found to be elevated in people with an unstable work career (Kivimäki, Vahtera et al 2003).

A recent systematic review of work stressors and mental disorders, as indicated by depressive symptoms, identified 14 independent cohort studies on this topic (Netterstrom et al 2008). The relative risks were consistently higher than one regarding job strain (three independent studies available) and high work demands (seven studies) but inconsistent for job control. For other work stressors, the number of studies meeting the quality filter was low. Another recent systematic review, that examined major depression defined using clinical criteria as well as depressive symptoms, identified 16 studies and similarly found higher risks in the three studies that provided data on job strain, particularly among men. Although the review found job control, social support and job demands were consistently associated with an excess risk of depression or depressive symptoms, it concluded that it could not rule out with confidence that observed associations between self-reported psychosocial work characteristics and poor mental health outcomes are biased or confounded (Bonde 2008).

Very recent research on job demands has managed to overcome uncertainty related to the self-reported measurement of job demands. For example, a study of hospital ward personnel determined demands using administrative records of monthly bed occupancy rates (Virtanen et al 2008). Daily data on purchased antidepressant prescriptions for employees were derived from national registers. The study found a dose-response between increasing bed occupancy and an increasing likelihood of antidepressant use. No support was found for alternative interpretations, such as reverse causality (ie depression leading to ward overcrowding). Thus, these findings confirm the association between work demands and reduced mental well-being with objective measures of both the exposure and outcome.

An objective description of the exposure has been used very rarely in relation to other stressors, probably because of the difficulties in finding a suitable objective indicator for these stressors with relevant documentation available. Some studies have constructed ecological measures where the degree of exposure is based on reports from people with the same types of jobs in particular work units, in order to reduce subjectivity bias (Kivimäki, Elovainio et al 2003). However, this may have happened at the expense of measurement precision, for example, work stressors may vary within work units.

Finally, few studies have focused on other adverse aspects of the work environment, such as bullying, but those that have suggest it is associated with both depression and depressive symptoms (Wieclaw et al 2006; Kivimäki, Virtanen, et al 2003).

Conclusions and implications

Whitehall II has been one of the leading sources of observational data in which to examine effects of workplace factors on health and mental well-being with standardized repeated measures. The evidence from Whitehall II and other studies demonstrates an association between self-reported job insecurity and poorer mental health. However, the status of objective job insecurity as a causal risk factor for poor mental health remains uncertain. In a similar vein, there is a clear association between work stress and mental well-being, but definite proof for causality is still lacking despite the large body of observational studies in this field.

Given all the evidence, we believe that there is a true association between high work demands or heavy workload and poorer mental health outcomes; a genuine relationship not entirely explained by chance, bias, or confounding. This is because for high work demands the evidence is consistent across self-reported and objective measures, across different settings and operationalizations of the exposure variable. A dose-response relationship and correct temporal order between work demands and mental well-being have been shown. Thus, measures to prevent high work demands appear to have the potential to protect mental health and well-being.

To be sure that a putative psychosocial risk factor is actually involved in the causal chain of disease development, it is necessary to show that eliminating or reducing exposure to the risk factor will lower the likelihood of the disease (Pickering 2001). Thus, to strengthen the basis for evidence-based public health guidance and standards, there is a need for large-scale intervention studies to investigate the extent to which the adverse effects of high work demands and other risk factors for mental well-being in the workplace can be prevented by implementing prevention strategies. Suggested approaches include prevention strategies at the level of the organization and workplace, such as new policies and job redesign, and, to an extent, a focus on individual concerns such as coping strategies.

Future challenges may therefore include:

1 Development of standardized, reproducible, and simple measurement instruments to identify and monitor harmful workplace factors.

A considerable amount of progress towards addressing this challenge has been made through the Management Standards for work-related stress developed by the UK Health and Safety Executive (HSE) in the late 1990s and early 2000s (Mackay et al 2004). Based on research from Whitehall II and similar studies the standards comprise a series of 'states to be achieved', which are statements of good practice in six key stressor areas: demands, control, support, relationships, role and organizational change. For example, the standard for support is (1) employees indicate that they receive adequate information and support from their colleagues and superiors; and (2) systems are in place locally to respond to any individual concerns (<www.hse.gov.uk/stress/standards/>). For each stressor there is also a 'statement' that outlines the main aims to be achieved by the organization. This statement may include a target percentage of employees finding that the organization meets the standard. To implement the Management Standards approach an organization must first assess the existing states for the six standards. This is followed by liaison with workers in focus groups to enable further exploration of any issues raised. This stage is sometimes followed by an intervention stage after which states for the standards are reviewed. The Management Standards are not legally enforceable rather it is the aim of the HSE that the Standards and the associated methodology will enable organizations effectively to tackle work-related stress.

2 Developing and testing clearly defined population interventions aimed at removing workplace risk factors.

Currently there is a distinct lack of knowledge on how organizational interventions, especially at the population level should be carried out. However, a series of case studies (Parker et al 1998) on a smaller scale have examined the impact of organizational interventions in the shape of job redesign (typically using quasi-experimental designs) on health and organizational measures. All these studies have examined important psychosocial work characteristics (eg control, demands) and mental health outcomes. In summary, these studies show that where job redesign is introduced with active employee involvement (which is a prerequisite), significant improvements in mental health can accrue (Parkes 1982; Parkes et al 1986). In addition to evidence of the benefits of positive change, one of the case studies exemplifies the effect of change from a more desirable to a less desirable state. The reintroduction of a repetitive moving line which decreased control was shown to result in poorer mental health outcomes (Parkes and Sparkes 1998).

However, taken together the evidence drawn from the evaluation of organizational interventions to date presents a mixed picture and it is not yet possible to give an unequivocal 'Yes' to the question 'Do organizational interventions work?' (Parkes and Sparkes 1998). While some commentators have drawn pessimistic conclusions (Briner and Reynolds 1997; Reynolds 2000), few negative findings have been reported, although intervening in complex organizations will always run the risk of these (Semmer 2003). Where studies have employed strong designs, focused on a significant work stress problem, and used a range of different outcome measures, encouraging results have been obtained. An important future challenge will be to evaluate the effectiveness of such interventions in a rigorous and systematic way.

Bibliography

Blumenthal, J. A., Sherwood, A., Babyak, M. A., Watkins, L. L., Waugh, R., Georgiades, A., et al (2005) 'Effects of exercise and stress management training on markers of cardiovascular risk in patients with ischemic heart disease: a randomized controlled trial' *Journal of American Medical Association—JAMA* 293: 1626–34

Bonde, J. P (2008) 'Psychosocial factors at work and risk of depression: a systematic review of the epidemiological evidence' *Occupational and Environmental Medicine* 65: 438–45

Bradburn, N. M. (1969) *Structure of Psychological Wellbeing*. Chicaco: Aldine

Briner, R. B., and Reynolds, S (1997) 'The costs, benefits, and limitations of organizational level stress interventions'. *Journal of Organizational Behavior* 20: 647–67

Burgard, S., Brand, J., and House, J. S. (2008) *Perceived Job Insecurity and Worker Health in the United States*. Michigan: Population Studies Center, University of Michigan

Cabinet Office: Next Steps Team (1997) *Next Steps Briefing Notes*. London: Cabinet Office

Chandola, T., Ferrie, J., Sacker, A., and Marmot, M. (2007) 'Social inequalities in self reported health in early old age: follow-up of prospective cohort study' *British Medical Journal* 334: 990–5

De Vogli, R., Ferrie, J. E., Chandola, T., Kivimäki, M., and Marmot, M. G. (2007) 'Unfairness and health: evidence from the Whitehall II Study' *Journal of Epidemiology and Community Health* 61: 513–18

Dekker, S. W. A. and Schaufeli, W. B. (1995) 'The effects of job insecurity on psychological health and withdrawal: A longitudinal study' *Australian Psychologist* 30: 57–63

Dooley, D., Rook, K. and Catalano R. (1987) 'Job and non-job stressors and their moderators' *Journal of Occupational Psychology* 60: 115–32

Elovainio, M., Kivimäki, M. and Vahtera, J. (2002) 'Organizational justice: evidence of a new psychosocial predictor of health' *American Journal of Public Health* 92: 105–108

Elovainio, M., Kivimäki, M., Vahtera, J., Keltikangas-Järvinen, L., and Virtanen, M. (2003) 'Sleeping problems and health behaviors as mediators between organizational justice and health' *Health Psychology* 22: 287–93

Elovainio, M., van den Bos, K., Linna, A., Kivimäki, M., Ala-Mursula, L., Pentti, J., and Vahtera, J. (2005) 'Combined effects of uncertainty and organizational justice on employee health: testing the uncertainty management model of fairness judgments among Finnish public sector employees' *Social Science and Medicine* 61: 2501–12

Everson, S. A., Maty, S. C., Lynch, J. W. and Kaplan, G. A. (2002) 'Epidemiologic evidence for the relation between socioeconomic status and depression, obesity, and diabetes'. *Journal of Psychosomatic Research* 53: 891–5

Feeney, A., North, F., Head, J., Canner, R. and Marmot, M. (1998) 'Socioeconomic and sex differentials in reason for sickness absence from the Whitehall II Study' *Occupational and Environmental Medicine* 55: 91–8

Ferrie, J. E., Head, J., Shipley, M. J., Vahtera, J., Marmot, M. G. and Kivimäki, M. (2006) 'Injustice at work and incidence of psychiatric morbidity: the Whitehall II study' *Occupational and Environmental Medicine* 63: 443–50

Ferrie, J. E., Martikainen, P., Shipley, M. J., Marmot, M. G., Stansfeld, S. A. and Davey Smith, G. (2001) 'Employment status and health after privatisation in white collar civil servants: prospective cohort study' *British Medical Journal* 322: 647–51

Ferrie, J. E., Shipley, M. J., Davey Smith, G., Stansfeld, S. A. and Marmot, M. G. (2002) 'Change in health inequalities among British civil servants: the Whitehall II study' *Journal of Epidemiology and Community Health* 56: 922–6

Ferrie, J. E., Shipley, M. J., Marmot, M. G., Stansfeld, S. and Davey Smith, G. (1995) 'Health effects of anticipation of job change and non-employment: longitudinal data from the Whitehall II study' *British Medical Journal* 311: 1264–9

Ferrie, J. E., Shipley, M. J., Marmot, M. G., Stansfeld, S. A. and Davey Smith, G. (1998a) 'The health effects of major organisational change and job insecurity' *Social Science & Medicine* 46: 243–54

Ferrie, J. E., Shipley, M. J., Marmot, M. G., Stansfeld, S. A. and Davey Smith, G. (1998b) 'An uncertain future: the health effects of threats to employment security in white-collar men and women' *American Journal of Public Health* 88: 1030–6

Ferrie J. E., Shipley, M. J., Stansfeld, S. A. and Marmot, M. G. (2002) 'Effects of chronic job insecurity and change in job security on self reported health, minor psychiatric morbidity, physiological measures, and health related behaviours in British civil servants: the Whitehall II study'. *Journal of Epidemiology and Community Health* 56: 450–4

Ferrie, J. E., Westerlund, H., Virtanen, M., Vahtera, J. and Kivimäki, M. (2008) 'Flexible labour markets and employee health' *Scandinavian Journal of Work, Environment and Health* 6 (Suppl): 98–110

Fuhrer, R., Stansfeld, S. A., Chemali, J. and Shipley, M. J. (1999) 'Gender, social relations and mental health: prospective findings from an occupational cohort (Whitehall II study)'. *Social Science & Medicine* 48: 77–87

Garratt, A., Schmidt, L., Mackintosh, A. and Fitzpatrick, R (2002) 'Quality of life measurement: bibliographic study of patient assessed health outcome measures' *British Medical Journal* 324: 1417–22

Goldberg D. P. (1972) *Detecting Psychiatric Illness by Questionnaire.* London: Oxford University Press.

Goldberg, D. and Williams, P. (1988) *A Users Guide to the General Health Questionnaire.* Windsor, Berkshire: NFER-Nelson Publishing Co

Griffin, J. M., Greiner, B. A., Stansfeld, S. A. and Marmot, M. (2007) 'The effect of self-reported and observed job conditions on depression and anxiety symptoms: a comparison of theoretical models' *Journal of Occupational Health Psychology* 12: 334–49

Harper, S., Lynch, J., Hsu, W. L., Everson, S. A., Hillemeier, M. M., Raghunathan, T. E., et al (2002) 'Life course socioeconomic conditions and adult psychosocial functioning' *International Journal of Epidemiology* 31: 395–403

Head, J., Ferrie, J. E., Alexanderson, K., Westerlund, H., Vahtera, J. and Kivimäki M. (2008) 'Diagnosis-specific sickness absence as a predictor of mortality in the Whitehall II prospective cohort study' *British Medical Journal* 337: a1469

Head, J., Kivimäki, M., Martikainen, P., Vahtera, J., Ferrie, J. E. and Marmot, M. G. (2006) 'Influence of change in psychosocial work characteristics on sickness absence: The Whitehall II Study' *Journal of Epidemiology and Community Health* 60: 55–61

Head, J., Kivimäki, M., Siegrist, J., Ferrie, J. E., Vahtera, J., Shipley, M. J., et al (2007) 'Effort-reward imbalance and relational injustice at work predict sickness absence: the Whitehall II study' *Journal of Psychosomatic Research* 63: 433–40

Head, J., Stansfeld, S. A. and Siegrist, J. (2004) 'The psychosocial work environment and alcohol dependence: a prospective study' *Occupational and Environmental Medicine* 61: 219–24

Hemingway, H., Nicholson, A., Stafford, M., Roberts, R. and Marmot, M. (1997) 'The impact of socioeconomic status on health functioning as assessed by the SF-36 questionnaire: the Whitehall II Study' *American Journal of Public Health* 87: 1484–90

Hemingway, H., Stafford, M., Stansfeld, S., Shipley, M. and Marmot, M. (1997) 'Is the SF-36 a valid measure of change in population health? Results from the Whitehall II Study' *British Medical Journal* 315: 1273–9

Hill, A. B. (1965) 'The Environment and Disease: Association or Causation?' *Proceedings of the Royal Society of Medicine* 58: 295–300

Huppert, F. A. and Whittington, J. E. (1995) 'Symptoms of psychological distress predict 7-year mortality' *Psychological Medicine* 25: 1073–86

Jahoda, M., Lazarsfeld, P. and Zeisel, H. (1972) *Marienthal: The Sociography of an Unemployed Community.* London: Tavistock

Johnson, J. V., Hall, E- M. and Theorell, T. (1989) 'Combined effects of job strain and social isolation on cardiovascular disease morbidity and mortality in a random sample of the Swedish male working population' *Scandinavian Journal of Work, Environment and Health* 15: 271–9

Karasek, R. and Theorell, T. (1990) *Healthy Work: Sress, Productivity, and the Reconstruction of Working Life.* New York: Basic Books

Kessler, R. C., Berglund, P., Demler, O., Jin, R., Merikangas, K. R. and Walters, E. E. (2005) 'Lifetime prevalence and age-of-onset distributions of DSM-IV disorders in the National Comorbidity Survey Replication' *Archives of General Psychiatry* 62: 593–602

Kinnunen, U. and Nätti, J. (1994) 'Job Insecurity in Finland: Antecedents and Consequences'. Jyväskylä: Gummerus

Kivimäki, M., Elovainio, M., Vahtera, J., Virtanen, M. and Stansfeld, S. A. (2003) 'Association between organizational inequity and incidence of psychiatric disorders in female employees' *Psychological Medicine* 33: 319–26

Kivimäki, M., Ferrie, J. E., Brunner, E., Head, J., Shipley, M. J., Vahtera, J., et al (2005) 'Justice at work and reduced risk of coronary heart disease among employees: the Whitehall II Study' *Archives of Internal Medicine* 165: 2245–51

Kivimäki, M., Head, J., Ferrie, J. E., Shipley, M. J., Vahtera, J. and Marmot, M. G. (2003) 'Sickness absence as a global measure of health: evidence from mortality in the Whitehall II prospective cohort study' *British Medical Journal* 327: 364–41

Kivimäki, M., Shipley, M. J., Ferrie, J. E., Singh-Manoux, A., Batty, G. D., Chandola, T., Marmot, M. G. and Davey Smith, G. (2008) 'Best-practice interventions to reduce socioeconomic inequalities of coronary heart disease mortality in UK: a prospective occupational cohort study' *Lancet* 372: 1648–54

Kivimäki, M., Vahtera, J., Virtanen, M., Elovainio, M., Pentti, J. and Ferrie, J. E. (2003) 'Temporary employment and risk of overall and cause-specific mortality' *American Journal of Epidemiology* 158: 663–8

Kivimäki, M., Virtanen, M., Vartia, M., Elovainio, M., Vahtera, J. and Keltikangas-Jarvinen, L. (2003) 'Workplace bullying and the risk of cardiovascular disease and depression' *Occupational and Environmental Medicine* 60: 779–83

Kokko, K. and Pulkkinen, L. (2000) 'Aggression in childhood and long-term unemployment in adulthood: a cycle of maladaptation and some protective factors' *Developmental Psychology* 36: 463–72

Kuper, H., Singh-Manoux, A., Siegrist, J. and Marmot, M. (2002) 'When reciprocity fails: effort-reward imbalance in relation to coronary heart disease and health functioning within the Whitehall II study' *Occupational and Environmental Medicine* 59: 777–84

Mackay, C. J., Cousins, R., Kelly, P. J., Lee, S. and McCaig, R. H. (2004) '"Management Standards" and work-related stress in the UK: Policy background and science' *Work and Stress* 18: 91–112

Marmot, M. G., Davey Smith, G., Stansfeld, S., Patel, C., North, F., Head, J., et al (1991) 'Health inequalities among British civil servants: the Whitehall II study' *Lancet* 337: 1387–93

Marmot, M. G., Shipley, M.J. and Rose, G. (1984) 'Inequalities in death–specific explanations of a general pattern?' *Lancet* 1: 1003–6

Martikainen, P., Stansfeld, S., Hemingway, H. and Marmot, M. (1999) 'Determinants of socioeconomic differences in change in physical and mental functioning' *Social Science & Medicine* 49: 499–507

McHorney, C. A., Ware, J. E., Jr., Lu, J.F. and Sherbourne, C. D. (1994) 'The MOS 36-item Short-Form Health Survey (SF-36): III Tests of data quality, scaling assumptions, and reliability across diverse patient groups' *Medical Care* 32: 40–66

McHorney, C. A., Ware, J. E., Jr. and Raczek, A. E. (1993) 'The MOS 36-Item Short-Form Health Survey (SF-36): II Psychometric and clinical tests of validity in measuring physical and mental health constructs' *Medical Care* 31: 247–63

Melchior, M., Caspi, A., Milne, B. J., Danese, A., Poulton, R. and Moffitt, T. E. (2007) 'Work stress precipitates depression and anxiety in young, working women and men'. *Psychological Medicine* 37: 1119–29

Moorman, R. H. (1991) 'Relationship between organizational justice and organizational citizenship behaviors: Do fairness perceptions influence employee citizenship?' *Journal of Applied Psychology* 76: 845–55

Netterstrom, B., Conrad, N., Bech, P., Fink, P., Olsen, O., Rugulies, R., et al (2008) 'The relation between work-related psychosocial factors and the development of depression' *Epidemiological Reviews* 30: 118–132

Parker, S. K., Jackson, P. R., Sprigg, C. A. and Whybrow, A. C. (1998) *Organisational interventions to reduce the impact of poor work design.* Sudbury: HSE Books

Parkers, K. A., Anastiasades, P., Broadbent, D. E., Johnston, O., Rendall, D., Matthiews, J., et al (1986) *Occupational stress among driving examiners: a study of the effect of workload reduction.* Oxford: HSE

Parkes, K. R. and Sparkes, T. I. (1998) *Organizational interventions to reduce work stress: Are they effective.* Colegate: HMSO

Parkes, K. R. (1982) 'Occupational stress among student nurses: a natural experiment' *Journal of Applied Psychology* 67: 784–96

Pevalin, D. J. (2000) 'Multiple applications of the GHQ-12 in a general population sample: an investigation of long-term retest effects' *Social Psychiatry and Psychiatric Epidemiology* 35: 508–12

Pickering, T. (2001) 'Job stress, control, and chronic disease: moving to the next level of evidence'. *Psychosomatic Medicine* 63: 734–6

Platt, S., Pavis, S. and Akram, G. (1998) *Changing Labour Market Conditions and Health: Systematic Literature Review (1993–1998).* Dublin: European Foundation for the Improvement of Living and Working Conditions

Prince, M., Patel, V., Saxena, S., Maj, M., Maselko, J., Phillips, M. R., et al (2007) 'No health without mental health' *Lancet* 370: 859–77

Qin, P., Agerbo, E. and Mortensen, P. B. (2003) 'Suicide risk in relation to socioeconomic, demographic, psychiatric, and familial factors: a national register-based study of all suicides in Denmark, 1981–1997'. *American Journal of Psychiatry* 160: 765–72

Radloff, L. S. (1977) 'The CES-D scale: A self-report depression scale for research in general population' *Applied Psychological Measurement* 1: 385–94

Reid, D. D., Brett, G. Z., Hamilton, P. J., Jarrett, R. J., Keen, H. and Rose, G. (1974) 'Cardiorespiratory disease and diabetes among middle-aged male Civil Servants A study of screening and intervention' *Lancet* 1: 469–73

Reynolds, S. (2000) 'What works and what doesn't' *Occupational Medicine* 50: 315–19

Roskies, E. and Louis-Guerin, C. (1990) 'Job insecurity in managers: Antecedents and consequences' *Journal of Organizational Behavior* 11: 345–59

Semmer, N. K. (2003) 'Job stress intervention and organization of work' in C. QJ, Tetrick LE (eds) *Handbook of occupational psychology*. Washington, DC: American Psychological Association

Siegrist, J. (1996) 'Adverse health effects of high-effort/low-reward conditions' *Journal of Occupational Health Psychology* 1: 27–41

Stansfeld, S. A., Fuhrer, R., Head, J., Ferrie, J. and Shipley, M. (1997) 'Work and psychiatric disorder in the Whitehall II Study' *Journal of Psychosomatic Research* 43: 73–81

Stansfeld, S. A., Fuhrer, R., Shipley, M. J. and Marmot, M. G. (1999) 'Work characteristics predict psychiatric disorder: prospective results from the Whitehall II Study' *Occupational and Environmental Medicine* 56: 302–7

Stansfeld, S. A., Head, J., Fuhrer, R., Wardle, J. and Cattell, V. (2003) 'Social inequalities in depressive symptoms and physical functioning in the Whitehall II study: exploring a common cause explanation' *Journal of Epidemiology and Community Health* 57: 361–7

Stansfeld, S. A., Head, J. and Marmot, M. G. (1998) 'Explaining social class differences in depression and well-being' *Social Psychiatry and Psychiatric Epidemiology* 33: 1–9

Stansfeld, S. A. and Marmot, M. G. (1992) 'Social class and minor psychiatric disorder in British Civil Servants: a validated screening survey using the General Health Questionnaire' *Psychological Medicine* 22: 739–49

Stansfeld, S. A., North, F. M., White, I. and Marmot, M. G. (1995) 'Work characteristics and psychiatric disorder in civil servants in London' *Journal of Epidemiology and Community Health* 49: 48–53

Stansfeld, S. A., Rael, E. G., Head, J., Shipley, M. and Marmot, M. (1997) 'Social support and psychiatric sickness absence: a prospective study of British civil servants' *Psychological Medicine* 27: 35–48

Sverke, M., Hellgren, J. and Naswall, K. (2002) 'No security: a meta-analysis and review of job insecurity and its consequences' *Journal of Occupational Health Psychology* 7: 242–64

Swaen, G. M., Bultmann, U., Kant, I. and van Amelsvoort, L. G. (2004) 'Effects of job insecurity from a workplace closure threat on fatigue and psychological distress' *Journal of Occupational Environmental Medicine* 46: 443–9

Virtanen, M., Kivimäki, M., Elovainio, M., Vahtera, J., Kokko, K. and Pulkkinen, L. (2005) 'Mental health and hostility as predictors of temporary employment: evidence from two prospective studies' *Social Science & Medicine* 61: 2084–95

Virtanen, M., Kivimäki, M., Joensuu, M., Virtanen, P., Elovainio, M. and Vahtera, J. (2005) 'Temporary employment and health: a review' *International Journal of Epidemiology* 34: 610–22

Virtanen, M., Pentti, J., Vahtera, J., Ferrie, J. E., Stansfeld, S. A., Helenius, H., et al (2008) 'Overcrowding in hospital wards as a predictor of antidepressant treatment among hospital staff' *American Journal of Psychiatry* 165: 1482–6

Ware, J. E., Jr. and Sherbourne, C. D. (1992) 'The MOS 36-item short-form health survey (SF-36). I. Conceptual framework and item selection' *Medical Care* 30: 473–83

Wieclaw, J., Agerbo, E., Mortensen, P. B., Burr, H., Tuchsen, F. and Bonde, J. P. (2006) 'Work related violence and threats and the risk of depression and stress disorders' *Journal of Epidemiology and Community Health* 60: 771–5

Chapter 18

Improving population health through area-based social interventions: generating evidence in a complex world

Steven Cummins

Introduction

Targeted interventions to improve population health have long been a feature of public health practice in high-income nations. Area-based interventions focused on improving the health of deprived communities have been a particularly important part of government policy since 1997. Such an approach has coincided with an increasing recognition of the role of 'context' in shaping individual health outcomes. The idea that risk factors for poor health and health inequality are not just properties of the individual but are also properties of neighbourhoods, schools, workplaces, and other environmental settings is a welcome one. However, the challenge for researchers, practitioners, and policy makers is to populate a sparse evidence base for the effectiveness of environmental interventions targeted at specific communities. Drawing on the evaluation of a 'natural' community experiment to improve diet in Glasgow—the Glasgow Superstore Project—this chapter outlines some of the challenges of generating evidence for the effectiveness of area-based strategies for heath improvement.

Place matters

The existence of long-standing spatial inequalities in health and life chances has led to a resurgence of interest in the idea that where you live matters for health independently of personal characteristics. Over the last two decades investigations of 'area' effects on health and health inequalities (also variously known as neighbourhood, place, contextual, ecological and environmental effects) have become increasingly common as a result of a revitalization of interest in understanding the social determinants of health (Diez Roux 2007). Area of residence, as an independent risk factor, has been observed for a wide range of health outcomes and behaviours, including cardiovascular disease, psychological well-being, smoking, diet, and physical activity (Macintyre et al 2002; Riva et al 2007).

Research on area effects has tended to focus on the role of compound community social and material disadvantage as the aggregate, contextual, risk factor through which disease and health inequalities were generated and maintained. Macintyre and colleagues

(Macintyre et al 1993; Macintyre et al 2002) have described the mechanism by which area effects are hypothesized to contribute to poor health as one of 'deprivation amplification'—where individual or household level deprivation is further amplified by area-level deprivation (Macintyre 2007). Residents of deprived areas are therefore doubly disadvantaged by a lack of access to health-related environmental resources, with the provision of these resources often inversely associated with population need. Poorer access to these locally available 'opportunity structures' in deprived areas is further compounded by increased exposure to environmental stressors which directly and indirectly impact on health behaviours and outcomes. For example, poorer access to green space for leisure activity and fewer local opportunities for walking and cycling may restrict opportunities to be physically active (Panter and Jones 2008). This in turn may be compounded by a greater presence of environmental stressors and incivilities such as noise, crime, graffiti, and litter which may further prevent the use of local neighbourhoods for active living (Poortinga 2006; Harrison et al 2007).

This new focus on the local environment as an independent causal agent in producing poor health has inevitably lead researchers and policy makers to consider interventions and policies that might ameliorate these area-level risks. A policy focus on area characteristics might involve trying to improve the geographical distribution of and access to health promoting amenities and resources, via mechanisms such as urban regeneration, planning, and zoning regulations (Macintyre 2007). However, the challenge when delivering such interventions is to provide better evidence of their effectiveness. Many area-based interventions have been developed and delivered with little knowledge about the public health effects of such initiatives. The Wanless report (Wanless 2004) spoke of the almost complete lack of evidence base on the cost-effectiveness of public health interventions and the need to seize every opportunity to generate evidence for current policy and practice.

Why might area-based interventions be good for health?

In recent years large-scale social programmes that tackle entrenched social deprivation through improvements in living conditions have become an increasing feature of the policy landscape. Such interventions have usually taken the form of large-scale urban regeneration and neighbourhood renewal programmes which are in a particularly good position to tackle health inequalities as they tend to focus on the wider social determinants of physical and mental health (Thomson 2008). In the last 20 years alone spending on such schemes in the UK has reached £11 billion (Thomson et al 2006). Many of these schemes are area-based and thus involve the targeting of places that are considered to be in the greatest social and economic need, emphasizing a focus on 'place poverty' rather than 'people poverty' (Powell et al 2001). As Thomson describes (Thomson 2008) these area-based initiatives target areas of multiple deprivation and commonly comprise of investment in the key socio-economic determinants of health, for example employment, housing, education, income, and welfare. In addition there may also be wider benefits through additional infrastructural improvements to the built environment such as better transport links, provision or upgrading of retail space, parks and public areas and general aesthetic improvement through the provision of street lighting, furniture and pedestrianization schemes. Even though area-based regeneration initiatives were often not designed to specifically target health and health inequalities, health gain was often routinely cited as a justification for investment. More recently however, in the post-Acheson world, links between wider social programmes and the fundamental social determinants of health have been made explicit leading to clearer and more explicit policy links between area-based investment and population health (Thomson 2008; HM Treasury 2002).

Area-based social programmes that tackle deprivation are popular among policy makers because they are assumed (perhaps incorrectly) to efficiently target deprived people, provide an opportunity for local involvement in identifying problems, and solutions, and recognize that 'area' matters and has a real effect (Stafford et al 2008; Lupton 2003). In terms of tackling health inequalities area-based initiatives may improve the health of the most disadvantaged in absolute terms, narrow health inequalities between deprived and affluent groups by improving health of the worst off at a relatively faster rate, or tackle the health gradient across whole populations (Graham 2004). Though, as Stafford et al recognizes, even though the aggregate health status of residents of poor areas may improve relative to the rest of the population, health inequalities may widen within areas if there is differential uptake of interventions locally by differing social and economic groups (Stafford et al 2008).

More recently area-based interventions have not just focused on tackling deprivation but have begun to have a specific health mandate. Early area-based initiatives such as Sure Start and Health Action Zones (HAZ) were explicitly focused on improving the health and life chances of vulnerable groups and communities. One more recent example of an explicitly area-based approach that tackles the environmental determinants of health is the Healthy Communities Challenge Fund (HCCF). The HCCF was set up to encourage the development of healthier lifestyles through improving opportunities to consume a healthy diet and increase physical activity in nine towns across England. These priorities are a key aim of current health policy in order to meet the Government's recent Public Service Agreement to reduce obesity to 2000 levels by 2020 (HM Government 2007). The HCCF was established to pilot and test a series of social and environmental interventions aimed at tackling the 'obesogenic' environment in England as part of the wider Change4Life national health promotion movement (Department of Health 2009). Thus, increasingly we can see that area-based public policy approaches have moved from a situation of having health as an associated or secondary benefit to one where health improvement is a central policy goal.

Have area-based interventions improved population health in the UK?

Despite compelling evidence for the importance of social and environmental factors in the production of poor health and health inequalities there remains limited evidence for the effectiveness of interventions aimed at modifying these risk factors (Macintyre et al 2001). A recent review of the available evidence generated from national evaluations of

UK area-based urban regeneration initiatives implemented since 1980 has synthesized the published evidence for direct and indirect effects on health and the socio-economic determinants of health (Thomson et al 2006). The authors identified 35 published reports of which 18 reported impacts on health or socio-economic circumstances. Overall, there were positive impacts on employment, education attainment, and household income. Impacts on health were also reported with some evidence for a very modest improvement in mortality rates. What is notable is that many of these evaluations were not directly comparable but instead reported impacts on a wide variety of outcomes including self-reported health, mortality, employment, educational attainment, income, and housing quality making it difficult to draw any firm conclusions about the impacts of area-based initiatives. In particular, there was a paucity of evidence on direct impacts on health, with only three evaluations measuring health outcomes prospectively. Even in these limited prospective evaluations the evidence was very mixed with both positive and negative impacts on health reported (Thomson et al 2006).

The ongoing evaluation of the health and socio-economic impacts of the New Deal for Communities (NDC) programme (Stafford et al 2008) has found minor (though non-statistically significant) improvements in psychological well-being, limiting long-term illness (LLTI), fruit and vegetables consumption and smoking cessation. Importantly, even though overall effects were small they were differentially distributed by socio-economic and demographic characteristics, particularly education (for LLTI and smoking cessation) with women in particular appearing to become more physically active. However, even though health of residents in NDC areas improved across a variety of domains there was also a similar level of improvement in individual health in non-NDC comparison areas. It is difficult, therefore, to infer that the NDC programme had any causal effect on health.

Sure Start and Health Action Zones: a tale of two initiatives

The above-mentioned area-based programmes were not set up with health improvement as a primary focus but rather prioritized tackling area deprivation through initiatives that promoted local social and economic development. However, there have been two flagship government projects with health improvement as their primary aim, Sure Start and Health Action Zones (HAZ). These programmes were explicitly area-based, targeted at deprived areas, and characterized the early part of the Labour government's social policies. Health Actions Zones in particular have been described as trailblazing 'third-way' area-based social policies with the express purpose of tackling health inequalities (Powell and Moon 2001). Both of these programmes have been subject to robust (and ongoing) evaluation of impacts.

Sure Start was developed in order to improve the health and well-being of young children in deprived neighbourhoods with the aim of breaking the cycle of poverty and social exclusion and thus increasing social mobility (Melhuish and Hall 2007). In its original conception Sure Start programmes were area-based, with residents of the 20% most deprived areas in England as selected targets for intervention (Melhuish et al 2008). Sure Start was unusual in that a high degree of autonomy was granted locally with service priorities developed in conjunction with local residents. Initial controlled, quasi-experimental evaluations of the original area-based Sure Start programmes found small and limited effects on family functioning, with some indication of better parenting skills and less chaos at home. These outcomes varied by relative social deprivation with relatively less socially deprived families benefiting from Sure Start programmes but outcomes for relatively more vulnerable residents (for example teenage mothers) worsening (Belsky et al 2006). Interestingly, health-led Sure Start programmes appeared to be the most effective. Later evaluations of fully implemented Sure Start programmes found that children had better social development, more positive social behaviour and greater independence and families had less negative parenting, provided a better home learning environment and used more services (Melhuish et al 2008). In contrast with the earlier evaluation, there was no evidence of any adverse effects on the most disadvantaged groups within Sure Start areas with reported positive impacts evenly distributed across population subgroups. This indicated that increased duration of exposure to Sure Start programmes has a beneficial effect and that effect of programmes themselves may take longer in some groups compared to others. However, despite positive impacts on these broad psychometric measures, effects on more focused health outcomes were mixed with negative impact on residents of Sure Start areas in terms of childhood immunization rates, childhood accidents and maternal smoking (Kane 2008).

In comparison to Sure Start programmes which had (and still have) sustained government support, the experience of Health Action Zones was very different. HAZs were the first area-based intervention instituted by the New Labour Government and were announced just 8 weeks after they were elected to power in 1997 (Powell and Moon 2001). HAZs were multi-agency partnerships explicitly set up to focus on area-based initiatives to tackle health inequalities and were, initially at least, very high profile nationally and internationally (Benzeval and Judge 2005). In total HAZs were set up in 26 areas of England in two waves between 1998 and 1999 and were originally scheduled to have a life of seven years, but in fact ceased meaningful operation in early 2003 (Judge and Bauld 2006). The national evaluation of HAZs was a process evaluation of the development and implementation of local partnerships and strategies, it was not designed to evaluate 'effectiveness' of the initiative on population health outcomes. In terms of health improvement and the reduction of health inequalities based on evidence available there appeared to be little measurable impact over the truncated lifespan of HAZs (Judge and Bauld 2006). The 'policy failure' of HAZs can be attributed, in part, to changes in government policies and the over-ambitious expectations of local and national policy makers. Despite the lack of a direct impact on health, partnership working by a variety of local agencies was much strengthened along with awareness and knowledge of the health inequalities agenda (Judge and Bauld 2006; Sullivan et al 2004).

Generating better evidence for the effectiveness of area-based interventions

As briefly outlined above, despite substantial investment in area-based programmes and policies, the overall success of area-based interventions in improving health is difficult to gauge with any certainty. Though evaluations of area-based initiatives that tackle health indirectly, by focusing on social deprivation, or directly, by focusing on changing health behaviours have been undertaken in the UK and elsewhere much of the work is fraught with methodological difficulties. Evaluations that are often found in the non-peer reviewed grey literature, do not directly assess the health impact of area-based programmes or focus on 'audit' oriented outcomes that document what money has been spent and the process of interventions rather than its impacts (Thomson 2008).

Evaluations of area-based interventions are inherently 'natural experiments', experiments where the evaluator has very little control over the nature and delivery of the intervention. It is often the case that not one single intervention or a single health outcome is being evaluated. In fact area-based interventions are themselves often inherently complex and multi-factorial and are being implemented on complex and diverse populations. These can lead to many methodological problems for example; attribution of causality (what aspect of the area-based intervention may causally relate to which outcome), definitions of the populations being exposed (not all local residents will be equally affected or participate in the overall intervention or programme), and adequate capturing of the context of an area that has already probably been subject to multiple interventions in its history. What, then, is required to generate better evidence of the effectiveness of area-based interventions? Below, is a brief description of some of the main issues arising from the Glasgow Superstore Study, a quasi-experimental evaluation of a natural experiment to improve diet in Springburn, Glasgow.

Learning from the Glasgow Superstore Study

The Glasgow Superstore Study was a Department of Health funded prospective, controlled evaluation of the impact on diet and psychological health of the opening of a major food superstore in Springburn, Glasgow, one of the most socio-economically deprived locations in the United Kingdom. The study compared changes in diet and self-reported psychological health in the area where the new supermarket was built (the intervention area), with a comparison area matched by deprivation, using a quasi-experimental study design. In addition, changes in food retail structure in both areas were assessed through pre- and (repeated) post-intervention shop count surveys. Qualitative data on diet, the neighbourhood, and the impact of the store were collected by means of focus groups.

The food superstore development was seen locally by policy makers as having the potential to make a significant contribution to ongoing area-based urban regeneration initiatives through providing long-term training and employment opportunities for local people, with estimates of up to 450 jobs being created (Brindle 1999; Tesco 2002). The superstore operator (Tesco) pledged to train local unemployed people in basic and retail skills with the promise of a job at the end of the training period. This reflected Tesco's wider corporate strategy of forming regeneration partnerships with the public sector. In the case of Springburn, this involved links with Glasgow Chamber of Commerce, a local training college, and regeneration companies (among others).

The supermarket was a legitimate subject for assessment of public health impact through two hypothesized causal mechanisms. Firstly, through a direct environmental influence on diet through improving local food accessibility and affordability in a previously underserved area; and secondly through influencing the social and psychosocial determinants of health through increased opportunities for employment and the psychosocial impact of highly visible inward investment in a previously resource poor setting (Cummins et al 2005b; Cummins et al 2008a). This chimed well with the general literature at the time and the policy rhetoric that inequalities in food retail access may contribute to diet-related health inequalities (Wrigley 2002; Cummins and Macintyre 2002).

The evaluation itself found little evidence that the opening of the food supermarket had any major effect on diet. Crucially, while there was an increase in fruit and vegetable consumption in the intervention area of around a third of a portion per day, a similar increase was observed in the control area making the attribution of change to the supermarket, rather than any wider secular change, difficult (Cummins et al 2005a). Contrary to the expectations of local shopkeepers, the development appeared to have little knock-on effect on structural aspects of the existing local food retail economy in the intervention area (Cummins et al 2008b).

Despite the failure of the study to demonstrate an independent effect of an area-based food retailing intervention on diet, the study led to further reflection on the complex methodological and conceptual issues involved in evaluating complex area-based interventions (Petticrew et al 2007; Petticrew et al 2005). Four broad issues emerged (i) the need for adequate control groups, (ii) triangulating quantitative and qualitative assessment of actual impacts and exposures, (iii) lack of control over the intervention, and (iv) the need for a robust underlying conceptual model of change to drive the evaluation. These are considered in turn below.

The need for adequate control groups in monitoring impacts

In any assessment of the impact of an area-based intervention, one needs to consider the counterfactual, what would have happened in the absence of the proposed intervention. In the Glasgow Superstore Study, without a control area, it is likely that we would have attributed the small change in diet observed in the intervention area to the new supermarket; yet similar positive improvements were also observed in the control area. This corroborates the view that it is not enough to predict impacts using approaches such as Health Impact Assessment (HIA), or even to monitor outcomes before and after the intervention is implemented—monitoring the intervention site alone may introduce bias (Petticrew et al 2007). Robust monitoring of health impacts thus requires assessment of change in both the affected area and in the control area in order to infer causality.

Controlled evaluations of 'natural' area-based interventions such as these may be complicated by the likelihood that the people and place characteristics of control and intervention areas differ at baseline in important ways that may be related to the outcomes that the evaluators are interested in (Petticrew et al 2005). In contrast to the gold-standard randomized control trial, where known and unknown confounding factors are distributed at random, evaluations of area-based interventions need to adequately account for these baseline differences through matching areas as far is possible. This is further complicated by the fact that it is unlikely that perfect matching can ever occur (the real world is a complex, messy place) and area-based differences may be not be easily identified, adjusted for, or even observed (Petticrew et al 2005). Thus, a defining feature of evaluations of area-based interventions is the difficultly in establishing 'true' causality and as such studies should be treated as indicative rather than conclusive (Macintyre 2003).

Triangulating quantitative and qualitative assessments of impacts and exposures

Many evaluations of the health impacts of area-based interventions only consider quantitative evaluation, however qualitative data is also important for robust evaluation as 'not everything that is important can be quantified' (Mindell et al 2001). Qualitative data is rarely used longitudinally to monitor the impacts of interventions. The Glasgow Supermarket Study used both conventional observational quantitative epidemiological techniques and qualitative data collection, which was carried out post-intervention (after the building of the superstore). A repeated retail survey was also carried out to collect information about the impact of the store in the local retail sector. This involved baseline survey work to 'map' the retail structure and then repeat surveys on six-monthly intervals to assess change. Existing secondary sources (eg data from local authority surveys and trade bodies) were used, but 'ground-truthing' these data by direct observation techniques in both areas identified errors, omissions, and changes from these secondary sources.

In the case of the superstore study, analysis of qualitative data suggested a lack of impact of the new store which was corroborated by similar findings from the quantitative arm of the study. It also allowed us to investigate the impact of the store on local people's perceptions of the quality and range of food available to them, and to explore attitudinal and other barriers to use of the hypermarket. Defining the affected population was also difficult. A new supermarket is not just used by the local population and conversely local people may use other retailers (see section 3.1.4). This problem of defining who is exposed also causes problems of contamination where some area-based interventions cannot be limited to those who reside in that specific area—this highlights the need for multi-method approaches where qualitative material can help explore process and mechanism and (in)validate quantitative data.

Lack of control over the intervention

The majority of area-based interventions can be viewed as 'natural experiments', interventions where the researcher has very little control over the content, timing, and implementation of the intervention. In the superstore study, local stakeholders in our initially selected intervention area successfully blocked planning permission for the development. Instead, the superstore was built in our control area resulting in a pragmatic decision to switch intervention and control areas, a difficulty probably not often encountered in true experiments. Timing was another problem, as delays in the planning process inevitably lead to delays in the opening of the new superstore. Political and budgetary considerations (as exemplified by the experience of HAZs) can interfere with the successful evaluation of interventions. Even with well-established lines of communication between research team and providers, timetables are not always followed which in turn has implications for research management and the maintenance of funding streams. In evaluating area-based interventions, if possible, flexibility should be built into evaluation protocols that allow for unforeseen changes in design and timing.

The need for a robust underlying conceptual model

On the basis of existing theory about the environmental determinants of diet, and past observational research, we would have realistically expected to observe some small changes in diet in the community where the store was built. However, the qualitative elements of the evaluation revealed flaws in our underlying conceptual model about how the intervention might work. Interviews with local residents in the intervention area raised questions of boundary and ownership of neighbourhood food resources; that is, what constituted local and appropriate food access for different individuals (Cummins 2007; Cummins et al 2008a). Though the new provision was acknowledged to have improved the range, choice, and quality of food locally, there were also concerns over the temptation to spend beyond household economic means. Even the construction of what was the local area for food shopping differed. In one case, a respondent reported that their 'local' shopping was several miles from their current address as this was where the respondent had grown up and lived for many years (Cummins et al 2008a). For this individual, though, the neighbourhood food resource was physically distant it was socially proximate, and thus any change in local provision had little impact on food shopping behaviour and thus diet. Such findings demonstrate the importance of incorporating qualitative work in evaluation designs to assess the impact of area-based interventions and having a clear and robust conceptual model of how the causal pathways from intervention to outcome are thought to operate.

Conclusion

On one level this chapter has documented the somewhat disappointing track record, in terms of the health impact, of area-based interventions in the United Kingdom, based on the evidence available. However, this should not necessarily persuade the reader that area-based interventions do not work, as definitive conclusions about effectiveness cannot realistically be drawn from the limited nature of the evidence for health impact. In order to populate the evidence base, evaluations of area-based 'natural experiments' are likely to provide the best and most realistic opportunities, at least in the short term, to estimate impacts on health and health inequalities.

An opportunity to undertake an evaluation of a naturally occurring area-based intervention to improve diet using a quasi-experimental design allowed us to reflect on the difficulties of generating evidence for the effectiveness of area-based programmes. Effective evaluation needs to be realistic and pragmatic with a clear definition of control and experimental conditions, exposed populations, and the flexibility to deal with the practical difficulties of evaluating area programmes that are inherently complex and dynamic, and often changing in response to external influences outside of the evaluator's control. Having a clear and rigorous *a priori* specification of the underlying conceptual causal models and pathways that drive area-based interventions is crucial and could be aided by the incorporation of qualitative approaches in testing and refining these models.

Complaints from researchers, practitioners, and policy makers about the scarcity and quality of the available evidence should provide sufficient justification for ensuring that the evaluations of area-based interventions are routinely undertaken. Only then will useful evidence be generated which can be translated into designing and implementing effective area-based interventions to improve population health.

Acknowledgments

The Glasgow Superstore Project was funded by the Department of Health under their Reducing Health Inequalities Research Programme. Steven Cummins is currently supported by a National Institute of Health Research Fellowship. I would like to acknowledge the many contributions of Mark Petticrew and Hillary Thomson whose work and insight provide the basis for many of the points made here. Any errors or omissions are entirely my own.

Bibliography

Belsky, J., Melhuish, E., Barnes, J., Leyland, A. H., Romaniuk, H. and Natl Evaluation Sure Start, R. (2006) 'Effects of Sure Start local programmes on children and families: early findings from a quasi-experimental, cross sectional study' *British Medical Journal* 332: 1476

Benzeval, M. and Judge, K. (2005) 'The Legacy Of Health Inequalities' in Barnes, M., Bauld, L., Benzeval, M., Judge, J., Mackenzie, M. and Sullivan, H. (eds), *Health Action Zones. Partnerships for Health Equity*. Abingdon, Routledge

Brindle, D. (1999) 'Tesco pioneers work skills in food desert' *The Guardian*. London

Cummins, S. (2007) 'Neighbourhood food environment and diet—Time for improved conceptual models?' *Preventive Medicine* 44: 196–7

Cummins, S., Findlay, A., Higgins, C., Petticrew, M., Sparks, L. and Thomson, H. (2008a) 'Reducing inequalities in health and diet: findings from a study on the impact of a food retail development' *Environment and Planning A* 40: 402–22

Cummins, S., Findlay, A., Petticrew, M. And Sparks, L. (2008b) 'Retail-led regeneration and store-switching behaviour' *Journal of Retailing & Consumer Services* 15: 288–95

Cummins, S. and Macintyre, S. (2002) '"Food deserts"—evidence and assumption in health policy making' *British Medical Journal* 325: 436–8

Cummins, S., Petticrew, M., Higgins, C., Findlay, A. and Sparks, L. (2005a) 'Large scale food retailing as an intervention for diet and health: quasi-experimental evaluation of a natural experiment' *Journal of Epidemiology and Community Health* 59: 1035–40

Cummins, S., Petticrew, M., Sparks, L. and Findlay, A. (2005b) 'Large scale food retail interventions and diet' *British Medical Journal* 330: 683–4

Department of Health (2008) *Change4Life—eat well, move more, live longer*. London: Department of Health

Diez Roux, A. V. (2007) 'Neighborhoods and health: where are we and were do we go from here?' *Rev Epidemiol Sante Publique* 55: 13–21

Graham, H. (2004) 'Tackling inequalities in health in England: Remedying health disadvantages, narrowing health gaps or reducing health gradients?' *Journal of Social Policy* 33: 115–131

Harrison, R. A., Gemmell, I. And Heller, R. F. (2007) 'The population effect of crime and neighbourhood on physical activity: an analysis of 15 461 adults' *Journal of Epidemiology and Community Health* 61: 34–9

HM Government (2007) 'PSA Delivery Agreement 12: Improve the Health and Wellbeing of Children and Young People' Norwich: HMSO

Judge, K. and Bauld, L. (2006) 'Learning from policy failure? Health action zones in England' *European Journal of Public Health* 16: 341–3

Kane, P. (2008) 'Sure Start Local Programmes in England' *Lancet* 372: 1610–12

Lupton, R. (2003) *Neighbourhood Effects: Can we measure them and does it matter?* CASE Papers. London: Centre for the Analysis of Social Exclusion, London School of Economics & Political Science

Macintyre, S. (2003) 'Evidence based policy making—Impact on health inequalities still needs to be assessed' *British Medical Journal* 326: 5–6

Macintyre, S. (2007) 'Deprivation amplification revisited; or, is it always true that poorer places have poorer access to resources for healthy diets and physical activity?' *International Journal of Behavioral Nutrition and Physical Activity* 4: 32

Macintyre, S., Chalmers, I., Horton, R. and Smith, R. (2001) 'Using evidence to inform health policy: case study' *British Medical Journal* 322: 222–5

Macintyre, S., Ellaway, A. and Cummins, S. (2002) 'Place effects on health: how can we conceptualise, operationalise and measure them?' *Social Science & Medicine* 55: 125–39

Macintyre, S., Maciver, S. and Sooman, A. (1993) 'Area, Class and Health: Should we be Focusing on Places or People?' *Journal of Social Policy* 22/2: 213–34

Melhuish, E., Belsky, J., Leyland, A. H., Barnes, J. and Natl Evaluation Sure Start Res, T. (2008) 'Effects of fully-established Sure Start Local Programmes on 3-year-old children and their families living in England: a quasi-experimental observational study' *Lancet* 372: 1641–7

Melhuish, E. and Hall, D. (2007) 'The policy background to Sure Start' in Belsky, J., Barnes, J. and Melhuish, E. (eds), *The national evaluation of Sure Start: does area-based early intervention work?* Bristol: Policy Press

Mindell, J., Hansell, A., Morrison, D., Douglas, M., Joffe, M. And Quantifiable, H. I. A. D. G. (2001) 'What do we need for robust, quantitative health impact assessment?' *Journal of Public Health Medicine* 23: 173–8

Panter, J. R. and Jones, A. P. (2008) 'Associations between physical activity, perceptions of the neighbourhood environment and access to facilities in an English city' *Social Science & Medicine* 67: 1917–23

Petticrew, M., Cummins, S., Ferrell, C., Findlay, A., Higgins, C., Hoy, C., Kearns, A. and Sparks, L. (2005) 'Natural experiments: an underused tool for public health?' *Public Health* 119: 751–7

Petticrew, M., Cummins, S., Sparks, L. and Findlay, A. (2007) 'Validating health impact assessment: Prediction is difficult (especially about the future)' *Environmental Impact Assessment Review* 27: 101–7

Poortinga, W. (2006) 'Perceptions of the environment, physical activity, and obesity' *Social Science & Medicine* 63: 2835–46

Powell, M., Boyne, G. and Ashworth, R. (2001) 'Towards a geography of people poverty and place poverty' *Policy and Politics* 29: 243–58

Powell, M. and Moon, G. (2001) 'Health Action Zones: the "third way" of a new area-based policy?' *Health & Social Care in the Community* 9: 43–50

Riva, M., Gauvin, L. And Barnett, T. A. (2007) 'Toward the next generation of research into small area effects on health: a synthesis of multilevel investigations published since July 1998' *Journal of Epidemiology and Community Health* 61: 853–61

Stafford, M., Nazroo, J., Popay, J. M. And Whitehead, M. (2008) 'Tackling inequalities in health: evaluating the New Deal for Communities initiative' *Journal of Epidemiology and Community Health* 62: 298–304

Sullivan, H., Judge, K. And Sewel, K. (2004) '"In the eye of the beholder": perceptions of local impact in English Health Action Zones' *Social Science & Medicine* 59: 1603–12

TESCO (2002) 'Tesco Regeneration Partnerships—The Story So Far' Cheshunt: TESCO

Thomson, H. (2008) 'A dose of realism for healthy urban policy: lessons from area-based initiatives in the UK' *Journal of Epidemiology and Community Health* 62: 932–6

Thomson, H., Atkinson, R., Petticrew, M. and Kearns, A. (2006) 'Do urban regeneration programmes improve public health and reduce health inequalities? A synthesis of the evidence from UK policy and practice (1980–2004)' *Journal of Epidemiology and Community Health* 60: 108–15

Treasury, H. (2002) *Tackling Health Inequalities: summary of the 2002 cross-cutting spending review.* London: HM Treasury and Department of Health

Wanless, D. (2004) *Securing good health for the whole population.* London: HM Treasury and Department of Health

Wrigley, N. (2002) '"Food deserts" in British cities: Policy context and research priorities' *Urban Studies* 39: 2029–40

Chapter 19

Built environment: walkability of neighbourhoods

Klaus Gebel, Adrian E Bauman, and Fiona C Bull

Introduction

Epidemiological studies have consistently demonstrated the numerous health benefits of regular moderate-intensity physical activity (Haskell et al 2007). However, in most Western countries large proportions of the population do not accumulate the recommended 150 minutes per week of moderate physical activity (Sjöström et al 2006). For instance, in the United Kingdom two in three men and three in four women are not sufficiently active, and rates of physical activity have not changed substantially at the population level (Stamatakis et al 2007).

Initial approaches to interventions to promote physical activity assessed the evidence from well-designed intervention studies that focused on individual behaviour change. From these studies, evidence-based recommendations could be made regarding 'what works in individual-level physical activity promotion' (Kahn et al 2002, National Institute for Health and Clinical Excellence (NICE) 2006). Much of this research focused on interventions aimed at individual and interpersonal correlates of physical activity (Marcus et al 2006), but rarely was any assessment made of the impact on population rates of inactivity. In recent years, emphasis has been placed on exploring the relationship between the physical environment and physical activity (Brug et al 2006). In the 19th century, public health approaches resulting in amelioration of social and living conditions (in the physical environment) led to reductions in communicable disease (Jackson 2005). The 21st century is characterized by epidemics of non-communicable diseases, and public health practice returns to the physical environment, in this instance, to promote physical activity, create healthy food environments, and to regulate environments where people smoke. It has been noted that physical activity has been engineered out of the daily life for many people and sedentariness and obesity are regarded as a 'normal' reaction to an 'abnormal' environment rather than vice versa (Egger and Swinburn 1997). As a consequence, individual-change programmes may be insufficient for population change.

Ecological models of health behaviour posit that intra-individual, social, and physical environmental factors all influence physical activity and are interrelated to each other. If environmental attributes are related to physical activity then environmental interventions might be an effective strategy to increase activity levels. Moreover, as such interventions would be relatively permanent, they would have wider reach and would be more likely to achieve a sustainable outcome (Saelens et al 2003; Giles-Corti et al 2005). The potential for environmental modifications to influence health has interested decision makers and has already elicited a substantial policy response. However, policy makers are most concerned that they invest in (these relatively expensive) environmental interventions only if they show promise in increasing population levels of physical activity, in addition to their established contribution to other urban and social environmental benefits.

Conceptual frameworks derived from a socio-ecological perspective suggested that various aspects of the environment, such as presence of walking and cycling paths, or proximity to shops and other places of interest, might facilitate physical activity, while others, such as heavy traffic or low urban density ('suburbanization' or urban sprawl) and poor street connectivity, could discourage active living behaviours (Owen et al 2000). As well, it has been argued that neighbourhoods that are more 'physical activity friendly' are also associated with higher social capital and community cohesion and lower rates of obesity, traffic congestion, crime, and less air pollution (Transportation Research Board 2005).

This chapter reviews the progress and issues in generating an evidence base to inform policy and practice in the area of environmental interventions and physical activity.

Initially, we review some of the broader issues related to the nature of evidence and research in this field. We then describe a framework of 'evidence', specifically:

- summarizing the available evidence using recent review papers and original studies published in the peer reviewed literature; and

- considering other 'forms of evidence' that might be available and usually missed by reviews based solely on publications in the peer reviewed literature.

We reconsider the 'evidence base' and the reasons for the recent policy response. Gaps in research evidence in this area of public health are also presented to provide both direction to what future research is needed, but also to highlight the limitations of the current evidence base.

Challenges in building the evidence base on the physical and social environment and physical activity

Any scientific review of the evidence on public health interventions starts with categorizing published scientific evidence, with studies ranked according to the strength of evidence, strongest research designs, and those that have minimized selection, measurement, and confounding bias; in addition, studies are ranked according to their appropriateness for a specific research question (Tang et al 2008). The strongest research designs, namely randomizing individuals or settings, may not be possible or feasible in answering many public health questions (Petticrew et al 2005; Victora et al 2004). In a scientific review, one would give more credence to cohort study data, where people were measured longitudinally 'before and after' an intervention, than evidence from cross-sectional study designs. In the field of environment-changing interventions, more opportunistic evaluation of natural experiments has been suggested for evidence generation (Petticrew et al 2005, Ogilvie et al 2006; Ramanathan et al 2008). However, these are associated with some problems and limitations. Environmental change is often developed by professionals from urban planning and transportation sectors, and better cooperation with public health researchers in the areas of evaluation designs and measurement could improve the quality of evidence collected (Ewing 2005).

There are several methodological challenges in evaluating the effects of environment-changing interventions. Figure 19.1 presents a framework for physical activity environmental interventions. One issue is the difficulty in defining the population exposed to an environmental intervention. For example, a new cycling trail might be used by people living nearby, or accessed by people living in other environments (Petticrew et al 2005). Second, research designs may need to be flexible, and using quasi-experimental designs may be the most feasible; however, even finding a suitable quasi-experimental control region can be problematic due to differences between towns or neighbourhoods (Ogilvie et al 2006, Reger-Nash et al 2006). For instance, people residing in more walkable neighbourhoods might value physical activity more than those who choose to live in more car dependent environments (Petticrew et al 2005, Saelens et al 2003).

The next methodological issue is measurement of exposure, and its relationship to physical activity outcomes. For many environmental studies, true cohort data may not be possible, due to often short timeframes of announcing proposed changes; however, alternative approaches have been proposed, including assessment of people's physical activity before and after they relocate to a neighbourhood with a different level of walkability (Krizek 2000, Giles-Corti et al 2008). However, an important limitation of 'relocation' studies is the challenge of disentangling the contribution of specific environmental attributes to behavioural changes.

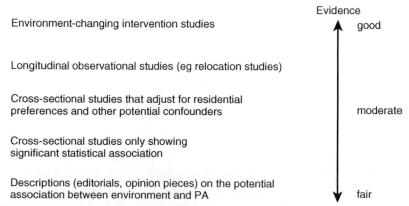

Fig. 19.1 Framework for evidence-based public health in physical environments and physical activity

A summary of the evidence on physical activity and the environment

In the last few years there has been a rapid increase in studies and concomitant review articles that have synthesized the emerging literature on the relationship between the physical environment and physical activity (Frank and Engelke 2001; Humpel et al 2002; Owen et al 2004; Lee and Moudon 2004; Heath et al 2006; Saelens and Handy 2008; Gebel et al 2007). These reviews have summarized the results of more than one hundred articles published since 1980, the majority showing consistent cross-sectional associations. We carried out a synthesis of the current evidence, drawing on three primary sources: (1) the pool of individual studies identified by previous literature reviews; (2) the recent systematic reviews conducted for national governments in the UK (National Institute of Health and Clinical Excellence, <http://www.nice.org.uk>) and the USA (US Guide to Community Preventive Services, <http://www.thecommunityguide.org>); and (3) the literature database from the Active Living Research group (www.activelivingresearch.org). The inclusion criteria were limited to studies published in peer-reviewed journals in English; studies were included if they reported associations between the physical environment and measures of physical activity. This summary is restricted to studies with participants aged 18 years or over. We excluded intervention studies where physical environmental change was not central, but was only a part of a multi-component intervention and studies in indoor environments, such as studies promoting stair use. We present the findings by study design to emphasize the nature of the evidence available, firstly a short summary of the large number of studies using cross-sectional research designs, followed by a detailed review of the few relocation and cohort studies.

Summary findings from cross-sectional studies

To date, most of the published research on the relationship between physical environments and physical activity is from cross-sectional studies and therefore does not provide causal evidence (Bauman 2005). Cross-sectional designs can only identify correlates, which are not necessarily the same as determinants of physical activity (Brug et al 2006; Bauman et al 2002). The results are however useful in generating hypotheses about potential pathways and mechanism of influence.

Overall, the findings from these studies show that physical activity was consistently associated with mixed land use, residential density, street connectivity, and the presence of footpaths and trails (Owen et al 2004; Gebel et al 2007). In addition, proximity to various destinations, such as shops, and recreation facilities, was significantly associated with increased physical activity. Less consistent associations were reported for aesthetic features, topographic factors, and perceptions of safety from crime and traffic.

These findings immediately point towards potential areas for action and intervention, such as improving access to shops and retail areas, provision of better infrastructure for walking and cycling; however, there are some important limitations to be considered before decision makers act. Most notably is that identified differences in physical activity levels between neighbourhoods could be due to direct effects of the physical environment or due to selection effects in the preferences of people who choose to live in more walk-able areas. If in fact the observed associations between neighbourhood walkability and higher levels of walking were mainly due to a self-selection bias, this implies that environ-mental interventions might only have minor effects. It is only recently that some cross-sectional studies have included questions on residential preferences (Handy et al 2006; Owen et al 2007; Frank et al 2007). By statistically adjusting for such preferences these studies have better isolated the direct effect of environments on physical activity (Schwanen and Mokhtarian 2005; Cao et al 2006; Owen et al 2007).When the investiga-tors adjusted for residential preferences, such as the neighbourhood being conducive to utilitarian or leisure walking, walkability was still associated with higher walking levels (Schwanen and Mokhtarian 2005; Cao et al 2006; Owen et al 2007).

Summary findings from retrospective 'relocation' studies

One of the limitations to evidence from cross-sectional study designs is the lack of any temporal relationship, in this case between the environment and the behaviour. In other words, we do not know if a change in the intervention preceded a change in the behav-iour. To date, there have been only two published studies that have attempted to address this issue by exploring behaviour before and after a move in residential address and there are other relocation studies underway (Giles-Corti et al 2008).

One prospective study from the US (Krizek 2000) reported on the influence of people moving between neighbourhoods on travel behaviour including modal split. Density, street patterns, and land use mix were objectively assessed and geocoded and these were summarized in a composite measure called Less Automobile Dependent Urban Form (LADUF). A limitation was that the only physical activity-related mode of transport was a composite measure called 'alternative mode', consisting of using public transport, cycling, and walking. The results revealed that only people relocating from a high to a medium LADUF score neighbourhood showed a significant change (decrease) in the percentage of trips by alternative mode. In a later publication Krizek (2003) showed that moving to neighbourhoods with higher accessibility was associated with fewer kilometres travelled by car, but no increase in walking.

In a retrospective relocation study from the US, Handy et al (2006) examined the asso-ciation between changes in the built environment and changes in walking and cycling amongst residents across 8 neighbourhoods (4 = 'traditional' design and 4 = 'suburban' design) in Northern California. Participants who relocated to more walkable environ-ments showed larger increases in walking frequency than those who moved to less walkable neighbourhoods. This also applied after controlling for residential preferences.

The retrospective cohort study design provides weaker evidence as it relies on recall of behaviour and therefore does not provide conclusive evidence on which to base action (decision and policy making). However, they provide better evidence than cross-sectional studies alone, indicate areas for further exploration, and are useful to help justify the expense and resources to conduct the necessary studies using more robust study designs.

Summary findings from environment-changing intervention studies

To date, there are few published studies reporting the results from actual changes to the environment. There are two typical research designs: those reporting results from retrospective analysis of behaviour and those that employed a pre/post-study design with or without a control or comparison group. In this area, there have been two recent review processes, both undertaken with national government support, which reviewed the intervention literature broadly. One was conducted in the UK and the other in the USA (<http://www.NICE.org.uk>; <http://www.thecommunityguide.org/pa>). The CDC Guide to Preventive Services reviewed the literature under three broad areas defined by scale or scope: the urban scale; the street-scale; and transport or travel-related policies. Despite the intent of the review to focus on 'environment changing interventions', only two of 11 studies included in the review reported testing an environmental change, the remainder were cross-sectional studies and were therefore prone to the previously reported limitations (Heath et al 2006).

However, to demonstrate both the paucity and diversity of peer-reviewed publications of intervention studies, we present a more detailed examination of specific examples of environment changing interventions below. This is not a complete systematic review, but does cover most of those obtainable from the peer-reviewed literature.

Brown and Werner (2007) used an uncontrolled, before-and–after, study design to evaluate the impact of a new light rail stop in Salt Lake City in the US on walking behaviour. Local residents were surveyed for the number of times they had used the light rail over the previous two weeks. After the new stop was launched light rail use increased significantly from 50% to 68.75% among local residents. The longitudinal analysis was limited by the small sample size ($n = 51$), but suggested that walks to the new light rail stop contributed to bouts of moderate physical activity above the levels before the intervention.

In a cross-sectional study from the US, Brownson and colleagues (2000) assessed the impact of newly built walking trails on walking behaviour of adults (n=1269). Among participants with access to the trails 38.8% had made use of them. Among these 55.2% stated that they had increased their walking levels since starting using the trail, with greater increases reported by women and by those from lower income groups.

With a cross-sectional design Cope et al (2003) analysed the impact of the UK National Cycle Network (NCN) on physical activity and health, social inclusion, and sustainable recreation and tourism. Intercept surveys of users of the cycle paths were carried out. Interestingly, a large proportion of users of the NCN were from population groups that are typically inactive. Of the surveyed adults 42% stated that the NCN has helped them to increase their physical activity levels by a large amount, and 30% declared that the NCN did not affect their activity levels. In three sites cycling and pedestrian activity were monitored in 1998 and again in 2001. Here, the number of users increased by between 29.7% and 50.1%. A limitation of this study is the lack of information on previous physical activity levels of NCN users.

In an uncontrolled before-and-after study from the US, Evenson and colleagues (2005) assessed the impact of a newly built rail trail. A randomly selected sample of 366 adults living within two miles of the trail was surveyed before and two months after the trail launch. Outcome measures included walking, cycling, moderate, vigorous, and transportation activity. Among trail users there was no significant change in any physical activity domain compared with those who did not make use of the trail.

Gordon et al (2004) interviewed 414 adults using two newly constructed trails in West Virginia. Participants were asked about current and previous trail usage and physical activity. Of the new trail users 23% were 'newly active'. Gordon concluded that providing new trails might be an effective strategy to promote physical activity especially among the inactive. This retrospective recall attempts to use 'previous recalled physical activity' to generate a quasi-cohort, but is strictly speaking cross-sectional in design.

In a before-and-after study from Australia, Merom et al (2003) investigated the impact on levels of walking and cycling of a local media campaign to promote a newly constructed rail trail. Residents living within 1.5km of the trail, and bike owners living within 5km of the trail were surveyed three months before and after the opening of the trail. Additionally, at four sites bike counters were used to monitor cycling activity, and showed significant increases after the launch of the trail. Only bicycle owners with a non-English speaking background who lived within 1.5km of the trail showed any significant increase in minutes of self-reported cycling. No changes were reported for self-reported walking.

In a prospective study, Morrison (2004) evaluated the impact of traffic calming schemes in Glasgow, Scotland. The scheme included raised platforms on the road to slow car drivers, zebra crossings, and parking bays. After the introduction of the traffic calming scheme 20% of the participants stated that they walked more in the area as a result of it. Only 3.8% reported to cycle more. Apart from one site, observed pedestrian activity increased for children, adults and pensioners.

In an English study with an uncontrolled before-and-after design, Painter (1996) evaluated the effects of street lighting improvements in three sites on crime and pedestrian street use. On-street pedestrian surveys were carried out six weeks before and after the intervention. In all three intervention sites the number of pedestrians using the streets increased by between 34–101% for both men and women.

Overall, the totality of findings from intervention studies published in the peer reviewed scientific literature provides a limited evidence base for policy makers, and one which might easily be regarded as insufficient on which to base action and resource investment. Indeed, the review here identified few published *intervention* studies in areas around transport system change (Brown and Werner 2007), a (national) cycling network (Cope et al 2003), traffic calming (Morrison et al 2004), street lighting (Painter 1996) and finally, several projects that showed a significant improvement in physical activity in association with trail / path development projects (Brownson et al 2000; Gordon et al 2004).

Extending the evidence base: using multiple sources of evidence

The peer-reviewed published evidence, particularly around environment-changing interventions, is relatively sparse. Although more and higher quality studies would help the evidence base (Brug et al 2006), other ways of generating evidence for action have been explored. Nonetheless, there is a high level of government interest in implementing an evidence-based public health response to address physical inactivity and rising levels of obesity. Therefore, reviews have been commissioned with a broader remit requesting the 'best available evidence' to be sought and considered, for example, by the National Institute of Health and Clinical Excellence (NICE). Recently commissioned work on the built environment and physical activity (National Institute for Health and Clinical Excellence (NICE) 2008) used inclusion criteria which allowed for government and non-government reports, case studies, and other summations of interventions or programmes to be included. Such literature is usually excluded in the criteria stipulated by scientific reviews and is often referred to as 'grey literature' (or 'fugitive literature' in the USA). Taking such an approach may be warranted where the evidence base is insufficient, and using traditional exclusion criteria based on study design simply leaves no evidence to review. Moreover, many public health interventions do not use optimal evaluation designs, and may be published only in government reports and the 'grey literature', yet these experiences and projects can still offer important lessons and contribute to the knowledge base around possible approaches to environment change (Ogilvie et al 2005).

The review undertaken for NICE identified some relevant additional studies aimed at environmental changes at street-level improvements, traffic calming, pedestrianization, road closures, and road usage (congestion) taxes that had not been identified in any other review. Table 19.1 shows a summary of some of these studies that may add to the evidence base, and illustrate new examples of potential areas for environmental intervention. In addition to extending the breadth of literature included in this review, the standardized approach to the development of national guidance on public health interventions includes inviting stakeholder comments on the literature and draft guidelines as well as a phase of community (field work) consultation (National Institute for Health and Clinical Excellence (NICE) 2007). This approach was innovative and the final NICE Guidance (published in March 2008) (National Institute for Health and Clinical Excellence (NICE) 2008), was well received by a wide audience in both the health and non-health sectors but it remains too early to evaluate if this approach to the evidence was in any way 'better' or more effective than other approaches.

Conclusions

Developing the evidence base for environment-changing interventions to promote physical activity is a slow process, and is limited by pace of research efforts and publication processes in the scientific literature. Overall, there is some evidence that improving the built environment (street connectivity in neighbourhoods, mixed land use, promoting pedestrian access to city centres, and traffic calming) may influence incidental physical

Table 19.1 Additional evidence on environmental interventions to promote physical activity: Using a narrative review and the 'grey literature' (case studies from the UK[1,2])

Area of evidence	UK studies investigated and methodological limitations
Street level improvements; micro-environmental changes	In addition to the street lighting improvement study by Painter (1996), work has been carried out on Home Zones in Leeds, that might have contributed to increased outdoor street play by children (Layfield et al 2003); others have examined 'pedestrianization' through the re-design and increasing the pedestrian usage of road networks, bridges, and green space (Space Syntax Ltd 2002, Space Syntax Ltd 2004b, Space Syntax Ltd 2004a) but their impact on physical activity is not clear.
Traffic calming studies	In addition to the Morrison et al (2004) study, others have reported interventions targeting street calming and traffic reduction, including 20mph zones (Babtie Group 2001, Kirby 2001) and speed humps (Silcock 1999, Webster et al 2006, Social Research Associates 2001); limitations include lack of descriptions of the interventions, and limited population physical activity outcome measurement, but some studies reported small increases in walking and cycling.
Trails	Additional trail-development interventions have demonstrated increased usage following road improvements (Sustrans 2005, Sustrans 2006); however this may reflect more frequent use by people already cycling or walking rather than changes in inactive populations.
Road closure and congestion taxes	These are *policy interventions* that potentially impact upon environments relevant to physical activity. Road closures or efforts to discourage car use might influence walking (as an example of international experiences in Bogota, Colombia, see: Shilton et al (2007). Congestion taxes in Central London resulted in increases in public transport, and in walking and cycling to work (Transport for London 2006).

[1] National Institute for Health and Clinical Excellence (NICE) Public Health Collaborating Centre—Physical Activity (2006) *Physical activity and the environment review one: transport.* London, National Institute for Health and Clinical Excellence

[2] National Institute for Health and Clinical Excellence (NICE) Public Health Collaborating Centre—Physical Activity (2006) *Physical activity and the environment review two: urban planning and design.* London, National Institute for Health and Clinical Excellence

activity, and there is stronger evidence that trails and path development may influence total physical activity levels. In particular, the evidence tentatively points to these interventions fostering 'incidental' or lifestyle activity, and these effects may be reaching marginalized and disadvantaged groups (Brownson et al 2000; Cope et al 2003; Merom et al 2003; Gordon et al 2004). This is of major public health significance, as many physical activity interventions reach the more educated in the population, often already with high intentions to exercise.

Despite the substantial increases in the number of published studies about physical environments and physical activity, many methodological issues and gaps remain and should be addressed in future research to improve the strength of evidence generated. These are summarized in Box 19.1 and include methodological issues, further areas for analysis, research design issues, and issues relevant to the evidence.

Box 19.1 Gaps in the evidence and methodological considerations for further research

♦ The additional information from studies identified in the 'grey literature' (illustrated in Table 19.1) provide new areas for investigation, and for further evidence generation, especially around the urban renewal and pedestrianization projects, and around road closures and policy-related restrictions on car usage.

♦ Most published studies are cross-sectional and of limited use for evidence generation; further correlational studies would not be likely to contribute to evidence generation.

♦ Additional methodological limitations were noted in the intervention studies, including the use of retrospective designs (recall and social desirability bias); also many studies only used one type of physical activity (such as walking or cycling) as the outcome measure, rather than the public health interest (total physical activity), and it may be that populations compensate for increases in 'active living' by reducing leisure time physical activity.

♦ The majority of studies emanate from urban environments in the US, Australia, and the UK, and studies from other countries, in socially and geographically variable environments, would add to the evidence base.

♦ Mostly research has been focused on micro-environmental aspects and there is a lack of evidence for macro-environmental influences (such as urban form and transport system patterns) on physical activity (and here, the grey literature has provided several examples, but with insufficient rigour to generate evidence). The CDC review (Heath et al 2006) further pointed out that transport-related interventions provided an insufficient number of studies for policy development.

♦ Physical activity may be differently associated with objective and perceived measures of the environment. Further, research is identifying different correlates between self-reported and objectively measured attributes of physical environments (Boehmer et al 2006; Gebel et al 2009).

♦ There are several measurement issues in this research area: most studies used self-reported measures of physical activity; more objective outcome measures, such as accelerometers or pedometers, should be considered. Measurement of the environment is at an early stage and important aspects of the environment might not yet be considered or assessed.

♦ While it is hypothesized that environmental interventions are likely to achieve sustainable outcomes, no long-term evaluations have been carried out so far.

Gaps in the evidence and methodological considerations for further research *(continued)*

+ Very few studies have used multilevel models with clear theoretical frameworks to determine the relative contributions of the physical environment on physical activity compared with intra-individual and social environmental factors (Bauman 2005; Brug et al 2006; Saelens and Handy 2008). All may be needed, in varying combinations, to induce population change (Giles-Corti and Donovan 2002; Giles-Corti and Donovan 2003). Research is needed to determine whether supportive physical environments, by themselves, are sufficient to achieve significant increases in population physical activity.

+ Little is known about the cost-effectiveness of environmental interventions; here researchers should not only look at physical activity outcomes, but also at other outcomes, including air quality, traffic hazards and noise, and social capital.

The plethora of cross-sectional associations has highlighted the agenda, but the paucity of longitudinal-designed intervention studies makes the evidence base less clear. Given the limited evidence, and the already burgeoning policy response, it is incumbent on public health researchers to advocate for ongoing collection of evidence, through opportunistic studies and natural experiments to further evaluate new physical environment-changing interventions for their impact on physical activity. These partnerships could permit better research designs, and incorporate additional elements such as multiple communities and multiple baselines (Bauman and Koepsell 2006), in order to further strengthen the scientific base for guiding practice and policy (Petticrew et al 2005).

In addition, other ways of looking at the evidence need to be considered, as policy makers may not wait for definitive science to catch up with the practice-perceived need for environmental interventions (Ogilvie et al 2005). The other non-health outcomes will drive environment-changing interventions anyway, such as reducing traffic, improving air quality, and possibly enhanced social capital in communities. Public health accepts these outcomes are also health-promoting, but needs to continue to enhance the evidence base around specific health outcomes of interest, in this case physical activity. One way of improving the evidence base is to allow the range of studies and their sources to be broadened, and this was the remit of reviews such as the NICE report (NICE 2008). This allows additional studies to be considered, and new areas to be explored, but even greater vigilance should be paid to careful appraisal of the internal and external validity of this research (Ogilvie et al 2005) as it is not in peer-reviewed publications. Nonetheless, it broadens thinking around this area, and increases policy maker confidence that the evidence base is at least modestly encouraging.

Others have used alternate methods to make the case. The CDC review of evidence on environmental interventions to promote physical activity compared cross-sectional studies, and approximated effect sizes (in terms of percentage differences in physical activity behaviours in those in exposed and unexposed environments (Heath et al 2006). This provides an effect size estimator although derived from cross-sectional studies, and has much in common with propensity analysis use in public health (Yanovitsky et al 2005).

In summary, research on environments and physical activity is still in its infancy. Nonetheless, there has already been a substantial policy response in this area, which may have exceeded the evidence base. The reasons for this policy response include increased policy and community attention to physical inactivity (and obesity), and the desire to 'do something' in response to political and community pressures. Clearly, changing the physical environment is an expensive and intersectoral (cross-cutting) policy issue, with ramifications for health, social and community cohesion, the 'green' environmental movement, and urban planning. The dissonance between 'actual evidence to date' and the policy response is an important message for public health practice, with strong advocacy required for ongoing evidence generation, and to broaden the range of interventions that are opportunistically evaluated, and range of studies considered as providing useful evidence (Ogilvie et al 2005). Even in the absence of clear causal evidence policy makers have to make decisions and advocate for interventions (Ramanathan et al 2008). There is not yet sufficient evidence that investments in environmental changes will produce major population changes in physical activity. However, in public health it is generally accepted that the pursuit of advocacy for obviously needed environmental and social changes cannot wait for final, conclusive scientific evidence to be available. The evidence base is not strong yet, but it is sufficient for initial action.

Acknowledgements

Klaus Gebel is supported by postgraduate scholarships of Sport Knowledge Australia and the Australian Housing and Urban Research Institute.

Bibliography

Babtie Group (2001) *Urban street activity in 20 mph zones: final report.* London: Department for Transport, Local Government and the Regions

Bauman, A. (2005) 'The physical environment and physical activity: moving from ecological associations to intervention evidence' *Journal of Epidemiology and Community Health* 59: 535–6

Bauman, A.E. and Koepsell, T.D. (2006) 'Epidemiologic issues in community interventions' in R. Brownson, and D. Petiti (eds), *Applied epidemiology: theory to practice*, pp 164–206. 2nd edn. New York: Oxford University Press

Bauman, A.E., Sallis, J.F., Dzewaltowski, D.A. and Owen, N. (2002) 'Toward a better understanding of the influences on physical activity: the role of determinants, correlates, causal variables, mediators, moderators, and confounders' *American Journal of Preventive Medicine* 23: 5–14

Boehmer, T., Hoehner, C., Wyrwich, K., Ramirez, L. and Brownson, R. (2006) 'Correspondence between perceived and observed measures of neighborhood environmental supports for physical activity' *Journal of Physical Activity & Health* 3: 22–36

Brown, B.B. and Werner, C.M. (2007) 'A new rail stop: tracking moderate physical activity bouts and ridership' *American Journal of Preventive Medicine* 33: 306–9

Brownson, R.C., Housemann, R.A., Brown, D.R., et al (2000) 'Promoting physical activity in rural communities: walking trail access, use, and effects' *American Journal of Preventive Medicine* 18: 235–41

Brug, J., van Lenthe, F.J. and Kremers, S.P. (2006) 'Revisiting Kurt Lewin: how to gain insight into environmental correlates of obesogenic behaviors' *American Journal of Preventive Medicine* 31: 525–9

Cao, X., Handy, S.L. and Mokhtarian, P. (2006) 'The influences of the built environment and residential self-selection on pedestrian behavior: evidence from Austin, TX' *Transportation Quarterly* 33: 1–20

Cope, A., Cairns, S., Fox, K., et al (2003) 'The UK National Cycle Network: an assessment of the benefits of a sustainable transport infrastructure' *World Transport Policy and Practice* 9: 6–17

Egger, G. and Swinburn, B. (1997) 'An "ecological" approach to the obesity pandemic' *British Medical Journal* 315: 477–80

Evenson, K.R., Herring, A.H. and Huston, S.L. (2005) 'Evaluating change in physical activity with the building of a multi-use trail' *American Journal of Preventive Medicine* 28: 177–85

Ewing, R. (2005) 'Building environment to promote health' *Journal of Epidemiology and Community Health* 59: 536–7

Frank, L.D. and Engelke, P.O. (2001) 'The built environment and human activity patterns: exploring the impacts of urban form on public health' *Journal of Planning Literature* 16: 202–18

Frank, L.D., Saelens, B.E., Powell, K.E. and Chapman, J.E. (2007) 'Stepping towards causation: do built environments or neighborhood and travel preferences explain physical activity, driving, and obesity?' *Social Science & Medicine* 65: 1898–914

Gebel, K., Bauman, A.E. and Owen, N. (2009) 'Correlates of non-concordance between perceived and objective measures of neighborhood walkability' *Annals of Behavioral Medicine* 37: 228–38

Gebel, K., Bauman, A.E. and Petticrew, M. (2007) 'The physical environment and physical activity: a critical appraisal of review articles' *American Journal of Preventive Medicine* 32: 361–9

Giles-Corti, B. and Donovan, R.J. (2002) 'The relative influence of individual, social and physical environment determinants of physical activity' *Social Science & Medicine* 54: 1793–812

Giles-Corti, B. and Donovan, R.J. (2003) 'Relative influences of individual, social environmental, and physical environmental correlates of walking' *American Journal of Public Health* 93: 1583–9

Giles-Corti, B., Knuiman, M., Timperio, A., et al (2008) 'Evaluation of the implementation of a state government community design policy aimed at increasing local walking: design issues and baseline results from RESIDE, Perth Western Australia' *Preventive Medicine* 46: 46–54

Giles-Corti, B., Timperio, A., Bull, F. and Pikora, T. (2005) 'Understanding physical activity environmental correlates: increased specificity for ecological models' *Exercise and Sport Sciences Reviews* 33: 175–81

Gordon, P., Zizzi, S. and Pauline, J. (2004) 'Use of a community trail among new and habitual exercisers: a preliminary assessment' *Preventing Chronic Disease* 1: 1–11

Handy, S.L., Cao, X. and Mokhtarian, P.L. (2006) 'Self-selection in the relationship between the built environment and walking—empirical evidence from Northern California' *Journal of the American Planning Association* 72: 55–74

Haskell, W.L., Lee, I.-M., Pate, R.R., et al (2007) 'Physical activity and public health: updated recommendation for adults from the American College of Sports Medicine and the American Heart Association' *Medicine & Science in Sports & Exercise* 39: 1423–34

Heath, G., Brownson, R., Kruger, J., et al (2006) 'The effectiveness of urban design and land use and transport policies and practices to increase physical activity: a systematic review' *Journal of Physical Activity and Health* 3: S55–S71

Humpel, N., Owen, N. and Leslie, E. (2002) 'Environmental factors associated with adults' participation in physical activity: a review' *American Journal of Preventive Medicine* 22: 188–99

Jackson, R.J. (2005) 'Commentary on active living research' *American Journal of Preventive Medicine* 28: 218–9

Kahn, E.B., Ramsey, L.T., Brownson, R.C., et al (2002) 'The effectiveness of interventions to increase physical activity. A systematic review' *American Journal of Preventive Medicine* 22: 73–107

Kirby, T. (2001) '20mph Zones in Kingston Upon Hull' *Managing vehicle speeds for safety: latest developments*. Aston University

Krizek, K. (2000) 'Pretest-posttest strategy for researching neighborhood-scale urban form and travel behavior' *Transportation Research Record* 1722: 48–55

Krizek, K.J. (2003) 'Residential relocation and changes in urban travel: does neighborhood-scale urban form matter?' *Journal of the American Planning Association* 69: 265–81

Layfield, R., Chinn, L. and Nicholls, D. (2003) *Pilot home zone schemes: evaluation of the Methleys*. Leeds: Transport Research Laboratory

Lee, C. and Moudon, A.V. (2004) 'Physical activity and environment research in the health field: implications for urban and transportation planning practice and research' *Journal of Planning Literature* 19: 147–81

Marcus, B.H., Williams, D.M., Dubbert, P.M., et al (2006) 'Physical activity intervention studies: what we know and what we need to know: a scientific statement from the American Heart Association Council on Nutrition, Physical Activity, and Metabolism (Subcommittee on Physical Activity); Council on Cardiovascular Disease in the Young; and the Interdisciplinary Working Group on Quality of Care and Outcomes Research' *Circulation* 114: 2739–52

Merom, D., Bauman, A.E., Vita, P. and Close, G. (2003) 'An environmental intervention to promote walking and cycling—the impact of a newly constructed Rail Trail in Western Sydney' *Preventive Medicine* 36: 235–42

Morrison, D.S., Thomson, H. and Petticrew, M. (2004) 'Evaluation of the health effects of a neighbourhood traffic calming scheme' *Journal of Epidemiology and Community Health* 58: 837–40

National Institute for Health and Clinical Excellence (NICE) (2006) *Four commonly used methods to increase physical activity: brief interventions in primary care, exercise referral schemes, community-based exercise programme for walking and cycling. Public health Intervention Guidance Number 2.* London: National Institute for Health and Clinical Excellence

National Institute for Health and Clinical Excellence (NICE) (2007) *Public health programme guidance process manual.* London: National Institute for Health and Clinical Excellence

National Institute for Health and Clinical Excellence (NICE) (2008) *Promoting and creating built or natural environments that encourage and support physical activity. Programme Guidance 4.* London: National Institute for Health and Clinical Excellence

Ogilvie, D., Egan, M., Hamilton, V. and Petticrew, M. (2005) 'Systematic reviews of health effects of social interventions: 2. Best available evidence: how low should you go?' *Journal of Epidemiology and Community Health* 59: 886–92

Ogilvie, D., Mitchell, R., Mutrie, N., Petticrew, M. and Platt, S. (2006) 'Evaluating health effects of transport interventions: methodologic case study' *American Journal of Preventive Medicine* 31: 118–26

Owen, N., Cerin, E., Leslie, E., et al (2007) 'Neighborhood walkability and the walking behavior of Australian adults' *American Journal of Preventive Medicine* 33: 387–95

Owen, N., Humpel, N., Leslie, E., Bauman, A.E. and Sallis, J.F. (2004) 'Understanding environmental influences on walking: review and research agenda' *American Journal of Preventive Medicine* 27: 67–76

Owen, N., Leslie, E., Salmon, J. and Fotheringham, M. (2000) 'Environmental determinants of physical activity and sedentary behavior' *Exercise and Sport Science Reviews* 28: 153–8

Painter, K. (1996) 'The influence of street lighting improvements on crime, fear and pedestrian street use, after dark' *Landscape and Urban Planning* 35: 193–201

Petticrew, M., Cummins, S., Ferrell, C., et al (2005) 'Natural experiments: an underused tool for public health?' *Public Health* 119: 751–7

Ramanathan, S., Allison, K.R., Faulkner, G. and Dwyer, J.J.M. (2008) 'Challenges in assessing the implementation and effectiveness of physical activity and nutrition policy interventions as natural experiments' *Health Promotion International* 23: 290–7

Reger-Nash, B., Bauman, A.E., Cooper, L., Chey, T. and Simon, K.J. (2006) 'Evaluating communitywide walking interventions' *Evaluation and Program Planning* 29: 251–9

Saelens, B.E. and Handy, S.L. (2008) 'Built environment correlates of walking: a review' *Medicine & Science in Sports & Exercise* 40: S550–66

Saelens, B.E., Sallis, J.F. and Frank, L.D. (2003) 'Environmental correlates of walking and cycling: findings from the transportation, urban design, and planning literatures' *Annals of Behavioral Medicine* 25: 80–91

Schwanen, T. and Mokhtarian, P.L. (2005) 'What affects commute mode choice: neighborhood physical structure or preferences toward neighborhoods?' *Journal of Transport Geography* 13: 83–99

Shilton, T., Bauman, A.E., Bull, F. and Sarmiento, O. (2007) 'Effectiveness and challenges for promoting physical activity globally' in D. McQueen, and C. Jones (eds), *Global perspectives on health promotion effectiveness,* pp 87–106. New York: Springer

Silcock, R. (1999) *The community impact of traffic calming schemes. Final report.* Edinburgh: Scottish Office

Sjöström, M., Oja, P., Hagströmer, M., Smith, B. and Bauman, A.E. (2006) 'Health-enhancing physical activity across European Union countries: the Eurobarometer study' *Journal of Public Health* 14: 291–300

Social Research Associates (2001) *Gloucester City Council. Safer City Project—2000, 2001.* Leicester: Social Research Associates

Space Syntax Ltd (2002) *Millennium Bridge and environs: pedestrian impact assessment study.* London: Space Syntax Ltd

Space Syntax Ltd (2004a) *Paternoster Square: comparative study of pedestrian flows following the re-design of the public space.* London: Space Syntax Ltd

Space Syntax Ltd (2004b) *Trafalgar Square: comparative study of space use patterns following the re-design of the public space.* London: Space Syntax Ltd

Stamatakis, E., Ekelund, U. and Wareham, N.J. (2007) 'Temporal trends in physical activity in England: the Health Survey for England 1991 to 2004' *Preventive Medicine* 45: 416–23

Sustrans (2005) *Monitoring report 2005. Case study: Ford Green.* Stoke: Sustrans

Sustrans (2006) *Survey of cycling and walking activity at Stedfastgate.* Edinburgh: Sustrans

Tang, K.C., Choi, B.C. and Beaglehole, R. (2008) 'Grading of evidence of the effectiveness of health promotion interventions' *Journal of Epidemiology and Community Health* 62: 832–4

Transport for London (2006) *Central London congestion charging impacts monitoring. Fourth annual report.* London: Transport for London

Transportation Research Board (2005) *Does the built environment influence physical activity? Examining the evidence.* Washington DC: Transportation Research Board

Victora, C.G., Habicht, J.P. and Bryce, J. (2004) 'Evidence-based public health: moving beyond randomized trials' *American Journal of Public Health* 94: 400–5

Webster, D., Tilley, A., Wheeler, A., Nichols, S. and Buttress, S. (2006) *TRL report 654. Pilot home zone schemes: summary of the schemes.* Crowthorne: Transport Research Laboratory

Yanovitzky, I., Zanutto, E., Hornik, R. (2005) 'Estimating causal effects of public health education campaigns using propensity score methodology' *Evaluation and Program Planning* 28: 209–20

Chapter 20

Fiscal policy and health related behaviours

Anne Ludbrook

Introduction

Public health is concerned with both the protection of people from harm and the promotion of health improvement. Government policies may affect individual health behaviours directly or indirectly, by affecting the context in which individual decisions are made. In this chapter, consideration is given primarily to the effect of fiscal policy (taxation). Fiscal policy is defined as the direct manipulation of prices through the tax system; however, this is only one way in which the cost, more broadly defined, of health behaviours could be affected by government. The time and effort required to purchase goods can be influenced by the regulatory or licensing framework. The cost of harmful behaviours, such as drink-driving, can be increased by changing the sanctions that apply and the extent of enforcement activity. It may also be relevant to consider mechanisms for subsidizing health improving behaviours. These other interventions cannot be entirely set aside because the effectiveness of fiscal interventions may be altered by coexisting policies and this will be discussed in reviewing the evidence.

In principle, fiscal interventions could be applied to most areas of health-related behaviour. In this chapter, most of the evidence examined comes from tobacco control[1] and alcohol, which are areas where government intervention using fiscal measures has been most established. In the UK, taxation has been increased on tobacco products, and more recently on alcohol, for explicit public health purposes. However, the cost of acquiring tobacco or alcohol, in terms of time and effort, can also be affected by a range of licensing restrictions and these have been used more widely in other countries.

The application and evaluation of policy in different areas of health behaviour can be complicated by the different goals which are being pursued and different ways of measuring outcomes. Although with tobacco the overall aim of reducing the prevalence of smoking is fairly clear, the effect of interventions are frequently measured in terms of aggregate consumption of tobacco. Cutting down on tobacco consumption may have some health benefits but not smoking at all produces the most health gain. With alcohol, moderate levels of consumption may have some health benefits and policy is mainly concerned

---

[1] Most studies relate to cigarettes, as this is the dominant form of tobacco consumption, and these terms will tend to be used interchangeably.

with reducing excessive consumption. However, self-reported consumption is not an entirely reliable indicator. At a population level, alcohol-related harms are correlated with aggregate alcohol consumption and this may be a better indicator for evaluating interventions.

This chapter addresses the evidence concerning the impact that fiscal policy has on health behaviour and also the relative effectiveness of fiscal policy and other interventions. The evidence will be set out first for the case of tobacco control and will consider results from the literature and the application of fiscal policy in the UK. This will address questions relating to the impact of fiscal policy on overall smoking prevalence and on socio-economic inequalities in smoking prevalence. This example will then be compared with the situation relating to alcohol and other health behaviours. Before turning to the evidence, the following sections consider the theoretical basis for fiscal interventions and how evidence of the effectiveness and efficiency of such interventions is generated.

Theoretical basis for intervention

Public health interventions should have a theoretical basis as well as an evidence base. In this chapter, the effects of the interventions being considered are examined in the context of economic theory as it relates to individual decision making. People purchase a range of goods and services, or undertake a range of activities, based on their costs and the benefit (utility) they derive from them. Although this analysis is usually presented in economics textbooks on the basis of price, this is generally understood as a proxy for cost. Cost can include the time and effort expended on purchasing a good or undertaking an activity. It is on this basis that policy interventions which restrict (or make easier) access to certain products or activities can be considered to increase (decrease) the cost even if the price is unchanged. The key elements of price theory are set out in Box 20.1.

It should be noted that the theory does not depend on *all* consumers *actually* behaving this way *all* of the time. The purpose of the assumption is to allow robust predictions to be made about aggregate market demand. Consumers will buy less of a good when the price goes up because they can get more benefit by switching their expenditure to other products where the price has stayed the same. Consumption will also be reduced because a price increase reduces the real value of the income available (income effect). However, if there is an increase in real income, more will be purchased of most goods and activities.

A negative price elasticity shows that the effect of a price increase is to reduce consumption, as expected. If the price elasticity is less than −1, then the reduction in the amount purchased will be less than proportional to the size of the price increase. Thus, for example, if the relationship between price and tobacco consumption shows the price elasticity to be −0.5, then the percentage reduction in consumption will be half the percentage increase in price. Income elasticities are positive, except for inferior goods. In the case of cigarettes, the income elasticity has changed in developed countries over time and more recent studies show that cigarettes are an inferior good (Wasserman et al 1991; Townsend et al 1994).

The analysis of demand for products such as tobacco has become more sophisticated than simple price and quantity relationships based on aggregate market data. One factor

---

Box 20.1 Basics of price theory

Consumers behave *as if* they aim to maximize the benefit they derive subject to the constraint of their available budget and other constraints such as time.

Consumers equalize the additional (marginal) benefit they derive from expenditure on each good or activity.

General predictions:

- the amount of a product purchased, or activity undertaken will increase (decrease) as the cost (money price or time) goes down (up); *price effect*

- the amount of a product purchased, or activity undertaken will increase (decrease) if income goes up (down); *income effect*

- the amount of a product purchased, or activity undertaken will increase (decrease) if the benefit (utility) goes up (down).

The size of the price effect (price elasticity) can be estimated from the gradient of the relationship between price and quantity (income fixed).

The size of the income effect (income elasticity) can be estimated from the gradient of the relationship between income and quantity (prices fixed).

---

to be taken into account is that tobacco consumption is addictive and this can be taken into account in a number of ways, with assumptions about whether or not consumers factor this into their decision to start smoking. Habit formation is also important in considering demand for alcohol. Studies using individual data allow for modelling the consumer decision about whether or not to smoke and then consider demand for tobacco contingent on this first decision. Some models have considered the impact that other interventions may have on the decision to smoke and the amount of tobacco consumed.

How effectiveness is assessed: generating evidence

When considering fiscal and regulatory interventions, this is an area where 'experimental' evidence is rare, in the sense of randomized or other controlled designs. (A notable exception was the negative income tax experiment in the US.) It is the nature of these interventions that they are applied across populations; therefore the only basis for measuring effects is comparison with other populations (cross-sectional studies) or with the same population over different time periods (time-series or cohort studies) usually on the basis of natural experiments rather than planned comparisons. The data available for analysis usually come from secondary sources; that is, they are routinely collected for various purposes and not specifically collected to address the research question of interest. The data may be at an aggregate market level, such as total expenditure per time period, or individual level data. The type of data available is a limiting factor in the analysis that can be undertaken and study designs have to be carefully implemented to ensure that confounding factors and other sources of bias are controlled for. Potential confounding factors include differences in the population characteristics, differences in social or legislative context, and interactions with other policy or economic changes taking place at the same time. Such studies can strictly only show relationships between price or regulatory intervention and consumption rather than causality; however, where such relationships are found consistently and have a clear theoretical basis, the evidence can be considered sound.

However, a critical issue to consider is how fiscal measures, regulation, and other interventions may interact. Whilst both theory and empirical evidence (see below) support the effectiveness of taxation in influencing consumption via price, the size of the effect may be related to the use of other interventions which may either enhance or reduce the effect of tax policies. Thus, for example, health promotion campaigns and direct interventions such as smoking cessation services might increase of the impact of a tax increase (and vice-versa) and it may be more difficult to obtain sufficient data to attribute the effects accurately. Similarly, strict regulation of supply may reduce the impact of taxation because price becomes a smaller component of total cost.

Evidence for the long-run effects of tax or price is mostly drawn from studies of time series data relating aggregate consumption to price and income data although cross-sectional studies have also been carried out. Analysis of individual level data has also allowed estimates to be made of the effect of price on both the decision to smoke and the amount smoked and can be used to consider the impacts on different sections of the population (age, gender, ethnicity, or social class). Studies of regulatory interventions are most frequently conducted on a cross-sectional basis although some studies use time series data and the effect of the regulation can be tested as a dummy variable. Time series analysis provides challenges in dealing with correlations among the independent variables and it is important that good estimation techniques are used to produce reliable estimates. Studies across different populations may introduce confounding factors which must be carefully controlled. Studies have been conducted on a cross-sectional basis in the USA to compare the effects that different taxation and regulatory regimes have and to consider the interaction between taxation and other regulatory interventions. The USA has the advantage for researchers of having different tax and regulatory mechanisms at state level, whilst confounding factors due to population characteristics are lessened (although not absent) in comparison to cross-country studies.

Case study on tobacco

Smoking is one of the areas where the most extensive use has been made of fiscal instruments and other policy interventions. The effectiveness of government intervention can be assessed by considering both the prevalence of smoking and the amount of tobacco consumed, as continuing smokers may smoke less. Survey-based estimates of cigarette smoking prevalence show that this has fallen from 65% of the male population aged 16 and over in 1948 to 22% in 2007 (41% to 20% for the female population) (Figure 20.1). This long-term trend displays interesting phases; relatively little change up to 1968 followed by a

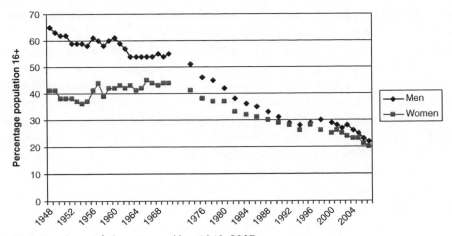

Fig. 20.1 Prevalence of cigarette smoking 1948–2007
Sources: <http://info.cancerresearchuk.org> and ONS General Household Survey

sustained downward trend that flattened out in the 1990s but has picked up again in the current decade.

The fall in smoking prevalence is mirrored by declining (legal) tobacco sales; HM Revenue & Customs figures on tobacco clearances fell from over 10 million kgs in 1986/7 to 4.6 million kgs in 2005/6 and household expenditure on tobacco, valued at constant prices, has been declining since 1974.

These prevalence figures also indicate that the target of 20% for smoking prevalence by the year 2000 set in The Health of the Nation (Department of Health 1992) was not achieved as the declining prevalence rates stalled in the mid 1990s. Smoking Kills (Department of Health 1998) aimed to re-establish the downward trend and to achieve a prevalence of 24% by 2010. The strategy involved a range of tobacco control measures but there was also explicit recognition that despite past increases in taxation, tobacco had become more affordable over time and there was a commitment to raise tax by 5% in real terms year on year.

Evidence relating to price and income effects

Scale of price effects

Numerous studies have estimated the price elasticity of demand for tobacco and one review of this literature gives estimates of the size of the price effect as a fairly wide range of –0.14 to –1.23 (Chaloupka and Warner 2000). However, the majority of results were in a narrower range of –0.3 to –0.5 and it should be noted that all of the estimates are negative; ie price does reduce demand but the effect of a 10% price increase may range between 1.4% and 12.3%. Given that studies cover different countries and different time periods, and use different modelling approaches based on different data sets, it is perhaps not surprising that the effect size varies. Particular differences in estimation have been found when using individual rather than aggregate data and when controlling for the impact of other tobacco control interventions (Wasserman et al 1991).

The results also depend on the extent to which data can be adjusted to account for tax avoidance through (legal) cross-border purchasing and smuggling. Some estimates suggest that taking smuggling into account may reduce the size of price elasticity estimates by half (Lanoie and Leclair 1998). Recent estimates for the UK show the price elasticity of total tobacco demand varying between −0.47 and −0.87 depending on how the model is specified. Furthermore, the effect on purchases of duty paid tobacco is estimated to be more than −1.0, whilst the price elasticity for smuggled and cross-border purchases are both positive (Cullum and Pissarides 2004).

Most evidence on the effect of price relates to aggregate consumption and this combines both reductions in prevalence and reductions in quantity smoked by continuing smokers. The effect on prevalence alone has been less studied and considering that this is only part of the effect the relationship is likely to be weaker. However, the health benefits from quitting are substantially greater than those from cutting down. Studies using individual level data, rather than aggregate data, are able to consider the effect of price on both the decision to smoke and the amount to smoke. These studies suggest that both are affected although by different amounts; for example, a price elasticity of smoking participation of −0.26 compared with price elasticity overall of −0.42 (Lewit et al 1981; Lewit and Coate 1982).

Relationship between tax and price

The questions of whether or not tax increases raise the price faced by consumers and by how much are fairly critical to the effectiveness of fiscal policy. Both in theory and in practice, this reflects the nature of competition in the market and the assumptions about consumer demand. The tobacco industry is heavily concentrated and there is some evidence that prices may increase more in response to tax increases possibly because the industry seeks to increase the profit margin on a smaller total demand. In the US, a one cent increase in the state cigarette tax was found to generate a 1.11 cent increase in the retail price (Keeler et al 1996).

Tobacco prices and taxation in the UK

The evidence above relates to general findings from the literature. In this section consideration is given to the application of fiscal policy in the UK and its relationship to the falling prevalence of smoking. Over the whole post-war period, tobacco has not actually become less affordable. The price has increased relative to all other goods (represented by the retail prices index (RPI)) but not by as much as the increase in real incomes. However, taxation has had an important role in keeping prices higher than they would otherwise have been and there has been a sustained increase in prices more recently.

Table 20.1 provides some data for the UK on price trends for premium brand cigarettes. This shows that pre-tax prices have been increasing by more than inflation, which may reflect both increasing costs and profit margins. There has been an even higher

Table 20.1 Prices for premium brands of cigarettes

	1981	2005	Index 1981=100
Pre-tax price	23.9	104.6	438
Tax	67.1	377.4	562
Total price	91	482	530
All price index (inflation)			257
Relative price index (total price index adjusted for inflation)			206
Real income index			194
Affordability (relative price adjusted for growth in income)			94

increase in taxation and the total price for these cigarettes has risen more than twice as fast as the general level of price increases. However, because real incomes have nearly doubled over the same time period, the affordability of premium brand cigarettes has fallen only slightly since 1981. Nonetheless, the effect of taxation has been to prevent cigarettes becoming more affordable; if taxation had only increased in line with general price inflation over this period then the tax levied would have been more than £2 lower in 2005.

In the period from 1980 to 1990, tobacco prices rose by 53% more than RPI: from 1990 to 2004 prices rose 3.5 times as fast as RPI. Sustained higher tax increases from 1997 onwards do appear to have promoted a return to the downward trend in prevalence and the achievement of the target for smoking prevalence set in Smoking Kills (24% or less by 2010). However, the tax increases have also been accompanied by increased support for smoking cessation services.

What contribution has fiscal policy made to reducing smoking prevalence compared with other interventions?

Disentangling the effects of fiscal policy from other tobacco control policies is difficult because these are frequently applied together. Higher taxation is often accompanied by other measures and increasing action on tobacco may also be observed in communities where there is greater anti-smoking sentiment. Econometric studies which attempt to separate out these effects have shown, for example, that regulation on smoking in public places had a significant effect on adult and teenage smoking in the US and the price effects were lower than in other studies (Wasserman et al 1991). A second study, in Canada, using an index of all tobacco control measures showed that total consumption responded to price but smoking prevalence responded to regulation (Lanoie and Leclair 1998).

The long-term trend in smoking prevalence in Great Britain is suggestive that other factors are involved as prevalence has fallen when cigarettes were becoming more afford-able. A UK study (Townsend et al 1994) showed that both price and the health message have effect on consumption but the size of price effect was greater. However, the model used did not include income.

Unintended consequences

There is some evidence that smokers respond to across the board tax increases by switching to cigarettes that are higher in tar and nicotine, which would reduce any health benefits of lower consumption (Evans and Farrelly 1998) and might point to taxation based on content rather than uniform levies. Studies of individual commodities fail to take account of the consequences of changes in demand for other health affecting commodities. Studies that have considered this issue have found both substitution effects and complementarity between such goods. For example, Dee (1999) found that higher cigarette taxes reduced both teenage smoking and the prevalence of teenage drinking and Farrelly et al (2001) found similar effects for marijuana use.

Price effects on different population groups

Another issue frequently raised is whether or not price rises will impact on particular groups of concern, such as younger (and possibly underage) smokers. Here the evidence would seem positive although the studies that have been carried out are largely in the USA, where the variation in prices and other regulatory matters across different states makes it easier to conduct research.

Most studies of demand for cigarettes that have considered age effects find an inverse relationship between price elasticity and age; for example, a price elasticity for younger people (20–25) which was double those over 25 (Lewit and Coate 1982). Most of the price effect was estimated to relate to the decision to smoke (participation elasticity –0.74). Similar but slightly higher estimates have been made for 12- to 17-year-olds (Lewit et al 1981). These findings have been replicated by other studies but when restrictions on access to tobacco are introduced the effect was not statistically significant (Wasserman et al 1991). For college students, however, price had a stronger effect than restrictions on smoking in public places (Chaloupka and Weschler 1997). Conflicting evidence on the impact of price on smoking initiation in youth in the US may be explained by high tax rates acting as a proxy for anti-smoking sentiment.

Another issue of concern is the impact that taxation has on different social groups, and particularly those on low incomes. There are two aspects to this: whether the taxes are regressive, imposing an unfair burden on lower social classes, and whether taxation is effective in reducing smoking prevalence in lower social classes and contributes to reducing health inequalities. These two issues are linked in the sense that if poor smokers reduce their smoking sufficiently more than richer smokers then they may pay relatively less following a tax increase (Remier 2004). Furthermore, if smokers want to quit/cut down and higher prices help them to do this then the regressive effect of taxation may be reduced (Gruber and Koszegi 2004).

UK evidence

Long-term trends in prevalence by social class can be difficult to monitor because of changing definitions over time. Figure 20.2 uses the highest and lowest social class, as defined at each point in time. The figures for 1968 are for all smokers; all other years

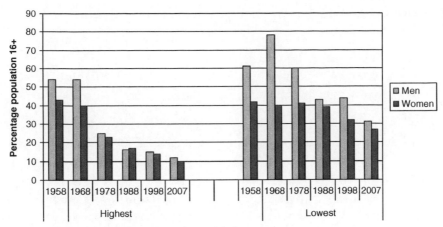

Fig. 20.2 Trends in smoking prevalence by social class
Sources: Todd (ed) (1959; 1969) ONS General Household Survey

relate to cigarette smokers. Without this variation, there would be a clear downward trend for the highest social group over the whole period. However, for the lowest social class, the downward movement in prevalence is only observed from 1988 for women and from 1998 for men. As a result, socio-economic inequalities in smoking had been widening but this trend has been reversed. Smoking Kills set a target for smoking prevalence to fall faster in manual groups than non-manual groups and this has already been achieved for men but not for women.

Only one study has directly assessed the effects of price on different groups in the UK (Townsend et al 1994). Price had a significant effect for men aged 25–34 and for women of all ages whereas health publicity was significant for all men except the oldest age group (60+) but was only significant for women 25–34 and 60+. Income had a positive (negative) effect for younger (older) men and a negative effect for older women. Price effects on smoking prevalence were higher for lower socio-economic groups and more recent survey results show that lower socio-economic groups more likely to report cost as a reason for quitting (Vangeli and West 2008). The study by Townsend et al used data from 1972–1990. Given the more sustained tax increases over recent years, this analysis would be worth repeating.

What about other health related behaviours?

The case study above has looked at tobacco control and has documented the general evidence that increasing prices reduce consumption and the contribution that higher taxes have made towards achieving policy objectives for smoking. Another area in which there is considerable evidence of price affecting consumption is alcohol. The price elasticity for alcohol has been estimated for various time periods and settings and, as with tobacco, the estimates are variable (Booth et al 2008). Price elasticities are generally estimated for different types of alcoholic drinks and sometimes for different drinking locations,

Table 20.2 Estimates of own-price elasticity for various types of alcoholic drink

	UK estimates	Range reported from literature
Beer: on sales	−0.48	
Beer: off sales	−1.03	
Beer		−0.09 to −3.2
Wine	−0.75	−0.30 to −2.30
Spirits	−1.31	−0.49 to −2.42

Source: Huang 2003

as consumer preferences may vary. For the UK, robust estimates are produced by the Government Economic Service for use in forecasting the yield of proposed tax increases. The most recent estimates of own-price elasticity for various types of alcoholic drink are shown in Table 20.2 and these lie within the range reported from other studies:

Price is also associated with alcohol related harms (Herttua et al 2008) and there is some evidence on under-age and youth drinking (Grossman et al 1994; Moore and Cook 1995). Frequent or heavy drinkers amongst youth are more price sensitive; high taxes reduce consumption and probability of excessive drinking.

In the UK, in contrast with the falling consumption of tobacco, there has been increasing consumption of alcohol as it has become more affordable despite increases in taxation. Recent attempts to apply above inflation increases in taxation, explicitly for public health purposes, may not have been passed on in full in a highly competitive market. In constant prices, reported expenditure increased by around 25% between 1976 and 2004 but has shown a small decline in the past three years. As the strength of alcoholic drinks has also been increasing over time, the amount of pure alcohol purchased has increased rather more quickly. Expenditure increased by 14% between 1986 and 2007 but the volume of alcohol cleared by HMRC[2] increased by 32%. Although recent survey data suggest that the proportion of the population drinking to excess may not have increased significantly, there is widespread under-reporting of alcohol consumption. Survey data on alcohol consumption accounts for only around half of the alcohol cleared for sale by HMRC (Department of Health and Home Office 2007) and household expenditure estimates are also only about half the total value of the UK market. Alcohol-related harms have been increasing and are probably a better indicator of alcohol misuse than self-reported consumption or expenditure.

The health issue for alcohol is more complex than with tobacco; it is not consumption per se that presents a problem but excess consumption. As a result, there has not been the same concerted use of the full range of policy instruments to restrict consumption.

[2] The volume of alcohol cleared by HMRC includes sales to visitors to the UK but excludes alcohol brought into the country by UK residents. These factors will tend to cancel each other out in estimating levels of alcohol consumption.

Fiscal policy has not been applied sufficiently to be effective. Even more complex is the growing problem of obesity, where there has been little or no interest in applying fiscal interventions. Some states in the US levy small taxes on soft drinks and some sweets and snacks but this is for revenue raising rather than public health reasons and it has been argued that they are too small to have any impact (Jacobson and Brownell 2000).

Economic theory tells us that price manipulation should influence dietary and physical activity behaviours. A few studies have modelled what these effects might be but with a tendency to focus on single issues, such as taxing high fat foods (Leicester and Windmeijer 2004). These studies show the expected effects on consumption behaviour but also demonstrate regressive impacts on low income families. Little if any attention has been given to a more systematic approach of taxing some foods and subsidizing others. Recognition also has to be given to existing producer subsidies to certain food items via agricultural policies. Additional empirical analysis is required in this area, however, much more attention should be given to the underlying model of consumer choice, as decisions relating to food and physical activity are far more complex than decisions relating to tobacco and alcohol.

Conclusions

Fiscal policy (taxation) has been applied to tobacco and alcohol and evidence suggests that these products respond to price. In the case of tobacco, above inflation rises in the UK have ensured that prices remain high and this has contributed to declining smoking prevalence and aggregate consumption. However, not all of the effect can be attributed to price; consideration has to be given to all the other interventions that have taken place. The fact that income elasticity has changed from positive to negative over time points to a change in consumer attitudes towards tobacco and may be indirect evidence of an education effect. There is evidence from North American studies that other tobacco control regulations are also effective and it may be difficult to determine precisely the relative contributions. In contrast, although alcohol duties have increased over time in the UK, they have not increased sufficiently to reduce the affordability of alcohol. There has also been an absence of other restrictions on availability of alcohol. Whilst fiscal policy may not be the only intervention that can change health-related behaviour, it would appear to be an important factor in an overall strategy.

Acknowledgements

The Health Economics Research Unit receives core funding from the Chief Scientist Office, Scottish Government Health Directorates, and from the University of Aberdeen. All opinions expressed are those of the author and should not be attributed to any funding body.

Bibliography

Booth A, Brennan A, Meier P et al (2008) *The Independent Review of the Effects of Alcohol Pricing and Promotion. Summary of evidence.* Accessed online at: <http://www.dh.gov.uk/en/Publichealth/Healthimprovement/Alcoholmisuse/DH_085390>

Chaloupka FJ and Warner KE (2000) 'The economics of smoking' in Culyer A J and Newhouse J P (eds), *Handbook of Health Economics*. Elsevier: Amsterdam

Chaloupka FJ and Weschler H (1997) 'Price, tobacco control policies and smoking among young adults' *Journal of Health Economics* 16: 359–73

Cullum P and Pissarides CA (2004) *The Demand for Tobacco Products in the UK*. Government Economic Service Working Paper 150. London: HM Customs and Excise

Dee TS (1999) 'The complementarity of teen smoking and drinking' *Journal of Health Economics* 18(6): 769–93

Department of Health (1992) *The Health of the Nation*. White Paper. London: HMSO

Department of Health (1998) *Smoking Kills—A White Paper on Tobacco*. Cm 4177. London: The Stationery Office

Department of Health and Home Office (2007) *Safe, Sensible, Social: The next steps in the national alcohol strategy*. London: Department of Health and Home Office

Evans WN and Farrelly MC (1998) 'The compensating behaviour of smokers: Taxes, tar and nicotine' *RAND Journal of Economics* 29/3: 578–95

Farrelly MC, Bray JW, Zarkin GA, and Wendling BW (2001) 'The joint demand for cigarettes and marijuana: evidence from the National Household Surveys on Drug Abuse' *Journal of Health Economics* 20/1: 51–68

Grossman M, Chaloupka FJ, Saffer H, and Laixuthai A (1994) 'Effects of alcohol price policy on youth: A summary of economic research' *Journal of Research on Adolescence* 4: 347–64

Gruber J and Koszegi B (2004) 'Tax incidence when individuals are time-inconsistent: the case of cigarette excise taxes' *Journal of Public Economics* 88: 1959–87

Herttua K, Mäkelä P, and Martikainen P (2008) 'Changes in alcohol-related mortality and its socioeconomic differences after a large reduction in alcohol prices: a natural experiment based on register data' *American Journal of Epidemiology* 168: 1110–8. Advance Access published online 20 August 2008 Doi:10.1093/aje/kwn216

Huang CD (2003) *Econometric Models of Alcohol Demand in the United Kingdom* Government Economic Service Working Paper 140. London: HM Customs and Excise

Jacobson MF and Brownell KD (2000) 'Small taxes on soft drinks and snack foods to promote health' *American Journal of Public Health* 90: 854–7

Keeler TE, Hu T-W, Barnett PG, Manning WG, and Sung HY (1996) 'Do cigarette producers discriminate by state? An empirical analysis of local cigarette pricing and taxation' *Journal of Health Economics* 15: 499–512

Lanoie P and Leclair P (1998) 'Taxation or regulation: Looking for a good anti-smoking policy' *Economics Letters* 58: 85–9

Leicester A and Windmeijer F (2004) *The 'Fat Tax' Economic Incentives to Reduce Obesity*. London: Institute for Fiscal Studies

Lewit EM, Coate D, and Grossman M (1981) 'The effects of government regulation on teenage smoking' *Journal of Law and Economics* 24/3: 545–69

Lewit EM and Coate D (1982) 'The potential for using excise taxes to reduce smoking' *Journal of Health Economics* 1/2: 121–45

Moore MJ and Cook PJ (1995) *Habit and heterogeneity in the youthful demand for alcohol*. Working Paper No 5152. Cambridge, MA: National Bureau of Economic Research

ONS (Office of National Statistics) (various years) *General Household Survey*. Available at: <http://www.statistics.gov.uk>

Remier DK (2004) 'Poor smokers, poor quitters, and cigarette tax regressivity' *American Journal of Public Health* 94: 225–9

Todd GF (ed) (1959) *Tobacco Manufacturers' Standing Committee Research Papers No 1 Statistics of Smoking*. 2nd edn. Table 18. London: Tobacco Manufacturers' Standing Committee

Todd GF (ed)(1969) *Tobacco Research Council Research Paper No 1 Statistics of Smoking in the United Kingdom*. 5th edn. Tables 21a and 21b. London: Tobacco Manufacturers' Standing Committee

Townsend JL, Roderick P, and Cooper J (1994) 'Cigarette smoking by socioeconomic group, sex, and age: Effects of price, income, and health publicity' *British Medical Journal* 309/6959: 923–6

Vangeli E and West R (2008) 'Sociodemographic differences in triggers to quit smoking:findings from a national survey' *Tobacco Control* 17: 410–15

Wasserman J, Manning WG, Newhouse JP, and Winkler JD (1991) 'The effects of excise taxes and regulations on cigarette smoking' *Journal of Health Economics* 10: 43–64

Part 4

Synthesizing evidence and developing guidance

Chapter 21

The process of systematic review of public health evidence: quality criteria and standards

Mark Petticrew

Introduction

> Decision makers need to assess and appraise all the available evidence irrespective as to whether it has been derived from RCTs or observational studies, and the strengths and weaknesses of each need to be understood if reasonable and reliable conclusions are to be drawn. Nor, in reaching these conclusions, is there any shame in accepting that judgements are required about the 'fitness for purpose' of the components of the evidence base. On the contrary, judgements are an essential ingredient of most aspects of the decision-making process.
>
> (Rawlins 2008)

Assessing 'study quality' is a key component of the systematic review process which is much contested. Systematic reviewers would argue that the purpose is to ensure that the final synthesis of evidence is based on the most robust studies—that is, those least susceptible to bias. A range of appraisal tools and checklists are often employed to ensure that attention is duly given to the main sources of bias, but to the non-initiated this approach often seems formulaic and narrowly-focused, and risks privileging a few key aspects of internal validity over other important aspects of research, such as its utility and generalizability. Moreover, for critics, the process of quality assessment seems to reduce the task of reviewing evidence to a series of box-ticking exercises, as opposed to an appraisal of the usefulness of research for decision-making purposes. Even the phrase 'study quality' itself is contentious.

The application of quality criteria becomes particularly difficult when reviewing public health evidence because the range of types of evidence to be included is potentially wide. In this context excluding studies on grounds of 'validity' or 'quality' alone may inadvertently introduce further biases. This chapter gives examples of this problem drawn from public health systematic reviews in the fields of tobacco control, transport, and physical activity.

Despite such potential pitfalls, systematic reviews do need to include an assessment of the risk of bias posed by each study, without taking it to extremes. This chapter also describes some of the challenges.

Assessing the quality of evidence on effectiveness of interventions

A key component of systematic reviews (or ideally, any evidence synthesis process) is the assessment of the quality or strength of the evidence presented. This, along with a comprehensive search for relevant evidence, and clear and transparent methods, is one of the defining characteristics of a systematic review. The particular and distinctive approach adopted by systematic reviewers in the early days of evidence-based medicine was one which involved identifying the key sources of bias to which research studies were prone, and using this information to develop a method of critically appraising the methods and findings of research studies, often guided by a checklist. The aim of this was primarily to ensure that the assessment of the methodological quality of individual studies was conducted in a systematic fashion; meaning that the use of a formal, often checklist-based approach removed the subjective element on the part of the reader and thus limited the scope for personal biases (for example, biases against particular studies, hypotheses, authors, institutions, and so on). It also ensured that sources of bias were not overlooked, and thus ensured that the appraisal criteria used did not vary from study to study. This approach was often contrasted with the more '*ad hoc*' approach adopted by traditional (non-systematic) literature reviews (Petticrew and Roberts 2006).

The importance of critical appraisal has been established through a number of meta-analyses which have shown that in the case of trials that aspects of study design (and study quality) are significantly related to study outcomes. In other words, study quality is an important determinant of study findings. In particular, lower quality studies have been shown to produce different results from higher quality studies, other things being equal.

This has been shown in meta-epidemiological studies of RCTs which have quantified the relationship between study quality and effect size. Wood et al (2008) for example have recently shown that the average bias associated with lack of adequate allocation concealment or lack of blinding was less for trials with objectively assessed outcomes (such as mortality) than for trials with subjectively-assessed outcomes, and less for trials with all-cause mortality as the outcome, than for trials with other outcomes (Wood et al 2008). In other words, biases in outcome assessment may affect effect sizes. They suggested that systematic reviewers should routinely assess the risk of bias in the results of included trials, and that such assessments should be outcome-specific, because of the greater risk of bias in subjectively-assessed outcomes.

Other studies have also suggested that flaws in study design are associated with inflated effect sizes (Schulz et al 1995). This is similar to what has been referred to as the 'stainless steel' law of evaluation, one of the 'metallic' laws of evaluation drawn up by American sociologist Peter Rossi, and derived from a 19th century practice of naming physical laws after substances of varying durability (Rossi 1987). According to Rossi, the 'stainless steel' law states that the better designed the outcome evaluation, the less effective the intervention seems. Hence, a close examination of the study design (as a proxy for study 'quality') tells us whether the findings on effectiveness are to be believed, or not. The same is likely to apply to quantitative studies which address issues other than effectiveness.

Positive and negative aspects of checklists

Perhaps one of the main (non-scientific) drawbacks of checklists is not a methodological one, but a presentational one: that is, they involve systematic reviewers assessing the quality of other researchers' studies and as such give off the unintended impression of (methodological) superiority and inflexibility. Researchers of course do not set out to do methodologically-flawed research, but every study has some flaws, however minor. These may have implications for the interpretation of the findings. In any case methodological purity is hard to attain, and the researcher's hope and intention is that the study nonetheless makes some useful contribution to knowledge. When someone who knows little of the context within which the study was conducted, or of the practical and financial hurdles which the research team faced, appears to appraise years of research by means of a tick-the-box exercise, then it is not surprising that checklist-based appraisal is sometimes seen as simplistic, mechanistic, and unhelpful. (Worse, the process is probably unfortunately reminiscent of 'having one's homework marked' by a slightly superior older pupil.)

The process of critical appraisal therefore often appears to separate studies simplistically into 'wheat' and 'chaff', that is, studies are labelled either informative or non-informative. Critics of systematic reviews would argue, however, that we should be more concerned with what studies can tell us, than with what they can't, and that every study, however flawed, probably has some useful insights hidden therein.

Systematic reviewers would probably agree, but would argue that there is a risk that these insights are hidden among other misleading or biased information. They would also argue that critical appraisal aims to help by identifying the main methodological flaws so that the research user is aware of them, while limiting opportunities for the reader's own biases to come into play. This is done by ensuring that a core set of methodological criteria are identified for different study designs, and each study is then systematically assessed against these basic common criteria. In the case of quantitative studies these criteria tend firstly to include descriptions of the core aspects of the methodology. For randomized controlled trials, for example, items relating to the randomization are key (such as whether there was potential for the randomization to be subverted; Jadad 1998) for trials and other evaluative study designs, whether an intention to treat analyses was conducted, and whether blinding, if possible, is adopted (this criterion may be applicable of course to trial and non-trial designs, and to non-evaluative studies). These criteria tend to cover problems that could have arisen in the course of the study, and those which may occur later at the analysis and reporting stages, such as the exclusion of relevant data (eg data on participants may be missing at follow-up, or from the analysis). Finally, critical appraisal tools often point the reader towards descriptive information on the study—who is in the sample, and whether the numbers actually add up.

Sometimes, however, there is confusion between study quality, and the quality of reporting of a study which can be difficult to deal with. That is, it is not clear whether the study has been done appropriately, but then reported inaccurately or incompletely. In such situations, contacting the original authors sometimes sheds further light, but often it doesn't; the original data sometimes has been destroyed, or the lead author understandably cannot remember after 20 years the reasons why three people were lost to follow-up, or how the randomization was conducted. Huwiler-Müntener, Juni, and colleagues (2002) examined this issue in a review of 60 RCTs, in which they analysed the association between a quantitative measure of reporting quality, and various indicators of methodological quality (Huwiler-Müntener et al 2002). They concluded that reporting quality is associated with methodological quality, but that similar quality of reporting may hide important differences in methodological quality, and even well-conducted trials may be reported badly.

Use of checklists in this way is no protection against bias of course. Jüni and colleagues (1999) have warned that very different results may obtained by scoring the same studies with different checklists (Jüni et al 1999). They used 25 different scales to score 17 RCTs and examined the relationship between summary scores and pooled treatment effects in a series of meta-analyses. The results showed that, depending on the scale used, very different (even opposite) results could be obtained. They concluded that it is more important to examine the methodological aspects of studies individually, rather than in summary form. This emphasizes again that the purpose of assessing study quality is not to simplistically identify good or bad studies, but to aid reviewers understand the biases which may affect a particular study, and to use this information to inform the overall synthesis.

From study quality to study designs

The systematic reviewer's concern with 'study quality' extends from individual aspects of study methods, to general categories of study design, so that in the case of studies of effectiveness, RCTs are likely to produce less biased estimates of effect than non-randomized designs, including observational studies. This has been previously formalized into a 'hierarchy of evidence', referring to the ability of different types of study design to provide unbiased answers to questions about the effectiveness of interventions. However, this has probably been widely misunderstood as an attempt to place all studies into a general, all-purpose hierarchy, signifying their value more generally. Although this was not the original purpose, attempts to assess study quality, and to place studies within hierarchies in the ways described above continue to generate suspicion and remain a sticking point for non-systematic reviewers, and sometimes review users.

This is not surprising because in some cases setting narrowly-defined inclusion criteria which admit only RCTs for consideration risks overlooking many relevant studies. Narrow and restrictive criteria will, for example, exclude most upstream interventions, which are of most relevance to reducing health inequalities. Most population-level interventions have not yet been subject to randomized (or even non-randomized, controlled) studies. Despite this there is often an evidence base which can be utilized, taking account of any methodological and other biases. For example, a recent systematic review of the effects of tobacco pricing on smoking behaviour found that studies on this important topic have not been subjected to controlled studies, but instead rely largely on observational methods, in particular cross-sectional or longitudinal survey data (Thomas et al 2008;

Main et al 2008). Nine of 42 such studies conducted to date have examined different aspects of equity (eg by comparing lower income versus higher income smokers, and manual versus professional occupations); these suggest that pricing may have a greater effect in those on lower incomes. This observational evidence base is quite informative about the differential effects of a major tobacco control intervention, whereas reviewing the evidence from RCTs alone would produce an 'empty review'—a review with little to say about such policies. In considering study quality, systematic reviewers therefore also need to consider study 'fitness for purpose', and the extent to which any study can provide meaningful evidence on the topic of interest. This will obviously vary from review to review; a review focused on synthesizing evidence on the experiences of intervention users will draw on different sources of evidence compared with a review which is more closely focused on issues of effectiveness (see Table 21.1).

This is not of course an argument against the greater use of RCTs of policies and other social interventions, as it is unarguable that experimental designs represent the strongest evidence of effectiveness because of their ability to control for both known and unknown confounders, and they remain much underused in the evaluation of social interventions (Oakley 2000). Instead it is an argument for ensuring that we make efficient use of the evidence available to us, and in some cases, this derives from non-randomized studies, and other types of evidence.

This can be illustrated with reference to a recent systematic review of the effectiveness of interventions in promoting a population shift from using cars towards walking and cycling, in order to promote physical activity (Ogilvie et al). The review found only three RCTs, and if it had included only these three studies the review would only have been able to include evidence about two small categories of intervention: targeted behaviour change programmes for commuters, and school travel coordinators. It would have meant excluding evidence on population-wide health promotion activities, 'environmental' engineering or transport service developments, or financial incentives. Extending the review criteria to include non-RCT designs allowed evidence about a much larger range of interventions to be incorporated. Observational studies are not simply failed RCTs.

Difficulty in its application to qualitative research

Quality appraisal has been particularly problematic in the case of qualitative research. Pope et al (2007) suggest that the debate has centred on two issues: whether the concepts of methodological quality should be similar to, or different from those used in the appraisal of quantitative research; and whether the judgement about study quality should be made before or during the synthesis of findings (Pope et al 2007). In the latter case, it is argued by some commentators that the value of some studies may only emerge during the synthesis process. Pope and colleagues conclude that it is important that reviewers have some sense of the rigour of the included studies and take account of this in the synthesis (as is common/best practice in the synthesis of quantitative studies). However, there is little consensus to allow a single approach to be prescribed, although potentially useful frameworks exist (eg Spencer et al 2003).

Table 21.1 Appropriate of research methods to particular questions

Research question	Qualitative research	Survey	Case-control studies	Cohort studies	RCTs	Quasi-experimental studies	Non-experimental evaluations	Systematic reviews
Effectiveness				+	++	+		+++
Process of service delivery	++	+					+	+++
Does it matter?	++	++						+++
Acceptability	++	+			+	+	+	+++
Cost-effectiveness					++			+++
Appropriateness	++	++						++
Satisfaction with the service	++	++	+	+				+

Source: Petticrew and Roberts (2003)

Part of the problem with quality assessment may lie in the use of the term 'quality assessment' with its pejorative overtones. The phrase 'critical appraisal' may be a better descriptor of the process—that is, it is an objective, critical assessment of the extent to which the findings of a particular study provide a credible answer to a particular question. This aim is surely common to qualitative and quantitative research and the goals are similar: to assess the study methods (including sampling and analytic methods) in order to determine what credence should be placed on them, and whether the findings as reported by the researcher are a credible answer to the research question. In both cases this can be facilitated by formal checklists and frameworks, without simply using the findings to include or exclude studies in the review.

Public health evidence

The difficulties in quality-assessing evidence are compounded in the case of more complex interventions, such as those which are encountered in public health settings, for two reasons. Firstly, as noted above, studies which have adopted robust experimental designs may not be available. Evaluations of policies have relatively infrequently adopted randomization, and so many evaluations involve observational methods, in particular controlled and uncontrolled designs (such as Interrupted Time Series designs). This may not be a result of a methodological choice made by the researchers of course; it may simply be because the intervention was rolled out across an entire region or country, and this was not in the researcher's control; and so randomization to a separate area or region was not politically or practically feasible. The same may also be likely to be the case for interventions delivered at community level; randomization is most easy to achieve at the level of the individual.

Secondly, evaluations of complex interventions may have deliberately adopted non-experimental methods in order to accommodate complexity—thus they may have involved a range of qualitative and quantitative methods, rather than a straightforward and randomized design, which may be easier to interpret. The assessment of quality for such a study is therefore itself more complex, and may involve a number of different approaches within the same review.

The recently revised MRC Guidance on Complex Interventions (Craig et al, 2008) also notes the place of non-experimental methods, and points to some situations in which non-experimental study designs may be appropriate, for example because the intervention is irreversible, necessarily applies to the whole population, or because large-scale implementation is already under way. The Guidance notes that non-experimental designs are most useful where the effects of the intervention are large or rapidly follow exposure, and where the effects of selection, allocation, and other biases are relatively small. It also emphasizes the importance of drawing on supporting evidence where possible, such as a consistent pattern of effects across studies, the presence of a dose-response relationship in which more intensive variants of the interventions are associated with larger effects, and evidence from other types of study for a causal mechanism that can explain the observed effect.

The GRADE approach

It would be simple if the challenges of incorporating different types and qualities of evidence could be addressed by simply calling for greater inclusiveness, but of course this may still leave the reviewer with the problem of having to use this information on study quality to inform recommendations about practice or policy. The GRADE approach is a useful illustration of how this can be done in the case of clinical evidence, and a similar approach may be of value in public health (Guyatt et al 2008). GRADE allows judgements about study quality to be incorporated with other criteria (alluded to earlier). It considers both factors that can reduce, and increase the quality of the evidence. In the former category are the methodological study limitations, if any; any inconsistency of findings across studies; indirectness of evidence; imprecision; and the existence of publication bias. Factors that can *increase* the quality of the evidence relating to a particular outcome in a systematic review include a large magnitude of effect; evidence of a dose-response gradient; and whether all plausible confounding would reduce the observed effect (or increase the effect, if no effect was observed).

These factors increase, or decrease the summary of the quality of evidence. Crucially, it is possible in this approach for observational studies to be upgraded to moderate/high quality, just as it is possible for RCTs to be downgraded. Hence, observational studies with no threats to validity yielding very large effects, and observational studies with no threats to validity and evidence of a dose-response gradient are graded 'high' and 'moderate' quality respectively. To achieve transparency and simplicity, the GRADE system classifies the quality of evidence in one of four levels—high, moderate, low, and very low:

+ high quality: *further research is very unlikely to change our confidence in the estimate of effect*;

+ moderate quality: further research is likely to have an important impact on our confidence in the estimate of effect and may change the estimate;

+ low quality: further research is very likely to have an important impact on our confidence in the estimate of effect and is likely to change the estimate;

+ very low quality: any estimate of effect is very uncertain (Guyatt et al 2008).

It is possible that the application of the GRADE approach as it stands to many complex public health interventions would be rather dispiriting; it might simply result in the repeated conclusion that the evidence is of 'low quality'. However, the development of 'GRADE-type' approaches may be of value in public health systematic reviews, and would help with the incorporation of judgements about study quality into policy and practice recommendations.

Conclusion

The issue of study quality is not a simple 'tick-the-box' exercise which can be conducted in isolation. The assessment of study quality cannot be divorced from the research question, and study design is often a crude indicator of study quality. One would not want to advocate the adoption of non-randomized methods where RCTs are clearly superior and possible; however, in the evaluation of some interventions, non-RCT designs represent best available evidence and reviewers need to work with the evidence that is available to them. However, methodological quality is only part of the appraisal. Reviewers may also need to assess whether the intervention (as opposed to the study used to evaluate it) meets accepted quality standards, and the quality of an intervention should not be confused with the quality of the design used to evaluate it; an RCT of a poorly implemented intervention tells us little about the quality of the intervention and its delivery (Hawe et al 2004). Finally, whatever study designs are eventually included in a review, reviewers do need to include a formal assessment of the risk of bias posed by each study, without taking it to extremes (Woolf 2000).

Bibliography

Craig, P., Dieppe, P., Macintyre, S., Michie, S., Nazareth, I. and Petticrew, M. (2008) *Developing and evaluating complex interventions: new guidance*. London: Medical Research Council. <http://www.mrc.ac.uk/complexinterventionsguidance>

Guyatt, G., Oxman, A., Vist, G., Kunz, R., Falck-Ytter, Y., Alonso-Coello, P., Schünemann, H. and the Grade Working Group (2008) 'GRADE: an emerging consensus on rating quality of evidence and strength of recommendations' *British Medical Journal* 336: 924–6

Hawe, P., Shiell, A. and Riley, T. (2004) 'Complex interventions: how "out of control" can a randomised controlled trial be?' *British Medical Journal* 328: 1561–3

Huwiler-Müntener, K., Jüni, P., Junker, C. and Egger, M. (2002) 'Quality of reporting of randomized trials as a measure of methodologic quality'. *Journal of the American Medical Association* 287: 2801–4

Jadad, A. (1998) *Randomised controlled trials: a users guide*. London: BMJ Books

Jüni, P., Witschi, A., Bloch, R. and Egger, M. (1999) 'The hazards of scoring the quality of clinical trials for meta-analysis' *Journal of the American Medical Association.* 282: 1054–60

Main C, Thomas S, Ogilvie D, Stirk L, Petticrew M, Whitehead M, Sowden A. (2008) 'Population tobacco control interventions and their effects on social inequalities in smoking: placing an equity lens on existing systematic reviews' *BMC Public Health* 8: 178

Oakley, A. (2000) *Experiments in knowing: gender and method in the social sciences*. Cambridge: Polity Press

Ogilvie, D., Egan, M., Hamilton, V. and Petticrew, M (2005) 'Systematic reviews of health effects of social interventions. 2: Best available evidence: how low should you go?' *Journal of Epidemiology and Community Health* 59: 886–92

Petticrew M, Roberts H. (2003) 'Evidence, hierarchies and typologies: horses for courses' *Journal of Epidemiology and Community Health* 57/7: 527–9

Petticrew, M. and Roberts, H. (2006) *Social science systematic reviews: a practical guide*. Oxford: Blackwell

Pope, C., Mays, N. and Popay, J. (2007) *Synthesizing qualitative and quantitative health research: A guide to methods*. Oxford: Oxford University Press

Rawlins M. (2008) *De Testimonio: On the evidence for decisions about the use of therapeutic interventions*. The Harveian Oration of 2008. London: The Royal College of Physicians

Rossi, P. (1987) 'The iron law of evaluation and other metallic rules' *Research in Social Problems and Public Policy* 4: 3–20

Schulz, K., Chalmers, I., Hayes, R. and Altman, D. (1995) 'Empirical evidence of bias. Dimensions of methodological quality associated with estimates of treatment effects in controlled trials' *Journal of the American Medical Association* 273: 408–12

Spencer, L., Ritchie, J., Lewis, J. and Dillon, L. (2003) 'Quality in Qualitative Evaluation: A framework for assessing research evidence' London: Government Chief Social Researcher's Office

Thomas, S., Fayter, D., Misso, K., Ogilvie, D., Petticrew, M., Sowden, A., Whitehead, M. and Worthy, G. (2008) 'Population tobacco control interventions and their effects on social inequalities in smoking: systematic review' *Tobacco Control* 17: 230–7

Wood, L., Egger, M., Gluud, L., Schulz, K., Jüni, P., Altman, D., Gluud, C., Martin, R., Wood, A. and Sterne, J. (2008) 'Empirical evidence of bias in treatment effect estimates in controlled trials with different interventions and outcomes: meta-epidemiological study' *British Medical Journal* 336: 601–5

Woolf S. (2000) 'Taking critical appraisal to extremes' *Journal of Family Practice* 49/12: 1081–5

Chapter 22

Assessing evidence and prioritizing clinical and public health guidance recommendations: the NICE way

Peter Littlejohns, Kalipso Chalkidou, Jeremy Wyatt, and Steven D Pearson

Introduction

The National Institute for Health and Clinical Excellence (NICE) is the independent organization responsible for providing national guidance on promoting good health and preventing and treating ill health in England and Wales. It was established as a special health authority in 1999 to offer NHS healthcare professionals guidance on how to provide their patients with the highest attainable standards of care and to reduce variation in the quality of care (Rawlins 1999). In 2005 its remit was expanded to include health promotion and disease prevention. All NICE guidance is based on the best available evidence; but there is often no consensus about the nature and content of the 'best available evidence'. There is a continuing debate about issues such as internal and external validity, reliability, and 'fitness for purpose' (Wailoo, Roberts et al 2004). Furthermore, the fact that developing guidance based on the 'best available evidence' also requires value judgements to be made (Rawlins and Culyer 2004), is often ignored.

The Institute has written extensively on its role in identifying the 'gaps' in the evidence base (Chalkidou, Culyer et al 2008; Chalkidou, Lord et al 2008; Chalkidou, Walley et al 2008; Dhalla, Garner et al 2009) and how to stimulate research to address them, but this chapter concentrates on how to assess the evidence as a precursor to developing recommendations.

The drive to produce evidence-based guidance has placed the critical appraisal process under scrutiny; and has led to the development of a variety of approaches to ranking evidence and the strength of the recommendations derived from it (Lohr 2004; Scottish Intercollegiate Guidelines Network 2002). But so complex have these processes become that decision makers have now reached a crossroads: either to extend, improve, and standardize current evidence hierarchies; or abandon them, and their associated levels of evidence, altogether (Glasziou, Vandenbroucke et al 2004).

In its various programmes NICE has adopted different approaches to the use of hierarchies of evidence. The Institute's clinical guidelines programme has, since its inception, used a formal approach to grading evidence (Table 22.1) (National Institute for Health

Table 22.1 Categories of evidence for interventional studies (11)

Level of evidence	Type of evidence
1++	High-quality meta-analyses, systematic reviews of RCTs, or RCTs with a very low risk of bias
1+	Well-conducted meta-analyses, systematic reviews of RCTs, or RCTs with a low risk of bias
1−	Meta-analyses, systematic reviews of RCTs, or RCTs with a high risk of bias*
2++	High-quality systematic reviews of case-control or cohort studiesHigh-quality case-control or cohort studies with a very low risk of confounding, bias, or chance and a high probability that the relationship is causal
2+	Well-conducted case-control or cohort studies with a low risk of confounding, bias, or chance and a moderate probability that the relationship is causal
2−	Case-control or cohort studies with a high risk of confounding, bias, or chance and a significant risk that the relationship is not causal*
3	Non-analytical studies (for example case reports, case series)
4	Expert opinion, formal consensus

*studies with a level of evidence '−' should not be used as a basis for making a recommendation

and Clinical Excellence, Clinical Guidelines Development Methods 2006) and, until recently, incorporated these grades into its recommendations. By contrast, NICE's appraisals and interventional procedures programmes have avoided the formal grading of evidence according to a predetermined hierarchy (National Institute for Health and Clinical Excellence 2004). These differing approaches across NICE's traditional guidance programmes, as well as its new responsibility for producing guidance for public health (Littlejohns and Kelly 2005), have stimulated the Institute to review its practices. This paper describes the deliberations that have led to the adoption, by NICE, of a set of generic principles, consistent across all its programmes, to govern the processes of assessing evidence and classifying recommendations. These principles reinforce the importance of basing decision making on good quality meta-analyses and reviews of studies designed to minimize systematic error. They also hold that, whatever the hierarchy or typology used to assess evidence, it should not be the sole factor driving the decision-making process; and the evidence 'rank' should be considered separately from the strength of the recommendation(s) it supports.

How responsive are evidence hierarchies to the needs of the guidance developer?

The concept of hierarchies of evidence originated in the late 1970s when the Canadian Task Force introduced a classification, and applied it to grade its recommendations for preventative interventions (Canadian Task Force on the Periodic Health Examination 1979). Since then, the notion that evidence should be assessed in a hierarchical fashion has been driven by a desire to emphasize the importance of internal validity in the interpretation of evidence. As a result, most hierarchies place meta-analyses of randomized controlled trials (RCTs) at their apex. By doing so, they assume that these studies constitute the best quality evidence: that is, their conclusions are least likely to be affected by bias or chance. However, this can prove to be a misleading assumption. Evidence hierarchies do very little to help identify the effects of chance or inadequately controlled biases on research findings (Stampfer and Colditz 1991; Schairer, Lubin et al 2000; Posthuma, Westendorp et al 1994).

Conventional hierarchies focus on the effectiveness of therapeutic interventions with meta-analyses of RCTs as their 'gold standard'. However, randomization (the sole distinguishing design characteristic of RCTs) does not itself protect against all other sources of bias. The beneficial effects of randomization can, for example, be negated when intention-to-treat analyses have not been undertaken. Moreover, RCTs are rarely able to demonstrate external validity or to answer clinically important questions about diagnostic accuracy or less common adverse (or beneficial) effects of treatments (Wyatt 2000). And, they are sometimes unnecessary or impossible to undertake. No-one, for example, doubts the effectiveness of thyroxine in the treatment of myxoedema, or of arthroplasty for osteoarthritis of the hip. Nor would it seem realistic or ethical to expect RCTs to confirm the relationship between lung cancer and smoking.

From the Institute's perspective, hierarchies have three distinct limitations. First, they are usually indifferent to the clinical or public health question under consideration. Such a 'one-size-fits-all' approach has inherent weaknesses that are particularly relevant to organizations such as NICE with a broad remit ranging from prevention and health improvement to treatment and rehabilitation.

Second, when indiscriminately applied, hierarchies can have awkward consequences. When the benefits of an intervention with modest, but unequivocal, health gain has been demonstrated in one or more RCTs, rigid application of an evidence hierarchy may assign disproportionate importance to its use relative to other measures that are likely to achieve equal or greater health gain. Alternatively, interventions that have not been examined by formal RCTs may be inappropriately discounted. This also highlights the wider question of why researchers and research funders fail to respond to the needs of patients and decision makers.

Finally, the use of hierarchies of evidence conveys a false sense of consistency. Their objective nature can be illusory because there are significant judgemental components in all grading schemes. In Table 22.1, for example, the distinctions between grades 1^{++} and 1^{+}, and between 1^{+} and 1, will be largely based on the judgements of those involved in allocating grades and may not be highly reproducible (Petticrew and Roberts 2003; Lohr and Carey 1999; Centre for Evidence Based Medicine 2009; Atkins, Best et al 2004; Harris, Helfand et al 2001).

When the quality of evidence trumps clinical or public health importance and budget implications

Some of the difficulties and inconsistencies observed when the strength of recommendations is based on grades of evidence can be seen in Table 22.2. These examples are taken

Table 22.2 NICE guideline recommendations and their associated grades of evidence

Recommendation	Grade of evidence	Grade of recommendation
In the treatment and management of superficial uncomplicated injuries of 5 cm or less in length, the use of tissue adhesive should be offered as a first-line treatment option. (230)	1+/++	A
Intravenous acetylcysteine should be considered as the treatment of choice for paracetamol overdose (30)	3	C
Patients should be informed that all psychological treatments for binge eating disorder have a limited effect on body weight. (31)	1+/++	A
Immediate [same day] specialist referral is indicated for patients presenting with dyspepsia together with significant gastrointestinal bleeding (32)	4	D
Consider the need for specialist investigation of patients with signs and symptoms suggesting a secondary cause of hypertension. Accelerated [malignant] hypertension and suspected phaeochromocytoma require immediate referral (33)	4	D

from the Institute's own guidelines. Those responsible for the adoption of guideline recommendations could be forgiven for assuming that it is more important to implement a recommendation based on the highest quality evidence than one supported by lower quality of evidence, regardless of the effect size or other factors that may determine its actual impact on health or its cost implications.

The option of converting the existing hierarchies into more sophisticated instruments has been explored in a range of initiatives. In 2001, the British Thoracic Society (BTS 2001) published a guideline where systematic reviews of cohort studies, and not RCTs, occupied the highest level of evidence for questions about prognosis or prevalence. The Oxford Centre for Evidence Based Medicine has proposed a similar approach. The GRADE group (Atkins et al 2004) is working on a scheme that accounts for factors additional to internal validity (such as generalizability, the appropriateness of the study design, and the balance of risks and benefits) for grading the quality of evidence and strength of recommendations. The US Preventive Services Task Force also considers other factors when deciding on the strength of recommendations, including disease burden and characteristics of the intervention (Harris et al 2001). In both these latter approaches, however, RCTs continue to occupy a pre-eminent position.

A tested alternative to traditional evidence hierarchies

The continued use of both traditional, and more recent, evidence hierarchies has posed serious challenges to the Institute. It has been time consuming and frustrating to engineer a solution for each occasion that the hierarchical approach is unsuitable or inappropriate. The expansion of the Institute's programmes into public health, and the variety of evidence (including health economic models) that NICE must consider, makes it difficult for the Institute to sustain a similar approach in the future. Prior to their functions being transferred to NICE in 2005 the Health Development Agency had commissioned research around the implications of the hierarchy approach as part of its preparation for collaborating with NICE on the production of the obesity guideline. It seemed that having to engineer a solution on every occasion when the hierarchy approach is unsuitable or inappropriate would be both frustrating and time consuming. Indeed, the expansion of the Institute's work programme and the variety of evidence, including health economic models, that is likely to be included in the future makes it difficult to see that how this general approach is sustainable.

In its technology appraisals programme, the Institute has adopted a decision-analytic framework to synthesize and assess the evidence presented to its advisory committees. This was, in part, made possible because of the relatively narrow scope of appraisals compared to clinical guidelines; and the requirement from the beginning of the process to produce comprehensive estimates of cost-effectiveness in a consistent and robust way. Within such a framework, all evidence, from RCTs to qualitative research, is combined to inform the economic model. Poor quality is usually reflected in the degree of uncertainty surrounding a study's conclusions, while probabilistic sensitivity analysis allows the advisory committees to assess the importance of different input values on the final model output. However, this approach is not without limitations: the 'model' has been likened to a black box making it impossible for stakeholders to understand the extent, the evidence and rationale behind the committees' conclusions. Despite its weaknesses, however, the example of the technology appraisals programme demonstrates that, within a decision-analytic framework, evidence-based decision making is possible without strict adherence to hierarchies.

To abandon quality assessment of the evidence would not only threaten the Institute's core principles of scientific robustness and transparency but also seriously compromise its role as an evidence-based healthcare decision maker. As the appraisal example illustrates, what is needed is for the connection between the outputs of the systematic review and the model inputs to be reinforced further.

A NICE change

The Institute has established two overarching principles for assessing evidence:

1 Pre-ordained evidentiary hierarchies, and their accompanying quality scales, will no longer be routinely used to inform decision making in the guidance development process (Juni, Witschi et al 1999). Instead, NICE's advisory bodies will apply the basic tenets of research methodology and critical appraisal in their decision-making process within a transparent and explicit framework developed by the Institute's Centres.

2 The Institute has decided to end the confusion between evidence grades and strength of recommendations. No quality scores will be published alongside Clinical Guidelines and Public Health Programme recommendations. Instead, a set of criteria for identifying key priorities for implementation will be developed by the Centres

To achieve the above objectives, the Institute has adopted the following stepwise approach:

Step 1 Define the clinical or public health question: This refers to all clinical or public health questions formulated by the Institute at the scoping phase of the development of guidance. These questions reflect the remit negotiated by the Institute for each individual piece of guidance, and will drive the next stages of the guidance development process.

Step 2 Identify the evidence: Relevant studies will be assessed for their internal and external validity and the extent to which they contribute to addressing the question(s) agreed in Step 1. To assess internal validity, quality assessment criteria will be applied mainly where these are evidence-based, ie when the quality indicator has been empirically shown to be strongly associated with effect size or diagnostic odds ratio (eg Lijmer, Mol et al 1999; Schulz, Chalmers et al 1995). Advisory bodies and guideline developers may still wish to use evidence grading tools to assist them in evaluating the evidence; the primary issue, however, should be the extent to which the study designs and analyses are 'fit for purpose' and to minimize the effect of bias and chance on the results.

Step 3 Synthesize and assess the body of evidence: This is where NICE's advisory bodies decide the extent to which the totality of the evidence answers the clinical or public health question(s). Factors such as consistency, balance of risks and benefits, completeness of the causal pathway, reproducibility of the study protocol across more than one centre, and (sometimes) evidence of dose-response relationship, will be taken into account within a transparent decision-making framework. The rationale behind these assessments will be made explicit in the form of a short narrative or single adjective (eg good, fair, poor) that is available to all guidance users. This will prevent the downgrading of data that, whilst regarded within hierarchical systems as 'methodologically weak', are nevertheless of critical importance in addressing relevant questions.

Step 4 Issue the recommendations: No quality scores will be published alongside NICE recommendations in any of the NICE products. Instead, for the guidelines programme, where there are often large numbers of recommendations, 'high priority' ones will be identified on the basis of criteria such as the degree of impact on patients' outcomes, current practice, and the efficient use of NHS resources (National Institute for Health and Clinical Excellence 2004).

Conclusion

NICE is committed to unlocking the critical assessment process by replacing hierarchies with the collective expertise, judgement, and wisdom of its advisory groups. It is these groups that must determine whether the evidence presented to them—in the form of a systematic review or a decision-analytic model—is fit-for-purpose in developing guidance; and then to explain their interpretation and use of the data.

Following a period of public consultation, the NICE guidelines programme has updated its methods manual. The *Urinary Incontinence* guideline was one of the first guidelines to omit recommendation grades (Rawlins 2008). This new approach could be perceived by some as compromising the principles of evidence-based decisions. Our experience, especially in the appraisals programme, suggests that this is not the case. Moreover, we believe that NICE's core principles of transparency and stakeholder involvement will safeguard the methodological integrity of our approach. We are confident that, in addition to removing a long-standing misconception about the relationship between the grading of evidence and the strength of recommendations, this measure will also improve implementation by facilitating prioritization at a local level.

When the theory underlying this new approach was presented as the basis of the Harveian Lecture at the Royal College of Physicians in 2008 (Rawlins 2008), its thesis was warmly received. The direction that the Institute is moving in de-emphasizing the use of formal hierarchies of evidence parallels the approach of drug regulatory authorities such as the US Food and Drugs Administration and the European Medicines Agency. Whilst drug regulatory bodies give considerable weight to the results of RCTs, the findings from these trials may well be less important in a final regulatory judgment if the results of observational studies show unacceptable harms, or if even a single case report reveals manufacturing defects.

Acknowledgements

This paper is the result of discussions between staff within the Institute, NICE board members, and the Institute's national collaborating centres. We particularly thank Professor Valerie Beral and the late Sir Richard Doll for stimulating the debate, and the comments of Sir Iain Chalmers and the NICE Technical Forum.

Bibliography

Atkins D, Best D, Briss PA, Eccles M, Falck-Ytter Y, Flottorp S, et al (2004) 'Grading quality of evidence and strength of recommendations' *British Medical Journal* 328/7454: 1490

British Thoracic Society Standards of Care Committee (2001) 'BTS Guidelines for the Management of Community Acquired Pneumonia in Adults' *Thorax* 56/4: IV1–64

Canadian Task Force on the Periodic Health Examination (1979) 'The periodic health examination' *Canadian Health Association Journal* 121: 1193–1254

Centre for Evidence Based Medicine (2009) *Levels of evidence and grades of recommendations.* Oxford: Centre for Evidence-based Medicine

Chalkidou K, Culyer T, Littlejohns P et al (2008) 'Imbalances in R&D funding in the UK: can NICE research recommendations make a difference?' *Evidence and Policy* 4/4: 355–69

Chalkidou K, Hoy A, Littlejohns P (2007) 'Making a decision to wait for more evidence: when the National Institute for Health and Clinical Excellence recommends a technology only in the context of research' *J R Soc Med* 100/10: 453–60

Chalkidou K, Lord J, Fischer A, Littlejohns P (2008) 'Evidence based decision making in healthcare: when should we wait for more information?' *Health Affairs* 27/6: 1642–53

Chalkidou K, Walley T, Littlejohns P, Culyer A (2008) 'Evidence-informed evidence-making' *Journal of Health Service Research and Policy* 13: 167–73

Dhalla I, Garner S, Chalkidou K, Littlejohns P (2009) 'Perspectives on NICE's recommendations to use health technologies only in research' *Int J Technol Assess Healthcare* 25/3: 272–80

Glasziou P, Vandenbroucke JP, Chalmers I (2004) 'Assessing the quality of research' *British Medical Journal* 328/7430: 39–41

Harris RP, Helfand M, Woolf SH, Lohr KN, Mulrow CD, Teutsch SM, et al (2001) 'Current methods of the US Preventive Services Task Force: a review of the process' *Am J Prev Med* 20/3: 21–35

Juni P, Witschi A, Bloch R, Egger M (1999) 'The hazards of scoring the quality of clinical trials for meta-analysis' *Jama* 282/11: 1054–60

Lijmer JG, Mol BW, Heisterkamp S, Bonsel GJ, Prins MH, van der Meulen JH, et al (1999) 'Empirical evidence of design-related bias in studies of diagnostic tests' *Jama* 282/11: 1061–6

Littlejohns P, Kelly M (2005) 'The changing face of NICE: the same but different' *Lancet* 366/9488: 791–4

Lohr KN, Carey TS (1999) 'Assessing "best evidence": issues in grading the quality of studies for systematic reviews' *Jt Comm J Qual Improv* 25/9: 470–9

Lohr KN (2004) 'Rating the strength of scientific evidence: relevance for quality improvement programs' *Int J Qual Health Care* 16/1: 9–18

National Institute for Health and Clinical Excellence (2006) *Clinical Guidelines Development Methods.* Cited August 2006. London: NICE. Available at: <http://www.nice.org.uk/guidelinesmanua>

National Institute for Health and Clinical Excellence (2004) *Guide to the Methods of Technology Appraisal.* Cited August 2006. London: NICE. Available at: <http://www.nice.org.uk/page.aspx?o=201973>

National Institute for Health and Clinical Excellence (2006) *Clinical Guideline: Urinary incontinence: the management of urinary incontinence in women (under consultation).* London: NICE

Petticrew M, Roberts H (2003) 'Evidence, hierarchies, and typologies: horses for courses' *J Epidemiol Community Health* 57/7: 527–9

Posthuma WF, Westendorp RG, Vandenbroucke JP (1994) 'Cardioprotective effect of hormone replacement therapy in postmenopausal women: is the evidence biased?' *British Medical Journal* 308/6939: 1268–9

Rawlins M (1999) 'In pursuit of quality: the National Institute for Clinical Excellence' *Lancet* 353/9158: 1079–82

Rawlins M (2008) 'De Testimonio: on the evidence for decisions about the use of therapeutic interventions' *Lancet* 372: 2152–6

Rawlins MD, Culyer AJ (2004) 'National Institute for Clinical Excellence and its value judgments' *British Medical Journal* 329/7459: 224–7

Schairer C, Lubin J, Troisi R, Sturgeon S, Brinton L, Hoover R (2000) 'Menopausal estrogen and estrogen-progestin replacement therapy and breast cancer risk' *Jama* 283/4: 485–91

Schulz KF, Chalmers I, Hayes RJ, Altman DG (1995) 'Empirical evidence of bias. Dimensions of methodological quality associated with estimates of treatment effects in controlled trials' *Jama* 273/5: 408–12

Scottish Intercollegiate Guidelines Network (2002) *A Guideline Developers Handbook.* Cited August 2006. Edinburgh: Scottish Intercollegiate Guidelines Network. Available at: <http://www.sign.ac.uk/>

Stampfer MJ, Colditz GA (1991) 'Estrogen replacement therapy and coronary heart disease: a quantitative assessment of the epidemiologic evidence' *Prev Med* 20/1: 47–63

Wailoo A, Roberts J, Brazier J, McCabe C (2004) 'Efficiency, equity, and NICE clinical guidelines' *British Medical Journal* 328/7439: 536–7

Wyatt JC (2000) 'Knowledge for the clinician. 1. Clinical questions and information needs' *J R Soc Med* 93: 168–71

Chapter 23

Social values in developing public health guidance

Nick Doyle

Introduction

The role of health care and public health guidance developers is to make recommendations for policy and practice that are based on the best available evidence. An assumption—though often an unstated one—is that the ideal circumstances would be those where all issues about a recommendation could be resolved by scientific evidence derived from high quality research into the effectiveness and/or cost-effectiveness of an intervention. In reality, and even in rare situations of abundant scientific evidence, such decisions can never be purely technical, as the problems to be addressed arise in a particular social, economic, and political context, as do solutions and the means of arriving at them.

The significance of social values will be more apparent in decisions the less there is public, professional, and political consensus on the route to be taken. Social values may also seem particularly important when evidence is in short supply, of poor quality, or arises from disciplines whose basic values and approaches diverge. Social values are thus an important factor in decision making and it is essential to have a process for identifying significant social value issues as they arise, and for considering their relevance to the guidance in hand in a systematic way.

NICE took on responsibility for producing public health guidance relatively recently. This means that it has had to accommodate a new perspective as well as values associated with public health that differ in significant ways from those it applies to the production of clinical guidance. This chapter examines how well these sets of values have been integrated and some of the as yet unresolved dilemmas and tensions. It first discusses the ethical, or social value, considerations affecting NICE guidance of all kinds, and their relationship to the specific set of social value principles which NICE has published as formal advice to the advisory bodies that make NICE guidance recommendations (NICE 2008a). It then considers how well the social value principles established to date cover the particular ethical questions that arise in public health. It highlights gaps and uncertainties, looking in particular at the issue of health inequalities, and using the ethical framework provided by the 'stewardship model' as a reference point (Nuffield Council on Bioethics 2007). The chapter concludes by looking at NICE's use of equality impact assessment as a means of meeting the public sector duties on eliminating discrimination and promoting equality, and the potential for the 'capabilities' approach to provide a supportive framework for NICE guidance recommendations concerned with inequality.

Ethical considerations in NICE guidance

Formal advice provided by NICE to its advisory bodies on applying social value judgements in the course of developing guidance makes a distinction between scientific value judgements, which are about interpreting the quality and significance of the evidence available, and social value judgements, 'which relate to society rather than science' (NICE 2008a).

In fact, the advice illustrates well that there is no absolute distinction between the two types of value judgement. It demonstrates that NICE's scientific judgements are framed by broader ethical, policy, and legal considerations, which always apply in some form, quite apart from specific social value questions that may arise with any given item of guidance. These considerations fall into a number of distinct categories.

Long-standing ethical and philosophical principles

The first category relates to widely accepted ethical and philosophical principles that underpin medicine and public health practice: respect for autonomy, non-maleficence, beneficence, and distributive justice. The problem of distributive justice is particularly important for NICE, given its role in the system of allocating resources for health care. NICE does not fully subscribe to either a utilitarian or egalitarian ethical approach to this problem. Instead, it aims to act according to principles of 'procedural justice', ie by ensuring that it can be held to account for the reasonableness or otherwise of its decisions by making the processes of decision making transparent, by involving patients, the public, and other interested parties, by giving reasons for its recommendations, and by publicizing what it is doing and publishing all documentation.

NICE's operating principles

The second category comprises NICE's fundamental operating principles. These derive from the role and functions of NICE set out in legislation and expressing democratically-endorsed social purposes such as promoting clinical and public health excellence and the effective use of NHS resources, and, in the case of public health, developing the evidence base on reducing health inequalities (Secretary of State 2005). By extension, these include procedural principles that overlap with the procedural justice principles noted above and include scientific rigour, independence of judgement, openness to challenge, and timeliness.

Legal requirements on equality and human rights

The third category derives from legislation on equality and human rights that applies to all public authorities. In very general terms, this requires NICE, in performing its functions, to have regard to the need to comply with the Human Rights Act 1998 and to eliminate various forms of discrimination and promote equality. The impact of these duties is discussed below.

The NHS's principles and objectives

The fourth category comprises the objectives and principles of the NHS, which apply to NICE as an NHS organization. NICE thus supports and acts on long-standing NHS values and principles and shorter-term priorities, such as those contained in the NHS constitution and three-year or annual service priorities, as expressed in the government's policy statements on public service agreements and the NHS operating framework. These include NHS commitments to improving health, tackling health inequalities, promoting equality, and ending the 'postcode lottery' in access to treatment.

Key principles

NICE has also highlighted a number of specific principles (see box below) and statements of policy that should inform decision making by its advisory bodies. These form a further category and comprise distillations of particularly important considerations concerned with NICE's scientific and methodological approach (such as the role of evidence and the requirement to consider both costs and benefits, and the manner of doing so), and statements of the approach to be applied to social value issues that recur in considerations of individual guidance recommendations or which have emerged as sensitive or important either within NICE or in the eyes of professionals or the public.

Often, they are issues on which NICE has sought advice from its Citizens Council, a 30-strong and broadly representative group of members of the public who have been independently recruited to deliberate as a 'citizens' jury' on problematic social value questions. To date, the Citizens Council has given its view on mandatory public health measures (NICE 2005a), the weight NICE's advisory bodies should give to health inequalities (NICE 2006a), the circumstances in which the age of a person should be taken into account (NICE 2004), as well as more clinically orientated issues such as ultra-orphan drugs (NICE 2005b), the 'rule of rescue' (NICE 2006b), quality-adjusted life years (QALYs), and severity of illness (NICE 2008b).

Box 23.1 Social values principles

1 NICE should not recommend an intervention (that is, a treatment, procedure, action, or programme) if there is no evidence, or not enough evidence, on which to make a clear decision. But NICE's advisory bodies may recommend the use of the intervention within a research programme if this will provide more information about its effectiveness, safety, or cost.

2 Those developing clinical guidelines, technology appraisals, or public health guidance must take into account the relative costs and benefits of interventions (their 'cost-effectiveness') when deciding whether or not to recommend them.

3 Decisions about whether to recommend interventions should not be based on evidence of their relative costs and benefits alone. NICE must consider other factors when developing its guidance, including the need to distribute health resources in the fairest way within society as a whole.

Social values principles *(continued)*

4 NICE usually expresses the cost-effectiveness of an intervention as the 'cost (in £) per quality-adjusted life year (QALY) gained.' This is based on an assessment of how much the intervention costs and how much health benefit it produces compared to an alternative. NICE should explain its reasons when it decides that an intervention with an Incremental Cost Effective Ratio (ICER) below £20,000 per QALY gained is not cost-effective; and when an intervention with an ICER of more than £20,000 to £30,000 per QALY gained is cost-effective.

5 Although NICE accepts that individual NHS users will expect to receive treatments to which their condition will respond, this should not impose a requirement on NICE's advisory bodies to recommend interventions that are not effective, or are not cost-effective enough to provide the best value to users of the NHS as a whole.

6 NICE should consider and respond to comments it receives about its draft guidance, and make changes where appropriate. But NICE and its advisory bodies must use their own judgement to ensure that what it recommends is cost-effective and takes account of the need to distribute health resources in the fairest way within society as a whole.

7 NICE can recommend that use of an intervention is restricted to a particular group of people within the population (for example, people under or over a certain age, or women only), but only in certain circumstances. There must be clear evidence about the increased effectiveness of the intervention in this subgroup, or other reasons relating to fairness for society as a whole, or a legal requirement to act in this way.

8 When choosing guidance topics, developing guidance, and supporting those who put its guidance into practice, the Institute should actively consider reducing health inequalities including those associated with sex, age, race, disability, and socio-economic status.

Social value principles and public health

The stated bioethical principles underpinning NICE's decision making mainly derive from traditional medical ethics and, while not inappropriate to public health guidance, do not take account of additional principles that over the years have come to be particularly associated with public health—for example, commitments to tackling health inequalities (or inequity), multi-sectoral action, participation, and empowerment, and to a focus on the social determinants of health, which derive from a succession of, mainly international, policy statements from the Ottawa Charter for Health Promotion (WHO 1986) to the recent report of the Commission on Social Determinants of Health (CSD 2008), but which include also the Acheson report in England into inequalities in health (Acheson 1997).

Similarly, while NICE is not entirely dogmatic about its approach to economic evalua-tion and the priority attached to cost-utility analysis, there is little acknowledgement that it also uses a 'cost-consequence' approach in public health guidance so that it can better take account of the complexity and multidimensional character of public health interven-tions and programmes, and ensure that issues such as equity and distribution, which are key to public health policy, can be used to inform the economic analysis (NICE 2006c). The account of the ethical or social value principles pertaining particularly to NICE's public health guidance, and how they sit alongside those that are more relevant to clinical medicine, is therefore somewhat underdeveloped.

There are several reasons for this. First, NICE took on responsibility for producing public health guidance relatively recently (in 2005), so it is not surprising that the join between its clinical and public health perspectives is not entirely seamless. Second, NICE's social value principles have emerged over time and mainly in response to problems or controversies around decision making which NICE's public health guidance has not so far aroused. Third, there are significant formal differences between NICE's remits for clinical and public health guidance: for example, the 2005 directions establishing NICE state that public health guidance should be concerned with reducing health inequalities, whereas there is no such explicit requirement for clinical guidance. Also, public health guidance has a societal economic perspective whereas the economic perspective for clini-cal guidance is that of the NHS and adult social care. (The latter may change following the Department of Health's commitment in the 2009 pharmaceutical price regulation scheme to explore the economic perspective it sets for NICE (Department of Health 2008).)

Despite these shortcomings, NICE recognizes that the mainly population focus of public health interventions raises ethical problems in guidance development that differ from those raised by the individual focus of health care interventions, and that health inequalities are an important factor for consideration.

NICE's social value principles and the stewardship model of public health

NICE, assisted by the Citizens Council (NICE 2005a), has considered the social value principles that would surround any recommendation for a mandatory public health measure, and so has tackled the central ethical question about the balance to be struck between individual liberty and the well-being of the community. It identified several issues that NICE's advisory bodies should take account of when considering any recom-mendation requiring an element of compulsion. These cover balancing benefits and costs; evidential standards in the event of a national emergency; the importance of respect-ing individual choice as far as possible; proportionality; the requirement to reduce health inequalities; potential adverse effects on vulnerable members of society; the need to ensure that mandatory measures are monitored, evaluated, and (as required) discontin-ued so as to avoid harmful consequences; and the importance of consultation with the broader community and explanation.

This approach is compatible with the stewardship model of public health intervention proposed in the report of the Nuffield Council on Bioethics on ethical issues in public health, particularly the ethical dimensions concerned with constraints or conditions to limit state action (Nuffield Council on Bioethics 2007, Krebs and Schmidt 2009 this volume).

In fact, the stewardship model is a useful reference point in considering NICE's public health approach more generally. As interpreted by the Nuffield Council on Bioethics, the model is based on the idea that a liberal state has responsibilities to look after important needs of people both individually and collectively, and an obligation to provide conditions that allow people to be healthy, especially in relation to reducing health inequalities, and to take an active role in promoting the health of the public.

The stewardship model defines appropriate means of achieving public health goals that are highly relevant to NICE's purpose—promoting health through programmes to support behaviour change as well as by providing information and advice; aiming to ensure that it is easy for people to lead a healthy life through changes in the physical and social environment; ensuring that people have access to medical services; and obligations in relation to health inequalities.

There are evident uncertainties in how NICE views the objectives of its guidance in relation to health inequalities, and about the contribution public health guidance makes to tackling health inequalities compared with that of clinical guidance. When the Citizens Council considered NICE's role in reducing health inequalities it concluded that, where feasible, NICE should support strategies that improve the health of the population while offering particular benefit to the most disadvantaged so as to reduce health inequalities, particularly in the context of public health (NICE 2006a). NICE's board was less definitive, taking the view that advisory bodies should try to ensure that implementing NICE guidance will not widen existing inequalities. The principle emerging from this discussion (principle 8 in the box above) states that, 'when choosing guidance topics, developing guidance and supporting those who put its guidance into practice, the Institute should actively consider reducing health inequalities including those associated with sex, age, race, disability and socioeconomic status'.

The somewhat tentative nature of this principle may be because of the differences noted above in the weight to be attached to reducing health inequalities in the mandates for NICE's public health and clinical guidance, but also basic differences between the public health and clinical outlooks.

One of the aims of public health, as illustrated by the stewardship model, is to ensure that people have equal access to the health services they need. NICE is itself a public health initiative for ensuring that high quality, cost-effective treatments are equally available in every locality. However, although they contribute to the definition of what should be locally available, individual items of NICE clinical guidance—whether technology appraisals or clinical guidelines—have not until fairly recently reflected systematic consideration of how guidance on treatments for individuals could contribute to reducing health inequalities. On the other hand, NICE's public health guidance has always in principle as well as according to remit been concerned with health inequalities, and as a consequence the approach to public health guidance development reflects a deeper analysis of what is meant by 'tackling health inequalities' (see for example Graham 2004).

Also, the principle covers not only reducing health inequalities related to socio-economic status but also those associated with sex, age, race, and disability in the context of NICE's legal duties to avoid discrimination and promote equality. Bringing related but also distinct types of inequality together in this way might suggest that NICE has not yet fully integrated them into a coherent policy framework. In fact, it has made significant progress in doing so in practice.

Public sector duties to promote equality

NICE, like all other public authorities, is under legal duties (sometimes called 'the public sector duties') to give due regard to the need to eliminate discrimination and promote equality in relation to sex, gender identity, sexual orientation, race (ie ethnicity), disability, religion or belief, and age. These duties apply in varying degrees to these 'equality characteristics'. NICE meets the duties chiefly by carrying out equality impact assessments at the various stages of guidance development (guidance scoping, evidence assessment, guidance recommendations, and research recommendations) and by trying to ensure that consultation and patient involvement processes result in useful information about the potential impact of guidance on the various groups with these equality characteristics (NICE 2007).

The equality impact assessment model that underpins the approach taken by each of NICE's guidance centres covers not just the equality characteristics protected by legislation but also inequality associated with socio-economic status or closely-related factors such as the impact of living in a deprived area, or inequality not necessarily associated with socio-economic or other circumstances, such as being in the population subgroup of looked after children.

This means that the model gives little weight to the distinction between equality characteristics recognized in legislation and characteristics that are not so recognized, such as socio-economic status, or covered only to a limited degree, such as age. It also means that NICE considers the potential to promote equality of opportunity to achieve health and well-being in all instances and not just in the legally defined instances of sex, race, and disability.

The strengths of the approach are that it requires NICE's guidance-producing centres to be proactive in identifying potentially negative impacts of guidance on equality and considering any measures that could lead to positive impacts. Thus, where before health inequalities might only have been under active consideration from the start of the public health guidance development process, they now have similar priority in all NICE guidance development processes.

This approach is in tune with wider developments in thinking about how equality and inequality should be conceptualized and how it should be treated in legislation. The 2007 Equalities Review proposed a definition of equality based on the capabilities approach developed by Amartya Sen and others[1], and a framework for measurement based on a list

---

[1] 'An equal society protects and promotes equal, real freedom and substantive opportunity to live in the ways people value and would choose, so that everyone can flourish. An equal society recognizes people's different needs, situations and goals and removes the barriers that limit what people can do and can be.'

of capabilities (sometimes described as 'central and valuable freedoms', 'substantive freedoms', or 'real opportunities') to be used by all public bodies to agree priorities, set targets, and evaluate progress towards equality (Equalities Review Panel 2007).

The capabilities are the things, in the view of the review, that 'members of our society feel it is most important they are *enabled* to do', and encompass opportunity (ie whether everyone has the same substantive freedom to flourish), agency (ie the degree of choice and control individuals have to do and achieve the things they value), and process (ie whether discrimination or some other barrier causes or contributes to a particular inequality). The review's recommendations have been accepted by government and have strongly influenced the work of the Equality and Human Rights Commission and proposals for a single equality bill.

From NICE's point of view there are several significant features of the capabilities approach and the measurement framework. First, the list of capabilities brings the capability to be healthy—including being able to achieve certain health outcomes, gain access to health care, be treated with respect, maintain a healthy lifestyle, and live in a healthy and safe environment—together with capabilities that substantially overlap with what, from a public health perspective, would be termed broader determinants of health and health inequalities. Second, the measurement framework includes socio-economic status alongside other equality characteristics.

And third, the capability approach could clarify some of the issues for decision makers when they consider how to promote equality, such as those where, under current public sector duties, NICE's advisory bodies must have due regard to the need to promote equality of opportunity, including in the case of disability equality, treating disabled people more favourably. This is because the capability approach establishes the relevance of differences in need to the conceptualization and measurement of inequality: it focuses attention on the fact that people can need more or different resources to achieve the same substantive freedoms (Vizard 2007).

The capability approach is well developed theoretically but experience of its application in practice is limited. Also, NICE will need to consider in more detail its implications, given that it arises from dissatisfaction with some of the economic theories that inform its social value principles, such as utility-based models in which utility is interpreted as subjective well-being, happiness, and preference-satisfaction (Vizard 2007).

Conclusions

NICE recognizes that complex and varied social value considerations arise in the course of producing guidance. It has produced formal advice on certain social value principles to help its advisory bodies to take systematic account of these considerations. For reasons such as the relatively recent inclusion of public health guidance in NICE's functions, differences in the statutory remits of public health and clinical guidance, and the contrasting perspectives of public health and clinical medicine, the social value principles concerning public health guidance are less well developed than those for clinical guidance, and they are unevenly integrated. The treatment of the role of NICE guidance in tackling health inequalities is an example. The stewardship model proposed by the Nuffield Council on Bioethics (2007) provides a framework that could be helpful in making NICE's social value principles concerned with public health more coherent. NICE's own response to meeting public sector duties on equality—for example, use of equality impact assessment techniques—means that its practice on equality is in some ways ahead of its advice on social value principles. The capability approach to conceiving of and acting on equality, which is influential on government thinking, could also help NICE in achieving more coherence.

Bibliography

Acheson D (1998) *Independent inquiry into inequalities in health: Report.* Norwich: The Stationery Office

Commission on Social Determinants of Health (2008) *Closing the gap in a generation: health equity through action on the social determinants of health, Final report.* Geneva: World Health Organization, Geneva

Department of Health and Association of the British Pharmaceutical Industry (2008) *The pharmaceutical price regulation scheme.* London: Department of Health

Equalities Review Panel (2007) *Fairness and freedom: the final report of the equalities review panel.* London: The Cabinet Office

Graham H and Kelly MP (2004) *Health inequalities: Concepts, frameworks and policy, Briefing paper.* London: Health Development Agency

NICE (2004) *NICE Citizens Council report on age* London: NICE

NICE (2005a) *NICE Citizens Council report: Mandatory public health measures.* London: NICE

NICE (2005b) *NICE Citizens Council report: Ultra orphan drugs.* London: NICE

NICE (2006a) *Report on NICE Citizens Council meeting: Inequalities in health.* London: NICE

NICE (2006b) *NICE Citizens Council report: Rule of rescue.* London: NICE

NICE (2006c) *Methods for development of NICE public health guidance.* London: NICE

NICE (2007) *NICE's equality scheme and action plan.* London: NICE

NICE (2008a) *Social value judgements. Principles for the development of NICE guidance.* 2nd edn. London: NICE

NICE (2008b) *Report on NICE Citizens Council meeting: Quality Adjusted Life Years (QALYs) and the severity of illness.* London: NICE

Nuffield Council on Bioethics (2007) *Public health: ethical issues.* London: Nuffield Council on Bioethics

Secretary of State for Health (2005) *Directions and consolidating directions to the National Institute for Health and Clinical Excellence 2005.* London: Secretary of State for Health

Vizard P and Burchardt T (2007) *Developing a capability list: Final recommendations of the Equalities Review Steering Group on Measurement, CASE/121.* London: Centre for Analysis of Social Exclusion

WHO (1986) *The Ottawa Charter for Health Promotion.* Geneva: World Health Organization

Chapter 24

A nudge in the right direction: developing guidance on changing behaviour

Catherine Swann, Lesley Owen, Chris Carmona, Michael P Kelly, Clare Wohlgemuth, and Jane Huntley

Introduction

In 2005, NICE was asked by the Department of Health to develop guidance on the effectiveness of different approaches and models aimed at changing knowledge, attitudes, behaviour, at individual, community and population level. This was in the context of the Government's national strategy—*Choosing Health*—that emphasized the role and responsibility of individuals in making healthier choices, within a supportive environment across different sectors of society (Department of Health 2004).

   This chapter describes the theories used to provide the conceptual framework for the development of the guidance, sets out the guidance development process, the range and nature of evidence considered, and outlines the areas covered by the recommendations.

A conceptual framework for changing health behaviours

For the purposes of the guidance, human behaviour (which was the target of any intervention aimed at change) was defined as 'the product of individual or collective human actions, seen within and influenced by their structural, social and economic context'. These actions produce observable social, cultural, and economic patterns which limit—or enable—what individuals can do.' (NICE 2007). Attempts to improve public health are generally founded on the assumption that there are links between health knowledge, health attitudes, health behaviours, and health outcomes (see, for example, Azjen 2001; Conner and Norman 2005). Some commentators assume that there are direct causal relationships between these, but others see the links as more tenuous. Many public health interventions—whether they focus on the individual, community, whole populations, or the environment—seek in some way to change knowledge, attitudes, and/or behaviours in relation to health, in order to influence health outcomes (Halpern et al 2004).

   It is well established (Ellis and Grey 2003; Jepson 2000; Roe et al 1997; Swann et al 2003) that some interventions aimed at influencing attitudes, beliefs, and behaviours tend to be more effective when they are planned and delivered within the framework of a considered theoretical approach, particularly in the areas of sexual health and nutrition.

There are many models and approaches within public health and related disciplines (including health psychology, and the sociology of health and medicine) that attempt to articulate the relationships between these factors and predict behavioural outcomes (for example, the Health Belief Model (Rosenstock 1966) and the Theory of Reasoned Action (Fishbein and Ajzen 1975)). Indeed, a significant amount of health promotion and public health practice incorporates elements of at least one popular model into their planning and delivery.

However, many of these models and approaches have been criticized for their inability to consider the context and environment within which health is experienced and enacted (Swann 2002). When the referral for his piece of guidance was received from ministers, it was—and still is—far from clear which theoretical model(s) or approaches are the more appropriate or effective, with whom, or in which circumstances—or indeed whether effectiveness is influenced by the model or approach itself or by the planning processes associated with adapting interventions to theoretical models and approaches (Halpern et al 2004). The ability of theoretical models and approaches to predict health behaviours and outcomes at all has also been questioned (Nora and Zimmerman 2005).

Health beliefs and behaviours in context

The individual

Health is experienced—and produced—at different levels. People experience health and health outcomes (positive or negative) at an individual level, through their bodily symptoms and sensations, and in the way they interpret these against the background of what they understand to be good or poor health—taken both from their own experiences, and what their immediate context 'tells' them should constitute health. An individual's sense of their own good or bad health, the actions they take as a consequence of their perceptions, and their knowledge, beliefs, and attitudes, are produced by an interaction between individual biological factors and predispositions and the external world.

The influence of these factors differs between individuals, depending on their life experiences, the resources available to them, their context, and the ways in which they make sense of those experiences, resources, and context. In experiencing conscious life, people engage day-to-day in creating and recreating their own 'life-worlds' (the constellation of things that are important to them and make up their daily 'reality') (Kelly 2006). Their experience of health and illness, and their ability to change, will, at least in part, be influenced by their 'life-world' and the salience that people attach to different outcomes, behaviours, and 'health states'.

Some health promotion and public health approaches target people at an individual level, to try to influence attitudes, beliefs and, ultimately, behaviours, and are often based on the premise that if you populate a person's lifeworld with 'real facts' about risk behaviours then that person will 'choose' the healthier behaviour. Arguably, the 2004 strategy 'Choosing health' marked a return to an emphasis on individually-focused approaches to changing health. It appeared to signal a shift away from a commitment to tackling health inequalities and addressing the 'broader determinants' of health. The individual is conceptualized as operating—and making free choices—within a market-based system.

The community

Communities—a category used here to refer to social or family groups defined by networks, geographical location, or other common marker (for example, a shared behaviour or trait)—respond as a group to contexts, environments, vulnerabilities, and shared (or different) behaviours and exhibit community-level health outcomes. These can be measured through the identification and monitoring of community-level health 'indicators', such as local availability of healthy food, or the assessment of community morbidity and mortality using geographical information systems. Some health promotion and public health interventions attempt to influence health attitudes, beliefs, and behaviours at this level by altering community-level structures and opportunities. One example is providing free leisure facilities within a community to promote physical activity. Other examples of interventions at this level include: school- or workplace-based policies, programmes and interventions, local enforcement of national legislation, and area-based community and regeneration programmes and initiatives.

Populations

Whole populations, like communities, also exhibit health behaviours and outcomes, which are expressed through population trends and mortality and morbidity statistics. At this level, it is usually possible to measure the different beliefs, attitudes and outcomes experienced by groups within a population (for example, the differences between men and women, or between different ethnic groups) and to ascertain how (if at all) these differ from the 'average'. Sometimes it is possible to use statistics to understand why health outcomes differ within populations (for example, the effect of average dietary habits of different ethnic groups on rates of coronary heart disease).

Interventions aimed at the whole population tend to focus on altering legislation and macro-level policy, both nationally and internationally, in order to influence knowledge, behaviours and/or attitudes, and ultimately health outcomes. Examples of public health interventions at this level include: legislation to make seatbelt-wearing compulsory, introduction of speed limits, and the use of safety cameras, and the introduction of specific health and welfare policies to influence health behaviours and outcomes in school-age children.

Interaction and impact across levels

Whether an intervention or programme is delivered to individuals, in community or family settings, or at population level, the effects are rarely restricted to one level. For example, a brief primary care intervention aimed at reducing alcohol consumption among individuals could have an impact: on an individual's behaviour (for example, level of alcohol consumption), on the local community (for example, local alcohol sales), or at

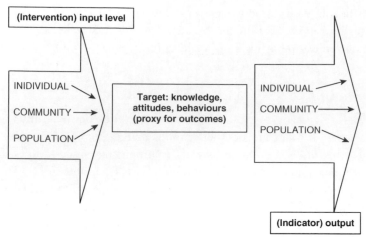

Fig. 24.1 Levels of intervention and impact on health

population level (for example, demographic patterns of liver cirrhosis). Whichever level an intervention targets, its impact may be tracked across these other levels.

Interventions aimed at individuals, communities, and populations may have an impact at levels other than the intervention point: for example, individuals may benefit (or be harmed by) a community-level intervention. An example of this is the creation of a new play area, which may benefit young residents' physical health, but, at the same time, may increase levels of accidental injury and falls. A broader example is the government policy recommendation that people should eat two portions of fish each week, one of which should be an oily fish. This recommendation may have health benefits for the population, but concerns have been raised about the impact of increased consumption on fish stocks.

Life-course and interventions

Health and illness are experienced throughout the life-course, and an individual's experience of them is the result of the interplay of biological, psychological, social, and economic factors. Key life changes and transition points render individuals, communities, or populations particularly vulnerable to negative health outcomes (Graham and Power 2004; Hertzman et al 2002; Hertzman and Wiens 1996; Keating and Hertzman 1999; Kuh et al 1997; Power and Hertzman 1997, 2004). Life changes and transitions like pregnancy or changing jobs, present opportunities for intervention and positive change at some or all of the levels described above since they are often the stimulus for individuals 'taking stock'. These transition points are also times when people may be more likely to make contact with public services. Other approaches to life-course work consider the accumulation of 'advantages' and 'deficits' over the life-course as the key to identifying 'turning points' or points of intervention (see, for example, Graham and Power 2004).

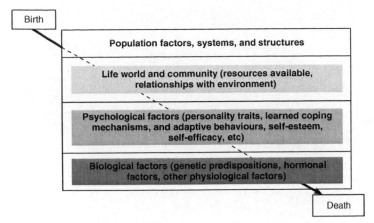

Fig. 24.2 Life course and behaviour change

A range of different personal, social, and environmental resources are available to individuals, communities, and populations to use at different life stages. One of the issues tackled by the evidence reviews—which the discussions in the advisory group (called the Programme Development Group or PDG) that developed the guidance also attempted to capture—was an understanding of the ways in which these resources can be deployed to enable otherwise vulnerable people to demonstrate 'resilience' to ill health or other crises. Such resources include 'social capital' (a resource based on trust and reciprocity that exists within communities and appears to promote better health outcomes (Morgan and Swann 2004)) and other assets for health, such as individual and community resilience. These resources—conceptualized as existing within community and network 'bonds'—have proven to be vital for thriving populations, and difficult to harness for the purpose of health or social improvement.

The process of developing the guidance

Within this framework the PDG and the supporting NICE technical team, working with various review teams, set about developing the guidance. NICE has a set method for producing public health guidance through independent committees and with widespread consultation, with registered stakeholders and representatives of those that will be expected to implement the guidance (NICE 2006, 2009). Systematic reviews of the evidence of effectiveness and cost-effectiveness are considered alongside other types of evidence, including expert testimony from practitioners, evidence from qualitative research (such as the views of a target audience), and economic models. NICE and its public health advisory committees base their decisions on the best available evidence, embedding their decisions within a clear account of whatever scientific and social value judgements have been made. The process for developing the guidance used in this piece of work is shown in Figure 24.3. (See Littlejohns et al 2009 this volume.)

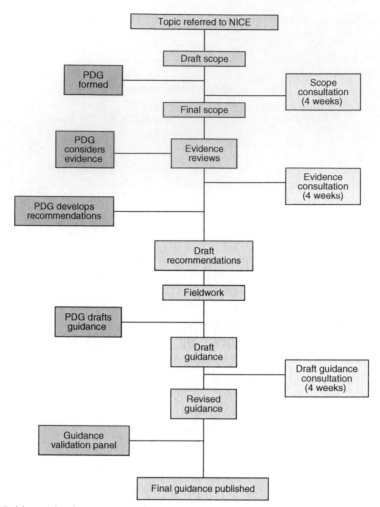

Fig. 24.3 Guidance development process

The knowledge and evidence from different disciplines are very different in the concepts they use, the assumptions they make about cause and explanation, and (sometimes) the methods that they favour. Consequently, combining knowledge and evidence from different levels—such as the social and the individual—is extremely difficult. To ensure that as broad a range as possible of knowledge and evidence was taken into account, the PDG adopted a pluralistic approach that acknowledged the value of different forms of evidence and research methods.

The evidence

The empirical evidence about behaviour change varies widely, in terms of methodological approach and quality. It also inhabits a wide range of different academic disciplines, most of which 'speak' different languages about the nature of behaviour, change, and society. The search for the evidence initially followed standard NICE processes. However, as relatively little of the evidence identified addressed effectiveness or cost-effectiveness, the searches were extended to cover theoretical, descriptive, and empirical studies of a type not previously reviewed for NICE guidance.

Six reviews, one expert report and an economic analysis which comprised a review of cost-effectiveness and an economic model were conducted. Full details are on the NICE website, <http://www.nice.org.uk>:

- Review 1 included systematic reviews and meta-analyses which focused on public health, health promotion or primary care-led interventions which contained an educational or behavioural component (Jepson et al 2007).

- Review 2 included reviews of intervention studies that evaluated the effectiveness of road safety interventions. Part two included reviews of intervention studies that evaluated the effectiveness of 'pro-environmental behaviour' (Stead et al 2007)

- Review 3 included reviews that provided an overview of conceptual, theoretical or research issues in relation to resilience, coping, and salutogenesis. It also included reviews of interventions explicitly linked to one of these theories. Part two included reviews of empirical evidence on positive adaptation in conditions of social-structural adversity (Harrop et al 2007).

- Review 4 included reviews of four behaviour change models—the health belief model (HBM), the theory of reasoned action (TRA), the theory of planned behaviour (TPB), and the trans-theoretical model (TTM) to study and predict health-related behaviour change (Taylor et al 2007).

- Review 5 included reviews of empirical data on the effectiveness of interventions designed to change knowledge, attitude, intention, and behaviour with respect to smoking, physical activity, and healthy eating. Specific attention was focused on whether or not effectiveness was influenced by the individual's position in the life course, the intervention's mode of delivery, or the social and cultural context (Taylor et al 2007).

- Review 6 included reports on the strategies used by marketeers to influence low-income consumers and any evidence of effectiveness (Stead et al 2007).

- Expert report: 'Evidence for the effect on inequalities in health of interventions designed to change behaviour' (Blaxter 2007).

- Economic analysis: The economic analysis consisted of a review cost-effectiveness and an economic model. The cost-effectiveness review focused on interventions designed to promote healthier lifestyles and to reduce the risk of developing CHD. A model was developed to determine the cost-effectiveness of a population-based behaviour change intervention (Fox-Rushby et al 2007).

The goals of the reviews varied and included consideration of efficacy, effectiveness, the theoretical 'soundness' and construction of different models, implementation issues, and programme evaluation. Studies included in the reviews contained all or some of these elements. All of the reviews completed in developing this guidance considered inequalities in health, and taking an overview of all the work completed it is clear that there is a lack of good-quality reviews of the evidence on behaviour change and its impact on social and health inequalities. There is, however, some evidence that the uptake of interventions or response to health education messages differs by social circumstances, and this has, historically, widened the health inequalities gap. Ultimately, evidence about interventions intended to narrow the health inequalities gap had to be drawn from the outcomes and methods described in other sorts of literature.

In addition to the reviews described above, the guidance was influenced by the PDG's knowledge and discussion about a number of different theories, concepts, and accounts of behaviour and behaviour change, drawn from the social and behavioural sciences. These include: resilience, coping, self-efficacy, planned behaviour, structure and agency, 'habitus', and social capital (Ajzen 1991, 2001; Antonovsky 1985, 1987; Bandura 1997; Bourdieu 1977, 1986; Conner and Sparks 2005; Giddens 1979, 1982, 1984; Lazarus 1976, 1985; Lazarus and Folkman 1984; Morgan and Swann 2004; Putnam 2000). As the evidence accumulated, the PDG (working with the NICE technical team) were able to sort and sift their ideas into key themes and concepts, and these in turn helped to structure the recommendations.

The guidance

The guidance itself focused on three main areas involved in changing behaviour: planning, delivery, and evaluation (see <http://guidance.nice.org.uk/PH6/guidance/pdf/english>).

Planning

The starting point for behaviour change is planning. The PDG recommended that those planning behaviour change initiatives should endeavour to work in partnership with individuals, communities, organizations, and—crucially—the populations whose behaviour is the focus of supposed change. This should involve a needs assessment and detailed understanding of the target audience. It is of paramount importance that interventions take account of the circumstances in which people live (especially the socio-economic and cultural context). Very importantly the plan should set out an explicit account of the way the target population, community, or group will be involved in the development, implementation, and evaluation of the intervention, and it should aim to develop—and build on—the skills talents and capacity of the people whose behaviour is the target.

Changing behaviour may not be a priority for the individuals being targeted. People do not necessarily make their own long-term health a priority and may want to focus on other, more immediate needs and goals (for example, relieving stress, or complying with peer pressure). Some damaging and, therefore, apparently negative health behaviours may provide positive psychological, social, or physical benefits for individuals in certain social and cultural contexts. For example, smoking cigarettes may provide 'time out' for people in difficult circumstances. To be effective, therefore, interventions must be planned to take account of the social, cultural, and economic acceptability of the intervention and the target group's attitudes toward the behaviour.

The PDG recommended that behaviour change interventions should be as specific as possible about their content. So what is to be done, to whom, in what social and economic context, and in what way should be made as clearly and precisely as possible.

Very importantly, the PDG argued for being explicit about which underlying theories articulate the causal links between actions and outcomes (Davidson et al 2003; Pawson 2006; Weiss 1995) and developing a logic model or conceptual framework to describe the presumed causal chain.

They also recommended that the training of practitioners involved in behaviour change should focus on generic competencies and skills, rather than on specific models. These competencies include the ability to: evaluate critically the evidence for different approaches to behaviour change; design valid and reliable interventions and programmes, that take account of the social, environmental, and economic context of behaviours; identify and use clear and appropriate outcome measures to assess changes in behaviour; employ a range of behaviour change methods and approaches, according to the best available evidence; and, regularly review the allocation of resources to interventions and pro-grammes in light of current evidence.

The PDG argued that the appropriate national organizations (for example, the Faculty of Public Health, the British Psychological Society, the Chartered Institute of Environmental Health, and the Nursing and Midwifery Council) should consider devel-oping standards for these competencies and skills. The standards should take into account the different roles and responsibilities of practitioners working both within and outside the NHS. In turn these ought to ensure fair and equitable access to education and train-ing, to enable practitioners and volunteers who help people to change their health-related behaviour to develop their skills and competencies. The responsible bodies should review current education and training practice in this area, and disinvest in approaches that lack supporting evidence.

Efforts to use policy and legislation to change behaviour were considered (although relatively little evidence on legislation was identified). It was observed that such measures tend to work via combinations of awareness-raising, compulsion, and enforcement which provide legislative or environmental 'structure' to the decisions people make about their behaviour. Legislation is often assumed to be a simple and powerful tool, and the evidence suggests that introducing legislation, in conjunction with other interventions, can be effective at the individual, community, and population levels. However, there is also a risk that legislation may be subject to contingencies and side effects, including criminalization, compensating or displaced behaviour, and lack of public support (Gostin 2000; Haw et al 2006; WHO 2005).

Delivery

The psychological literature is extensive and provides a number of general models of health behaviour and behaviour change. Close attention was paid in developing the guid-ance to the psychological models that attempt to show relationships between knowledge, attitudes, and behaviour. The PDG noted that for some actions the links between intentions and behaviour can be described very precisely. However, simple models do not capture more complex or population-level dynamics in the behaviour change process. Although the evidence on psychological models was found to be limited, a number of concepts drawn from the psychological literature were regarded by the PDG as very helpful when planning work on behaviour change with individuals. When used in conjunction with recommendations in the guidance on planning and social context, these concepts can be used to structure and inform interventions. They include: outcome expectancies (helping people to develop accurate knowledge about the health consequences of their behaviours); personal relevance (emphasizing the personal salience of health behaviours); positive attitude (promoting positive feelings towards the outcomes of behaviour change); self-efficacy (enhancing people's belief in their ability to change); descriptive norms (promoting the visibility of positive health behaviours in people's reference groups—that is, the groups they compare themselves to, or aspire to); subjective norms (enhancing social approval for positive health behaviours in significant others and reference groups); personal and moral norms (promoting personal and moral commitments to behaviour change); intention formation and concrete plans (helping people to form plans and goals for changing behaviours, over time and in specific contexts); behavioural contracts (asking people to share their plans and goals with others); relapse prevention (helping people develop skills to cope with difficult situations and conflicting goals).

At community level, investment in interventions and programmes that identify and build on the strengths of individuals and communities and the relationships within communities was recommended. These include interventions and programmes to: promote and develop positive parental skills and enhance relationships between children and their carers; improve self-efficacy; develop and maintain supportive social networks and nurture relationships (for example, extended kinship networks and other ties); support organizations and institutions that offer opportunities for local people to take part in the planning and delivery of services; support organizations and institutions that promote participation in leisure and voluntary activities; promote resilience and build skills, by promoting positive social networks and helping to develop relationships; and, promote access to the financial and material resources needed to facilitate behaviour change.

At population level, policies, interventions, and programmes tailored to change specific, health-related behaviours should be based on information gathered about the context, needs, and behaviours of the target population(s). They could include: fiscal and legislative interventions; national and local advertising and mass media campaigns (for example, information campaigns, promotion of positive role models and general promotion of health-enhancing behaviours); point of sale promotions and interventions (for example, working in partnership with private sector organizations to offer information, price reductions, or other promotions); ensuring that population-level interventions and programmes aiming to change behaviour are consistent with those delivered to individuals and communities. In this regard it is important to ensure that interventions and programmes are based on the best available evidence of effectiveness and cost-effectiveness; that the risks, costs, and benefits have been assessed for all target groups; and that time and resources should be set aside for evaluation. The PDG insisted that the size and nature of the intervention, its aims and objectives, and the underlying theory of change used should determine the form of evaluation.

The PDG concluded that the population-level interventions have the greatest potential when supported by government and implemented effectively, from population down to individual level (legislation on the compulsory use of seatbelts was one example considered by the PDG). Epidemiological theory suggests that even small degrees of change, over time, can result in significant improvements in population-level health (Rose 1985), which implies that population-level interventions—with their small and steady gains—can be an effective and cost-effective way of changing behaviour. It was noted that a wide range of policies and the actions of a range of government and non-governmental organizations impact directly and indirectly on health. (Relevant policies and actions include those related to taxation, the licensing laws and the benefits system.) This could be explicitly acknowledged by carrying out routine health impact assessments on how a policy, law, or system affects people's health-related behaviour.

Evaluation

The guidance notes that the distinction between monitoring and evaluation is important. Monitoring involves routinely collecting information on a day-to-day basis and using shared information resources and statistics to keep local and national health activity under surveillance. It is part of quality and safety assurance. Evaluation, on the other hand, is the formal assessment of the process and impact of a programme or intervention. The PDG argued that where an intervention is employed that has already been rigorously evaluated and demonstrated to be effective in equivalent conditions, then monitoring, rather than a full evaluation, is likely to be sufficient.

Complex public health interventions can be systematically evaluated based on the relevant theory and evidence, if they use a well-planned, 'staged' approach to evaluation. Formal outcome and process evaluation can be challenging, but it is an important way of assessing efforts to change behaviour. An effective evaluation is based on clearly defined outcome measures—at individual, community, and population levels, as appropriate. Qualitative research looking at the experience, meaning, and value of changes to individuals may also be appropriate. Methods and outcome measures should be. The PDG recommended that interventions should specify their 'programme theory' (or reason why particular actions are expected to have particular outcomes) and use a framework of 'action–reason–outcome' to guide evaluation (Campbell et al 2000; Campbell et al 2007; Flay 1986; Nutbeam 1998; Pawson 2006).

The recommendation here was to ensure that funding applications and project plans for new interventions and programmes include specific provision for evaluation and monitoring. The PDG recommended that wherever possible, the following elements of behaviour change interventions and programmes should be evaluated using appropriate process or outcome measures: effectiveness, acceptability, feasibility, equity, and safety. All interventions need to be developed and evaluated in stages, using an established approach such as the Medical Research Council's framework for the development and evaluation of complex interventions (Campbell et al 2000; Craig et al 2009 this volume; see also Campbell et al 2007; Flay 1986; Nutbeam 1998). Such an approach will help ensure interventions are based on the best available evidence of feasibility, acceptability, safety, effectiveness, efficiency, or equity.

Finally, the guidance recomended collecting data for cost-effectiveness analysis, including quality of life measures. Where practicable, estimating the cost savings (if any) when researching or evaluating behaviour change interventions and programmes. This is particularly pertinent for research: on mid- to long-term behaviour change; comparing the effectiveness and efficiency of interventions and programmes delivered to different population groups (for example, low- versus high-income groups, men versus women, young versus older people); and comparing the cost-effectiveness of primary prevention versus clinical treatment for behaviour-related diseases.

Conclusions

The guidance was published in late 2007 (NICE 2007), to relatively little fanfare, perhaps because on reading the principle there was a sense of 'So . . . what's new?' And yet, in considering such a vast and varied literature, the guidance managed to bring together experts and ideas from across several academic and practice divides, challenging some of the sacred cows of public health in the process.

Many of the challenges to confront the PDG and NICE team are encountered in any process which seeks to determine what constitutes the best or most appropriate evidence, and use or apply it in the real world. There were, however, some special issues with which this PDG had to deal. For instance, as we noted earlier, it became apparent as work progressed that what is meant by the terms 'scientific' or 'evidence' differs across psychology, economics, sociology, and medicine. Each discipline contained different assumptions about, and constructions of, the individual and their place in a social, economic, and health giving context. For example, psychology places the process of behaviour change in individual cognitions, processing, and motivation, while sociological accounts lean towards a broader conception of change that is located within the relationship that exists between society and the individual. These differences were real parts of the discourse of the committee.

Breaking free of these disciplinary boundaries was part of the challenge facing the committee. All the economic, behavioural, and social sciences are products of the Enlightenment. The central issues here, such as the nature of the self, the role of mind, the relation between society and the individual, and the role of economic forces in shaping human affairs were all articulated in recognizably modern form in that period. So, too, were the conceptual bases of the way economics, sociology, and psychology now provide the answers. What is especially interesting is that, whilst our post-Enlightenment disciplines have drawn and still police these boundaries, the key Enlightenment figures who first developed their ideas around these fundamental questions placed no boundaries around their thinking at all. They do not feature in the writings of Adam Smith, David Hume, George Berkeley, or Immanuel Kant. These writers range from mind and self to society quite comfortably. Even Smith, author of what is generally considered to be the foundation text in economics, is no 'narrow utilitarian': his thesis in the *Wealth of Nations* covers the state, civil society, and mind as well as market mechanisms and commerce. For these writers the key division was instead between rationalism and empiricism, which they treated as different forms of knowing and not as different epistemological positions. The key question for these writers was, could knowledge be derived *a priori* from certain logical precepts or was knowledge only possible on the basis of experience—empirically.

Happily, our post-Enlightenment limitations did not prove to be an insurmountable barrier to progress, as rather than adopt a discipline-bound approach to considering the evidence, the PDG managed to negotiate a path that did not privilege one or other of the disciplines and engage in 'synthetic' thinking, about concurrent and sometimes conflicting ideas, and develop a new account. It produced guidance which very importantly used both rationalist *a priori* thinking and empirical evidence together to produce a theoretically coherent and genuinely 'synthetic' piece of work.

The principles that have come out of this programme of work may seem to some to be common sense, yet they contain significant challenges both for government and the workforce. They speak of the need for well-planned, quality interventions, based on evidence from research and practice, stemming from careful legislation and an integrated national structure, delivered locally by trained professionals. The guidance acknowledges the place of individuals and choice in creating health behaviours, but it also reminds us that these individuals move within communities, systems, and structures that encourage, nudge, or even push them in particular directions. And it tells us that, if we want to change health, we need to tackle the job fairly and properly, from system to street, from family to individual child. We—the technical team that supported the PDG—believe this was worth saying, and saying it in the context of NICE guidance gives these principles an opportunity to make a difference. Since its publication, it has quietly and gradually begun to be taken up within public health service provision and practice, in a variety of different ways—for example, as the basis of the winning local project for the 2008 NICE 'shared learning' award, see <http://www.nice.org.uk/usingguidance/sharedlearningimplement ingniceguidance/examplesofimplementation/eximpresults.jsp?o=183>. And although we cannot claim to have found the final solution to the vexed issue of behaviour change—not least because the solutions are multiple—the NICE guidance has certainly given it a nudge, in the right direction.

Bibliography

Ajzen I (1991) 'The theory of planned behaviour' *Organisational Behaviour and Human Decision Processes* 50: 179–211

Ajzen I (2001) 'Nature and operation of attitudes' *Annual Review of Psychology* 52: 27–58

Antonovsky A (1985) *Health stress and coping.* San Francisco: Jossey Bass

Antonovsky A (1987) *Unravelling the mystery of health: how people manage stress and stay well.* San Francisco: Jossey Bass

Bandura A (1997) *Self-efficacy: the exercise of control.* New York: Freeman

Bourdieu P (1977) *Outline of a theory of practice.* Cambridge: Cambridge University Press

Bourdieu P (1986) *The forms of capital. In Richardson J, editor Handbook of theory and research for the sociology of education.* New York: Greenwood Press

Campbell M, Fitzpatrick R, Haines A et al (2000) 'Framework for design and evaluation of complex interventions to improve health' *British Medical Journal* 321: 694–6

Campbell NC, Murray E, Darbyshire J et al (2007) 'Designing and evaluating complex interventions to improve health care' *British Medical Journal* 334: 455–9

Conner M, Norman P (2005) *Predicting health behaviour: research and practice with social cognition models.* Maidenhead: Open University Press

Conner M, Sparks P (2005) 'Theory of planned behaviour and health behaviour' in M Conner and P Norman, *Predicting health behaviour: Research and practice with social cognition models.* Maidenhead: Open University Press

Davidson K, Goldstein M, Kaplan RM et al (2003) 'Evidence-based behavioral medicine: what it is and how do we achieve it?' *Annals of Behavioral Medicine* 26: 161–71

Department of Health (2004) *Choosing health: Making healthier choices easier*. London: HMSO

Ellis S and Grey A (2003) *STI infection: A review of reviews*. London: Health Development Agency

Fishbein M and Ajzen I (1975) *Belief, attitude, intention and behaviour: an introduction to theory and research*. Reading: Addison-Wesley

Fox-Rushby J, Griffith G, Vitsou E, Buxton M (2006) *The cost effectiveness of behaviour change interventions designed to reduce CHD: A thorough review of existing literature. NICE cost effectiveness review*. London: NICE. Available at: <http://www.nice.org.uk/guidance/index.jsp?action=download&o=34613>

Fox-Rushby J, Griffith G, Buxton M (2007) *The cost effectiveness of population level interventions to lower cholesterol and prevent CHD: Extrapolation and modelling results on promoting healthy eating from Norway to the UK. NICE modelling report*. London: NICE. Available at: <http://www.nice.org.uk/guidance/index.jsp?action=download&o=38510>

Flay BR (1986) 'Efficacy and effectiveness trials (and other phases of research) in the development of health promotion programmes' *Preventive Medicine* 15: 451–74

Giddens A (1979) *Central problems in social theory: action, structure and contradiction in social analysis*. Berkeley: University of California Press

Giddens A (1982) *Profiles and critiques in social theory*. London: Macmillan

Giddens A (1984) *The constitution of society: outline of the theory of structuration*. Berkeley: University of California Press

Graham H, Power C (2004) *Childhood disadvantage and adult health: a lifecourse framework*. London: NICE. Available at: <http://www.nice.org.uk/page.aspx?o=502707>

Gostin L (2000) *Public health law*. California: University of California Press

Halpern D, Bates C, Mulgan G and Aldridge S (2004) *Personal responsibility and changing behaviour: the state of knowledge and its implications for public policy. Strategy Unit Discussion Paper*. London: UK Cabinet Office

Harrop E, Addis S, Elliot E and Williams G (2006) *Resilience, coping and salutogenic approaches to generating and maintaining health: A review. NICE evidence review*. London: NICE. Available at: <http://www.nice.org.uk/guidance/index.jsp?action=download&o=34609>

Haw S, Gruer L, Amos A et al (2006) 'Legislation on smoking in enclosed places in Scotland' *Journal of Public Health* 28: 24–30

Hertzman C and Wiens M (1996) 'Child development and long-term outcomes: a population health perspective and summary of successful interventions' *Social Science and Medicine* 43: 1083–95

Hertzman C, McLean SA, Kohen DE, Dunn J and Evans T (2002) *Early Development in Vancouver: Report of the Community Asset Mapping Project (CAMP)*. Vancouver: Human Early Learning Partnership (HELP), University of British Columbia, <http://www.earlylearning.ubc.ca>

Jepson R (2000) *The effectiveness of interventions to change health-related behaviours: a review of reviews*. MRC Social & Public Health Sciences Unit Occasional Paper No 3. Glasgow: MRC Social & Public Health Sciences Unit.

Jepson R, Harris F, Macgillivray S, Kearney N and Rowa-Dewar N (2006) *A review of the effectiveness of interventions, approaches and models at individual, community and population level that are aimed at changing health outcomes by changing knowledge, attitudes and behaviours. NICE evidence review*. London: NICE. Available at: <http://www.nice.org.uk/guidance/index.jsp?action=download&o=34610>

Keating C and Hertzman DP (1999) 'Modernity's paradox' in C Keating and DP Hertzman (eds), *Developmental Health and the Wealth of Nations*. London/New York: Guilford Press.

Kelly MP (2006) 'Mapping the life world: a future research priority for public health' in A Killoran, C Swann, MP Kelly (eds), *Public Health Evidence: Tackling Health Inequalities*, pp 553–74. Oxford: Oxford University Press

Kiernan K (1997) 'Becoming a young parent: a longitudinal study of associated factors' *British Journal of Sociology* 48/3: 406–28

Kuh D, Power C, Blane D and Bartley M (1997) 'Social pathways between childhood and adult health' in DL Kuh and Y Ben-Shlomo (eds), *A Life Course Approach to Chronic Disease Epidemiology: tracing the origins of ill health from early to adult life*. 1st edn. Oxford: Oxford University Press

Lazarus R (1976) *Patterns of adjustment*. New York: McGraw Hill

Lazarus RS (1985) The costs and benefits of denial. In Monat A, Lazarus R (eds), *Stress and coping: an anthology*. New York: Columbia University Press

Lazarus R, Folkman S (1984) *Stress, appraisal and coping*. New York: Springer

Morgan A and Swann C (eds) (2004) *Social capital for health: issues of definition, measurement and links to health*. London: Health Development Agency

Nora SM and Zimmerman RS (2005) 'Health Behavior Theory and cumulative knowledge regarding health behaviors: are we moving in the right direction?' *Health Education Research* 20/3: 275–90

Nutbeam D (1998) 'Evaluating health promotion—progress, problems and solutions' *Health Promotion International* 13: 27–44

Pawson R (2006) *Evidence based policy: a realist perspective.* London: Sage

Power C and Hertzman C (1997) 'Social and biological pathways linking early life and adult disease' in MG Marmot and MEJ Wadsworth (eds), Fetal and early childhood environment: long-term health implications. *British Medical Bulletin* 53/1: 210–21

Power C and Hertzman C (2004) 'Health and human development from life course research' in M Barer, R Evans, C Hertzman, and Heyman J (eds), *Population Health: Policy Dilemmas.* Oxford: Oxford University Press

Putnam R (2000) *Bowling alone: the collapse and revival of American community.* New York: Simon & Schuster

Roe L, Hunt P, Bradshaw H and Rayner M (1997) *Health promotion interventions to promote healthy eating in the general population: A review.* London: Health Education Authority

Rose G (1985) 'Sick individuals and sick populations' *International Journal of Epidemiology* 14: 32–8

Rosenstock IM (1966) 'Why people use health services' *Millbank Memorial Fund Quarterly* 44: 94–124

Stead M, McDermott L, Broughton P, Angus K and Hastings G (2006) *Review of the effectiveness of road safety and pro-environmental interventions. NICE evidence review.* London: NICE. Available at: <http://www.nice.org.uk/guidance/index.jsp?action=download&o=34608>

Stead M, McDermott L, Angus K and Hastings G (2006) *Marketing review. NICE evidence review.* London: NICE. Available at: <http://www.nice.org.uk/guidance/index.jsp?action=download&o=34615>

Swann CJ (2002) 'Psychosocial theory, public health and the gendered body' *The Psychologist* 15: 4

Swann CJ, Bowe K, McCormick G and Kosmin M (2003) *Teenage pregnancy and parenthood: A review of reviews.* London: Health Development Agency

Taylor D, Bury M, Campling N, Carter S, Garfied S, Newbould J, Rennie T (2006a) *A review of the use of the health belief model (HBM), the theory of reasoned action (TRA), the theory of planned behaviour (TPA) and the transtheoretical model (TTM) to study and predict health related behaviour change. NICE evidence review.* London: NICE. Available at: <http://www.nice.org.uk/guidance/index.jsp?action=download&o=34606>

Taylor D, Bury M, Carter S, Garfied S, Newbould J, Rennie T (2006b) *The influence of social and cultural context on the effectiveness of health behaviour change interventions in relation to diet, exercise and smoking cessation. NICE evidence review.* London: NICE. Available at: <http://www.nice.org.uk/guidance/index.jsp?action=download&o=34605>

Wanless D (2004) *Securing good health for the whole population: final report.* London: HM Treasury

Weiss CH (1995) 'Nothing as practical as good theory: exploring theory-based evaluation for comprehensive community initiatives for children and families'. in Connell JP, Kubisch A, Schorr LB et al (eds), *New approaches to evaluating community initiatives: concepts, methods and context.* Washington DC: Aspen Institute

WHO (2005) *Seventh futures forum on unpopular decisions in public health. Regional office for Europe.* Geneva: World Health Organization. Available at: <http://www.euro.who.int/InformationSources/Publications/Catalogue/20050608_1>

Chapter 25

Promoting the emotional and social well-being of children in primary education: evidence-based guidance

Amanda Killoran, Antony Morgan,
and James Jagroo

Introduction

Promoting the social and emotional well-being of children is seen increasingly by policy makers as an important component of broader strategies designed to improve the outcomes of children and young people. This focus has the potential to minimize the health risks and negative social outcomes associated with 'modern' childhood and adolescence, including anti-social behaviour, binge drinking, and lack of involvement in training and employment (Feinstein and Sabates 2006).

The World Health Organization (WHO) identified positive mental health and well-being as assets for the growth and development of children and adolescents (WHO, 2008). Taking an asset approach, the promotion of social and emotional well-being provides the best chance for children and young people to achieve and sustain mental health and well-being in later life (Morgan and Ziglio 2007; WHO 2008).

Schools have a particular role in contributing to these goals. Investment in programmes that focus on the positive attributes of children and young people provide the building block for development of indicators of well being such as self esteem (WHO 2004; Weare, 2000). Such school based approaches aim to improve health through both organizational-wide changes as well as individually based methods, and represent 'complex social interventions'.

In the UK, the promotion of social and emotional well-being of children and young people has become an explicit feature of policies and targets, and identified as a way of protecting against poor outcomes. The Children's Plan (2008) states:

> Good social and emotional skills are vital for healthy personal development. They build resilience and reduce the likelihood of engaging in risky behaviour, and support educational achievement, employment and earnings, and relationships in adulthood.

> (Department for Children, Families and Schools 2008)

The National Institute of Health and Clinical Excellence (NICE) seeks to support such policies by producing evidence-based guidance which defines the key features of effective programmes and the conditions necessary for their successful implementation. The guidance serves to provide standards to support the development, monitoring and evaluation of evidence-based practice nationally.

This chapter summarizes the recommendations made by NICE to raise standards in the programmes and activities used to promote the social and emotional well-being of children specifically in relation to primary education. In doing so it highlights:

- the role of conceptual frameworks in defining emotional and social well-being and the rationale for interventions;
- the principles used by NICE for development of standards and guidance, taking account of the underdeveloped nature of the evidence; and
- issues for research, and for policy and practice, to ensure effective investments in improving the social and emotional well-being of children.

Conceptualizing social and emotional well-being

The rationale for intervention rests on a robust conceptualization of mental health and mental illness (see below). However the mental health of children and young people is a broad concept and there is no widely agreed standard definition. A deficit model has traditionally defined mental health as the absence of a psychiatric diagnosis (WHO 2004). However, ideas of positive mental health and emotional well-being are increasingly acknowledged as integral to the broad concept of mental health in children and young people. For example, good mental health in childhood and adolescence is indicated by:

- their capacity to enter into and sustain mutually satisfying personal relationships ('secure attachment behaviour');
- continuing progressing of psychological development;
- their ability to play and learn so that attainments are appropriate for age and intellectual level;
- the development of a sense of right and wrong; and
- any psychological distress or maladaptive behaviour being within the usual limits for a child's age and context (UK Mental Health Foundation 2001).

From a current UK policy perspective a wide range of terms are used with reference to mental health, often depending on professional standpoint. For example, terms such as 'mental health', 'mental health difficulties', and 'mental health disorders' are more commonly used within health and social care, whereas local authorities and schools increasingly use the term 'emotional health and well-being' in relation to both the care they take of pupils and the curriculum they provide (Ofsted 2005; Department of Health 2004). In addition, the term 'emotional and behavioural difficulties' is a term used for children experiencing, and externalizing in school, mental health problems arising from adverse early experiences, difficult family relationships, or ineffective behaviour management (Department for Education and Skills 2001).

A broad and positive definition of mental well-being was adopted for the purpose of development of NICE guidance. This was based on the life course perspective that defines social and emotional well-being as a critical asset in a child's development and also future life chances. Furthermore this positive definition (and language) supported the positioning of the guidance within educational policies and reform.

Mental well-being was defined as encompassing the following:

+ emotional well-being (including happiness and confidence, and the opposite of depression);

+ psychological well-being (including autonomy, problem solving, resilience, attentiveness, and involvement); and

+ social well-being (good relationships with others, and the opposite of conduct disorder, delinquency, interpersonal violence, and bullying).

The life course approach provides a strong theoretical rationale for investing in promoting the emotional and social well-being of children. The life course perspective is concerned with how social and biological factors interact through the stages of life and generations (Kuh et al 2003). Evidence indicates that cumulative exposure to adverse social circumstances increases a child's risk of emotional and behavioural problems during childhood, but also their health and social prospects in later life. Children with emotional and behavioural problems have increased likelihood of school exclusion, anti-social behaviour, drug misuse, and alcohol in adolescence, as well as mental illness in later life (Buchan and Hudson 2000). Graham and Power model how poor social circumstances influence physical, emotional, cognitive and social development and produce trajectories of risky health behaviours and social identities (such as teenage parenthood) that compromise health and social position in adulthood (Graham and Power 2004). Furthermore, these pathways sustain social patterning of health inequalities at a population level.

Evidence from cross-sectional and longitudinal studies has established the specific factors that increase risk of poor emotional and social development and behavioural problems. Table 25.1 shows the range of risk factors (many linked to poor social circumstances). It is hypothesized that the more risk factors a child or young person experiences, the more likely they will experience poorer social and health outcomes. Protective factors, such as solid family bonds and the capacity to succeed in school, help safeguard young people from behavioural problems and addictive behaviours. However, exposure to even a substantial number of risk factors does not necessarily mean that a child will suffer behavioural problems. The presence of protective factors can reduce the likelihood that behavioural problems will develop. Among 'resilient' children protective factors appear to potentially mediate the negative impact of risk factors.

Risks and protective factors therefore provide an important intervention focus for prevention of negative outcomes. *Mostly individual protective factors are identical to features of positive social and emotional well-being,* and therefore interventions aimed at strengthening these 'assets' act to prevent behavioural disorders and mental health problems.

Table 25.1 Risk and protective factors for mental health in childhood and adolescence

	Individual	Family	Community
Risks	Male Learning disability Physical illness Academic failure Low self-esteem Developmental delay Communication problems	Parental conflict Family breakdown Inconsistent/unclear discipline Physical, sexual, or emotional abuse Parental mental illness Criminality or substance addiction Death or loss	Socio-economic disadvantage Homelessness Disaster Discrimination Unemployment Poor school
Protective Factors	Female Self-esteem and sense of self-identity and self efficacy Good communication and social skills School success	At least one good parent–child relationship Authoritative discipline Support for education Supportive marriage/absence of severe discord	Wider support networks Access to sport and leisure opportunities High standard of living Schools with strong academic and non-academic opportunities Good housing

The UK Government's commitment to improving social and emotional well-being clearly reflects a life course perspective (HM Treasury 2003, 2004, 2007). The policy notion of 'progressive prevention', responding to those at risk, draws on research that shows childhood problems (particularly behaviour difficulties) can be strong predictors of poor and costly adult outcomes (Feinstein and Sabates 2006). With respect to primary education, two specific programmes (Social and Emotional Aspects of Learning (SEAL) and Healthy Schools) are designed to promote social and emotional well-being. These programmes are discussed further below.

Development of evidence-based guidance: principles, processes, and methods

As noted above, many school-based approaches, concerned with improving health, aim to bring about organizational-wide changes in school systems and processes as well as individual level changes. Such approaches represent 'complex social programmes' and as such their evaluation pose methodological, practical, and ethical difficulties. The difficulty of conducting controlled trials in educational settings is well documented. In common with other areas of public health, there is a dearth of evidence on effectiveness and cost-effectiveness of school-based interventions and what evidence is available is of variable quality. Review work has highlighted important limitations and gaps in the evidence (Stewart-Brown et al 2006; Wells et al 2002). Evaluations of all the components of whole school approaches have not been conducted and the most rigorous studies are concerned with evaluation of indicated or targeted programmes (ie a deficit approach). Most of the evaluation studies and evidence are US-based. Few studies address issues of implementation and process evaluations are lacking. School-based interventions have not been subject to economic evaluation.

However, the development of NICE public health guidance is based on a set of principles, processes, and methods that recognize the underdeveloped nature of the evidence base on such complex interventions. The *best available evidence* is considered by independent advisory committees and judgements are made on the basis of this evidence as well as other factors to produce practical guidance that can be implemented in the English context. The key elements of this guidance development process are described below.

A logic model for school-based interventions

The development of a logic model was an important part of the scoping of this piece of guidance (Figure 25.1 below). It helped define what and how interventions might promote the social and emotional well-being of children in primary schools, and also identify what specific research questions should be addressed by evidence reviews. The logic model was also important in defining the local context for implementation of interventions, specifically the local governance mechanisms, strategies, and performance management arrangements.

Figure 25.1 shows the links between national and local policy drivers, school-based interventions and outcomes. These interventions operate at both the level of the whole school system, and at an individual level.

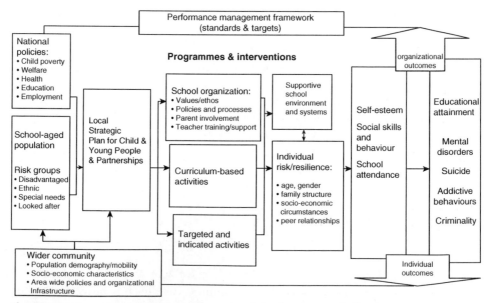

Fig. 25.1 Logic model: child social and emotional development and schools

Conceptually, interventions can be categorized as universal or indicated/targeted. Universal approaches aim to cover all children, and focus on the whole school context and not only on the behaviour of individual pupils. Such approaches include: management, ethos, communication, policies, physical environment, and relationships with parents and with the community. Universal approaches also include curriculum-based programmes concerned with developing social and emotional competences. *Indicated and targeted* interventions focus on pupils who are at risk of developing emotional and behavioural difficulties and mental disorders or already experience problems. Interventions explicitly address risks relating to poor mental health, or aspects of mental disorders.

In principle, these school based interventions can address a number of the important risk and protective factors identified in Table 25.1. For example schools can have an important influence on self-esteem, academic success, communication, and social skills (strengthening assets). But the model also responds to the needs of those children who are already experiencing difficulties (deficits).

In England there are two main school-based programmes that are concerned with improving health and well-being of children and young people. Social and Emotional Aspects of Learning (SEAL) provides a 'whole curriculum framework' for teaching social and emotional skills to children from the Foundation Stage to Year 6 (Department for Education and Skills 2005a; Department for Children, Schools and Families 2007). The evaluation of the pilot phase of the SEAL programme reported that it had a major impact (as perceived by teachers) on children's confidence, social and communication skills, and relationships (Hallam et al 2006). The National Healthy School programme emphasizes a holistic (whole-school) approach to promoting health (Department for Education and Skills 2005b). It links to work on Personal, Social and Health Education, and citizenship that have an important role in developing emotional and social competences and well being. The national evaluation of the National Healthy School Standard showed mixed results as measured by changes in health behaviours (Blenkinsop et al 2004).

Best available evidence

The principle of evidence that is 'fit for purpose' underpins the development of NICE public health guidance, ie it is the research questions that determine what type of evidence and methods are most appropriate. Experimental and quasi-experimental evidence are appropriate for evaluating the effectiveness of school-based intervention. However, application of experimental designs in the school setting involves methodological, practical, and ethical difficulties. Furthermore, questions about local implementation are more appropriately addressed through process and qualitative methods.

Systematic reviews of research evidence were commissioned by NICE to address the primary question:

> What universal and targeted approaches are effective in promoting the mental health of children (aged 4–11 years old) in primary schools?

Subsidiary questions were also considered relating to the content, the timing, and the person delivering the universal or targeted intervention.

In addition an economic appraisal was undertaken. This involved a review of economic evaluations and an analysis of the cost-effectiveness of interventions that were highlighted as effective by the review work.

The reviews comprised:

- effectiveness of universal approaches (non-violence related outcomes) to promote mental well-being in children in primary education (Adi et al 2007);
- effectiveness of universal approaches (violence related outcomes) to promote mental well-being in children in primary education (Adi et al 2007); and
- mental well-being of children in primary education using targeted/indicated activities (Shucksmith et al 2007).

The full reviews are available on the NICE website: <http://www.nice.org.uk>.

The studies that met the inclusion criteria were assessed for methodological rigour and quality using the NICE methodology checklist, as set out in the NICE manual 'Methods for development of NICE public health guidance' (NICE 2006). Studies included in the economic review were assessed for quality using a checklist based on the criteria developed by Drummond et al (1997).

The evidence was synthesized and used to produce 'evidence statements', ie summary statements that addressed the research questions. The statements reflected the strength (quantity, type, and quality) of evidence and its applicability.

The strongest evidence that *universal interventions* had positive effects was provided by a small number of good quality trials. These were evaluations of multi-component programmes that had a number of common features: curriculum to develop children's social skills, teachers' training in management of behaviour, and education of parents.

Examples included the Seattle Social Development Project (Hawkins 1991, 1999, 2005), which, at follow-up of students at 18 years of age, showed reduced levels of violent delinquent action and school misbehaviour. The LIFT programme (Linking Interests of Families and Teachers) reported reduced arrests at three years post-intervention (Reid et al 1999; Stoolmiller 2000; Eddy et al 2003).

Two large good quality RCTs of the Peace Builders programme (Krug 1997; Vazsonyi 2004) showed a clear positive effect on outcomes relating to violence and aggressive behaviour and social competences. Ethos and culture were important in changing values, attitudes, and behaviours of children and staff relating to their conduct of relationships. This was reinforced in the curriculum and work with parents.

The PATHS programme reported reduction in aggression and hyperactive disruptive behaviours and showed the importance of teacher training and universal class-based teaching of social and emotional development programmes (CPPRG 1999, 2004, 2004; Greenberg 1995).

A number of good quality RCTs demonstrated that targeted approaches that focused on groups of children at risk /or already showing signs of behavioural difficulties can have positive effects on measures of social skills.

Cognitive behavioural therapy (CBT)-based prevention programmes, delivered by therapists appeared to be effective in preventing anxiety disorders and depression.

Studies also showed that multi-component approaches could be effective in preventing violent and aggressive behaviours (including conduct disorders). These programmes combined use of CBT with children with other activities including teacher training and parent support. An example was the Incredible Years Intervention, reported by a group led by Webster-Stratton (Webster-Stratton et al 2001, 2003, 2004; Reid et al 2003).

The studies also indicated that application of these targeted approaches involved difficulties. Teachers found identification of 'at risk' children difficult.

The recruitment and sustained involvement of parents in the programmes was also problematic. These interventions were resource intensive, drawing on outside specialists to deliver the interventions (rather than school-based staff), while full potential benefits and cost savings were beyond the study periods.

Although a number of high quality randomized controlled trials were identified, the reviews showed substantial variation in the quality of the studies in this area. There were considerable difficulties involved in conducting such school-based evaluations. The criteria of randomization and blinding were not necessarily appropriate or feasible. However, other areas of weakness included lack of detailed description of interventions, failure to take account of cluster effects in analyses, and failure to report all outcomes (Adi et al 2007).

Shucksmith and colleagues observed that the targeted interventions and evaluation designs became increasingly sophisticated over time (Shucksmith et al 2007). Early interventions (early 1990s) used weak controls, and were small and underpowered, while later multi-component studies had larger samples leading to better powered analyses.

Economic modelling

The economic analysis aimed to assess the cost-effectiveness of universal and targeted interventions. Universal approaches produced an expected Incremental Cost Effectiveness Ratio (ICER) of between £5,000–£10,000 Quality Adjusted Life Years (QALYs), depending on the assumed level of impact. This QALY perspective did not take account of any sustained educational or socio-economic benefits of the interventions. However, the Advisory Committee acknowledged that evidence provided by observational studies had consistently indicated that interventions of this type were likely to have a wide range of benefits and effects in both the short and long term across multiple sectors. These covered educational attainment, mental, physical, and emotional health, socio-economic status and reduced involvement in the criminal justice system. Targeted approaches alone were more resource intensive and cost-effectiveness was judged to be dependent on the benefits realized over a number of years.

Members of the Advisory Committee used the evidence statements and the findings from the economic review to draft recommendations.

Testing guidance in context

These draft recommendations were tested through locally-based fieldwork (NICE 2007). The findings showed that teachers and other practitioners, governors, and parents all acknowledged that the academic performance of a school and the mental well-being of its pupils were inextricably linked. Furthermore, teachers and other practitioners endorsed the emphasis on prevention, but admitted that they tended to intervene reactively after a problem had occurred.

The findings indicated that the promotion of social and emotional well-being involved a challenging process of organizational development. Some schools were much more advanced in this process than others. Those schools had commitment at a senior level, with senior staff having designated responsibilities for this area; and the focus of Social and Emotional Aspects of Learning (SEAL) and Healthy Schools had supported adoption of a whole school approach. Some schools had also invested in specialist posts for example in pastoral care, and also had good access to wider specialist support, including clinical psychologists, educational psychologists, school nurses, social workers, counsellors, and therapists- working in child and adolescent mental health services, or primary care or local authority teams or the voluntary sector.

The final recommendations are set out in Table 25.2.

Table 25.2 Recommendations: promoting emotional and social well-being of children in primary education

	Who should take action	**What action should be taken**
Whole school approach	Commissioners and providers of services to children in primary education	Agree arrangements as part of strategic plan to ensure all primary schools adopt a comprehensive, whole school approach to children's social and emotional well-being. All primary schools should: ◆ Create an ethos and conditions that support positive behaviours for learning and for successful relationships ◆ Provide an emotionally secure and safe environment that prevents any form of bullying or violence ◆ Support all pupils ◆ Provide specific help for those most at risk ◆ Include social and emotional well-being in policies for attaining outcome targets ◆ Offer teachers and practitioners in schools training and support ◆ Put in place and evaluate coordinating mechanisms to ensure primary schools have access to the skills, advice, and support to deliver comprehensive and effective programmes Schools and local authority children's services should work closely with child and adolescent mental health and other services to develop and agree local protocols defining the role of schools and other agencies in delivering different interventions

Table 25.2 (continued) Recommendations: promoting emotional and social well-being of children in primary education

	Who should take action	What action should be taken
Universal activities	Teachers and practitioners working with children in primary education Those working in local authority education and children's services, primary care, child and adolescent mental health services and voluntary agencies	Provide a comprehensive programme to help develop children's social and emotional skills and well-being. This should include: ♦ A curriculum that integrates the development of social and emotional skills within all subject areas ♦ Training and development to ensure teachers and practitioners deliver this curriculum effectively Support to help parents and carers develop their parenting skills
Targeted activities	Teachers and practitioners working with children in primary education Those working in local authority education and children series, primary care, child and adolescent metal health services and voluntary agencies	Ensure teachers and practitioners are trained to identify and assess the early signs of anxiety, emotional distress, and behavioural problems among primary school children. Identify and assess children who are showing early signs of anxiety, emotional distress, or behavioural problems. Normally specialists should only be involved if the child has a combination of risk factors and /or the difficulties are recurrent or persistent. Discuss the options for tackling those problems with the child and their parents or carers. Agree an action plan Ensure parents or carers living in disadvantaged circumstances are given the support they need to participate fully in any parenting sessions that are offered

Actions at the local strategic level were recommended that would enable all primary schools to adopt a 'whole school' approach to children's social and emotional well-being. This approach should comprise both universal and targeted interventions. The components of universal approaches were defined, covering curriculum, training, and development, support to parents and carers and wider activities. The provision of targeted inventions involved the identification and assessment of those children who are at risk (or already showing early signs) of anxiety, emotional distress, or behavioural problems, and the agreement of an action plan according to the child's needs. This should be part of a multi-agency approach to support the child and their family.

In summary, the recommendations set out an integrated asset-based approach that could prevent negative behaviours and costly consequences for the NHS, social services, and the criminal justice system.

NICE's independent advisory committees consider a range of issues when making judgements about the evidence and preparing guidance for policy makers and practitioners.

These include ethical and equity concerns. With respect to this guidance, the Committee considered issues regarding the 'needs', 'rights', and 'quality of life' of children, and made explicit a number of these expectations. The Committee emphasized the importance of the creation by schools of a supportive and secure ethos and environment that could help avoid stigma and discrimination towards mental health, and social and emotional difficulties. It was also important to acknowledge that all children may demonstrate emotional, social, and behavioural difficulties during the normal experience of childhood. But such difficulties were not always indicative of a significant psychological or medical problem. Furthermore, it was important to ensure that social and emotional difficulties were not misinterpreted due to cultural differences. Programmes should be culturally sensitive, and take account of different socio-economic, cultural, and ethnic backgrounds.

The Committee also stated that school-based programmes could only be one element in a broader strategy designed to develop and protect the social and emotional well-being of children. Policies to improve the social and economic circumstances of children living in disadvantaged circumstances were critical to this goal. Nevertheless, lack of investment in mental health promotion in primary schools was likely to lead to significant costs for society. Children who experienced emotional and social problems were more likely to have lower prospects in life, including unemployment, and involvement in crime.

Conclusion

We conclude by highlighting how this NICE guidance on promoting the social and emotional well-being of children in primary education served to support implementation of education and health polices despite the limitations of the evidence in this area.

The process of guidance development described above demonstrates the underdeveloped nature of the evidence base and some substantial gaps, particularly the lack of UK-based high quality long-term evaluation studies. Much evidence is US-based and schools are operating in a very different social, cultural, and policy context. This raises questions of transferability to the English setting. Guidance development also highlighted the distinct challenges involved in evaluating 'public health' programmes based on change and management of 'organizational systems'. Effectiveness is likely to be dependent on the leadership and the management capabilities of governors and teachers, as well as teaching competencies. Nevertheless, despite these difficulties relating to the evidence, NICE principles allow use of the 'best evidence' that is available, as derived from the scientific literature. And these principles also ensure that the guidance is relevant and can be practically implemented, taking account of the policy and practice context. The scientific evidence is one element in the production of evidence-based guidelines, but other considerations are important relating to issues such as equity and implementation informed by expert knowledge and field research.

In England policy makers show a clear commitment to apply what works to improve the outcomes of children. As stated, programmes concerned with promoting social and emotional well-being in schools, as well as other national programmes are examples of practice informed by evidence. Consequently, this NICE guidance served to 'add value' by promoting national application of evidence-based standards and their monitoring through the performance management system.

Furthermore, guidance development also identified those significant gaps in research that need to be addressed to determine more precisely the types of interventions that could be effective in promoting the social and emotional well-being of young people. The Committee was able to define specific research questions that would improve the evidence base on social and emotional well-being in the future. It agreed that further work was required to develop indicators which better measure the social and emotional well-being of primary schoolchildren for monitoring and evaluation purposes. It was also important to consider the effectiveness and cost-effectiveness of interventions in terms of impact on multiple outcomes—educational, health, and social—over the longer term as well as short term. In addition, there needs to be greater understanding of the differential impact of different approaches according to the key dimensions of age, gender, and social disadvantage and ethnicity. While the principle of involvement of children in the development, implementation, and evaluation of interventions is well understood, we need to know more about the best approaches for achieving it. In summary, there is a considerable agenda for building the evidence base for effective practice in this area.

Acknowledgements

The guidance was prepared by the NICE Public Health Intervention Advisory Committee (PHIAC), supported by the NICE technical team. The Chair of the Committee was Professor Catherine Law. The reviews were undertaken by two collaborating centres: Warwick Medical School, University of Warwick; and School of Health and Social Care, University of Teesside. This guidance can be accessed at: <http://guidance.nice.org.uk/PH12>.

Bibliography

Adi Y, Killoran A, Janmohamed K, Stewart Brown S (2007) *Systematic review of the effectiveness of interventions to promote mental wellbeing in primary education.* Report 1: universal approaches which do not focus on violence and bullying. London: National Institute for Health and Clinical Excellence

Adi Y, Killoran A, Schrader McMillan A, Stewart Brown S (2007) *Systematic review of the effectiveness of interventions to promote mental wellbeing in children in primary education.* Report 3: universal approaches with a focus on prevention of violence and bullying. London: National Institute for Health and Clinical Excellence

Blenkinsop S, Eggers M, Schagen I, Schagen S, Scott E (2004) *Evaluation of the impact of the National Healthy School Standard.* Final Report. Slough: NFER and Thomas Coram Research Unit. Available at: <http://www.wiredforhealth.gov.uk/PDF/Full report 2004.pdf>

Buchanan A, Hudson B (2000) *Promoting Children's Emotional Wellbeing.* Oxford: Oxford University Press

Collishaw S, Maughan B, Goodman R et al (2004) 'Time trends in adolescent mental health' *Journal of Child Psychology and Psychiatry* 45/8: 1350–60

Conduct Problems Prevention Research Group (CPPRG) (1999) 'I Initial impact of the Fast Track prevention trial for conduct problems: II. Classroom effects. Conduct Problems Prevention Research Group' *Journal of Consulting & Clinical Psychology* 67/5: 648–57

Conduct Problems Prevention Research Group (1999) 'Initial Impact of the Fast Track Prevention Trial for Conduct Problems: I. The High-Risk Sample' *Journal of Consulting and Clinical Psychology* 67/5: 631–47

Conduct Problems Prevention Research Group (2002) 'Evaluation of the First 3 Years of the Fast Track Prevention Trial with Children at High Risk for Adolescent Conduct Problems' *Journal of Abnormal Child Psychology* 30/1: 19–35

Conduct Problems Prevention Research Group (2004) 'The Effects of the Fast Track Program on Serious Problem Outcomes at the End of Elementary School' *Journal of Clinical Child and Adolescent Psychology* 33/4: 650–61

Department for Children, Schools and Families (2007) *Guidance for schools on developing emotional health and wellbeing.* London: Department for Children, Schools and Families

Department for Children, Schools and Families (2008) *Children's Plan.* London: Department for Children, Schools and Families

Department for Education and Employment (2001) *Promoting children's. mental health within early years and school settings.* London: Department for Education and Employment

Department for Education and Skills (2004) *Healthy living blueprint for schools.* London: Department for Education and Skills

Department for Education and Skills (2005b) *Excellence and enjoyment: social and emotional aspects of learning.* London: Department for Education and Skills

Department for Education and Skills (2005c) *National healthy school status—a guide for schools.* London: Department of Health

Department of Health (2004a) *National service framework for children, young people and maternity services. Core standards.* London: Department of Health

Department of Health (2004b) *Choosing health: making healthier choices easier.* London: Department of Health

Drummond MF et al (1997) 'Critical assessment of economic evaluation' in Drummond MF et al, *Methods for the economic evaluation of health care programmes.* 2nd edn. Oxford: Oxford University Press

Eddy JM, Reid JB, Stoolmiller M, Fetrow RA (2003) 'Outcomes during middle school for an elementary school-based preventive intervention for conduct problems: follow up results from a randomised trial' *Behavior Therapy* 34/4: 377–84

Feinstein L, Sabates R (2006) *Predicting adult life outcomes from earlier signals: identifying those at risk.* Report for Prime Minister's Strategy Unit. London: Cabinet Office

Graham H, Power C (2003) *Childhood disadvantage and adult health: a lifecourse framework.* London: Health Development Agency.

Greenberg MT, Kusche CA, Cook ET (1995) 'Quamma JP. Promoting emotional competence in school-aged children: The effects of the PATHS curriculum' *Development and Psychopathology* 7/1: 117–36

Hallam S, Rhamie J, Shaw J (2006) *Evaluation of the Primary Behaviour and Attendance Pilot.* London, UK: Department for Education and Skills

Hawkins JD, Kosterman R, Catalano RF, Hill KG, Abbott RD (2005) 'Promoting positive adult functioning through social development intervention in childhood: long-term effects from the Seattle Social Development Project' [Erratum appears in Arch Pediatr Adolesc Med. 2005 May, 159/5: 469.] *Archives of Pediatrics & Adolescent Medicine* 159/1: 25–31

Hawkins JD, Catalano RF, Kosterman R, Abbott R, Hill KG (1999) 'Preventing adolescent health-risk behaviors by strengthening protection during childhood' *Archives of Pediatrics & Adolescent Medicine* 153/3: 226–34

Hawkins JD, Von CE, Catalano JRF (1991) 'Reducing early childhood aggression: Results of a primary prevention program' *Journal of the American Academy of Child & Adolescent Psychiatry* 30/2: 208–17

HM Government (2003) *Every child matters.* London: Department for Education and Skills

HM Government (2004) *Every child matters: change for children.* London: Department for Education and Skills

HM Treasury (2007) *Policy review of children and young people: a discussion paper.* London: HM Treasury

Krug EG, Brener ND, Dahlberg LL, Ryan GW, Powell KE (1997) 'The impact of an elementary school-based violence prevention program on visits to the school nurse' *American Journal of Preventive Medicine* 13/6: 459–63

Kuh D, Power C, Blane D et al (1997) 'Social pathways between childhood and adult health' in D Kuh and Y Ben-Shlomo (eds), *A life course approach to chronic disease epidemiology.* Oxford: Oxford University Press

Mental Health Foundation (2001) *What is mental health?* London: Mental Health Foundation

Morgan A, Ziglio E (2007) 'Revitalising the evidence base for public health: an assets model' *IUHPE Promotion & Education* Supplement 2: 17–22

National Institute for Health and Clinical Excellence (2007) *Promoting children's social and emotional wellbeing in primary education (12).* London: National Institute for Health and Clinical Excellence.

NICE (2006) *Methods for development of NICE public health guidance.* London: NICE. Available at: <http://www.NICE.org.uk>

NICE (2007) *Mental wellbeing of children -public health intervention guidance: fieldwork report (Dr Foster Intelligence).* London: NICE

Ofsted (2005) *Healthy Minds: promoting emotional health and wellbeing in schools.* London: Ofsted

Reid J, Webster-Stratton C, Hammond M (2003) 'Follow-Up of children who received the Incredible Years Intervention for Oppositional-Defiant Disorder: Maintenance and Prediction of 2-Year Outcome' *Behaviour Therapy* 34: 471–91

Shucksmith J, Summerbell C, Jones S, Whittaker V (2007) *Mental wellbeing of children in primary education: targeted/ indicated activities.* London: National Institute for Health and Clinical Excellence

Stewart-Brown S (2006). *What is the evidence on school health promotion in improving health or preventing disease and specifically, what is the effectiveness of the health promoting schools approach?* WHO Regional Office for Europe (Health Evidence Report). Copenhagen: WHO

Weare K (2000) *Promoting mental, emotional and social health: a whole school approach.* London: Routledge

Weare K, Gray G (2005) *What works in developing children's emotional and social competence and wellbeing?* Report for the Department for Education and Skills

Webster-Stratton C, Reid J, Hammond M (2001) 'Social Skills and Problem-solving Training for Children with Early-onset Conduct Problems: Who Benefits?' *Journal of Child Psychiatry* 42/7: 943–52

Webster-Stratton C, Reid J (2003) 'Treating Conduct Problems and Strengthening Social and Emotional Competence in Young Children: The Dina Dinosaur Treatment Program' *Journal of Emotional and Behavioural Disorders* 11/3: 130–43

Webster-Stratton C, Reid J, Hammond M (2004) 'Treating Children with Early-Onset Conduct Problems: Intervention Outcomes for Parent, Child and Teacher Training' *Journal of Clinical Child and Adolescent Psychology* 33/1: 105–24

Wells J, Barlow J, Stewart-Brown S (2003) 'A systematic review of universal approaches to mental health promotion in schools' *Health Education* 103/4: 220

WHO (2004) *Prevention of mental disorders: effective interventions and policy options. Summary report of the WHO dept of mental health and substance abuse.* Geneva: WHO

WHO (2008) *Social cohesion for mental wellbeing amongst adolescents.* Copenhagen: WHO

Vazsonyi AT, Belliston LM, Flannery DJ (2004) 'Evaluation of a School-Based, Universal Violence Prevention Program: Low-, Medium-, and High-Risk Children' *Youth Violence and Juvenile Justice* 2/2: 185–206

Chapter 26

What environmental changes can increase physical activity?

Hugo Crombie, Amanda Killoran,
and Bhash Naidoo

Introduction

This chapter discusses the development of NICE public health guidance on physical activity and the environment. The guidance was aimed at professionals whose activities within the NHS, local authorities and the wider public, private, voluntary, and community sectors could impact on the public's physical activity levels. Such actions would help increase levels of physical activity among local communities, to meet the physical activity recommendations of the Chief Medical Officer of England (Department of Health 2004).

The guidance was produced using the NICE process and methods (NICE 2006). NICE guidance is developed by independent advisory committees taking account of the best available evidence as well as other considerations. For this piece of work, the Committee included members from the diverse fields of public health, physical activity, transport, economics, natural environment, schools, architecture, planning, and local communities.

It addressed the question:

> What environmental interventions can increase levels of physical activity amongst the general population as part of daily life?

Both policy and research communities now recognize that strategies that focus on changing physical activity of individuals are unlikely to achieve the necessary population-wide impact to yield major health benefits. Policy and environmental measures are required to create the necessary conditions for behaviour change. However, what constitutes effective and cost-effective environmental measures for increasing levels of physical activity is uncertain.

In particular the development of this guidance highlights:

- the need for conceptual understanding of how the environment influences patterns of physical activity and what constitutes 'interventions'—modifications of the environment that can increase physical activity;

- the underdeveloped and variable nature of the evidence on the effectiveness and cost-effectiveness of 'environmental modifications' in increasing physical activity; and

◆ the potential for use of multi-sectoral governance mechanisms as levers for implementing evidence-based guidance on promoting environmental change.

This chapter first sets out the context in England for the development of guidance (low levels of physical activity and policy targets for improvements). We then document the principal NICE processes and methods involved in the development of the guidance: establishing a conceptual framework, identifying and synthesis of the best available evidence, developing and testing of recommendations, and facilitating implementation of the guidance. The lessons and implications are then considered.

The context for development of guidance

Trends in physical activity in England

In England, it is clear that the majority of the population are not currently active at a level to provide the general health benefits of physical activity. Figures from the Health Survey for England (HSE) suggest that around 65% of men and 75% of women do not achieve at least five episodes of at least moderate activity a week, the level advised by the CMO as the minimum for health benefits (Department of Health 2004).

Physical activity is a complex measure incorporating duration, frequency, and intensity, and trends over time are more difficult to discern precisely. The CMO report 'at least five times a week' notes that:

> Overall it appears that, over the past 20 or 30 years, there has been a decrease in physical activity as part of daily routines in England, but a small increase in the proportion of people taking physical activity for leisure. The overall reduction in population activity levels partly reflects other changes that have taken place in society. For example, compared with 30–40 years ago there are fewer manual jobs, and the physically active elements of housework, shopping and other necessary activities have diminished substantially in western society

> (Department of Health 2004)

The nature of the relationship between physical activity and social circumstances is somewhat complicated. Analysis has shown a clear gradient in the prevalence of low activity levels across the income quintiles for both men and women—with those in the lowest income quintile more likely to be in the low participation group than those in the highest income quintile (Information Centre 2008). For those who are more active, (meeting the recommendations for physical activity), a gradient exists for men but this is less clear for women.

It is clear that some areas and some people are more disadvantaged by poor or degraded environmental conditions than others (Social Exclusion Unit 2002). Exposure to dangerous roads in part explains the substantial difference in pedestrian injury and death rates between social classes. More than one quarter of child pedestrian injuries happen in the most deprived tenth of wards (Millward et al 2003). Some people, for instance those who are partially sighted, older people with mobility difficulties, or those encumbered with shopping or children are more likely to find environments challenging and to find routine physical activity less easy to incorporate into daily life.

Routine activity, including walking and cycling, are important sources of physical activity. Walking has been described as a 'near perfect' exercise:

> It is the most natural activity and the only sustained dynamic aerobic exercise that is common to everyone except for the seriously disabled or very frail . . . Unlike so much physical activity, there is little, if any, decline in middle age. It is a year-round, readily repeatable self-reinforcing habit-forming activity and the main option for increasing physical activity in sedentary populations

> (Morris and Hardman 1997)

In recent decades, levels of both walking and cycling have declined. Between 1975/76 and 2005 walking has declined from an average of 248 to 169 miles per person per year (Department for Transport 2007). Cycling for transport is now restricted in England to a relatively small section of the population. Bicycle use fell dramatically between the 1950s and 1970s, principally due to a reduction in numbers of regular cyclists rather than a reduction in distance travelled by cyclists. The change in walking seems not as dramatic as the change in cycling, but as a core human activity may be even more significant.

Policy context: physical activity as a cross-cutting issue

In responding to these trends, the promotion of physical activity has become an important focus of UK health policy over the last decade, in common with many other industrialized countries. This policy concern has been given impetus by the rising levels of obesity and predictions of the future health burden and costs to society associated with sedentary lifestyles.

The two Treasury-led reports on public health (Wanless 2003, 2004) indicated that major increases in levels of physical activity were central to future health gains in England.

Increasing the level of physical activity in the population was designated one of the six overarching priorities of the public health White Paper, *Choosing health: making healthy choices easier* (Department of Health 2004). The subsequent action plan, *Choosing Activity:* (2005), stated that a 'culture shift' was needed if physical activity levels in England were to increase; and the plan committed the Government to creating opportunities by 'changing the physical and cultural landscape—and building an environment that supports people in more active lifestyles'. (This environmental focus contrasts with previous national strategies that gave greater emphasis to public education campaigns and behaviour change at the individual level.)

Cross-government policy commitments to promote physical activity are evident in health, community safety, sustainable development, sustainable communities, neighbourhood renewal and social inclusion, 'liveability', and 'urban renaissance and rural revival', and transport (Killoran et al 2006). These commitments are reflected in a number of national targets (as shown in Box 26.1). Certain policy areas have shown an early and explicit commitment to physical activity. For example, the integrated transport White Paper (1998) identified transport as a health determinant, stating 'the way we travel is making us a less healthy nation' (Department for Transport, 1998). In other policy areas physical activity is an implicit or subsidiary outcome, although the potential impact could be significant.

Box 26.1 Examples of national targets (Public Service Agreements): physical activity and the environment

Physical environment of neighbourhoods: liveability

Lead the delivery of cleaner, safer, and greener public spaces and improvement of the quality of the built environment in deprived areas and across the country, with measurable improvement by 2008 (Department of Communities and Local Government).

By 2010–11, the ten largest urban areas will meet the congestion targets set in their Local Transport Plan relating to movement on main roads into city centres (Department for Transport).

Reduce the number of people killed or seriously injured in Great Britain in road accidents by 40% and the number of children killed or seriously injured by 50%, by 2010 compared with the average for 1994–98, tackling the significantly higher incidence in disadvantaged communities (Department for Transport).

Social environment: community safety and cohesion

Increase voluntary and community engagement, especially amongst those at risk of social exclusion (Home Office).

Health

Halt the year-on-year rise in obesity among children under 11 by 2010 in the context of a broader strategy to tackle obesity in the population as a whole. (DfES/Department of Health/Department of Culture, Media and Sport)

Access to facilities for sport

By 2008, increase the take-up of cultural and sporting opportunities by adults and young people aged 16 and above from priority groups by: increasing the number who participate in active sports at least twelve times a year, by 3%, and increasing the number who engage in at least 30 minutes of moderate intensity level sport at least three times a week, by 3% (Department of Communities and Local Government)

Most recently the Foresight report (2008) on obesity used the term 'passive obesity' to emphasize that the rise in obesity levels is primarily due to the 'obesogenic environments' created by modern industrialized society. Social and physical environments have produced patterns of living characterized by an excess energy balance (Government Office for Science 2008).

The Foresight report highlighted the opportunities for promoting physical activity through alignment to other related policy priorities. But the report also emphasized the policy tensions and contradictions that act as barriers to change. For example, interventions to promote cycling and walking may be offset by policies supporting road building and car usage. In many respects cross-government policies have been advanced despite the limited available evidence on their impact on physical activity. However, in the context of competing political interests, sustained investment in environmental measures at the scale that can impact on the whole population physical activity levels will require evidence-based arguments.

Conceptual perspectives on promotion of physical activity

Handy (2004) and others have commented that there is no consensus on a theoretical framework for understanding the influence of environmental factors on physical activity, and the potential for intervening to increase levels of physical activity. While much attention has been given to advancing theories of behaviour change at an individual level, it is clear that a broader perspective is required to understand the relationships between environment and individual physical activity. For example, King emphasizes the need to draw on a wider range of theories in order to understand how personal activity-related choices and decisions are shaped by the social and physical environments and policies operating at the meso and macro levels (King et al 2002).

An ecological approach has been advocated by a number of researchers as an overarching framework; bringing together behavioural theories and ecological principles and recognizing the interactions of physical and social influences with individual choices and actions (eg Stokols 1996; Owen et al 2004). The aim is to define the complexity of these relationships and possible pathways between environmental factors and patterns of physical activity. These pathways provide the rationale for design of interventions that modify these environmental factors in ways that can increase physical activity (eg Sallis 2001; Sallis et al 2004; Frank et al 2006). There is supporting evidence from observational studies that suggests for example how neighbourhood characteristics can affect patterns of physical activity, independent of individual-level factors. The ecological perspective has also been applied to encompass the links to obesity. For example, the International Obesity Task Force has set out a model that defines factors operating at different levels: global, national, regional, community, and individual (Kumanyika et al 2002).

A logic model for physical activity guidance development

The scoping stage of guidance development was informed by a conceptual map (logic model) of possible intervention options for increasing levels of physical activity, and specifically modifications of the environment.

This logic model (Figure 26.1) sets out the assumed links between the policies, local plans, and interventions and desired outcomes. It shows possible pathways between the different interventions at macro (policy), meso (settings) and personal levels and impact on individuals' decisions about physical activity and health and other related outcomes. It attempts to operationalize the conceptual thinking discussed above.

A range of factors drives national policies that are designed, *either implicitly or explicitly* to impact on physical activity and health. At regional and local levels, various governance mechanisms operate to promote implementation of government policies. Local strategic

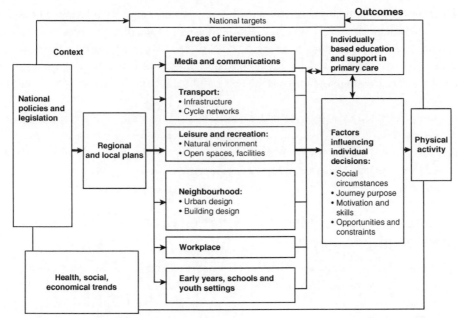

Fig. 26.1 Physical activity framework—logic model

partnerships (LSPs) and local area agreements (LAAs), are mechanisms that bring together local agencies from the public and other sectors to work on achieving national targets (Box 26.1) and local priorities.

Planned changes in the environment aim to create opportunities for physical activity as part of everyday life, and/or remove perceived or actual barriers to physical activity. A 'review of reviews' of environmental correlates of physical activity and walking showed what aspects of the environment are important in influencing physical activity and walking (Bauman and Bull 2007[1]). It showed consistent associations between access to physical activity facilities, convenient and proximate access to destinations, high residential density, land use and urban 'walkability' scores. There were also consistent associations between perceived safety, exercise equipment, pavement, and physical activity participation. There were less clear associations for aesthetic features of the environment, parks, and perceived crime. For children the most consistent associations were for the provision of pavements, destinations for walking, and low road traffic hazards, and also aspects of the recreation infrastructure (access to parks, playgrounds, and recreation areas).

The groups of interventions shown in Figure 26.1 are illustrative. Interventions involving environmental modification operate at different levels and within different settings. For example, at a policy level, zoning and land use regulations influence densities and mix of different functions and services, and leisure and recreation settings can provide access to open spaces and natural environments.

---

[1] Review commissioned by NICE to inform the development of the guidance.

The model also shows that important feedback loops operate. The interdependence of the decisions people make, for example about choice of mode of travel, means that such decisions have the potential to generate positive or negative externalities. One person's decision to drive to work or school may contribute to creating an adverse environment for active travel and therefore influence the probability that another person will decide to ride a bike.

It should be noted that the governance mechanism (including performance management systems) described above, offer important 'points of leverage' at macro, meso, and micro levels for securing environmental changes. National targets related directly or indirectly to physical activity (Box 26.1) act as incentives to local government and other local agencies, to take action through their Local Area Agreements (LAAs).

The best available evidence on what environmental changes impact on physical activity

NICE commissioned a series of reviews of evidence of effectiveness, to inform the development of the recommendations of the independent advisory group of experts. These reviews were carried out by NICE's Public Health Collaborating Centre (CC) for Physical Activity. The Collaborating Centre was an alliance between the British Heart Foundation Health Promotion Research Group (University of Oxford) and the British Heart Foundation National Centre for Physical Activity and Health (Loughborough University).

The effectiveness reviews covered five topics (highlighted in the logic model):

+ policy;
+ transport;
+ urban planning;
+ the built environment; and
+ the natural environment.

Extensive searches of databases, reference lists, and websites were carried out. In addition, experts in each topic area were used to 'fast track' the identification of the most relevant and significant material. Over all the five review areas, approximately 95,000 references were identified. The vast majority of these were not suitable for inclusion, and only 54 were finally included. It is important to note that of these 54 studies, 28 were identified through experts. This emphasizes the crucial element of involving experts in the identification of evidence in topics beyond the traditional public health fields of research.

For the purposes of the reviews it was agreed to focus primarily on studies which involved a change to the physical environment and an attempt to measure a dimension of physical activity and to ascribe this to the change. It was likely that few experimental studies (randomized controlled trials) would be available to provide evidence on the effect of environmental changes, given the difficulties of applying this design to complex interventions. The minimum requirements were, therefore, specification of an intervention which produced a change to the physical environment, and measurement of at least one outcome relating to physical activity. This outcome had to take the form of a measured behaviour, such as walking or cycling or an indication of a population level of activity such as modal transport share. Outcomes such as attitudes to physical activity or intentions were not included. For the policy review this was extended to the need for a policy change to be identified which had led to environmental modifications which in turn led to a measure of physical activity (Figure 26.2).

Findings of the reviews

Policy review

This review investigated the extent to which public policies on the environment, at either national or local level can influence changes in physical activity. Three studies met the inclusion criteria. These studies were cross-sectional post-only designs that described the implementation of policies and related this to levels of physical activity.

Pucher and Dijkstra (2003) is an example of one of the studies. It examined the relationship between national transport policies in the USA, Germany, and the Netherlands and levels of walking and cycling. Policies adopted in Germany and the Netherlands were characterized by better facilities for walking and cycling, traffic calming in residential neighbourhoods, and urban design orientated to people with restrictions on motor vehicle use. National travel data showed corresponding increases in levels of walking and cycling.

This review concluded that the studies suggest an association between specific national policies and levels of walking and cycling (measures related to environmental improvements, transport policies, and spatial planning).

Transport review

The transport review considered studies of all designs that assessed an intervention that related to modifying the transport environment and that had as an outcome of walking or cycling, rates or modal share. 26 studies met these criteria. The review noted that the

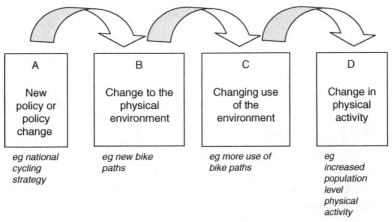

Fig. 26.2 Review of policy impact on physical activity
Source: Physical activity and the environment. Review Four: Policy (Cavill, Foster and Bull 2007, 10)

limited number of studies considering walking or cycling in part reflected the historical interest of transport professionals in motorized transport as the 'dominant and normative' form of travel. Six categories of transport interventions were identified:

+ traffic calming;

+ multi-use trails;

+ closing or restricting use of roads;

+ road user charging;

+ cycle infrastructure; and

+ safe routes to school.

The evidence suggested that these approaches could result in increases in physical activity.

Urban planning review

The review included studies that assessed the effect of an intervention involving a modification of the urban environment and used intervention study designs. Thirteen studies met these criteria. Most studies in these disciplines are 'natural experiments'; the use of controlled research designs is rare (and mostly impractical) and causality is consequently difficult to demonstrate.

The evidence suggested that changes in the urban infrastructure at street level could lead to increased levels of pedestrian activity. The evidence also suggested that other outcomes such as perceptions of safety and fear of crime and perceptions of attractiveness and pollution can be positively changed as a result of street level changes. Changes in the composition of the built environment at the community level (modification, upgrading, or redesign of features) can also have a positive impact on levels of walking and cycling. Studies of development and use of recreational spaces (trails, parks, and broadwalks) indicated a positive impact on levels of physical activity).

Building design review

This review examined interventions which change the design or amenities of buildings and the associated impact on levels of physical activity. Ten studies were included and covered four settings: workplaces, stair wells, school playgrounds, and school classrooms.

Overall, the evidence in workplaces, stairwells, and school playgrounds suggested that there were opportunities to increase physical activity. There was insufficient evidence in school classrooms to make any overall conclusions about effectiveness. In the studies looking at workplaces, it was interesting to note that none considered the effect of provision of facilities such as changing rooms or cycle storage.

Natural environment review

Only two studies were included in the review examining the effect of an intervention that involved a physical modification to the natural environment. The review concluded that there was insufficient evidence to draw conclusions about the effect on physical activity of interventions in these settings.

Quality of the evidence: what is the 'best available'?

The findings of the five reviews clearly raise questions about what constitutes appropriate evidence for judging the effectiveness of environmental interventions in increasing levels of physical activity. The available evidence varied in type and quality. The studies on school playgrounds included those with the highest overall 'quality assessment' score. These included randomization and objective measurement of heart rate using monitors, and were conducted by public health professionals. Although not without its challenges, it is more feasible to design and carry out controlled 'experiments' in a school environment than in a broader environmental setting (such as a street environment). It is clearly more difficult to evaluate the impact of complex and diffuse interventions involving urban design and transport infrastructure using randomized controlled trials. Consequently, the review findings were reliant on evidence from evaluations that observed changes in a less than controlled, experimental setting.

Overall, a range of methodological issues made it difficult to ascertain to what extent the interventions under examination were responsible for the observed changes in physical activity. In particular:

- less than 20% of studies used a comparison group;
- a substantial number of studies (35) only measured physical activity levels after an intervention;
- only a minority used an appropriate, overall measure of physical activity;
- follow-up was often short (at around eight weeks);
- few studies took into account any other factors that might have led to the results;
- most studies did not account for the fact that the intervention may have only had an impact on groups that were already active—and may not have affected the population as a whole; and
- changes in physical activity levels (an increase or decrease) were often an unintended outcome of the interventions studied and were not usually the main focus of evaluation which were sometimes more interested in traffic congestion or use of motor vehicles.

Furthermore, the economic analysis of environmental interventions posed a number of distinct difficulties. The established technique to assess cost-effectiveness of health-related interventions is to calculate a cost per quality adjusted life year (QALY), and this is the technique generally adopted by NICE. However, other professionals use different methods to value their activities. Transport professionals, for instance, rely on cost–benefit analyses. As this work crossed both professional areas it was judged appropriate to use both techniques to provide information in terms that the relevant professional groups would find familiar. The cost-effectiveness of specific environmental interventions that increased physical activity was therefore assessed using both cost–benefit analysis, (the method favoured by the transport sector), and cost–utility analysis (as traditionally undertaken by NICE).

Environmental interventions such as cycling infrastructure were found to have very favourable cost–benefit ratios (1:11) and incremental cost-effective ratios below the upper bound of the threshold used by NICE (£30,000 per QALY) to judge cost-effectiveness (Beale, Bending, and Trueman 2007).

However, it is debatable how much of the cost should be attributable to the health benefits accrued from increased physical activity, as often the main aim of the environmental interventions considered was not to increase physical activity, but rather to, for example, reduce accidents or congestions.

In addition, there are problems relating to comparability. The NICE approach requires that benefits are measured using a cost–utility analysis whereas other sectors of the economy tend to use cost–benefit analysis. This makes it difficult to compare, say, the valuation of a road death avoided with a QALY. Ideally, when estimating public health benefits all sectors of the economy should use common methods for attributing costs and valuing benefits. This would allow decision makers to prioritize interventions that cut across multiple sectors.

Making the recommendations

The recommendations are set out in Table 26.1. The Committee took account of strength and quality of the evidence provided by reviews and the economic modelling in making their recommendations, but also considered a number of other issues. The Committee acknowledged the range of economic, social, cultural, and environmental factors that influence physical activity levels and that the overall impact of changes in these may be synergistic rather than simply cumulative. It also recognized that the multiple players involved—the many organizations that own, manage, or otherwise influence the space used routinely by the public and so can influence people's ability to be physically active. These include public sector landowners and managers (such as local authorities, the education sector, and the NHS) as well as private, voluntary, and non-governmental organizations. Specific issues relating to equity were highlighted; it would be important to pay particular attention to the needs of people whose mobility is impaired. This included the needs of people with physical disabilities (including wheelchair users), frail older people, and parents or carers with small children. This was important, not only to ensure these groups benefit directly, but to get the largest possible increase in physical activity levels across the population as a whole.

The Committee also considered the gaps in the current evidence base and made two research recommendations (see Table 26.2).

Testing guidance and supporting implementation

Implementation of the guidance will be dependent on its integration within the local planning, management, and performance management processes (as shown in the logic model), especially within processes of spatial planning and urban design. Consequently, the fieldwork stage of the guidance development was used to test with key professional groups whether and how the guidance could be used within this local planning context. The fieldwork involved use of qualitative methods; a combination of focus groups and

Table 26.1 Physical activity and environment recommendations

Recommendation	Who should take action	What action should be taken
Recommendation 1: Strategies, policies, and plans	Those responsible for all strategies, policies, and plans involving changes to the physical environment: development, modification and maintenance of towns, urban extensions, major regeneration projects, and transport infrastructure.	◆ Involve all local communities and experts at all stages of the development. ◆ Ensure planning applications for new developments always prioritize the need for people to be physically active as a routine part of their daily life. ◆ Assess in advance what impact the proposals are likely to have on physical activity levels.
Recommendations 2 and 3: Transport	Those responsible for all strategies, policies and plans involving changes to the physical environment: including local transport authorities, transport planners, regional and local authorities.	◆ Ensure pedestrians, cyclists, and users of other modes of transport that involve physical activity are given the highest priority when developing or maintaining streets and roads. ◆ Plan and provide a comprehensive network for walking, cycling, and using other modes of transport involving physical activity.
Recommendation 4: Public open spaces	Designers and managers of public open spaces, paths and rights of way.Panning and transport agencies including regional and local authorities.	◆ Ensure public open spaces and public paths can be reached on foot, by bicycle, and using other modes of transport involving physical activity. ◆ Ensure public open spaces and public paths are maintained to a high standard.
Recommendation 5 and 6: Buildings	Architects, designers, developers, employers, and planners	◆ Those involved with campus sites, including hospitals and universities, should ensure different parts of the site are linked by appropriate walking and cycling routes. ◆ Ensure new workplaces are linked to walking and cycling networks.
	Architects, designers, and facility managers who are responsible for public buildings including workplaces and schools.	◆ During building design or refurbishment, ensure staircases are designed and positioned to encourage people to use them. ◆ Ensure staircases are clearly signposted and attractive to use.
Recommendation 7: Schools	Children's services, School Sport Partnerships, school governing bodies, and head teachers.	◆ Ensure school playgrounds are designed to encourage varied physically active play. ◆ Primary schools should create areas to promote individual and group physical activities.

Table 26.2 Physical activity and environment research recommendations

Recommendation	Who should take action?	What action should they take?
Recommendation 1	Research councils, research commissioners, and funders.	Fund studies, based on the most rigorous designs possible, to examine the impact that changes to the physical environment have on physical activity levels. Develop theoretical frameworks and methodologies for evaluating the economic benefits of environmental change to encourage physical activity. Develop reliable and valid impact assessment methods that can identify changes in physical activity levels resulting from changes to the physical environment.
Recommendation 2	Research councils, research commissioners, funders, and researchers.	Ensure public health outcomes can be identified and attributed as a standard part of research into the links between changes to the physical environment and physical activity levels. Consider the impact of environmental change on health inequalities: how it affects people's physical activity levels according to, for instance, their socio-economic status, age, gender, disability, ethnicity, religion, and sexual orientation. Examine the relative contribution of environmental factors and personal characteristics to variations in physical activity levels.

one–to-one interviews with 79 professionals (architects, transport planners, planners, and developers as well as public health specialists).

The findings revealed that although the recommendations were viewed as relevant there were real barriers to their implementation locally. The guidance provided the 'health rationale' for the work of transport planners, developers, and architects. It provided the weight as 'evidence-based health endorsement' of areas of existing guidance documents. However, professionals stated that the guidance would need to be made obligatory within a number of key policy guidance documents (Local Transport Plan, Local Development Frameworks, regional spatial strategies, planning guidance for transport, open space, sport and recreation). Furthermore, it was important to recognize that the arena of local planning involved competing interests and there were tensions between different areas of policy. For example, the recommendation on stairs potentially conflicted with existing guidance (building and health and safety legislation and the Disability Discrimination Act).

Despite these concerns, the professionals involved in the fieldwork viewed the guidance as a potential catalyst for discussion of active travel within the local multi-sectoral planning and decision-making processes. In response, NICE sought to actively facilitate this process through development of a number of practical support tools, including a 'checklist for health overview and scrutiny committees'. Overview and Scrutiny Committees of local authorities have the statutory power to promote the well-being of local communities through effective scrutiny of health care planning and delivery and wider health and social care issues. The guide aimed to help these Committees to scrutinize compliance of local processes and plans with the guidance on physical activity and environment. This was prepared in collaboration with the local authority support agency—the Centre for Public Scrutiny. This guide provided local politicians with a checklist of questions that could be used to assess whether the NICE recommendations were being adopted within joint community strategies, access plans, and local area agreements. For example, politicians could check whether planning applications for new developments gave priority to the need for people to be physically active as a routine part of their daily life. They could check whether measures had been introduced to give priority to walkers and cyclists (pavement widening, cycle lanes, road-user charging schemes, traffic-calming schemes, and safe routes to schools) and whether playgrounds were designed to encourage varied, physically active play.

Summary

Both policy and research communities now acknowledge the need to redesign and recreate environments that enable people to be physically active as part of their daily lives. Physical activity has been 'engineered out' not as a deliberate policy but as an unintended consequence of urbanization and development over decades. In the UK there has been increasing acceptance across government of the links between the environment and physical activity, (although commitments to environmental changes may be primarily driven by other policy goals). Rather than being evidence-based, policy development has been ahead of the evidence.

The development of this NICE guidance demonstrates the limited nature of the evidence on the effectiveness and cost-effectiveness of environmental changes. It raises a number of issues about what constitute environmental interventions and the best available evidence on effectiveness, and how evidence-based guidance can be used to inform actions designed to increase levels of physical activity.

The use of a 'conceptual framework' proved valuable in making explicit what environmental features (and modifications) can in principle shape individuals' attitudes, experiences, and decisions and that can yield public health outcomes. It also helped identify priority areas for review of evidence. Furthermore, it defined the context for implementing the guidance, within local governance and planning systems. Achieving change in relation to these factors requires action on the part of many players, many of whom have interests other than the health of the population as their prime concern. Identifying the relevant professional groups and developing an understanding of their motivations is important in achieving political support for change.

A multidisciplinary approach to research and evaluation in this area is urged (Handy 2004; Sallis et al 2004). The development of the guidance involved investigating what types of evidence and methods would be most appropriate for determining the effectiveness of 'upstream' interventions, (and testing the theoretical links). While experimental evaluation designs are the 'normal' gold standard for establishing effectiveness (based on randomized controlled studies) such designs are clearly difficult to apply to environmental interventions. Much of the research in transport, planning, and environmental literature comprised correlates: where outcomes are related to changes implemented these are frequently before and after measures at a limited number of sites. We relied on the small number of these observation studies (discussed above) as the best available evidence. Future evaluation research needs to be based on an explicit conceptual framework that recognizes environmental influences on physical activity if evidence gaps are to be filled.

Changes in the environment have by their nature a wider constituency of political and professional groupings involved in their effective implementation. These groups also have their own methods of assessing activities and of ascribing value to outcomes. It is not appropriate to assume that a health outcome is a suitable marker for these groups and reliance on an economic case that speaks only to those interested in comparisons with other health interventions would be unlikely to achieve the best outcomes.

Gaining the acceptance and commitment of this broad constituency is a key challenge to understanding the nature of 'upstream' factors and to the development and implementation of successful solutions that are 'win–wins'—yield both health and goals of 'sustainable communities'. Guidance must have resonance with these broader perspectives. This process will require creative thinking on the part of those involved in considering problems, such as funders and researchers, on the part of those involved in assembling and developing guidance and on the part of those implementing proposed changes. This will be based on an acceptance that we are dealing with complex, dynamic systems with many participants in which a variety of approaches to assess the changes are needed.

Acknowledgements

The guidance was produced by the NICE technical team following meetings of the Programme Development Group, an independent committee brought together specifically for the production of this guidance. The Chair was Professor Nanette Mutrie. Full membership of the group is given in the published guidance available at <http://www.nice.org.uk/Guidance/PH8/Guidance/pdf/English>. The reviews of effectiveness were carried out by the physical activity collaborating centre, an alliance between the British Heart Foundation Health Promotion Research Group [University of Oxford] and the British Heart Foundation National Centre for Physical Activity and Health [Loughborough University]. Reviews of literature relating to cost-effectiveness and the economic modelling work were carried out by the York Health Economics Consortium. This guidance can be accessed at: <http://guidance.nice.org.uk.PH8>.

Bibliography

Bauman A and Bull F (2007) *Expert report: Environmental correlates of physical activity and walking in adults and children: a review of reviews.* London: NICE

Beale S, Bending M and Trueman P (2007) *An economic analysis of environmental interventions that promote physical activity.* London: NICE

Beale S, Bending M, Trueman P and Yi Y (2007) *A Rapid review of economic literature related to environmental interventions that increase physical activity levels in the general population*. London: NICE

Booth et al (2001) 'Environmental and societal factors that affect food choice and physical activity. Report of the Working Group of the International Food Information Council 2001' *Nutrition Reviews* 59/3: 21–39

Bull F, Hutton C, Cavill N and Foster C (2007) *Physical activity and the environment review two: urban planning and design review*. London: NICE

Bull F, Hutton C, Cavill N and Foster C (2007) *Physical activity and the environment review five: building design review*. London: NICE

Buxton KE, Carr RE, Bull F, Cavill N and Foster C (2007) *Physical activity and the environment review three: natural environment review*. London: NICE

Cavill N, Foster C and Bull F (2007) *Physical activity and the environment review four: policy review*. London: NICE

Davis A, Foster C, Cavill N, Buxton KE and Bull F (2007) *Physical activity and the environment review one: transport review*. London: NICE

Department for Transport (2007) *National travel survey 2006*. London: Department for Transport

Department of Health (2004) *At least five a week: evidence on the impact of physical activity and its relationship to health*. London: Department of Health

Department of Health (2004) *Choosing Health*. London: Department of Health

Frank LD, Sallis JF, Conway TL, Chapman JE, Saelens BE, Bachman W (2006) 'Many Pathways from Land Use to Health: Associations between Neighborhood Walkability and Active Transportation, Body Mass Index, and Air Quality' *Journal of the American Planning Association* 72: 1

Government Office for Science (2008) *Tackling Obesities: Future Choices*. Foresight Project Report. London: Government Office for Science

Handy S (2004) *Critical Assessment of the Literature on the Relationships among Transportation, Land Use and Physical Activity*. Prepared for the Transportation Research Board and the Institute of Medicine Committee on Physical Activity, Health, Transportation, and Land Use. Washington DC, USA

Information Centre (2008) *Statistics on Obesity, Physical Activity and Diet: England*. London: Information Centre

Information Centre for Health and Social Care (2002, 2004, and 2006) *Health Survey for England*. London: TSO

Killoran A, Doyle N, Waller S, Wohlgemuth C, Crombie H (2006) *Transport interventions promoting safe cycling and walking: evidence briefing*. London: NICE

King AC et al (2002) 'Theoretical approaches to the promotion of physical activity' *Am J Prev Med* 23/2S: 15–25

Kumanyika S, Jeffrey RW, Morabia A, Ritenbaugh C, Antipastis V (2002) 'Public health approaches to the prevention of obesity. Working Group of the International Obesity Task Force. Obesity prevention: the case for action' *Int J Obes* 26: 425–36

Millward LM, Morgan A, Kelly MP (2003) *Prevention and reduction of accidental injury in children and older people: evidence briefing*. London: Health Development Agency

Morris JN, Hardman AE (1997) 'Walking to health' *Sports Medicine* 23: 306–32

Petersen S, Mockford C, Rayner M (1999) *Coronary heart disease statistics*. London: BHF

NICE (2009) *Methods for development of NICE public health guidance*. London: NICE. Available at: <http://www.nice.org.uk/phmethods>

Owen N, Humpel N, Leslie E, Bauman A, Sallis JF (2004) 'Understanding environmental influences on walking: Review and research agenda' *American Journal of Preventive Medicine* 27/1: 67–76

Pucher J and Dijkstra L (2003) 'Public health matters. Promoting safe walking and cycling to improve public health: lessons from the Netherlands and Germany' *American Journal of Public Health* 93: 1509–16

Sallis JF (2001) 'Progress in behavioural research on physical activity' *Ann Behav Med* 23: 77–8

Sallis JF, Frank LD, Saelens BE, Kraft MK (2004) 'Active transportation and physical activity: opportunities for collaboration on transportation and public health research' *Transportation Research* Part A/38: 249–68

Social Exclusion Unit (2003) *Making the connections: final report on transport and social exclusion*. Norwich: TSO

Stokols D (1996) 'Translating social ecological theory into guidelines for community health promotion' *American Journal of Health Promotion* 10/4: 282–98

Wanless D (2004) *Securing good health for the whole population. Final report*. London: HM Treasury

Wanless D (2002) *Securing our future health: taking a long-term view. Final report*. London: HM Treasury

Chapter 27

Developing evidence-based guidance for health technologies: the NICE experience

David Barnett, Andrew Stevens, Meindert Boysen, and Carole Longson

Introduction

The NICE approach to the evaluation of health care technologies has been a source of considerable interest in the UK, within the wider debate about National Health Service funding and resource allocation (eg Steinbrook 2008). In addition our methodological approach has generated substantial international interest with many attempts at emulation by other governments to assure quality and cost-effective use of scarce health care resources.

The NICE approach to appraisal of health care technologies was established in 1999 on the basis of three guiding principles:

- to provide guidance and standards to the NHS based on clinical and cost-effectiveness of methods of treating ill health;

- to resolve uncertainty amongst both health care professionals and patients regarding the best approach to therapy; and consequently

- to minimize inappropriate variation in clinical practice.

In addition there is an overall commitment to encourage innovation in health care but with due regard to cost-effectiveness.

It is important to note that NICE methods and processes for appraisal of health technologies are different from those used for public health guidance. Health technologies are principally individual interventions (most frequently pharmaceuticals), and this chapter provides a distinctive perspective on the assessment of effectiveness and cost-effectiveness that contrasts with the population-based perspective of public health interventions.

The recipients of NICE guidance are primarily clinical professionals, commissioners of health care as well as the patients and carers that use the NHS. However, the 'audience' for NICE guidance is much wider and includes the manufacturers, the media, politicians, the general public, and the international community. It is the interplay between these groups coupled with a funding direction for technologies receiving a positive recommendation from the NICE Technology Appraisal Programme that makes the production of guidance challenging and at times controversial. The evaluation of cost-effectiveness has been of paramount importance within the development of all NICE guidance. It is also the most contentious issue and subject to much criticism from clinical professionals, patients, the health care technologies industry, and the media (see for example Speight and Reaney 2009).

This chapter:

+ provides an overview of the processes and methods used to appraise health care technologies, typically a new drug;

+ illustrates the appraisal of cost-effectiveness of health technologies—using the 'reference case'; and

+ highlights the role of ethical, legal, media, and political influences on the development of health technologies guidance.

Process and methods for health technologies appraisal

The production of all NICE guidance products is based on the following general principles:

+ independent advisory committees develop the guidance, supported by the provision of expert contributions;

+ open and transparent process and decision making;

+ the review of an inclusive evidence base taken from multiple perspectives;

+ extensive consultation with all stakeholders and the general public; and

+ regular review to ensure the most up to date advice.

The methods and process for production of NICE technology guidance, although broadly similar to those used throughout the world (eg the Australian Pharmaceutical Benefits Advisory programme: *PBAC)*, are nevertheless flexible and continually evolving.

Between 2000 and 2004 NICE's appraisal methods were set by the prior and developing experience of academic technology assessment review teams and of the appraisal committee members. These were consolidated in 2004 into NICE's *Guide to the Method of Technology Appraisal.* And this guide was reviewed and revised in 2008 (NICE 2008). This evolution of our methods has taken account of three key factors:

+ academic methodological progress in health technology assessment—for example in methods for dealing with missing data and indirect comparisons, and methods on assessing the merits of making recommendations linked to the need for further evidence generation ie the 'only in research/coverage with evidence' recommendations;

+ increasing committee and evidence review group experience in dealing with ambiguity and uncertainty—which require the appraisal committee to take a view on the relevance and reliability of evidence which is sometimes only indirectly related to the technology or patient group under consideration; and

+ the development of overarching decision rules for appraisal concerning such issues as the law on discrimination, and social value judgements that institutions such as NICE might make (Social Value Judgements 2008). Such value judgements concern for example: whether all life years are of equal value (irrespective of the age at which they are enjoyed, or the productivity of the patient), whether patient choice should ever be allowed to override cost-effectiveness (and therefore displace potentially more cost-effective interventions), and whose costs should be measured in health technology appraisal.

Stakeholders in the appraisals process are drawn from a wide variety of interested parties. National organizations that represent patient or professional interests, as well as manufacturers or sponsors of health technologies, are known as 'consultees' to the process. Apart from being invited to participate in public consultation on the preliminary recommendations of the Appraisal Committee, the consultees are also invited to make evidence submissions, nominate clinical and patient experts (except for the manufacturers of health technologies), and are able to lodge an appeal against the final recommendations of the Appraisal Committee.

The topics for technology appraisals can be suggested through the NICE website and are initially screened against the following five criteria:

1 policy priority as determined by the Department of Health;

2 the specific characteristics of the population affected and the overall burden of disease;

3 the resource impact for the NHS;

4 identified variation in practice, uptake and current usage in the NHS; and

5 the need for timeliness/urgency in providing guidance.

All potential topics for appraisal are then assessed by advisory 'consideration panels' to inform which topics are formally referred to NICE by the Minister of State for Health.

The process of appraising the clinical and cost-effectiveness of health technologies at NICE is broadly comprised of five phases (see Figure 27.1) which may be followed by an appeal from consultees if they have legitimate grounds for contesting the appraisal committee's decision:

1 scoping;

2 evidence submission;

3 evidence assessment/appraisal;

4 appraisal and preliminary recommendations; and

5 consultation and final recommendations.

The scoping stage determines the key question to be addressed in the technology appraisal and secures input from interested parties on the range of issue that should be considered including the population of patients for whom the technology will be used, the comparators, the evidence base for possible subgroups and additional factors relevant for the economic analysis and the fulfilment of NICE's duties for equality of access. This phase predates the final referral from the Department of Health to ensure that the remit and scope of the appraisal are appropriate and fit for purpose.

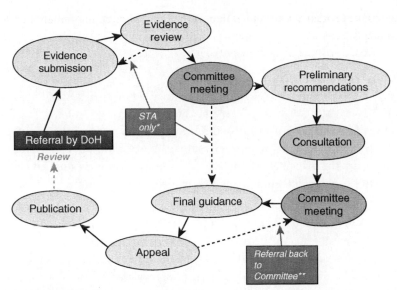

* The STA process allows for
  • a clarification step with the manufacturer between the evidence submission and the evidence review; and
  • bypass of the intermediate consultation period if guidance is recommending the technology without substantial deviation from the licensed indications.
** If an appeal is upheld the appraisal may be referred back to the Committee for further consideration.

Fig. 27.1 NICE technology appraisal process

Evidence is submitted from a variety of sources including the manufacturer of the technology, the relevant clinical specialists, and patient and carer organizations. In addition an independent academic group provide a full systematic review or economic analysis and/or a critique of the manufacturers' evidence submissions.

Evidence assessment/appraisal is undertaken by the Appraisal Committee in a preliminary meeting where expert advisors who have been nominated by the relevant clinical specialists and patient and carer organizations are invited to provide oral views and answer Committee questions.

Final recommendations are made by the Committee following a consultation on its draft recommendations (preliminary Appraisal Consultation Document).

Appeal against the recommendations by consultees is possible after publication of the Committee's final recommendations for guidance on the use of the technology on three possible counts:

1 the Institute has failed to act in accordance with its published processes and that this has been unfair and not allowed full engagement with consultees;

2 the final recommendations do not appropriately and fully reflect the evidence base submitted and thus the Institute has prepared Guidance which is perverse in the light of this evidence; or

3 the Institute has exceeded its powers as for example related to legal directives on human rights and transparency

The appraisal process can be undertaken via two separate mechanisms:

+ multiple technology appraisal (MTA)– in which several technologies for a specific area of health care are considered and the evidence submitted includes an independent systematic review and economic model; or

+ single technology appraisal (STA)—which is focused on the appraisal of single technologies (normally pharmaceuticals) that are for single indications and close to the granting of market authorization and release. For this purpose the manufacturer is considered to be the main repository of the primary supportive evidence base and thus provides the principal submission. This submission is critiqued by an external group but no independent assessment is made nor an alternative economic model provided.

It is important that guidance is issued to the NHS in as timely a fashion as possible to ensure, where appropriate, the uptake of new drug therapies close to the receipt of their marketing authorization for the EU/UK. This has led to establishment of the more rapid STA approach. The STA process may cut the time of initiation of appraisal for publication of the final recommendations to 27–35 weeks from an average of 52 weeks for MTA.

The Appraisal Committee does not normally make recommendations regarding the use of a drug outside the terms of its marketing authorization, as published in the manufacturer's summary of product characteristics unless specifically asked to by the Department of Health. It can, however, consider unlicensed comparator technologies if these are used regularly in the NHS. The Committee is not able to make recommendations on the pricing of technologies to the NHS and also NICE is not able to enter into direct price negotiation. The Committee can consider special schema proposed by the manufacturer that have the effect of reducing the cost-effectiveness of the technology under appraisal by altering the overall acquisition costs such response-rebate schemes as long as they are available nationally throughout the NHS, and are accepted in principle by the Department of Health.

Appraisal of health technologies: the reference case

The aim of health technology appraisal is to decide whether a health care technology, typically a new drug, represents acceptable value for money to the health service. Separate decisions can be made for distinct patient sub groups who may have different base-line risks, or different responses to treatment.

The judgement is based on:

+ clinical effectiveness—that is the judgement as to whether a new technology confers an overall health benefit, taking into account any harmful effects when comparing it with relevant alternative treatment; and

+ cost-effectiveness—that is technologies can be considered to be cost-effective if the health benefits are greater than the *opportunity costs* measured in terms of the health benefits associated with programmes that may be displaced to fund the 'new technology'. (Opportunity costs are the benefits for patients in the NHS which are foregone when paying for the benefits for those patients who may receive a technology of interest)

Cost-effectiveness is calculated as the incremental cost-effectiveness ratio (ICER) of a new technology (A) over what it will replace (B).

$$ICER = \frac{\text{Cost of Technology A} - \text{Cost of Technology B}}{\text{Benefits of Technology A} - \text{Benefits of Technology B}}$$

The definition of a cost-effectiveness threshold has been a source of continuous debate since the inception of NICE in 1999. The current approach to this issue (as detailed in the Technology Appraisal Methods Guide) has been that if the ICER falls below a threshold range currently set as £20,000–£30,000 per quality adjusted life year (QALY) it can be considered acceptable, and if it is above the band it is normally considered not acceptable as a cost-effective use of health care resources for the NHS.

The appraisal committee have some flexibility and are expected to exercise their judgement when considering ICERs within and beyond the threshold range, according to limited criteria as follows:

- the degree of certainty around the ICER, 'in particular the committee will be more cautious about recommending a technology where they are less certain about the ICERs presented';
- the innovative nature of the technology which means specifically that the innovation adds demonstrative and distinctive benefit which may not have been adequately captured in the assessment eg the measures of quality of life;
- some flexibility to give the benefit of the doubt in serious diseases where there are few treatment alternatives; and
- where benefits in terms of quality of life of persons other than the patients (eg carers) may not have been fully captured (eg where the patients are children or disabled and dependent).

Following public consultation (January 2009), the Institute has issued supplementary advice to the Appraisal Committees to be taken into account when appraising treatments which may be life-extending for patients with an otherwise short life expectancy. This has the effect of allowing additional flexibility to the Committee when considering innovative treatments (normally drugs) for which the best available evidence leads to an assessment of the ICER to be in excess of the normally accepted threshold range.

This supplementary advice is to be applied when the treatment is indicated for patients with a short life expectancy (normally less than 24 months) and the treatment offers an extension to life (normally of at least an additional three months). In addition, no alternative treatment with comparable benefits is available through the NHS.

Principally, this additional flexibility is aimed at the consideration of treatments that are licensed or otherwise indicated for small patient populations and for whom the innovative nature of the treatment provides a 'step up' in care not previously available in this group.

In these circumstances the appraisal committee may consider it appropriate to accept an additional weighting of the benefits to patients for life extending treatments at the end of life.

The implementation and impact of this supplementary advice on appraisals guidance will be evaluated by the Institute and amendments made as necessary.

Calculating the ICER

The ICER calculation, although in outline quite simple, is often very complicated. The inputs in terms of both the cost and the benefit sides of the equation can vary greatly with different assumptions, under different conditions, and over different time spans. ICERs for the same condition and the same patient group can also therefore vary considerably according to the assumptions made.

Appraisal deals with this in two ways: firstly by having a *'reference case'* for the estimation of data inputs (see Box 27.1), and secondly by every committee undertaking a process of interrogating the source and justifiability of each input.

Box 27.1 The Reference Case

Broadly the reference case constrains the following parameters such that the:

- *Technology*—is defined in the scope of the appraisal.

- *Population*—is set in the scope of the appraisal, although it is within the committee's brief to decide on plausible subgroups according to clinical logic and the evidence provided.

- *Comparators*—are the technologies most frequently used in the NHS which could be displaced by the technology under appraisal. Alternative comparators could include current best practice, which may not always be the same as technologies most frequently used.

- *Outcomes*—are defined as all health effects on individuals and is based on a systematic review of the evidence base.

- *Health related quality of life*—is that reported by patients and/or carers.

- *Valuation of health related quality of life*—derived from a representative sample of the public and not patients or carers or healthcare professionals.

- *Equity weighting*—is avoided; that is an additional QALY has the same weight regardless of the other characteristics of the individuals receiving the technology

- *Perspective on costs*—is NHS and Personal Social Services normally funded by the health service.

- *Cost information*—is based on published cost analyses or recognized publicly available databases or price lists and should be based on those nationally available throughout the NHS.

- *Discount rate*—is an annual rate of 3.5% for both costs and health effects.

- *Time horizon*—needs to be sufficiently long to reflect all important differences in costs or outcomes between the technologies being compared: this is normally considered to be a 'lifetime' horizon.

The reference case offers considerable scope for interpretation and compilation of data, and is not obligatory where a case can be argued to tackle a parameter in a different way. The assessment group and the committee therefore have a crucial role in interrogating every variable.

The importance of carefully interrogating the assumptions that feed a health technology assessment can be illustrated with a simple hypothetical example.

Table 27.1 sets out an illustration for a new technology (in this case a chemotherapeutic agent for cancer treatment) with an optimistic versus a realistic view of the parameters that would be considered in the appraisal.

The principal parameters in the example are:

- the time the patient is in a disease progression free state (PFS);
- the time they are in a deteriorating state during disease progression (PPS);
- the utility values estimated for both these states;
- the values estimated for side effects; and
- the various costs including drug cost and other treatment costs eg for side effects as well as the costs of best supportive care after progression.

The realistic and an optimistic ICER for Drug A compared to Drug B can be calculated by dividing costs (£s) by benefits (QALYs) as follows:

$$\text{Realistic} \quad \frac{12+2+4-4+2+4}{0.4+0.25-0.1-0.31+0.25-0.1} = \text{£89,000 per QALY}$$

$$\text{Optimistic} \quad \frac{12+4-4+3+4}{0.4+0.25-0.28+0.21-0.1} = \text{£19,000 per QALY}$$

Clearly the difference between the £89,000 calculated for the realistic ICER and the £19,000 calculated for the optimistic ICER is very important, given a threshold band of £20,000 to £30,000 per QALY; but it is not always straightforward to identify, particularly if only the optimistic parameter values have been submitted for appraisal.

Table 27.1 Hypothetical realistic and optimistic appraisal parameters (Drug A is the new technology and Drug B the main comparator)

States	PFS	PPS	Side effects (disutility)	Drug cost (£k)	Other costs (£k)	PPS cost (£k)
Utilities	0.8	0.5				
Realistic						
Drug A	26 wks	26 wks	0.1	£12k	£2k	£4k
Drug B	20 wks	26 wks	0.1	£4k	£2k	£4k
Optimistic						
Drug A	26 wks	26 wks	0	£12k	£0	£4k
Drug B	18 wks	22 wks	0.1	£4k	£3k	£4k

Appraisals experience has indentified numerous examples of uncertainties around the values associated with different parameters and is illustrative of the crucial role of the appraisal committee in its interrogation of the evidence and analysis.

Some examples are listed below which are taken from NICE's appraisal experience over the last ten years. Each example represents a dilemma concerning the provision of information and/or its interpretation:

1 Inconsistent clinical trial results and the emergence of new data. The emergence of new information either from clinical trials or observational/registry data during the course of an appraisal can be problematic. To avoid bias, there has to be an agreed cut-off point during the evaluation with emerging trials combined with a standard approach to the timing of the review for an appraisal

2 Indirect comparisons in the absence of head to head trials. The rules for using indirect comparison remain a grey area for appraisals. Mixed treatment comparisons have been suggested as a solution where there is RCT evidence that at least links an intervention to comparator through a third strategy eg best supportive care. The appraisal committee has, however, expressed concerns regarding the use of indirect comparisons for a number of reasons including:

   a trials undertaken at different times and in different patient groups are unlikely to be comparable (indeed careful patient selection may be undertaken in a later trial on the basis of what is known from earlier trials);

   b the network of trials which is used in a mixed treatment comparison is open to biased selection; and

   c different networks that can be compiled will generate different results.

The validity of the method crucially depends on objective systematic review and definition of networks, and on the careful scrutiny of the context of different trials undertaken at different times.

3 The estimation of health utility reflecting the quality life in different health states. The paradigm for assessing heath related quality of life for NICE is a two-stage process:

   a the assessment of health care states based on quality of life questionnaires from patients and carers; and

   b valuation of these health states to apportion a utility based on the perspective of the general public ie the 'tax payer'.

Thus the key to making the economic assessment, is the disutilities assigned to living with the condition in the different health states and the sources of this information. This source is preferably based on the primary clinical trials but frequently this data is absent or has not been collected. The alternatives, either assessing the value of quality of life from other disease states and extrapolating it to the condition being considered or the setting up of separate studies based on general public panels who make hypothetical judgements is fraught with difficulty and open to substantial uncertainty and potential bias.

4 Assessing the importance of side effects. It is unusual for any drugs, new or long-standing to be free of side effects. However it takes some time for the evidence of side

effects to accumulate reliably. This tends to discriminate against long-standing treatments in which the evidence has been well documented as opposed to new treatments for which only short-term trial results are available and appraisal has to factor in some allowance for this. When dealing with side effects, differential consideration should be given to those that are perceived by the individual as having an obvious and direct effect on their quality of life (eg alopecia, gastrointestinal disturbance, severe skin reactions) versus those that may not immediately effect the individual unless extreme (eg bone marrow suppression). A particularly unusual situation, however, is where a new treatment is accompanied not just by adverse side effects, but by beneficial ones too. An example is the drug raloxifene, licensed for the treatment of post-menopausal osteoporosis. A significant proportion of women in the raloxifene arm of the pivotal clinical trial had been shown to have lower incidence of breast cancer than in the control arm. Raloxifene has, however, not been licensed for breast cancer prevention, only for osteoporosis. Logic dictates that if negative side effects are factored into an ICER calculation so should positive ones. In the case of raloxifene, however, the positive 'side effect' dwarfed its benefits in the prevention of osteoporosis.

5 Choosing an appropriate time horizon for cost-effectiveness analysis. Although the reference case is very clear in that the time horizon for the assessment of cost-effectiveness must be sufficient to reflect all costs and all benefits (ie normally a lifetime horizon) the problem for appraisal is that the evidence from clinical trials, trial extensions, or observational data seldom stretches out much beyond a year or two. So, although benefits and costs can be projected indefinitely, the projections are just that; projections and not evidence. The NICE appraisal team is therefore frequently exposed to multiple, different ICER calculations depending on the degree of optimism in the extrapolation of the benefits of the technology. This key dimension in the production of ICERs calculations is therefore very much bound up with whether an objective and plausible case is presented rather than an unjustifiably optimistic one.

External influences on development of health technologies guidance

The Appraisals programme is subject to a range of external pressures that include:

- societal values relating to an individual's perception of 'health' and the availability of health care;
- the need to ensure equality of access to care in the NHS and the special nature of disability;
- medico-legal issues relating to the responsibilities of health care practitioners; and
- the influence of the media and politicians.

Societal values

When developing advice to the NHS, NICE bases its conclusions on the 'best available' evidence. However, this evidence is not always very good and is rarely (if ever) complete.

It may be of poor quality, lack critical elements, or both. Those responsible for formulating the Institute's advice about efficacy, effectiveness, cost-effectiveness, and safety are therefore inevitably required to make judgements both scientific and societal (ie social value judgements). Social value judgements relate to society rather than to basic or clinical science and they take account of ethical principles, preferences, culture, and aspirations that should underpin the nature and extent that society values health and the provision of health care.

The Institute has produced a series of guidelines to describe the social value judgements that should, generally, be incorporated into the processes and methods used to develop and be applied when preparing individual items of NICE guidance (Social Value Judgements 2008). It is recognized, however, that there will be circumstances when—for valid reasons—departures from these general principles are appropriate and for that reason these guidelines are advisory only.

The main principle underlying these judgements is that decisions about whether to recommend interventions should not be based on evidence of their relative costs and benefits alone. NICE must consider other factors when developing its guidance, including the need to distribute health resources in the fairest way within society as a whole. In this context the advisory committees are requested to consider factors that are:

◆ relevant if due to differences in clinical effectiveness, baseline risk or differential benefits/risk (eg age, gender, or sexual orientation); and

◆ relevant to clinical effectiveness (eg ethnic background, self inflicted illness).

In addition specifically recommended to the advisory Committees are:

◆ Social class or societal roles—should not be given any weight, positive or negative

◆ Individual choice—is important but does not override the need to consider clinical and cost-effectiveness and opportunity costs

◆ Disability—should require special note of the needs of disabled people, including obstacles that might prevent them from benefiting from NICE guidance, and consider whether it may be necessary to take positive steps to take account of these needs.

Equality of access to care

Consideration of equality of access to health care must be undertaken during the process of appraisal. This was tested during the Judicial Review of the guidance on the use of drugs for the treatment of Alzheimer's disease. In that case the courts instructed NICE to actively and positively identify those patients for whom the final recommendations were not accessible because of their 'disability'. It was argued that people with learning disabilities and people whose first language was not English would not respond in the same way to the diagnostic instrument used for assessing cognitive functioning which determined access to the drugs, and could therefore be discriminated against (Eisai (and Others) v NICE (2007).Thus in the preparation of appraisal guidance the Committee must demonstrate that it has taken steps to:

◆ eliminate unlawful discrimination ie treating someone less favourably because of their race, sex, religious belief, sexual orientation, or disability unless it can be shown that this recommendation is a 'proportionate means of achieving a legitimate aim'; and

+ promote equality of opportunity among racial groups, between disabled people and other people, and between men and women.

+ take account of the disabilities of disabled people, including consideration of more favourable treatment.

Medico-legal responsibilities of health care practitioners

NICE guidance, specifically appraisals and the link to the associated funding direction, has frequently been accused of inhibiting the freedom of clinicians to judge what is best for their patient and unreasonably restrict the choice of treatments. However, recommendations on the use of health care technologies have always been 'guidance' and not statute. Furthermore, the funding mandate that accompanies the guidance places the onus on commissioners of health care to make funding available for the technology, if appropriate, but does not direct practitioners to slavishly adhere to recommendations which might not be appropriate in individual clinical circumstances.

Hence all NICE technology guidance is published with the following proviso:

> This guidance represents the view of the Institute, which was arrived at after careful consideration of the evidence available. Healthcare professionals are expected to take it fully into account when exercising their clinical judgement. The guidance does not, however, override the individual responsibility of healthcare professionals to make decisions appropriate to the circumstances of the individual patient, in consultation with the patient and/or guardian or carer.

The specific challenges to health care professionals in implementing the guidance relate to circumstances of adherence to and deviation from guidance. Although to date there has not been a legal case where the decision of a clinician *not* to follow NICE guidance has been tested either in court or in front of the General Medical Council health care professionals are advised:

+ to be aware of NICE guidance and to follow it if, in their clinical judgement, to do so would be in the patient's best interest;

+ that it is unlikely that the General Medical Council would make an adverse finding against a doctor if his or her actions are supported by a responsible body of colleagues as per the 'Bolam principle' (ie health professionals who *follow* NICE guidance might be able to count on that fact to help their defence if challenged); and

+ that *deviation* from NICE guidance is not necessarily negligent. However, ignorance of NICE guidance may be a poor defence and a reasoned and reasonable decision to reject the guidance in an individual case should be accompanied by a good contemporaneous record.

The media and politicians

NICE has a very high profile both in the UK and internationally. It is therefore not surprising that the media attention given to our recommendations is very intense. The reports on individual sets of guidance vary from general acceptance to strong criticism.

Some journalists have taken up the cause of individual pressure groups, but for the most part the serious press comment is very supportive of the work of the appraisals programme, recognizing the need to provide unbiased advice on the rational use of the fixed level of resource available to the NHS.

As an 'arm's length body' NICE and the appraisals programme is divorced from political intervention. This is not always how it is perceived by the general or professional audience who receive the guidance. Sometimes political intervention has been presumed when a particularly unpopular recommendation at the consultation stage has been changed to more positive guidance at the final hurdle or when NICE guidance has seemed to be pre-empted by unguarded comments from individual politicians. However, this is not the case. NICE is very careful in preserving its independence from government and our guidance is released directly to the NHS. Indeed, the UK political establishment is overwhelmingly supportive of the Institute's work and, to date, no 'political' intervention has occurred for any of our guidance from either individual politicians or the Department of Health.

The NICE experience of appraising health technologies

Over the first ten years of its existence the success of NICE can be seen in the increasing acceptance both nationally and worldwide of:

- that assessment of cost-effectiveness as well as clinical effectiveness is valid and necessary to inform the rational use of health care resources;
- the importance of rigorous and consistent methodology in the assessment of clinical and cost-effectiveness;
- the need for transparency and clarity in decision making; and
- the need to take into account social as well as scientific value judgements.

The process of appraising the clinical and cost-effectiveness of health care technologies is a complex one which is challenging health care providers worldwide. It is also a dynamic process with the development of new approaches to methodology in part catalysed by this international interest. NICE has sought to learn from and respond to both scientific developments as well as external factors. The substantial interest in the work of NICE and the wish of international health care agencies to emulate in one form or other the processes and methods used in production of guidance is a testament to the success that NICE has had in this process of development.

Bibliography

Eisai (and Others) v *NICE* [2007] EWHC 1941, 10 August 2007. Available at: <http://www.judiciary.gov.uk/judgment_guidance/judgments/index.htm>

National Institute for Health and Clinical Excellence (2008) *Updated guide to the methods of technology appraisal 2008.* London: NICE. Available at <http://www.nice.org.uk>

National Institute for Health and Clinical Excellence (2008) *Social value judgments: principles for the development of NICE guidance.* London: NICE. Available at <http://www.nice.org.uk>

Speight, J and Reaney, M (2009) 'Wouldn't it be NICE to consider patients' views when rationing health care?' *British Medical Journal* 338: b85

Steinbrook, R (2008) 'Saying no isn't NICE—the travails of Britain's National Institute for Health and Clinical Excellence' *N Engl J Med* 359/19: 1977–81

Chapter 28

Supporting implementation of public health guidance: NICE experience

Val Moore, Nick Baillie, Annie Coppel, and Julie Royce

Introduction

The National Institute for Health and Clinical Excellence (NICE) first published public health guidance in March 2006. A series of public health evidence-based guidance covering a diverse range of public health topics have since been published. These topic areas include school-based interventions on alcohol, promoting physical activity in the workplace, community engagement, and maternal and child nutrition. This guidance aims to support national health policy development and implementation. It provides national standards for all those concerned with improving the health and well-being of their local populations—working in local government, health services, and other areas of public, voluntary, and private sectors. The impact of the guidance is clearly dependent on its implementation in policy and practice.

Ensuring that the guidance is relevant and can be implemented in different local contexts is a central concern throughout the process of development of guidance (as discussed in other chapters). For example, local stakeholders are consulted throughout the process, surveys of local practice may be undertaken to inform the guidance, and field testing of the draft guidance highlights both barriers and opportunities for implementation. This chapter however, focuses on the NICE strategy for supporting implementation of *published* guidance and builds on the guidance development process.

This implementation support strategy has sought to take account of the evidence on how to implement guidance effectively, but this evidence base is not well developed, particularly with regard to public health.

Kitson and colleagues (2008) emphasize that guideline implementation (and implementation of evidence more generally) requires whole systems change involving both the individual and organizational levels, and furthermore 'despite growing awareness that getting evidence into practice is a complex, multi-faceted process, there remains a lack of knowledge about what methods and approaches are effective, with whom and in what contexts'.

Greenhalgh and colleagues' systematic review of diffusion of innovations identified a number of important factors that influence the adoption process: the nature of the innovation, characteristics of adopters, modes of diffusion and dissemination, the readiness of the system to assimilate innovation, the structure of the system, the system's ability to adapt to and routinize innovation, and the 'outer' context (Greenhalgh et al 2004).

These two references highlight the range of factors that influence the translation of evidence into local practice and provide a useful summary of a number of key findings of evaluation of implementation processes. NICE has drawn on such evidence, from a number of different literatures (management and organizational change, innovation, and health services research) to establish its principles for supporting implementation. Local ownership and leadership in particular are shown to be vital. Consequently, the key components of NICE's strategy are concerned with helping develop local agencies' own capacity to manage the process of implementing guidance, within the context of the joint planning and performance management processes.

This chapter documents how this is undertaken. It covers:

◆ the local context for improving health and tackling health inequalities and how NICE seeks to use national 'levers' to support local implementation;

◆ the approaches and methods used to provide local support for implementation; and

◆ issues and challenges for future development of NICE's approach to supporting implementation of public health guidance.

Local public health context and national levers for change

As highlighted above, the implementation of NICE guidance is dependent on its integration within the national/local joint planning and performance management systems.

Nationally, targets relating to areas of public health are defined in Public Service Agreements (PSA) for each government department. Locally, primary health trusts and local authorities, and others, are expected to work in partnership to prepare and implement strategies that seek to meet national targets, as well as respond to local concerns. NICE seeks to use the opportunities provided by this system to secure the uptake of guidance. There is currently an important policy debate about the balance between central control and local autonomy, but a centrally determined framework benefits NICE by creating opportunities for influencing local implementation of NICE guidance.

Figure 28.1 sets out in more detail the main elements of this national/local joint planning and performance management system. The diagram provides an overview of the interactions among these various processes.

Locally, the focus for improving health and tackling health inequalities centres on the geographical area of administration of a democratically elected local authority or an NHS primary care trust (PCT). Sometimes these areas coincide and the local authority and PCT are said to be 'coterminous'. However, the areas sometimes overlap but do not coincide and therefore arrangements can be more complicated. At present there are around 380 local authorities in England and Wales and 150 PCTs in England, with upper tier local authorities and PCTs serving populations of around 300,000 on average.

The local authority has a duty to promote the health and well-being of the area, and the PCT and other public sector agencies, such as the police, are obliged to work in

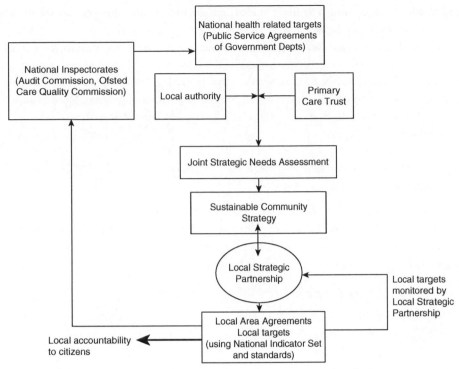

Fig. 28.1 National/local joint planning and performance management system
Adapted from: DCLG (2007) Delivering health and well-being in partnership: The crucial role of the new local performance framework

partnership with it. Local strategic partnerships are the key strategic forum, to fulfil these partnership duties.

The Government's policy for *Strong and prosperous communities* (Department for Communities and Local Government 2006) and the subsequent *Local Government and Public Involvement in Health Act 2007* served to strengthen local authority and PCT collaboration on improving health and well-being and tackling inequalities. PCTs and councils are now required to carry out a joint strategic needs assessment (JSNA) for their area, and NHS partners to participate in agreeing what should be included as *Local Area Agreement* targets in the strategy for the local area (*the Sustainable Communities Strategy*) and to take responsibility for their contribution to meeting them. LAAs are a statutory requirement.

JSNA is described as a 'systematic method for reviewing the health and well-being issues facing a population, leading to agreed commissioning priorities that will improve health and well-being outcomes and reduce inequalities'.

Local authorities and PCTs, and their other partners, are required to use the national indicator set (NIS), derived from the PSAs, to define their own local area agreement (LAA) priorities. The NIS data on progress towards LAA targets, together with established national standards (including NICE standards), are used by national inspectorate bodies (including the Audit Commission and Ofsted) as a major source of evidence on the performance of local agencies and, under the new comprehensive area assessment (CAA), in judgements about improvements in local quality of life collectively achieved by local agencies, and about an area's future prospects.

There is therefore a very clear opportunity to facilitate the implementation of evidence-based public health interventions through these processes and enable the cross sector and cross-organizational boundary working that is needed to deliver on this. The use of evidence-based cost-effective guidance can be seen as enhancing the likelihood of achieving the outcomes aspired to in local plans, and doing it in a manner that represents value for money.

NICE methods and approaches for facilitating and supporting local change

NICE has developed a range of methods and approaches for supporting the implementation of guidance within the local joint planning system—combining a 'consultancy function' with a menu of support tools. This multi-faceted approach is well founded in the literature as the most likely approach to achieving impact.

Field team consultancy

In 2006 NICE established a small field team of 'consultants' with the responsibility for facilitating implementation of NICE guidance, in public health and clinical areas. Their task is to promote the integration of NICE guidance within existing local systems for planning, management, audit, and evaluation of the local strategies for health and well-being (described above). The team's role is at an early stage with respect to public health. Initial experience has raised a number of questions and issues. The local public health context is complex, but in principle there are key 'entry points' for promoting the uptake of guidance—the local strategic partnerships, children's trusts, the performance management process and the scrutiny function. In practice, however, there is substantial variation in the 'robustness' (or stage of development) of the local systems. Although national policy clearly expects local government to deliver against health targets as part of community strategies, their organizational 'readiness' for change is variable. With respect to local authorities, the Healthcare Commission's assessment of their performance in 2006/07 indicated a mixed picture. The local councils that were improving the most had plans that took account of national priorities such as smoking and obesity, and also targeted activity for children and young people. Initiatives that transcended the traditional health agenda were rare, but some councils included health objectives within plans for regeneration, housing, and tackling crime (Healthcare Commission 2008).

The NICE field team, through local visits with key individuals (including Directors of Public Health and Directors of Children's services), are seeking to understand the local public health agenda. The field team is assessing the 'readiness' of local authorities and PCTs to implement NICE evidence-based guidance, and consequently their particular needs for different types of facilitation and support.

The field team role is consistent with the framework, proposed by Kitson and colleagues (2008), for successful implementation of evidence into practice. This conceptualizes the process of evidence implementation as the interplay of evidence, context, and facilitation. 'Appropriate facilitation and the role of the facilitator is dependent on the 'state of preparedness' of the local team in terms of their acceptance and understanding of evidence, the receptivity of their place of work, or context in terms of resources, culture and values, leadership style, and evaluation activity. Facilitators work with individuals and teams to enhance the process of implementation'. The field team's work to date has focused on 'diagnosis' of the local context, as well as helping local managers access a range of tools that are available to help support the local process of guidance implementation (and described below).

Implementation tools for local use

Reviews of implementation evidence commonly recommend that a diagnostic analysis (Effective Healthcare 1999) or work to understand the community context (Fixsen 2005) is undertaken as a first step in the implementation process. NICE provides a number of practical tools alongside the guidance via its website to support this process. A guide on *How to change practice* (NICE 2007) describes processes that can be used to identify barriers to change in different contexts. Implementation advice is published for public health guidance and helps to identify all stakeholders in the particular guidance, levers for change relating to that topic, and national agencies that may be able to provide help and support in different contexts. The *Guide to resources* (NICE 2008a) that accompanies the NICE guidance on physical activity and the environment, for example, highlights further national strategies and policies that can help to support the implementation of this guidance as well as sources of case studies which may help in planning new developments.

Costing of implementation of guidance

The Audit Commission (2005) reviewed the evidence of how health organizations were responding to NICE guidance and found that at the planning stage, organizations were struggling to consider the financial impacts of NICE guidance. NICE therefore now produces a costing tool for each piece of guidance. This allows organizations to calculate their local costs or savings in relation to specific pieces of guidance.

The tools in relation to guidance on smoking cessation in the workplace, for example, support any organization, be it private or public sector, to calculate the long-term savings that are made by implementing this guidance. The tool contains assumptions about the health benefits that can be expected in terms of smoking cessation and offsets the financial implications of this against those of supporting smoking cessation in the workplace. Additionally a forward planner is provided by NICE which highlights all forthcoming guidance and estimates of the likely financial impacts, thus facilitating longer term planning in terms of implementation of NICE guidance.

Proactive dissemination

Active rather than passive dissemination of guidelines is more likely to be effective (Effective Health Care 1994; Lomas 1991; Oxman et al 1995). Methods that have been shown to be more effective include using local opinion leaders (Doumit et al 2007), educational outreach visits (O'Brien et al 2007) and interactive educational meetings.

It is clear that multiple strategies are required for effective dissemination of evidence-based guidance that is targeted to local circumstances (Bero et al 1998; Effective Health Care 1999). In particular, some form of diagnostic analysis (described earlier in this chapter) can help inform the methods of dissemination and implementation (Hamilton et al 2007; Brownson et al 2007) but the quality of the analysis is important (Shaw et al 2005). A key part of the implementation strategy for NICE is therefore making support available to enable local leaders to take more proactive approaches to dissemination and ensure that awareness of the need to change is raised. Presenters' slides are made available to fulfil this function and support educational sessions and proactive methods of dissemination. Coupled with the implementation advice published by NICE identifying the key stakeholders in each piece of guidance, this is a key resource to form the basis of dissemination and implementation plans.

Auditing local changes in practice

Systematic reviews have indicated that the use of audit and feedback has been an effective tool. Jamtvedt and colleagues (2006) point out that the effects may be variable, but can be greatest when 'baseline adherence to recommended practice is low and when feedback is delivered more intensively'. NICE therefore provides audit support for the implementation of some public health guidance where appropriate.

In the development of this support it is acknowledged that traditional clinical audit and feedback may not be the most appropriate approach for the public health context. In response to this, several of the audit support packages have been published as checklists to support the planning process. For example, checklists have been developed to support the implementation of guidance on promoting physical activity for children and young people. Two practical tools aimed at schools and local authorities fulfil the same principles and function as clinical audit by reviewing current practice but have been designed to fit the context and language of public health communities more appropriately.

Strategic commissioning of public health interventions

The commissioning of health services is another process key to improving the health and well-being of communities and individuals and consequently can play an important role in the local implementation of evidence-based public health practice.

In recognition of this NICE now produces commissioning guides and tools across a range of topics to provide both support for the process and a mechanism to introduce evidence-based interventions. The web-based guides comprise a series of text-based web pages that signpost and provide topic-specific information on key clinical and service-related issues to consider during the commissioning process. Each guide contains a commissioning tool, which is an interactive resource that can be used to estimate and inform the level of service needed locally as well as the cost of local commissioning decisions. Topics addressed to date include peer-support programmes for women who breastfeed and smoking cessation prior to elective surgery.

Implementation issues and future developments

NICE's experience including the work conducted by the field team of implementation consultants, with local authorities, is informing the further development of its implementation support strategy. The consultant visits (as described earlier) involved discussions with local authority senior officers responsible for health, elected members involved in Scrutiny Committees, and Directors of Children's Services who have oversight, across all public sectors, of children and young people strategies for each locality. A number of key themes have emerged from this work discussed below.

Box 28.1 Implementation themes

The importance of NICE collaboration with other national organizations to support local authorities

NICE should work with organizations such as Improvement & Development Agency (IDeA), the Local Government Association, and the Social Care Institute that have a designated remit for working with and supporting local authorities.

Promoting the relevance of NICE guidance and methods to local authorities

The rigor of NICE 'evidence-based' guidance is valued. However, the relevance of the different pieces of guidance to local authority concerns and priorities needed to be clearly signalled.

Acceptability and accessibility of NICE guidance to key audiences

NICE guidance is 'NHS branded'; but this is viewed by some as a potential barrier to attracting the recognition and commitment of key decision makers in local authorities, and others beyond the NHS, and the effective uptake of the guidance.

Reaching and targeting of key individuals within local authorities

The intended audience of the guidance is diverse and covers those working at both strategic and operational levels. They include officers, elected councillors, those involved in local strategic partnerships, and those involved with commissioning and scrutiny.

Selection of topics for future public health guidance

The NICE process for selection of future topics seeks to ensure that local authoritiy public health priorities are considered. A range of methods for ensuring local authority views are considered and could be explored.

Strategic relationships

NICE recognizes that to ensure its public health guidance has an impact, it has to build its reputation and credibility in sectors outside the NHS to help sell the benefits. To achieve this, NICE has established strategic relationships with key national stakeholders who share the objective of promoting evidence-based practice, and have the respect of these non-NHS audiences. For example, strategic relationships have been established with the Department for Children, Schools and Families, National healthy schools programme, and OFSTED, to help promote uptake of NICE recommendations in schools, and with the Improvement and Development Agency and the Audit Commission in relation to local authorities. A further example is the way NICE works with national Skills Sector Councils in order to reach professional audiences on a topic specific basis, and to embed NICE recommendations into their training standards, thereby influencing future training provision.

Working with local authorities

In response to the recognition of the unique challenges in implementing public health guidance NICE has developed a 'how to guide' that aims to support local authorities with the implementation of NICE guidance (NICE 2008b). The guide is split into three parts:

- ◆ Part 1 discusses getting started with the process of implementing NICE guidance;
- ◆ Part 2 outlines the principles of implementation of NICE guidance; and
- ◆ Part 3 discusses the practical steps to implementation of NICE guidance.

In addition NICE has developed a document that maps out how the implementation of guidance can help local authorities to meet a number of LAA targets and Multi-Area Agreement (MAA) priorities <http://www.nice.org.uk/usingguidance/implementationtools/implementation_tools.jsp>.

New implementation tools

It has been highlighted earlier in the chapter that in some cases the provision of audit support by NICE has been revised to make it more appropriate to public health audiences. Further bespoke practical tools have also been developed in response to specific pieces of guidance. The wide range of stakeholders required to take action to implement NICE guidance on physical activity and the environment has been identified above. NICE therefore worked with the Centre for Public Scrutiny in the development of its support package for this guidance. Consequently, a checklist of questions has been produced for overview and scrutiny committees to ask when considering local proposals that may have an impact on the environment and delivery of this guidance. Furthermore, the wide range of public health guidance that has an impact on and requires action by those working in the education sector, has resulted in NICE developing a guide to these recommendations for schools. The guide also demonstrates how working towards and implementing these standards helps schools to meet policy requirements and targets from traditional advisory bodies in their field.

NHS Evidence

In the Darzi report 'High Quality Care for All' (Department of Health 2008) NICE was asked to establish NHS Evidence—a new single portal through which anyone will be able to access clinical and non-clinical evidence and best practice. The non-clinical information will include public health and social care evidence, systematic reviews, and practical support.

Is the NICE implementation strategy achieving local change?

The monitoring and evaluation of the NICE implementation strategy in relation to public health guidance presents a particular challenge. It is important to assess uptake of guidance for a number of reasons that are key to anyone working to deliver evidence-based public health care at any level. Firstly, it ensures that implementation activities are targeted in the areas that they are needed and secondly, it helps those with a vested interest in the work understand what the impacts have been.

This, however, is an issue for those working to implement evidence-based public health guidance as there are few if any national data collection systems and public health programmes are often delivered by a wide variety of stakeholders. Careful consideration therefore needs to be given amongst public health communities as to how data can be collected to measure the uptake of, and evaluate, these implementation projects.

The initial focus of the work of NICE in this area has therefore been to try and gather case studies which demonstrate the positive impact that public health guidance can have. NICE has therefore established a Shared Learning database on its website where organizations implementing guidance can share their experiences, impacts, and success of the processes as well as those aspects which may have been particularly challenging. Additionally an annual award is organized to celebrate the best of the submissions and includes a specific category focusing on those in the public health community working to implement guidance. The examples on the database and entrants to these awards have included diverse activities from a range of organizations such as projects by Staffordshire County Council to reduce alcohol consumption in young people; Bolton PCT to incorporate smoking cessation activity into pre-operative assessments; and Upstream (a charitable organization) working to encourage behaviour change amongst older people in the community to increase their well-being.

Conclusions

The delivery of evidence-based cost-effective public health programmes has the potential to make a significant impact on population health. NICE has successfully demonstrated the first step in this process by publishing evidence-based public health guidance on a number of topics. This in itself is not enough, and support for implementation also needs to be provided both nationally and locally. There are a wide range of approaches that can be utilized to implement change but research shows us that very few of these are universally successful and that multi-faceted strategies need to be employed. With limited resources NICE has developed an implementation strategy in response to this evidence base and whilst this chapter has demonstrated that some of the principles and approaches can still be utilized within the public health sector, it has also been demonstrated that there are unique aspects to working in the public health field and these need to be taken into account in implementation strategies. NICE has responded to these but there is still a need to evaluate and undertake more research to gain a fuller understanding of public health guidance implementation.

Unresolved challenges also remain with regards to how implementation and uptake can be assessed at a local level without the need for creating new data collection systems. In particular, from the perspective of NICE, there is interest in whether data can be collated to give an overview of implementation at a national level. The way that NICE has responded to the challenge of implementation also demonstrates that the largely clinical evidence base is transferable to the public health setting and that with due attention to the unique context of public health, effective support can be provided for implementation strategies at a local level.

Bibliography

Audit Commission (2005) *Managing the financial implications of NICE guidance*. London: Audit Commission

Bero L, Grilli R, Grimshaw J, Harvey E, Oxman A and Thomson MA (1998) 'Closing the gap between research and practice: an overview of systematic reviews of interventions to promote the implementation of research findings' *British Medical Journal* 317: 465–8

Brownson R, Ballew P, Brown K, Elliott M, Haire-Joshu D, Heath G and Kreuter M (2007) 'The effect of disseminating evidence based interventions that promote physical activity to health departments' *American Journal of Public Health* 97/10: 1900–7

Department for Communities and Local Government (2006) *Strong and prosperous communities*. London: The Stationery Office

Department for Communities and Local Government (2007) *Delivering health and well-being in partnership: The crucial role of the new local performance framework*. London: The Stationery Office

Department of Health (2008) *High Quality Care For All*. London: The Stationery Office

Doumit G, Gattellari M, Grimshaw J and O'Brien MA (2007) 'Local opinion leaders: effects on professional practice and health care outcomes' *Cochrane Database of Systematic Reviews* 1: CD000125. DOI: 10.1002/14651858. CD000125.pub3

Effective Health Care (1994) *Implementing clinical guidelines: can guidelines be used to improve clinical practice?* Leeds: University of Leeds

Effective Health Care (1999) *Getting Evidence Into Practice*. York: University of York

Fixsen D, Naoom S, Blase K, Friedman R and Wallace F (2005) *Implementation Research: A Synthesis of the Literature*. Florida: University of South Florida

Greenhalgh T, Robert G, Bate P, Macfarlane F and Kyriakidou O (2004) *Diffusion of innovations in health service organisations. A systematic literature review*. Oxford: BMJ books, Blackwell Publishing

Hamilton S, McLaren S and Mulhall A (2007) 'Assessing organisational readiness for change: use of diagnostic analysis prior to the implementation of a multidisciplinary assessment for acute stroke care' *Implementation Science* 2: 21. DOI:10.1186/1748-5908-2-21

Healthcare Commission (2008) *Are we choosing health?* London: Healthcare Commission

Jamtvedt G, Young JM, Kristoffersen DT, O'Brien MA and Oxman AD (2006) 'Audit and feedback: effects on professional practice and health care outcomes' *Cochrane Database of Systematic Reviews* 2: CD000259. DOI: 10.1002/14651858.CD000259.pub2

Kitson AL, Rycroft-Malone J, Harvey G, McCormack B, Seers K and Titchen A (2008) 'Evaluating the successful implementation of evidence into practice using the PARiHS framework: theoretical and practical challenges' *Implement Science* 3: 1

Lomas J (1991) 'Words without action? The production, dissemination, and impact of consensus recommendations' *Annual Review of Public Health* 12: 41–65

NICE (2007) *How to change practice: understand, identify and overcome barriers to change.* London: NICE. Available at: <http://www.nice.org.uk/usingguidance/implementationtools/howtoguide/barrierstochange.jsp>

NICE (2008a) *Physical activity and the environment: Guide to resources.* London: NICE. Available at: <http://www.nice.org.uk/usingguidance/implementationtools/supporttools/support_tool_doc.jsp?o=40287>

NICE (2008b) *How to put NICE guidance into practice and improve the health and wellbeing of communities: Practical steps for local authorities.* London: NICE. Available at: <http://www.nice.org.uk/usingguidance/implementationtools/howtoguide/HowNICEguidanceintopracticeandimprovethehealthandwellbeingof communitiespracticalstepsforlocalauthorities.jsp>

O'Brien MA, Rogers S, Jamtvedt G, Oxman AD, Odgaard-Jensen J, Kristoffersen DT, Forsetlund L, Bainbridge D, Freemantle N, Davis DA, Haynes RB and Harvey EL. (2007) 'Educational outreach visits: effects on professional practice and health care outcomes' *Cochrane Database of Systematic Reviews* 4: CD000409. DOI: 10.1002/14651858.CD000409.pub2

Oxman AD, Thomson MA, Davis DA and Haynes R (1995) 'No magic bullets: a systematic review of 102 trials of interventions to improve professional practice' *CMAJ* 153: 1423–31

Shaw B, Cheater F, Baker R, Gillies C, Hearnshaw H, Flottorp S and Robertson N (2005) 'Tailored interventions to overcome identified barriers to change: effects on professional practice and health care outcomes' *Cochrane Database of Systematic Reviews* 3: CD005470. DOI: 10.1002/14651858.CD005470

Part 5

Knowledge, evidence, and policy

Chapter 29

The individual and the social level in public health

Michael P Kelly

Introduction

This chapter identifies two distinct analytic levels—the 'individual' and the 'social' – for defining and explaining individual disease outcomes and population patterns of health and disease. An evidence-based approach to public health needs to recognize and address the causal pathways that operate at both these levels.

The arguments in this chapter draw on a number of disciplines and authors not usually associated with public health, but such thinking is relevant and necessary for understanding and explaining the social processes that give rise to patterns of heath and disease. These include David Hume (1748), Immanuel Kant (1781), Alfred Schutz (1964, 1967, 1970), George Herbert Mead (1934), Adam Smith (1776), and Emile Durkheim (1915, 1965, 1933, 1897). The ideas also draw heavily on the public health guidance producing activities of NICE (2007) and also NICE's contribution to the WHO Commission on the Social Determinants of Health (Bonnefoy et al 2007; Blas et al 2008; Kelly 2009, Kelly et al 2007, 2009).

The argument is that there are two distinct levels of analysis and corresponding causal pathways, and they explain different sets of processes. The mechanisms which occur at the individual level which lead to disease are real as are the consequence of pathologies in the human body. The mechanisms which operate at the social level are also real and so too are their consequences. These mechanisms operating at the individual and the social levels are, however, analytically separate and make different epistemological assumptions. The social level is not merely the aggregation of what happens at the individual level. It has a reality *sui generis*. The underlying reality at social level is observable or is represented empirically, for example, by the *patterns* of morbidity and mortality in the population. These patterns in the statistical data are the representation empirically of structural properties of the social level. The structural properties relating to disease are a subtype of broader patterns which exist at the social level usually called the social structure, for example, social class, gender and ethnic relations. These structures are real, and their forms are discernible empirically, in principle, in just the same way that pathology in the human body is discernible empirically.

The failure to acknowledge the different reality of these two distinct levels—individual and social—has confounded some arguments in public health and especially led to a needless debate between proponents of a biomedical and of a social approach to health. The suggestion that there is an irresolvable contradiction between the precepts of the medical model of health and the social model is not congruent with the explanation developed in this chapter. The difference between the two is best understood not as an irresolvable conflict, but as two separate levels of analysis which deal with two separate realities.

Public health needs both levels of analysis and explanation (McDowell 2008). The purpose therefore of this chapter is to draw out what is the distinct nature of the social or population level and to provide a more precise definition and description than is usually the case.

The powerful epistemology of modern medicine

The undoubted success of medicine and of the associated individually oriented medical model has powered an epistemology in which a number of principles predominate. The first is cause. The idea is that pathological events in the human body have preceding causes. These causes can take many forms from viruses, bacteria, and genes to physical trauma. The second principle is inferential reasoning. The idea is that the underlying events in the human body have external manifestations or symptoms that are revealed by observation or diagnostic tests from which underlying pathology can be inferred. The third principle is system. The argument is that the human body is made up of a series of interrelated systems and pathology can manifest itself as a malfunction of that system or systems. The fourth principle is of intervention. The principle is that if the underlying pathology can be recognized, then appropriate intervention can follow in the form of drugs, surgery, or other therapy. The epistemology here is grounded in reductionism in which individuals are reduced to their systems, cells, microbiology, biochemistry, and genetics.

In contemporary society there are few people who have not directly benefited from medical interventions based on these principles. A considerable proportion of the benefits to human health in contemporary western societies compared to two hundred years ago can be laid at the door of modern medicine (Bunker 2001). But at the same time as this reductionist epistemology has done its business to great effect, a more confusing socially oriented approach has grown up. The socially oriented approach may be traced mainly to the 19th century and the work of the great public health pioneers. The names of Duncan (Frazer 1947), Chadwick (Hamlin 1995), Farr (Hamlin 1995), Gairdner (1862) amongst others in Britain, and Virchow (Mackenbach 2008) in Germany are the most well known. Their contributions were many and are rightly celebrated (Webster 1990). However, these pioneers unintentionally shaped a very different and potentially non-reductionist epistemology which has never gained the prominence of the more powerful individualistic and reductionist medical model. This level of explanation is social.

Two levels of explanation of health and disease

Public health operates intellectually at two levels which in turn produce two distinct but overlapping epistemological approaches. On the one hand, public health, like medicine as a whole, using the powerful epistemological approach of modern medicine, is concerned with the causation of disease from various agents, with pathological outcomes in the individual human body being the centre of attention. On the other hand, it is also concerned with explanations of population level patterns of disease. Therefore, there are two conceptually distinct but overlapping explanations required, one dealing with individual pathology, the other with the patterning of those pathologies at the social level. It is clearly important to develop as precise an understanding of the social level of explanation as it is the individual level.

At the individual level this may be illustrated by the following examples. The Human Immuno Deficiency Virus is the biological agent, the vector of transmission is the sharing of infected drug injecting paraphernalia among illicit drug users and the host is the person who becomes HIV positive. All of this operates at the individual level. Very precise causal pathways conceptualized as residing in individual biology and behaviour can be defined. There are many diseases where the origins of disease may be explained similarly using this type of biomedical explanation. Sometimes those origins are distal. Mesothelioma is caused by asbestos fibres in the lung. The vector would be exposure to asbestos fibres. The reason for the exposure would be perhaps industrial or occupational. The ultimate cause, though, would reside in the job that person did. There might be an even more distal set of causes operating, in that the choice of occupation would have been driven by opportunity, education, and place of residence and the local presence of shipbuilding or lagging industries using asbestos. For each individual with mesothelioma there is an individual causal pathway unique to them in which the reasons for the presence of the disease can be plotted. It is also true of coronary disease and lung cancer. There will be an individual causal pathway producing a particular pathology in the individual human body.

The usual public health contribution is to acknowledge and to bring into the causal explanation the more distal factors which will be behavioural, social, or economic. Having identified the causal pathway, preventive action can follow by finding specific points along the pathway where the process could be blocked or arrested. This might be done by reducing exposure, as in much occupational health and safety or encouraging the use of clean needles and syringes amongst illicit drug users. The effort might be to produce immunity by immunization, or encouraging detection and early intervention in the form of screening for hypertension or elevated cholesterol. This is classic public health and is conventionally defined as either primary prevention (the protection from risk in the first place), or secondary prevention (stopping the progress of disease once it has begun). This type of approach has been aided by some of the classic epidemiological studies such as those linking smoking and lung cancer (Doll and Hill 1952), lack of exercise, and heart attack (Morris et al 1953), and asbestos and lung cancer (Doll 1955). It is relatively easy to see how individual actions located in particular social and economic contexts combine with specific pathogens to produce disease at the individual level.

However, public health operates at another distinct level of explanation which is social. The problem is that the social level sometimes gets obscured by the power of the biomedical approach. This has been a feature of public health since the first public health physicians wrestled with the relationship between social conditions and disease. The earliest practitioners identified the fact that social conditions were directly linked to epidemic prevalence. The first medical officer of health, in Liverpool, William Duncan, in his evidence to the Select Committee of the House of Commons, showed a very strong association at a population level between patterns of the outbreak of disease and local social conditions (Frazer 1947). William Tennant Gairdner (1862) the first Medical Officer of Health in Glasgow, based in part on data collected nationally by William Farr and in part on the basis of his observations in Glasgow, showed how social, environmental, and economic conditions demonstrated remarkable patterning. These public health pioneers described in vivid and sometimes lurid detail the lifeworlds of socially disadvantaged people in Victorian Britain. The lethal cocktail of filth, overcrowding, poverty, hunger, drunkenness, and sexual licence, is graphically and horrifically described. They could not necessarily detect the underlying causal factors—the bacteria and the viruses—empirically. However, they gathered enough other circumstantial evidence to demonstrate the association between poor social conditions and disease. What the pioneers failed to grasp was that there was not one explanatory real mechanism at work but two—individual and social. That is the patterning of outbreaks they observed were not just the aggregate of all the individual events they saw, it was a phenomenon in its own right requiring explanation.

The early public health practitioners made the connection between social conditions and poor health. What they observed pointed to a set of underlying causes which had to be real, even if they could not be empirically detected. The classic case is cholera where the early pioneers knew that there was an underlying cause probably located in the water but possibly also in the air. Their only recourse was to protect people from the water or the air. They did not have the observational tools to identify the bacteria (Gairdner 1862; Chave 1958). This in time has produced a view which sees it as self-evidently true that if people are poor, social conditions filthy, people live in dirty overcrowded insanitary hovels; it is inevitable that disease will be rife. And to some extent it is of course self-evident. However, it is really only self-evident once one has a grasp of the basic tenets of contagion—ie that disease can be spread from person to person, or from animals and insects to persons, from filth to the person by a variety of routes.

The risk approach and contagion approach which grew out of this are important and populations have benefited from measures introduced as a result of these understandings. So reducing the risks associated with dirty water or the presence of sewage has had profoundly beneficial effects. Likewise, improving general social conditions and providing benefits and support to the needy have produced healthier and fitter individuals and populations. However, beyond individual contagion, risk, and/or lifestyle, there is also a social phenomenon, ie the patterning of disease, not just the aggregation of all the individual level events, which requires an explanation. This type of explanation has been much less well developed in traditional public health. The potential power for sociological reasoning about the nature of social structure and individual human actions has been absent from the public health lexicon, or at least has not provided the insight that it might have been able to do. Although the potential for this sociological input is large, methodologically the impact of the discipline has been negligible.

Sociology operates at the level of the social and arranges its explanations around structures like the family, institutions, groups, and communities. Its premise is that each of these and other social units have properties and the potential to impact on individuals in ways that are just as tangible as the biochemistry of the cell. However, the ways this happens are often more difficult to discern.

It is nevertheless vitally important to tease out the social level as it potentially offers enormous scope for intervention. Our knowledge of the individual level pathways is a great deal more sophisticated than our knowledge of the social pathways. This reflects the dominance of the biomedical approach and the very sophisticated tools for empirical observation of biological phenomena. This description of the social level is potentially of great scientific importance because while the case for the social determinants is very well established, there remains a dearth of good theory to drive observation (CSDH 2008; Bonnefoy et al 2007; Kelly et al 2007, 2009; Blas et al 2008).

A sociologically based analysis sometimes appears to take all responsibility away from individuals and denies any kind of free will in favour of a socially determined reality writ large. No one has any responsibility for anything and human motive would have no role in the explanation of human behaviour. This form of extreme determinism is unhelpful (Kelly et al 2009). What is also unhelpful is to counterpose the individual and social levels as one being correct and the other not. A more subtle account of human behaviour is required. The basis for delimiting this is a consideration of the relationship between free will and determinism and agency and structure (Kelly et al 2009).

Free will and determinism and agency and structure

There are patterns in human behaviour and societies which seem to be so repetitive and common, that the idea that there is some kind of determinism operating seems highly plausible. Structures of inequalities in society, the operations of markets, conflict, competition, sexual conduct all follow discernible patterns which operate independent of human will or agency. And yet at the individual level individuality seems to be what is going on.

Various proxies are often used for social structure, such as measures of social class or other classifications of the population into groups for the purposes of collecting data about occupation or sickness or earnings or some other such feature. Sometimes social institutions like schools, families, and bureaucracies are seen as proxies or even component parts of the social structure. Still other ideas like culture are used to mean some aspect of social structure or as a synonym for it. These are all manifestations of the structural properties of society, but the idea of social structure is something more than this.

Social structures arise from human behaviour or agency and then in turn human behaviour is affected by social structures. Social structures are the patterns of social arrangements that arise naturally out of human conduct; they are patterns because they have a repetitive quality. They provide the limits to individual freedom and they determine lines of human conduct in turn. These patterns are part of human experience. They are part of the sensations and perceptions of human conduct. They are such a familiar part of human life that they are very difficult sometimes to notice or to see, in the way we can see a house or a wall or a flower. But they are real none the less. They are not concrete in a material sense.

The normal processes of socialization and emersion in the culture all around us, provides us with an awareness of social structures, albeit intuitively. Socialization is a process of experience. Therefore social structures are known through experience and very importantly they are taken account of by humans when taking actions. The social structure exerts an effect by virtue of its reality. People are also aware of social structure although not necessarily with complete clarity and then they deliberately orient their actions accordingly. This in turn generates the social structure (Giddens 1979, 1982, 1984).

These principles apply generally to social relations. They also apply to the public health problem of individual causation of disease and of the patterning of disease at population or community level. In daily life individual actors make choices about what they eat, how much alcohol they consume, how they will do their work, how often they clean their teeth, whether they will use a condom and so on, in a myriad of minor and major health related decisions and activities. At the same time managers and policy makers—other actors in the social system are making other choices and decisions about resource allocation, service development etc with a broad range of potential outcomes. At another level, national governments and supra-state formations act on national and global stages in ways which influence health, ranging from debt relief programmes, guaranteeing human rights, and providing basic services. Of course other actors will be making decisions and acting in ways that will damage health (Blas et al 2008). Still other actors in civil society engage in their own agendas and a vast array of human and organizational activity takes place.

This system clearly may be messy, chaotic, very complex, and made up of billions and billions of individual actions, but its endpoints are far from unclear and are highly structured. At its starkest, in health terms, there is very good empirical capture of health gradients measuring mortality and morbidity in different social groups. There are considerable inequities within and between societies in patterns of health, illness, and death, although the shape of these inequities varies from place to place (Blas et al 2008). These patterns show consistently that health state and health status are directly associated with social position. Further, these patterns are produced and reproduced generation upon generation. This was part of what Duncan and Gairdner in the 19th century exposed (Gairdner 1862; Frazer 1947). Interestingly, when Gairdner's lists of places in mid 19th century Britain which had high infant mortality are compared to the early 21st century areas with high levels of infant mortality, the overlaps are considerable. The causes of death may be different and the absolute rates lower, but the concentrations in particular localities, often the very same localities, are very striking. This in itself is reason to conceptualize the patterns as real and tangible. Amidst all the noise in the system, all the billions of human actions by diverse human actors, at the social level there are real mechanisms which have these effects—excess mortality—which can be observed epidemiologically.

We are quite good at observing these outcomes empirically in the form of epidemiological data about different rates of mortality and morbidity. However, our empirical grasp of the way these things work beyond the statistical measurement and hence what we might do about it is much less well developed. This is explored in the next section.

The concept of the social level

This idea of the patterns or structures at the social or population level which, it is being claimed, require explanation here, is a difficult concept to grasp. The structures of health differences are helpful in identifying the social level. The statistics describing population level blood pressure and the epidemiological data describing patterns of mortality and morbidity for cardiovascular disease for example, are the empirical representation of an underlying reality which is a social structure or pattern.

The reality is the biological variation and this patterning have causes separate from, although linked to, the causes of individual pathologies. These include a range of patterns of behaviour, shared social circumstances, and cultural habits operating through environmental, population, organizational and social factors interacting with human behaviour (Kelly et al 2009). However, not all structures are so amenable to empirical observation. This is because data are not collected about them, or they cannot be measured, or no one even thinks to measure them because they are so familiar and all around us that we scarcely notice them.

Mostly modern science directs us, and certainly modern medicine directs us to smaller and smaller units of analysis and explanation. We just do not use our analytic and observational faculties to observe the structures which make up the social level. The structures which make up the social level are for the most part difficult to see and difficult to capture empirically. Also, social structures are sometimes highly transient features of social life. However, the patterns or structures are all around us. They constrain and limit our lives in many different ways. An example is peer group pressure. It is a structural phenomenon arising out of behaviour and directly influencing behaviour. The social norms that dictate expected habits, rituals, and 'fashions' are other examples of structures that exert significant power over individuals. Structures are real even though they are difficult to discern empirically with very much precision. That means the empirical descriptions of these structures are limited except in the very specific cases like mortality, morbidity, or those things which are measurable or as manifested in legal and regulatory structures.

The intellectual or conceptual representation of the structures is not the same as the structures themselves. It is important not to commit the error of assuming those aspects of structure which are easy to measure are the same thing as the underlying reality that they represent. They are in that sense a representation, not the thing itself. In turn the thing itself, its empirical representation, has to be distinguished from theoretical ideas about both. So we posit (i) underlying real structures having real effects and being the product of human actions and having in turn an impact on them; (ii) empirical representations of the underlying reality like mortality and morbidity data, census data, legal codes; and (iii) theories about the social structure and what its empirical representation might look like in the form of ideas like peer group pressure, bureaucracy, social facts, etc.

The structures are not static. They do though persist through time. The capacity for some of the same structures to be reproduced through every generation provides for the stability and continuity in social systems. However, these structures not only reproduce they also change. They have the capacity to evolve gradually and some structures relating to say the relationships between men and women and sexual reproduction show that characteristic, while others change rapidly sometimes. The changes in fashion are a good example of that. The structures have a degree of permanence but they are not concrete and unchanging. This apparently self-contradictory observation is at the heart of two of the most enduring sociological questions at the centre of the concerns of the classical period of modern sociology. These are how it is that societies change and at the same time how is social order possible (Nisbet 1970; Neustadt 1965)? The answer to this statement is on closer reflection not so contradictory. It lies in the continuity of social structures, the fact that they produce and reproduce themselves over time so have that sense of continuity, but that they are also constantly changing and evolving. Both are the product of the billions and billions of individual human actions. Of course as classical sociology also well understood, such structures are the root of conflict in social systems, sometimes on a cataclysmic scale, but they are also the root of social order.

The social level is difficult to conceptualize and to describe. However, it is worth considering that some of the most notable contributions to social and economic theory have been made by individual social scientists and philosophers who grasped the idea of structure, although calling it many different things. These include Hume (1748) and Kant's (1781) conception of the general will, Durkheim's social facts (1897; 1965), Weber's ideal types (Gerth and Mills 1948), Smith's hidden hand of the market (1776), Parsons' pattern variables (1951), Merton's reference groups (Merton and Kitts 1982), Giddens' structuration (1979; 1982; 1984), Schutz's conception of lifeworld (1964; 1967; 1970), Marx's class consciousness (Marx and Engels 1967), Garfinkel's ethnomethodology (1967), Mead's generalized other (1934) and Bourdieu's habitus (1977; 1986). These are all outstanding examples of what has been referred to here simply as structures. What all these writers had in mind were the various patterns that emerge through the ordinary interaction of people with each other, meaning that the social system has within it a series of emergent properties, independent of individual will, which in turn impact on the individual will.

Conclusion

Using the specific conceptual framework developed by Kant in *the Critique of Pure Reason* (1781) it is possible to formalize these ideas a little more. Kant distinguished between noumena—meaning real things, and phenomena—meaning the way that we represent things in our minds conceptually. The real things at the individual level here are individual biological events in the human body and individual behaviours and individual lifeworlds (the individual experiences of biology and social life and the everyday stresses and anxieties). The real thing is also the individual lifecourse or accumulated costs and benefits in health terms accrued through life. Individual health outcomes are a conse-quence of the operation of these elements (Kelly et al 2009). The phenomena are what we are able to describe and measure using various instruments, such as the lipid levels in the blood.

At the social or population level, the real things are the structures of social life including collective and coalescing life worlds, and also the population differences in things like blood pressure, mortality, and morbidities in whole populations and sub-populations. The phenomena (or representations) of these are mortality rates; the bell shaped blood pressure curve, sickness rates, crime rates, as well as observable aspects of social life.

Phenomena require interpretation both to relate them back to the underlying noumena and to make theoretical and conceptual sense of them. The data or empirical evidence do not speak for themselves; they are a representation of reality and they require theoretical manipulation to understand them and make sense of them. We should treat empirical observations strictly speaking as 'matters of fact'. Our theoretical ideas about our empirical observations are separate. And both empirical observation and our theo-retical frameworks are distinct from the underlying reality.

For public health it is an important task to develop our understandings of the social level, because ultimately the types of intervention which will bring about large scale changes in the health of the public operate at that level. Understanding the causal rela-tionships at that level is therefore vital. Public health must also break free of the assump-tion that the population level is only the aggregate of the individual level. There are important individual level things for public health to do and much individual suffering can be alleviated. However, individual level interventions will not in themselves funda-mentally transform the health of the public.

The argument here is a realist one, ie it proceeds from the premise that both individual pathology and population patterns of pathology are things in themselves that are real. They can be observed empirically but the empirical observation is not the same as the reality, it is a representation of it. It also acknowledges that our empirical observation of these mechanisms may be faulty, imprecise, or incomplete and therefore we have to be content for the time being with partial empirical understandings of the processes involved. On the basis of our incomplete empirical observations it is, however, possible to develop theories which account for the observed relationships. The causal pathways are such theories. The theories are the basis for intervention.

Bibliography

Blas, E., Gilson, L., Kelly, M.P., Labonte, R., Lapitan, J., Muntaner, C., Ostlin, P., Popay, J., Sadana, R., Sen, G., Schrecker, T., Vaghri, Z. (2008) 'Addressing social determinants of health inequities: what can the state and civil society do?' *The Lancet* 372: 1684–9

Bonnefoy, J., Moran, A., Kelly, M.P., Butt, J., Bergman, V., with P. Tugwell, V. Robinson, M. Exworthy, J. Mackenbach, J. Popay, C. Pope, T. Narayan, L. Myer, S. Simpson, T. Houweling, L. Jadue (2007) *Constructing the evidence base on the social determinants of health: A guide.* Report to the World Health Organization Commission on the Social Determinants of Health, from Measurement and Evidence Knowledge Network, The hub coordinating the Measurement and Evidence Knowledge Network is run by: Universidad del Desarrollo, Chile and National Institute for Health and Clinical Excellence, United Kingdom. Available at; <http://www.who.int/social_determinants/knowledge_networks/add_documents/mekn_final_guide_112007.pdf>

Bourdieu (1977) *Outline of a Theory of Practice*. Cambridge: Cambridge University Press

Bourdieu, P. (1986) 'The forms of capital' in J Richardson (ed), *Handbook of Theory and Research for the Sociology of Education*. New York: Greenwood

Bunker, J. (2001) *Medicine Matters After All: Measuring the benefits of medical care, a healthy lifestyle, and a just social environment*. London: The Stationery Office/The Nuffield Trust

CSDH (2008) *Closing the Gap in a Generation: Health Equity Through Action on the Social Determinants of Health*. Geneva: WHO

Chave, S.W.P. (1958) 'John Snow, the Broad Street pump and after' *The Medical Officer* 99: 347–9

Doll, R and Hill, A.B. (1952) 'Smoking and carcinoma of the lung' *British Medical Journal* 2: 84–92

Doll, R. (1955) 'Mortality from lung cancer in asbestos workers' *British Journal of Industrial Medicine* 12: 81–6

Durkheim, E. (1897/1952) *Suicide: A Study in Sociology*. Trans J.A. Spaulding and G. Simpson. London: Routledge & Kegan Paul

Durkheim, E. (1915) *The Elementary Forms of the Religious Life: A Study in Religious Sociology*. Translated by Joseph Ward Swain. London: Allen & Unwin

Durkheim, E. (1965) *The Rules of the Sociological Method*. New York: Free Press

Durkheim, E. (1933) *The Division of Labour in Society*. Trans G. Simpson. New York: Free Press

Frazer, W.M. (1947) *Duncan of Liverpool: Being an Account of the Work of Dr W.H. Duncan Medical Officer of Health of Liverpool 1847–63*. London: Hamish Hamilton. Republished Preston: Carnegie in 1997

Gairdner, W.T. (1862) *Public Health in Relation to Air and Water*. Edinburgh: Edmonston and Douglas

Garfinkel, H. (1967) *Studies in Ethnomethodology*. New Jersey: Prentice Hall

Gerth, H and Mills, CW (eds) (1948) *From Max Weber: Essays in Sociology*. London: Routledge & Kegan Paul

Giddens, A (1979) *Central Problems in Social Theory: Action, Structure and Contradiction in Social Analysis*. Berkeley: University of California Press

Giddens, A (1982) *Profiles and Critiques in Social Theory*. London: Macmillan

Giddens, A (1984) *The Constitution of Society: Outline of the Theory of Structuration*. Berkeley: University of California Press

Hamlin, C. (1995) 'Could you starve to death in England in 1839? The Chadwick—Farr controversy and the loss of social in public health' *American Journal of Public Health* 85: 856–66

Hume, D. (1748/2007) *An Enquiry Concerning Human Understanding*. Ed and intro P. Millican. First published 1748. Oxford: Oxford University Press

Kant, I. (1781/2007) *Critique of Pure Reason*. Trans N. Kemp Smith, intro H. Caygill. Basingstoke: Palgrave Macmillan

Kelly, M.P., Morgan, A., Bonnefoy, J., Butt, J., Bergman, V., With J. Mackenbach, M. Exworthy, J. Popay, P. Tugwell, V. Robinson, S. Simpson, T. Narayan, L. Myer, T. Houweling, L. Jadue, F. Florenzano, (2007) *The social determinants of health: Developing an evidence base for political action*. Final Report to the World Health Organization Commission on the Social Determinants of Health, from Measurement and Evidence Knowledge Network, The hub coordinating the Measurement and Evidence Knowledge Network is run by: Universidad del Desarrollo, Chile, and National Institute for Health and Clinical Excellence, United Kingdom. Available at: <http://www.who.int/social_determinants/resources/mekn_report_10oct07.pdf>

Kelly, M. P., Stewart, E., Morgan, A., Killoran, A., Fischer, A., Threlful, A. Bonnefoy, J. (2009) 'A conceptual framework for public health: NICE's emerging approach' *Public Health*, doi:10.1016/j.puhe.2008.10.031. Public Health 123: e14–e20

Mackenbach, J.P. (2008) *Politics is Nothing but Medicine on a Larger Scale*. Rotterdam: Erasmus Medical Centre

McDowell, I. (2008) 'From risk factors to explanation in public health' *Journal of Public Health* 30: 219–23

Marx, K. and Engels, F. (1967) *The Communist Manifesto*, with an introduction by A.J.P. Taylor. Harmondsworth: Penguin

Mead, G.H. (1934) *Mind, Self and Society: from the Standpoint of the Social Behaviourist*. Chicago: Chicago University Press

Merton, R.K. and Kitts, A. (1982) 'Reference groups' in L Coser and B Rosenberg (eds), *Sociological Theory: A Book of Readings*. 5th edn. London: Collier Macmillan

Morris, J., Heady, J.A., Raffle, P.A.B., Parks, J.W. (1953) 'Coronary heart disease and physical activity at work' *Lancet* ii: 1053–7, 1111–20

Neustadt, I. (1965) *Teaching Sociology*. Leicester: Leicester University Press

NICE (2007) *Behaviour Change at Population, Community and Individual Levels*. NICE Public Health Guidance 6. London: NICE. Available at: <http://guidance.nice.org.uk/PH006>

Nisbet, R.A. (1970) *The Social Bond: An Introduction to the Study of Society*. New York: Alfred Knopf

Parsons, T. (1951) *The Social System*. London: Routledge & Kegan Paul

Schutz, A. (1964) *Collected Papers: II Studies in Social Theory*. The Hague: Martinus Nijhoff

Schutz, A. (1967) *The Phenomenology of the Social World*. Trans G. Walsh and F. Lehnert. Evanston Ill: North Western University Press

Schutz, A. (1970) *On Phenomenology and Social Relations: Selected Writings*. Chicago: Chicago University Press

Smith, A. (1776) *An Enquiry into the Nature and Causes of the Wealth of Nations*. Ed R.H. Campbell and A.S. Skinner. Oxford: Clarendon

Webster, C. (1990) *The Victorian Public Health Legacy: A Challenge to the Future*. London: Institution of Environmental Health Officers/Public Health Alliance

Chapter 30

Informing public health policy with the best available evidence

Laurie M Anderson and David V McQueen

Introduction

The use of research synthesis methods to form generalizations from a body of scientific literature has enjoyed considerable popularity over the past twenty years. The term evidence-based practice has become part of the professional vernacular. Books on the methodology of research synthesis became more widespread in the 1980's (Hedges and Olkin 1985; Hunter et al 1982; Light and Pillemer 1984) followed by specialized texts on applications in medicine, education, and the social sciences (Brownson et al 2003; Cooper and Hedges 1994; Petticrew and Roberts 2006; Sackett 1997). Scientific collaborations formed to establish standards for the conduct of high quality research syntheses, provide organizational infrastructure to support production of systematic reviews, and create portals to access the knowledge generated from these efforts. In 1993 the international Cochrane Collaboration was established to produce and disseminate systematic reviews of health care interventions. In 2000 the Campbell Collaboration was established to produce and disseminate systematic reviews in the fields of education, social welfare, and crime and justice. A profusion of publicly and privately sponsored organizations have since emerged to produce evidence-informed guidelines and recommendations for policy and practice across a variety of scientific disciplines.

The development of the evidence-based movement has not come without criticism. While many would agree that decisions concerning public policies and practices should be based on the best available evidence that they do more good than harm, how this evidence is accrued and applied remains debatable (McQueen 2007; McQueen and Anderson 2001). The decision to choose a quantitative and/or qualitative methodological approach that best captures any evidence that a programme or policy works, while also accounting for complexity and context, remains an open question. Most would agree, however, that evidence is more robust when it comes from a thorough and systematic assessment of a body of knowledge rather than a limited or predisposed selection.

In public health, the use of research synthesis in the interest of improving population health outcomes has gained wide acceptance, coupled with the recognition that meaningful translation and dissemination must also occur if new knowledge is to influence health policy and programme decisions. But an integrated approach to knowledge generation, synthesis, dissemination, uptake, and evaluation has yet to be realized in most public health settings. In this chapter we discuss the advantages of knowledge synthesis approaches to support public health decision making, perspectives on the translation of knowledge for different purposes, and the importance of creating institutional capacity to support evidence-informed public health policies.

Knowledge synthesis for health policy

Scientific knowledge is regarded as cumulative and contingent. We would argue that a reliance on the results of a single study to inform health policy decisions can be chancy. Publication bias, selective reporting of positive outcomes, and smaller or even contradictory results in later studies of similar interventions all suggest a careful and critical use of the scientific literature (Dwan et al 2008; Ioannidis 2005). Systematic reviews and the synthesis of research findings attempt to reduce the risk of biases by comprehensively searching for pertinent research evidence, compiling this body of information in a transparent manner, and assessing the contribution of individual studies in the context of all relevant information.

The steps in conducting a systematic review include assembling a multidisciplinary review team and stating the research question. At this stage, including those likely to be affected by the policy or programme, as well as those making decisions regarding its use, can enhance the relevancy of the review question and the likelihood that review findings will be used. Next, a comprehensive literature search is conducted to find all relevant studies. Information from eligible studies is coded and summarized either narratively or quantitatively (meta-analysis) to provide a sense of the impact of the intervention. Should the intervention literature be large enough, examination of the settings, populations, and intervention components can provide useful information on what works best for whom. Where there is a paucity of information, a well-articulated research question outlines where a gap in knowledge exists. In either case, the translation of findings into a meaningful message with purposeful dissemination is necessary if the effort is to advance an area of research.

One benefit of systematic reviews for research synthesis is that they take advantage of the temporal dimension of knowledge production. The production of scientific knowledge is a cumulative endeavour. Rather than being faced with a plethora of reports of individual studies, often with tentative or contradictory findings, the synthesis of research places new results in the context of similar studies over time (Chalmers et al 2002). Considerable resources are invested in health research. Knowing when additional research is no longer needed helps redirect resources to where knowledge gaps do exist. On the other hand, a cumulative assessment of the scientific literatures can identify significant underinvestment in particular areas of health research.

The contextual relevance of scientific information is also time-dependent. Programme effectiveness questions must be revised periodically because interventions found to be effective at one point in time may be less effective later if the conditions that contributed to their effectiveness change. For example, an intervention strategy to promote the use of a screening test may be less effective as baseline rates improve. Aside from temporal effects, contextual relevance and the legitimacy of making generalizations from a body of intervention literature to new situations needs careful consideration. The tension between the notion that scientific evidence is context-free versus the view that evidence has little meaning unless it is understood and adapted to the circumstances of its application (context-dependent) requires balanced consideration.

One laudable result of the widespread use of systematic reviews has been increased accountability in the reporting of health research. The review process calls not only for identification of all relevant studies that meet explicit criteria, but also an appraisal of their characteristics and potential for bias. Researchers and journal editors have joined together to establish standards to improve transparency in the conduct of health research and quality in reporting (Begg et al 1996; Des et al 2004; Vandenbroucke et al 2007). Research users can be more confident in the quality of published research as a consequence.

Knowledge tools and translation

It is important to distinguish that, aside from the issue of quality and availability of scientific information, knowledge use is a social process. Whether original research or a synthesis of research findings, the time it takes to get new knowledge into policies and programmes is often unacceptably slow (Contopoulos-Ioannidis et al 2008). As a result, what is already known to be beneficial quite often is not considered in policy and practice decisions, while ineffectual or sometimes harmful practices continue. Turning knowledge into action is a deliberate process that requires more than locating evidence of effectiveness. The knowledge to action cycle in Figure 30.1 illustrates this continuous process. Here Graham distinguishes between the stages of knowledge creation; selection and adaptation to local context; assessment of barriers to knowledge use and implementation in policies or programmes; monitoring knowledge use; and evaluating resulting outcomes to sustain the knowledge to action cycle (Graham et al 2006). Knowledge creation builds upon empirical research to improve our understanding of phenomena by uncovering new information, while knowledge synthesis attempts to improve understanding by amassing existing knowledge from various sources. Creation of knowledge, by itself, doesn't change policy. The knowledge to action cycle is complex and iterative and must be both deliberately employed and adequately resourced to be successful. Each phase is shaped by factors besides scientific evidence alone.

Dynamics of knowledge transfer and use

As the imperative to base public health decisions on sound evidence grows, it underscores the broader question of how different types of evidence can be useful. Compared to researchers, policy makers and other knowledge users may have different views on what constitutes useful evidence for decisions. Quite often there is a mismatch between the complex and nuanced health and social policy problems faced by policy makers and what is available in the form of evaluative knowledge produced by more narrowly focused research questions (Bensing et al 2003; Nutbeam and Boxall 2008). In general, published research describes correlates of health conditions rather than tested solutions that are

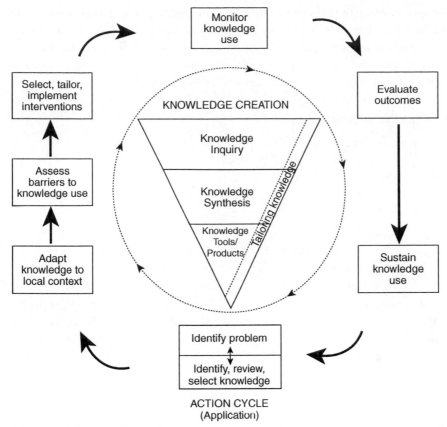

Fig. 30.1 Knowledge to action cycle
Source: Ian Graham 2006

more useful for policy decisions. Even when policy or programme solutions are evaluated for effectiveness, they typically focus on a single intervention or theoretically similar subset. Policy decisions, on the other hand, require weighing the pros and cons of a broad range of options to find the best fit within the constraints of public acceptability, institutional capacity, funding and opportunity costs. For example, if the problem is low birth weight in a population, should the solution focus on unintended pregnancy, prenatal care, women's health, sexually-transmitted diseases, stress, birth defects, or a combination of these? Seldom do systematic reviews provide information on a portfolio of solutions in a way that allows weighing the benefits and costs of each approach in a comparable metric.

Cost-effectiveness information is frequently missing from programme and policy evaluations; for decision makers this is essential information for selecting pragmatic solutions. Reducing uncertainties is at the basis of many policy decisions and this involves knowledge beyond that typically found in health research (eg political climate, public opinion, historical considerations, and leveraging resources). If public health research is to influence policy decisions, early collaboration between researchers and knowledge users (policy makers) is necessary. Research on facilitators and barriers to the use of research in policy-making points to the importance of personal contact; timeliness; and relevance of the research information; high quality research that reports effectiveness data; actionable findings with clear recommendations; and public demand for the use of evidence-informed policies and programmes (Innvaer et al 2002).

Models and lessons

There are numerous examples of knowledge synthesis and translation activities globally. We describe three examples here. The Cochrane Collaboration Public Health Review Group provides an avenue to produce and to locate high quality systematic reviews of public health interventions (Waters et al 2008). Initiatives such as the UN Millennium Development Goals have called for more evidence, within the international context, to inform policy decisions that affect population-level health outcomes. Global involvement by the public health community is necessary, particularly from researchers, practitioners, and policy makers in low-and middle-income countries. To that end, the Cochrane Public Health Review Group (PHRG) is establishing a registry that will include prospective registration of public health intervention studies, so potential reviewers can identify global sources of relevant evidence (Morgan et al 2008). The PHRG provides review authors editorial guidance throughout the review process. Effects of public health interventions to improve health and other outcomes are examined at the population level, rather than individuals, and include interventions aimed at macro-environmental and sociocultural factors that influence health.

The PHRG's priority topic areas and examples of interventions are listed in Table 30.1. Based upon the underlying principles of equity and social justice in public health, the PHRG seeks to gather the evidence needed to address root determinants of health inequalities. Of vital importance is the uptake of review findings by policy makers, practitioners, and the public. The Cochrane Collaboration Library provides a central site for review results with free access for low-income countries. In other countries a subscription to the Cochrane library is necessary and it typically can be accessed through universities and major health institutions. Each Cochrane systematic review is accompanied by a plain language summary and, more recently, a summary of findings table, to enhance translation and uptake by stakeholders.

In the United States, the Task Force on Community Preventive Services is a key source of recommendations for public health practice and policy interventions (Zaza et al 2000). Convened by the US Department of Health and Human Services in 1996, the fifteen-member, multidisciplinary Task Force is an independent decision-making body that oversees the production of systematic reviews on topics that align with national health objectives outlined in Healthy People 2010 (Anon 2000). Taking a step beyond synthesis of intervention research, the Task Force explicitly recommends for, or against, public health policy or programme interventions. Where systematic reviews uncover a paucity of scientific information on topics considered critical to the public's health, the Task Force issues a research agenda.

Table 30.1 Cochrane Public Health Review Group priority topics and example interventions

EMPLOYMENT and THE WORK ENVIRONMENT
Collaboration with council and workplaces to provide facilities (eg showers and bike racks) that encourage active transport
Collaboration with workplaces for introducing healthy staff canteen policy
Designated workplace health promotion staff for supporting colleagues in developing organization-wide health activities
Workplace and/or legislative interventions for addressing work-life balance in adults
Workplace interventions (eg flexible work hours, control over shift patterns) for improving employee health and well-being

INCOME DISTRIBUTION/FINANCIAL INTERVENTIONS
Business loans and other financial strategies for improving well-being (and other health outcomes) of women in developing countries
Cash transfer programmes for improving health and related outcomes
Equity funds financed by government for increasing health insurance coverage specifically for the poor
Financing mechanisms for improving access to health services for the poor
Provision of scholarships for improving health and related outcomes in economically vulnerable students
Childcare payments linked to administration of childhood immunization for improving immunization rates

HOUSING and THE BUILT ENVIRONMENT
Healthy cities, municipalities, or spaces projects for reducing health risk factors
Housing interventions for improved health and socio-economic outcomes
Interventions for minimizing the adverse health effects of urban sprawl
Slum upgrading strategies to improve living conditions in developing world cities

FOOD SUPPLY / ACCESS
Interventions addressing gender disparities in family food distribution for improving child nutrition
Interventions aimed at enhancing access for increased consumption of fruit and vegetables
Interventions focusing on adolescent girls for improving the nutritional status in women of child-bearing age prior to first pregnancy
Interventions for improving food security
Interventions for improving nutritional status in refugee and displaced populations
Pricing policies for increasing healthy food choices
Sales promotion strategies of supermarkets for increasing healthier food purchase

EDUCATION
Interventions for increasing school completion rates

HEALTH and RELATED SYSTEMS
Advocacy to increase the range of options for people with disabilities to use all public facilities, including sports and recreation programmes
Capacity-building interventions for health care professionals for promoting health
Contracting out primary health care services to NGOs for increasing uptake of services by the poor

PUBLIC SAFETY
Community-led advocacy for improving safety around schools
Legislation to ban drivers using cell phones

SOCIAL NETWORKS/SUPPORT
Enhancing/Building protective environments for reducing health risk behaviours in adolescents
Interventions to enhance development of social networks for promoting well-being
Transport schemes for improving social connectedness of adults
Community-building interventions to improve physical, social, and mental health

Table 30.1 (continued) Cochrane Public Health Review Group priority topics and example interventions

THE NATURAL ENVIRONMENT

Community-led advocacy for eliminating hazardous chemicals in local soils
Community-level educational strategies for preventing water-borne infections/food-borne infections
Environmental strategies for preventing water-borne infections/food-borne infections
Interventions that employ a combination of environmental, social, and educational strategies for increasing proper garbage disposal to promote health
Interventions that employ a combination of environmental, social, and educational strategies for preventing water-borne infections/food-borne infections
Social strategies for preventing water-borne infections/food-borne infections

TRANSPORT

Active transport initiatives for increasing physical activity
Increasing the supply/quality of public sidewalks and walking trails for increasing physical activity levels of communities
Segregated cycle facilities for increasing the use of active transport by adults and children
Transport schemes for improving social connectedness of adults

OTHER

Initiatives for promoting health among out-of-school youth
Introduction of restricted trading hours for gaming venues for reducing problem gambling
Mass media campaigns for promoting vaccinations at a community/population level
Health promotion for oral health

The Task Force on Community Preventive Services promotes the use of their recommendations by a variety of public health agencies and institutions. Main stakeholders are the fifty state health departments and the many local and county health departments within their jurisdictions who collectively are responsible for public health policies and programmes that span the United States. The Task Force encourages health departments to use their recommendations to implement state and local evidence-based public health improvement programmes and policies. Uptake of these recommendations is voluntary; no policy or regulatory mechanisms require their use. The recommendations and systematic review findings are accessible on the website <http://www.thecommunityguide.org> and are published in peer-reviewed journals. To evaluate the reach and relevance of the recommendations of the Task Force and to establish a benchmark for assessing changes in uptake, a survey of state and local public health decision makers was conducted in 2005 (Burrus et al 2006). Half of the respondents surveyed were familiar with the work of the Task Force; state health directors were twice as likely as local or county health directors to be aware. When asked what had the most influence on their programme and policy decisions, at both state and local levels the respondents reported that funding guidance from legislative authorities or federal funding sources had more influence than systematic reviews of the scientific literature. This suggests the importance of including in government funding guidance and legislative directives a call for the use of evidence that programmes and policies in fact work. Such a call for the use of the best available evidence requires a parallel investment by government funders in integrated approaches to knowledge generation, synthesis, dissemination, uptake, and evaluation.

Widespread and persistent global inequities in health provided the background rationale for the World Health Organization to establish a Commission on the Social Determinants of Health (CSDH) in 2005. Based on the widely accepted thesis that the health of individuals and of populations is determined to a large degree by social determinants that produce health inequities within and between societies, the Commission wanted to learn from existing information and apply that knowledge to global and national political and economic action (CSDH 2008). Nine Knowledge Networks were established consisting of academics and practitioners from universities and research institutions, government ministries, and international and civil society organizations around the world. Table 30.2 lists the Knowledge Networks and the focus of each in generating and summarizing the evidence where action on these social determinants of health was shown to be possible and effective. The Commission wanted their recommendations for action to be underpinned by an etiological conceptual framework; supported by a robust global evidence base that demonstrated favourable outcomes of action on social determinants of health and health inequities; supported by evidence of feasibility of implementation of programmes and policies under varying conditions; and supported by evidence of consistent effects in different population groups and countries with different levels of economic development (CSDH 2008).

In the process the Commission had to balance the use of different types of evidence. Global and national social and economic approaches and policies are rarely evaluated in the context of controlled trials. Matching research questions to the appropriate

Table 30.2 Knowledge Networks established by the WHO Commission on Social Determinants of Health

Early child development	Opportunities for young children that shape lifelong health and development status.
Employment conditions	Different types of jobs and effects of unemployment on workers' health.
Globalization	Globalization's dynamics and processes (eg trade liberalization, integration of production of goods) and health outcomes.
Health systems	Innovative actions on social determinants of health, particularly in countries with limited resources.
Measurement and evidence	Methodologies and tools for measuring the causes, pathways, and health outcomes of policy interventions.
Priority public health conditions	Programmes that increase access to health care for socially and economically disadvantaged groups.
Social exclusion	Relational processes that lead to the exclusion of groups of people from engaging fully in community, social life.
Urban settings	Broad policy interventions related to healthy urbanization and slum upgrading.
Women and gender equity	Mechanisms, processes, and actions that reduce gender-based inequities in health.

methodologies was the guiding principle and allowed the inclusion of evidence from observational studies, natural experiments, case studies, expert and lay knowledge, as well as community trials. In addition to fitness for purpose, a transparent and explicit process for appraising evidence, a means for taking into account risk of bias, and explicit thresholds of acceptability that were open to external scrutiny was considered fundamental (Kelly et al 2007). The culmination of the work of the Commission on Social Determinants of Health and the Knowledge Networks was the 2008 report, *Closing the gap in a generation: health equity through action on social determinants of health*. The extensive gathering and summarizing evidence of action on social determinants of health was distilled under three overarching themes: improving daily living conditions; tackling the inequitable distribution of power, money, and resources; and measuring and understanding the problems related to social determinants of health and the impact of action. Table 30.3 outlines the 12 key topics for action identified by the Commission and their final report details 56 specific recommendations for programme and policy approaches evaluated by the Commission and Knowledge Networks as feasible, transferable, and producing favourable outcomes (CSDH 2008).

Evidence gaps and uncertainty

In a recent paper Nutbeam contrasted the transfer of research knowledge into health policy and practice in England and Australia and concluded that the usefulness of available evidence depends largely upon the nature of data routinely produced by government (Nutbeam and Boxall 2008). Far more information was available on health disparities and socio-economic correlates of poor health in England because the country had collected data and studied the problem since the mid 19th century. Australia's public health surveillance systems focused more on behavioural determinates of health (ie behavioural

Table 30.3 Key action areas identified by the WHO Commission on Social Determinants of Health

Improve daily living conditions
Equity from the start
Healthy places healthy people
Fair employment and decent work
Social protection across the lifecourse
Universal health care
Tackle the inequitable distribution of power, money, and resources
Health equity in all policies, systems, and programmes
Fair financing
Market responsibility
Gender equity
Political empowerment—inclusion and voice
Good global governance
Measure and understand the problem and assess the impact of action
Social determinants of health: monitoring, training, and research

risk factors). As a consequence, England had a knowledge base for developing policies and programmes to tackle health inequalities, while Australia did not. Nutbeam concluded 'the way public health problems are defined and measured has a powerful influence on policy makers' perceptions of the challenges they face and the viable solutions' (Nutbeam and Boxall 2008).

In the United States, the Task Force on Community Preventive Services has been synthesizing information on the effectiveness of health promotion and disease prevention interventions for twelve years (Zaza et al 2000). More than two-hundred policy and programme interventions have been reviewed for evidence of effectiveness and feasibility. In some areas, such as preventing tobacco use, a robust literature to assess a variety of interventions was found. But early on it became clear that the evidence base for public health effectiveness was not evenly distributed across policies and programmes targeting leading determinants of population health. Approximately half of the systematic reviews on topics considered by the Task Force as key areas for health improvement have received the designation 'insufficient evidence to determine effectiveness' because few studies of adequate quality, and few studies reporting pertinent and comparable evaluation outcomes across the body of literature could be found (Anderson et al 2005). The Task Force found that some programme-effectiveness questions were easier to answer than others. Part of the challenge involves the level of impact of a programme or policy; interventions that work in a specific setting or small groups proved difficult to evaluate when implemented on a broader community scale where more complex social processes had to be taken into account. When social influences operate at different levels of analysis—family, social networks, organization, public policy, culture—it is difficult to evaluate cumulative effects (McLeroy et al 2003). Furthermore, some outcomes were more difficult to evaluate than others; where valid outcomes measures exist (eg immunization status in a medical record), evidence of intervention effect is easier to capture, but relevant and comparable measures are missing in important areas (eg health literacy, cultural competency). It was also more difficult to find studies reporting health outcomes in interventions aimed at broad, social determinants of health (eg community empowerment, income supplementation) that affect change across multiple intermediate and distal health outcomes. The recent work of the Commission on Social Determinants of Health, and particularly the Measurement and Evidence Knowledge Network, has advanced this effort considerably. But it is fair to say that while systematic reviews aim to reduce uncertainly by strengthening the evidence base, at the same time they often result in insufficient evidence to provide specific guidance for decision makers (Waters, Petticrew, Priest, Weightman, Harden, and Doyle 2008).

Better use of evidence for public health policies and programmes

This chapter has illustrated some of the strengths and weaknesses of producing evidence for public health use. Further development of this area, leading to a better use of evidence for public health policies and programmes, is contingent on factors outside the realm of the discussion to this point. There are needs that relate to: government resources and staff, academic infrastructure, intersectoral partnerships, and the engagement of civil society as informed consumers of scientific evidence. For example, it becomes clear in the whole discussion that in order to provide better evidence and to make sure that it is better used we need resources devoted specifically to the use of evidence, that is, the translation of knowledge to policy makers and into policies. To date, the efforts have been on the identification of the necessary evidence; resources now have to be given to making sure that best evidence is put into policy. In part this will be done through the engagement of diverse sectors of society through partnerships and the acceptance by major advocacy organizations, from NGOs to WHO, of using the best available evidence where it is available, and investing in satisfying the research gaps where it is not.

Clearly those global policy efforts affecting health, such as the Millennium Developmental Goals, the Commission on Social Determinants of Health, and other efforts of advocacy organizations to confront the challenges of globalization, and health inequities, would benefit from the best available evidence on how to effectively improve health at the population level. It has often been asserted that to manage the challenges of globalization, policy must be coherent across all levels of government, United Nations bodies, and other organizations, including the private sector. However, this is a hypothesis to be tested through synthesis of knowledge and explication of evidence. In reality we need to truly understand the limits of the established repertoire of proven effective strategies that need to be taken up. Without further investment in the infrastructure to understand and disseminate the best strategies little will change.

The conclusions in this paper are those of the author(s) and do not necessarily represent the official views of the Centers for Disease Control and Prevention.

Bibliography

US Department of Health and Human Services (2000) 'Office of Disease Prevention and Health Promotion—Healthy People 2010'. Available at: <http://www.healthypeople.gov/>

Anderson, L.M., Brownson, R.C., Fullilove, M.T., Teutsch, S.M., Novick, L.F., Fielding, J., and Land, G.H. (2005) 'Evidence-based public health policy and practice: promises and limits' *Am J Prev Med* 28/5 Suppl: 226–30

Begg, C., Cho, M., Eastwood, S., Horton, R., Moher, D., Olkin, I., Pitkin, R., Rennie, D., Schulz, K.F., Simel, D., and Stroup, D.F. (1996) 'Improving the quality of reporting of randomized controlled trials. The CONSORT statement' *JAMA* 276/8: 637–9

Bensing, J.M., Caris-Verhallen, W.M., Dekker, J., Delnoij, D.M., and Groenewegen, P.P. (2003) 'Doing the right thing and doing it right: toward a framework for assessing the policy relevance of health services research' *Int. J Technol. Assess. Health Care* 19/4: 604–12

Brownson, R.C., Baker, E.A., and Leet, T.L. (2003) *Evidence-based public health*. New York: Oxford University Press

Burrus, B., Dean, E., Flicker, L., Aiken, D., Heinrich, T., and Weizenkamp, D. (2006) *Surveillance Survey for the Guide to Community Preventive Services*. Research Triangle Park, NC, RTI Project 0208235.015

Chalmers, I., Hedges, L.V., and Cooper, H. (2002) 'A brief history of research synthesis' *Evaluation and the Health Professions* 25/1: 12–37

Contopoulos-Ioannidis, D.G., Alexiou, G.A., Gouvias, T.C., and Ioannidis, J.P. (2008) 'Medicine. Life cycle of translational research for medical interventions' *Science* 321/5894: 1298–99

Cooper, H. and Hedges, L. (1994) *The handbook of research synthesis*. New York, Russelll Sage Foundation

CSDH (2008) *Closing the gap in a generation: health equity through action on the social determinants of health. Final report of the Commission on Social Determinants of Health*. Geneva: World Health Organization

Des, J., Lyles, C., and Crepaz, N. (2004) 'Improving the reporting quality of nonrandomized evaluations of behavioral and public health interventions: the TREND statement' *Am J Public Health* 94/3: 361–6

Dwan, K., Altman, D.G., Arnaiz, J.A., Bloom, J., Chan, A.W., Cronin, E., Decullier, E., Easterbrook, P.J., Von, E.E., Gamble, C., Ghersi, D., Ioannidis, J.P., Simes, J., and Williamson, P.R. (2008) 'Systematic review of the empirical evidence of study publication bias and outcome reporting bias' *PLoS.ONE* 3/8: e3081

Graham, I.D., Logan, J., Harrison, M.B., Straus, S.E., Tetroe, J., Caswell, W., and Robinson, N. (2006) 'Lost in knowledge translation: time for a map?' *J Contin. Educ. Health Prof.* 26/1: 13–24

Hedges, L.V. and Olkin, I. (1985) *Statistical methods for meta-analysis*. Orlando, FL: Academic Press

Hunter, J.E., Schmidt, F.L., and Jackson, G.B. (1982) *Meta-analysis: cumulative research findings across studies*. Beverly Hills, CA: Sage

Innvaer, S., Vist, G., Trommald, M., and Oxman, A. (2002) 'Health policy-makers' perceptions of their use of evidence: a systematic review' *J Health Serv. Res Policy* 7/4: 239–44

Ioannidis, J.P. (2005) 'Contradicted and initially stronger effects in highly cited clinical research' *JAMA* 294/2: 218–28

Kelly, M.P., Morgan, A., Bonnefoy, J., Butt, J., Bergman, V., and Mackenbach, J. et al (2007) *The social determinants of health: developing an evidence base for political action*. Final report to the WHO Commission on the Social Determinants of Health. Measurement and Evidence Knowledge Network, Geneva. Available at: <http://www.who.int/social_determinants/resources/mekn_report_10oct07.pdf>

Light, R.J. and Pillemer, D.B. (1984) *Summing up: the science of reviewing research*. Cambridge, MA: Harvard University Press

McLeroy, K.R., Norton, B.L., Kegler, M.C., Burdine, J.N., and Sumaya, C.V. (2003) 'Community-based interventions' *Am J Public Health* 93/4: 529–33

McQueen, D.V. (2007) 'Evidence and theory; continuing debates on evidence and effectiveness' in DV McQueen and CM Jones (eds),*Global perspectives on health promotion effectiveness*. New York: Springer

McQueen, D.V. and Anderson, L.M. (2001) 'What counts as evidence: issues and debates' *WHO Reg Publ. Eur. Ser.* 92: 63–81

Morgan, H., Turley, R., Kavanagh, J., Armstrong, R., and Weightman, A. (2008) 'Developing a specialized register for the Public Health Review Group' *Journal of Public Health* 30/4: 508–9

Nutbeam, D. and Boxall, A.M. (2008) 'What influences the transfer of research into health policy and practice? Observations from England and Australia' *Public Health* 122/8: 747–53

Petticrew, M. and Roberts, H. (2006) *Systematic reviews in the social sciences*. Oxford: Blackwell Publishing

Sackett, D. (1997) *Evidence-based medicine: how to practice and teach EBM*. New York: Churchill Livingstone

Vandenbroucke, J.P., Von, E.E., Altman, D.G., Gotzsche, P.C., Mulrow, C.D., Pocock, S.J., Poole, C., Schlesselman, J.J., and Egger, M. (2007) 'Strengthening the Reporting of Observational Studies in Epidemiology (STROBE): explanation and elaboration' *Epidemiology* 18/6: 805–35

Waters, E., Petticrew, M., Priest, N., Weightman, A., Harden, A., and Doyle, J. (2008) 'Evidence synthesis, upstream determinants and health inequalities: the role of a proposed new Cochrane Public Health Review Group' *Eur. J Public Health* 18/3: 221–3

Zaza, S., Lawrence, R.S., Mahan, C.S., Fullilove, M., Fleming, D., Isham, G.J., and Pappaioanou, M. (2000) 'Scope and organization of the Guide to Community Preventive Services. The Task Force on Community Preventive Services' *Am J Prev Med* 18/1 Supp: 27–34

Chapter 31

Changing policy: reflections on the role of public health evidence

Virginia Berridge

Introduction

When reports on public health topics are published now, they are always accompanied by references to the 'evidence base' and are accompanied by a sheaf of footnotes. The report makes sure that the reader knows what the evidence is and that it has been published in 'high impact' journals. An evidence industry accompanies policy prescription. But before the 1960s or 1970s, this type of format was rarer. For medicine, the clinical impression rather than the research report held sway, and evidence in public health was just beginning its post-war rise. This chapter will look at the history of the rise of evidence, in public health but also in science and in policy making more generally. It will dissect the ways in which people have thought about the relationship between evidence and policy. And it will finish with a case study, that of the Black Report, which illustrates the different ways of thinking about the relationship.

The rise of evidence

When we consider the rise of evidence, there are some basic questions—what has counted as evidence in health and medicine and how and why has that evidence come to be considered as a prerequisite for policy making? We also need to consider what sort of evidence for what sort of policy arena. We can be talking about science; about health and medicine, or about social science. For public health, the developments really cover all three areas, and both qualitative and quantitative research styles.

For basic science the relationship between evidence and policy can be traced back as far as the 17th century to the emergence of governmental support for the Royal Observatory at Greenwich. So far as medicine is concerned, there was the use of statistical methods by British physicians and surgeons in assessing therapies for fevers, scurvy, and dropsy in the 18th century. This predated the later statistical evaluation of old and new treatments by Louis' numerical method in the Paris School in the 1830s. For social research, the social survey was established in the 19th century. Social research at that time was a leisure time activity conducted by amateurs, doctors, and others interested in social reform. Booth's surveys of London life or Seebohm Rowntree's study of York were examples; and the London School of Economics (LSE) was a unique example of early institutionalization, formed round the Fabian ideal of research-based permeation.

Early developments: 19th century

There were attempts to bring medicine and social science together from the mid Victorian period. Doctors were among the founders of the National Association for Social Science in 1856, which aimed to create a social science of government. Public health was an early user of evidence. The 19th century reliance on statistics, in particular in public health advocacy, was underpinned by the rise of empirical social research in Britain between 1800 and 1914. The establishment of the General Register Office, responsible since 1837 for registration of births and deaths and for conducting the census, was part of a general interest in surveys of social conditions, often conducted by local statistical societies, which fed into the public health movement. The London Statistical Society and the establishment of the Epidemiological Society were typical of this purpose. The 'rise of the expert' in various fields was part of the 19th century 'revolution in government'. The role of the 'medical expert' was part of those developments (McLeod 1988). Experts gave evidence in legal cases and the medico-legal side of medical work developed. They also began to work within government; the emergent role of the Chief Medical Officer, initially as the Medical Officer to the Privy Council, and to the Local Government Board, is the best known example and important for public health (Sheard and Donaldson 2005). More of these advisory positions developed in the early years of the 20th century. Forensic science was an important mediator of the relationship between professional research interests and government.

'Medicine as science' was increasingly important within government; and wider relationships between government and the sponsorship of science were also developing apace at the end of the century. The establishment of the National Physical Laboratory in 1899 was a significant change. Following German example, the Laboratory was devoted to the task of bringing scientific knowledge to bear upon everyday industrial and commercial practice, opening the way to substantial state support for research as opposed to the routine application of scientific techniques, as in the Laboratory of the Government Chemist. At the same time clinical and laboratory research were seen increasingly as the route to better health and the conquest of disease. Hospital-based research facilities, on the German model, began to percolate, although Britain was far behind developments in Germany and the USA. Full-time academic appointments did not develop in the London medical schools until after the First World War. However, the 1911 National Insurance Act made available a small amount of money to fund work on tuberculosis (TB). This expanded to form what eventually became the Medical Research Council (MRC), the government body funding scientific research (Austoker and Bryder 1989). Government sponsored developments were also taking place in the field of agriculture at the same time.

Wartime developments

The role of the First World War in strengthening research funding mechanisms within government was an important one. The Haldane committee's emphasis in 1918 on the need for government to have access to 'intelligence and research' lay behind a considerable development of the state/research machinery. It was in the wake of this report that the earlier Medical Research Committee was reconstituted as the Medical Research Council, the main vehicle for government funded medical research, although operating autonomously from government. Lord Zuckerman later considered that it was during this period that the world of scientific research developed into two distinct strands. The Royal Society, Research Council and University Science nexus operated independently, with greater prestige than the scientific laboratories of government departments or of industry. But as Pickstone has noted, although many of the wartime techno-scientific programmes evaporated, research institutions emerged stronger. The pharmaceutical industry and its inter-war development was a particular example of these networks, as was cancer research. Pickstone emphasizes the development of what he calls academic–industrial and medical complexes in the inter-war years (Pickstone 2000).

The Second World War marked another turning point in government/science relationships. Scientists, economists, and other experts were integrated into government planning in a way they had not been previously. Advice on biological warfare was formalized during the inter war years, with experts positing the threat which would result from a disrupted public health system (Balmer 2001). Here was the impetus which led to the wartime establishment of the Public Health Laboratory Service. Wartime production of penicillin led to the development of new antibiotics and to research-oriented pharmaceutical companies. The National Health Service became a major funder of medical research, including salaried clinical professors instead of the part-time appointees who had relied on private practice. Clinical research became common in all teaching hospitals, often with pharmaceutical or other industrial involvement. The wartime science advice role led into a post-war network of advisory committees, both for science and for the newly established National Health Service. The Central Health Services Council and its attendant standing committees were, for example, among the first locations in which the science/policy relationship for smoking, or for diet and heart disease, were played out in the 1950s.

Recent construction of the 'evidence base' for policy

These three strands of science; health and medicine; and social science also appear in the recent history of the 'evidence base'. There has been the rise of distinctive styles of public health research alongside medical research and the relation to policy; the role of social science in government policy making; and developments, building on the wartime structures, in science policy. The rise of a framework for government sponsorship of science and its research councils has been well covered and there are some recent histories of post-war science and technology policy (Edgerton 1996). The appointment in 1964 of Sir Solly Zuckermann as chief scientific adviser to the Cabinet was a measure of the increased importance accorded to science in the 1960s. For social science research, too, it was a period of great influence. Two distinct periods have been identified—one of close interaction between social scientists and political actors occurring in most countries at some time between the late 1950s and the early 1970s; and a period of state directed science policies in the 1970s and 1980s. Interaction in the first period was based on a consensus favouring both political and intellectual reform, a period which came to an end towards the end of the 1970s. The 1960s and 70s were in some sense a 'golden age' of social science research advocacy and interaction with government. But this period also saw a transformation of that state towards a more interventionist role to which the social sciences were increasingly exposed. The distance between the two spheres was reduced, with the devaluation of academic criteria in the funding of research and the substitution of criteria of relevance to government (Wagner et al 1991).

The work of the Government Statistical Service, growing rapidly in the 1960s, represented a significant extension of activity in the field of social intelligence, while university teachers of social administration, sociology, even history, were translated into government advisors. Research funding began to be channelled into social science research through the newly established Social Science Research Council (SSRC, established in 1965). Research-linked programmes in education and community development embodied a commitment to evaluate social action, a tendency which was also increasingly marked in donor programmes in Third World countries.

In the 1970s these developments took more government oriented directions. In 1972, the report produced by Lord Rothschild, head of the recently formed Central Policy Review Staff, on central government Research and Development clarified lines of accountability in Whitehall. The much publicized 'customer—contractor' principle specified a more utilitarian view of research funding. 'The customer says what he wants; the contractor does it (if he can); and the customer pays' (Rothschild Report 1972). The implementation of this principle brought consequences for the science research councils as some of their funds were transferred to the relevant ministries; it led to more formalized research funding machinery within departments and across government, with the establishment of Cabinet machinery for the coordination of advice on the research and development activities of government. It brought changes in the advisory machinery for the research councils as well through the establishment of the Advisory Board for the Research Councils (ABRC). Research liaison groups were established within departments but, as Kogan and Henkel's study of the Department of Health showed, the customer–contractor relationship was problematic and far from simple (Kogan, Henkel, and Hanney 2006).

The 'golden age' of free-ranging social science influence was to some extent over and nowhere was this more obvious than in the struggle over the future of the SSRC at the end of the decade. The incoming Conservative government as part of its rejection of the idea of post-war planning and its doubts about how much could be achieved by government, also expressed doubts about what the social sciences could achieve. The 1982 Rothschild report on the SSRC was asked to consider what aspects of its work could be done at the expense of the customer; social science had to prove its usefulness not just to society in general, but in a more specific and empirical way. The Committee's report came out in favour of the Council's continuation (albeit renamed as the Economic and Social Research Council) and recognized that there was little to which the concept of the 'ultimate user' of social science research could be applied. The concept of the 'user' of research became, however, more important in funding, serving, as Lewis has noted, both to depoliticize it and to elevate the supposedly value, free neutrality of quantitative research (Lewis 2003).

Public health evidence

Many of these developments had their parallels in health and public health research. The developing field of health research also began to rely on quantitative research. This tendency can be traced pre-war in the transmutation of eugenics, a doctrine with adherents from both ends of the political spectrum, with a concern for the quality of the population as a major public health concern. Post-war it was the bifurcation of social medicine which provided the impetus. The rise of social medicine was connected with the work of Richard Titmuss and Jerry Morris in an ambitious project, in which, as Dorothy Porter has noted 'statistical and other forms of social research could reshape both health policy and medical practice' (Porter 1997). Public health also began to open up to emergent medical sociology in the 1950s, as sociology struggled to establish its role in relation to the more dominant discipline of anthropology which had been important within an imperial culture. Post-war social medicine research went down two routes. It transmuted into chronic disease epidemiology, the new science of public health. The research which demonstrated the relationship between smoking and lung cancer in 1950 was a portent of a new style of public health research, although it was not until the 1960s the outside bodies, initially the Royal College of Physicians, began to promote the policy implications. In the 1970s, the formation of health activist bodies such as ASH (Action on Smoking and Health) began to play an important role in translating public health evidence into the policy domain (Berridge 2007). The focus of earlier social medicine epidemiological research on class and social factors changed during the 1950s into psychological explanation, placing greater emphasis on the role of personal responsibility; here was the underpinning of later changes within the reconceptualization of public health in the 1970s (Porter 2000). Research into occupational health was an important, if now often forgotten, component of the emergent field of social medicine/ public health research in the 1950s and 1960s.

Health services research

The other legacy of social medicine was research into health services (HSR), which became increasingly dominant. There was operational research in the early NHS. Research into the impact and utilization of health services developed in a number of centres in the 1960s. The central figure in the UK was Archie Cochrane, who argued that since health care resources would always be limited, these resources should be used to provide health services which have been shown to be effective. Cochrane's *Effectiveness and Efficiency* (1972) was an early and influential publication raising those issues, which led to the rise of the randomized controlled trial as the 'gold standard' of research (Cochrane 1999). The history of those developments, and of the later negotiations over government funding of HSR which went on in the 1970s and 1980s, has been little studied. The period was marked by tensions between MRC and the Department of Health about how such responsibility was to be divided. But also, as Klein has noted, until the end of the 1970s, there was consensus about many areas of NHS operation and therefore no real perceived need for research. The immunity of the medical profession from scrutiny and the relative acceptability of the lack of accountability and scrutiny provided little impetus for investigation (Klein 1990).

It was during the 1970s, too, that changes in the mechanisms linking science/ research/ government and the medical profession were put in place. A network of governmental advisory committees on specific subject areas, with a research and policy brief, largely supplanted the influence of the old NHS central committee machinery. The Advisory Council on the Misuse of Drugs, originally set up as the Advisory Committee on Drug Dependence in the late 1960s, and the Advisory Committee on Alcoholism (1978) were examples of these new departures. The 1980s and the arrival of the Conservative Government saw changes in the role of social science within government; and in the role of health research. The story of the Black Report in 1980, covered as a case study later, illustrates some of these changing relationships. The incoming government's rejection of the report on inequalities in health commissioned by the former Labour government was symbolic. It marked a break in the relationships which had sustained social and health-related academics outside government with politicians and civil servants inside government since the 1960s (Berridge and Blume 2003).

The latter part of the decade saw considerable impetus for health research and also for a greater degree of coordination in research, a tendency which affected science policy as well. The tensions round who 'owned' illicit drugs research prevented coordination in that area; shortly after, in the late 1980s the advent of AIDS as a perceived significant threat to the 'health of the nation' brought considerable amounts of government funding. There were AIDS initiatives and increased funding both for biomedical research and for social science. Research participants spoke in terms of a wartime situation where different interests were put aside for the common effort (Berridge 1996).

This model of applied and directed research also had its impact on health services research, where the late 1980s saw the acceptance of the case for more applied research by the House of Lords Select Committee on Science and Technology. Government decided to locate research at the heart of the NHS rather than funding it through an independent NHS Research Authority. There was a particular emphasis on health technology and the Standing Committee on Health Technology commissioned two new centres, the UK Cochrane Centre at Oxford and the York Centre for Reviews and Dissemination (Black 1997). The first five years of the NHS Research and Development programme was a 'golden age' of research so far as funding and extension of research activity was concerned—although critics of government health policy pointed out that there was little investigation of pilot projects of government changes in health services funding and policy. There, what Klein called 'ambiguous and partisan' evidence was used to bolster the perceptions of ministers. In general the late 1980s and first half of the 1990s saw increased funding for research and also for forms of research which appeared to provide 'user information' and to be value-free—health economics and RCTs were the most obvious examples.

That field was also marked by controversies about the sponsorship of research funding. In the 1970s and 1980s, there had been concern that government was becoming too dominant in its relationships with researchers and that autonomy and independence were being lost. In the 1990s, the focus, so far as public health went, was more on industry funding, and there were vehement debates about this, in particular over the industry funding of tobacco and alcohol research. Some spoke of a 'new McCarthyism' in science, arguing that government funding was as likely to skew research as was that from industry. The taken-for-granted alliance 40 years earlier between government, scientists, and industry was fragmented so far as public health industrial funding from tobacco or alcohol was concerned, although this was at a time when industrial funding and commercial connections with research in general were growing stronger.

The picture in the latter half of the 1990s began to change again. There were new arrangements for obtaining external medical and scientific advice in the Department of Health and the amalgamation of 'medical' and 'generalist' civil servant strands within the department. The medical civil servant had been a key 'gatekeeper' in the relationship with researchers outside the department. The BSE (Bovine Spongiform Encephalopathy in cattle) crisis and the crisis of scientific and governmental authority which it engendered brought more consideration of the ways in which government obtained scientific advice.

The evidence-policy relationship: schools of thought

This, of course, is only the British story. Writers on the research/policy relationships have been at pains to stress that different national cultures led to a differential set of relationships. The relationship between evidence and policy is not a simple one. There are different schools of thought which have looked at the relationship and we can now turn to look at some of these. Here, I categorize four main ways of talking about the relationship between evidence and policy; the evidence-based medicine/evidence-based health policy approach; the journalist school of thought; sociology of scientific knowledge (SSK); and finally science policy/policy science studies.

The *evidence-based medicine/health policy approach* lies behind the recent history of the relationship described above. This is what has been called the 'engineering' model of research impact on policy. Its advocates assume a rational model of evidence and policy and argue that all that is needed are technical adjustments to make the relationships work. This model implies that knowledge can indeed impact in a value-free way.

A more sophisticated was of looking at the dissemination and impact of research has come through the *enlightenment model* developed by Weiss (Weiss 1982). Here research is not seen as having a direct 'user' impact, but rather as feeding into the climate of policy making. This model was refined by Thomas who identified, from a study of the uses of social policy research, how policy makers actually did use research (Thomas 1985). The enlightenment model as described by Weiss, was essentially how 'generalisations and ideas from numbers of studies come into currency . . . through articles in academic journals, journals of opinion, stories in the media . . . lobbying by special interest groups, conversations of colleagues, attendance at conferences . . . and other uncatalogued sources.' The role of pressure groups and of the media was important in this context; the making of 'knowledge claims' by scientists and policy actors created public controversy, much of which has come to be played out through the media.

Analogous, but more narrowly channelled approaches to the science/policy relationship appear in the *journalist school*. This label is not just because it is practised by journalists, but because it embodies a way of looking at the world which often characterizes media agendas on science and policy. Here again, the relationship between evidence and policy is seen as desirable, but perhaps in a more partisan way. When some hiatus occurs in the relationship, the interpretation is in terms of conspiracy. The interruption is seen in terms of 'delay' and blame is attached to key participants. This 'heroes and villains' school of analysis is a conventionally accepted mode, even in academic circles, of looking at the nature of response, especially to public health issues. AIDS is a recent example, likewise BSE. Smoking is often seen only as a matter of industry 'villains' versus public health 'heroes'. Such analyses are readable. Yet they leave too many loose ends, not least the nature of science and evidence and the complexity of the structural interests which surround the relationship with policy development.

These are issues taken up in our third and fourth schools of thought. The *sociology of scientific knowledge* (SSK) is a field which has undergone rapid development over the past twenty or so years. Changes in scientific ideas cannot be understood, its proponents argue, as the simple pursuit of accurate accounts of 'external reality'. The closure of scientific debate cannot be understood as the result of discoveries about a world 'out there'. Closure of debate in science, the discovery of scientific facts must be studied as social processes, as socially constructed. This strand of investigation has focused on the creation of science within the laboratory as in Latour and Woolgar's observational study of *Laboratory Life* (Latour and Woolgar 1979). And Latour's *Science in Action* has provided an account of the 'actor networks' which sustain the research process: the strength of any scientific claim being based on the resources, whether people, organizations, other disciplines, or objects, from which its proponents are able to derive support. But the wider interactions with state and the formation of governmental policy (as opposed to clinical policy) are neglected in this type of work, as some of its protagonists recognize.

The perspectives of SSK nevertheless are of relevance to our fourth intellectual 'interest area', the *policy science interest in the research/policy relationship*. Here, the opposite is true. The policy dimension is to the fore and there is less interest in the 'construction' of scientific facts. Analysing policy networks has become a dominant approach for the study of policy-making processes in Britain, Europe, and North America. Such approaches emphasize the interaction and patterns of association between actors in different policy areas. These networks have been one of the most discussed and contested terms in political science. Richardson and Jordan developed the idea of the 'policy community' focusing on what they called 'the government, civil service—pressure group network'(Richardson and Jordan 1979). The relationship between all or part of government departments and external bodies is the central idea; policy formulation takes place in stable subsystems comprising government agencies and outside groups. The whole system is compartmentalized such that relationships between government and external groups vary for each policy area. The dominant role of the medical profession is a theme in many health policy analyses. Evans, in his review of Department of Health external advice mechanisms in the mid 1990s instanced a range of ways of seeking external advice; informal networking by civil servants; individuals in a formal relationship with the department, such as the Chief Medical Officer's (CMO) consultant advisors; advisory committees; and external bodies such as professional associations, medical Royal Colleges, and other public bodies such as the Public Health Laboratory Service (PHLS) (Department of Health 1995).

Work on the impact of science is relevant here, for example Jasanoff's emphasis on the 'co production' of knowledge (Jasanoff 1990). Dorothy Nelkin too has written of the symbiosis between political values and scientific facts. 'The boundaries of the problems to be studied, the alternatives weighed, the issues regarded as appropriate—all tend to determine which data are selected as important, which facts emerge' (Nelkin 1984). The American sociologist Hilgartner's recent work characterizes science and its formulation into expert advice as a form of drama. This perspective usefully marries the construction of scientific orthodoxy with the locations in which this process takes place, the advisory committees which present the public face of science. Other activities which go to make that consensus are hidden ' backstage'. Using three US National Academy of Sciences reports on diet and health which had very different policy impacts (one was very influential, one was largely discredited, and one was cancelled before publication), he shows how stage management techniques played a central role in shaping the credibility of science advice (Hilgartner 2000).

A public health case study: the Black Report

So the role of evidence in relation to policy is far from simple. If we take one key public health example, that of the Black Report of 1980, already mentioned above, we can see what it tells us about these analyses in action. The report was commissioned by the Labour Government of the 1970s but presented to the incoming Conservative Government in 1980. Its recommendations were less acceptable to the new government and the report was published on an August Bank Holiday in a limited number of copies. The resultant media furore gained the report great publicity: there was a rerun with another report on inequalities, *The health divide*, commissioned by David Player as the head of the Health Education Council in 1987 (Berridge and Blume 2003).

The Black Report episode seems at first glance to fit within two of our models of the relationship between evidence and policy. It could be seen as '*rationality thwarted*': the rational model could not be applied. Or it could be seen as an example of the '*journalist school*', with health heroes on the committee, confronting the political villains in the government.

But characterizing it in these two ways gives less than the full picture. At a 'witness seminar' in 1999 which gathered together most of the key protagonists, a different picture began to emerge. Firstly, the lesson of the evidence was not clear and was variously interpreted by key members of the committee, dependent on their perceptions. It was clear that there had been disagreements in the committee about the evidence and what it meant in terms of policy advice. Should the focus be on hospital services or on prevention and welfare? Jerry Morris and Peter Townsend, two members of the committee, exemplified opposing tendencies. As a result the report was delayed. More than twenty years later, the civil servants involved, Sir Arthur Buller the Chief Scientist, and Dr Elizabeth Shore, the deputy CMO, were clearly exasperated. They had been hoping for something which would have political utility prior to the expected change in government. Lord Jenkin, the Minister involved, on the other hand, mentioned that his civil servants had advised distance from the report when it was received. At this level, then, the genesis and reception of the report showed a more complex picture, which we can fit within *the science policy theories*. Evidence itself and its interpretation was fluid and fitted within networks linking researchers and interests in government. In this case it was the linkages between civil servants and health researchers which were potentially important, and those with politicians which did not operate. The role of the media was also important in disseminating a view of the report which has continued to have influence.

We can also see the Black Report as exemplifying *enlightenment theories* of the influence of research. Although the report itself was not the basis for political action, it continued and developed its influence throughout the years of Conservative Government in the 1980s and 1990s. A network of researchers on inequalities (renamed as 'variations on health') expanded during these years, ready for the revival of inequalities as a political issue which came with the election of a Labour Government in 1997. The Black Report was successful in enlightening opinion through a much lengthier process than the simple 'rational' model.

Conclusion

The recent history of the last ten years has seen a rapid sequence of developments for both public health and health services. For the latter the NHS research strategy has shifted from the service itself as the consumer of research to the patient as its consumer. Initiatives such as *Best research for best health* (2005) and the establishment of the National Institute for Health Research positioned patients in this role. The Cooksey review examined the whole system of health research in the UK including the NHS R and D programme and the MRC, where the traditional view of independent research had been strongest. Its focus was on 'knowledge transfer' and whether translation from 'bench to bedside' could be improved. This review aimed to consider the needs of all customers including industry (Hanney, Kuruvilla, Mays 2008). These developments have also impacted in the public health sphere. The Health Education Authority was reconstituted as the Health Development Agency quite early on, losing its public education focus and becoming instead the arbiter of the public health 'evidence base'. Its eventual amalgamation into the National Institute for Health and Clinical Excellence (NICE) brought public health and clinical aspects of evidence into a relationship. The role of such arm's length bodies has been characteristic of new developments in evidence and policy. The role of the National Treatment Agency (NTA) for drug use, applying evidence to practice, is another example. The Wanless Report on public health placed emphasis on the role of research.

There have been recent examples, for example, the 2004 Alcohol Harm Reduction Strategy, where the document summarizing research evidence was published separately because of its extensive nature. References to 'the evidence base' are common currency in a way in which our 19th century forebears would find strange. But the example of the Black Report cited here and of recent responses to policy formulation for alcohol both show that the nature of the interaction between evidence and policy is complex. Evidence must make its way through a thicket of sometimes competing, sometimes coalescing, interests. Political and electoral concerns, the media, health activism, industrial interests, civil servants, expert committees, and government agencies help determine the boundaries and the impact of evidence on policy.

Bibliography

Austoker, J. and Bryder, L. (eds) (1989) *Historical Perspectives on the role of the MRC*. Oxford: Oxford University Press

Balmer, B (2001) *Britain and Biological Warfare. Expert Advice and Science Policy 1930–65*. Basingstoke: Palgrave

Berridge, V (1996) *Aids in the UK: the making of policy, 1981–1994*. Oxford: Oxford University Press

Berridge, V (ed) (2005) *Making Health Policy. Networks in research and policy since 1945*. Amsterdam: Rodopi

Berridge, V (2007) *Marketing Health. Smoking and the discourse of public health, 1945–c.2000*. Oxford: Oxford University Press

Berridge, V and Blume, S. (2003) *Poor Health. Social inequality before and after the Black Report*. London: Frank Cass

Black, N (1997) 'National strategy for research and development: lessons from England' *Annual Review Public Health* 18: 485–505

Cochrane, AL (1992) *Effectiveness and Efficiency: Random Reflections on Health Services*. London: RSM Press, reprint of 1972 publication

Department of Health (1995) *Review of the Department of Health's Arrangements for Obtaining External Medical and Scientific Advice (Evans Report)*. London: Department of Health

Edgerton, D (1996) *Science, Technology and the British Industrial 'decline', c.1870–1970*. Cambridge: Cambridge University Press/Economic History Society

Hanney, S, Kuruvilla, S, and Mays, N (2008) 'Who needs what from health systems? Lessons from R and D reforms in England' submitted to *Health Research Policy and Systems*

Hilgartner, S (2000) *Science on Stage: Expert Advice as Public Drama*. Stanford: Stanford University Press

Jasanoff,S. (1990) *The Fifth Branch: Science Advisors as Policy Makers*. Cambridge: Harvard University Press

Klein, R (1990) 'Research, Policy and the National Health Service' *Journal of Health Policy, Politics and Law* 15/3: 501–22

Kogan, M, Henkel, M, and Hanney, S (2006) *Government and Research. Thirty years of Evolution*. Dordrecht: Springer

Latour, B and Woolgar, S (1979) *Laboratory Life: The Social Construction of Scientific Facts*. London: Sage

Lewis, J (2003) 'How useful are the social sciences?' *Political Quarterly* 74/2: 193–201

McLeod, R (1988) *Government and Expertise: Specialists, Administrators and Professionals, 1860–1919*. Cambridge: Cambridge University Press

Nelkin, D (ed) (1984) *Controversy: Politics of Technical Decisions*. Newbury Park: Sage

Pickstone, J (2000) *Ways of Knowing: A New History of Science Technology and Medicine*. Manchester: Manchester University Press

Porter, D (1997) *Social Medicine and Medical Sociology in the Twentieth Century*. Amsterdam: Rodopi

Porter, D (2003) 'From social class to social behaviour' in V Berridge and S Blume (eds), *Poor Health*, pp 58–80. London: Frank Cass

Richardson, JJ and Jordan, AG (1979) *Governing Under Pressure: The Policy process in a post parliamentary democracy*. Oxford: Martin Robertson

Rothschild Report (1972) *The Organisation and Management of Government Research and Development*. London: HMSO

Sheard, S and Donaldson, L (2005) *The Nation's Doctor; the role of the Chief Medical Officer 1885–1998*. Oxford: Radcliffe

Thomas, P (1985) *The Aims and Outcomes of Social Policy Research*. London: Croom Helm

Wagner, P, Weiss, C, Wittrock, B, and Wollman, H (eds) (1991) *Social Sciences and Modern States: National experiences and Theoretical Cross Roads*. Cambridge: Cambridge University Press

Weiss, C (1986) 'The many meanings of research utilisation' in M Bulmer (ed), *Social Science and Social Policy*, pp 31–59. London: Allen and Unwin

A synopsis: effectiveness and efficiency in public health

Amanda Killoran

Evidence-based public health is the *process involved in providing the best available evidence to influence decisions about the effectiveness of policies and interventions aimed at improving health and reducing health inequalities.*

This volume provides a guide to this process. The many contributors present and discuss the main elements of this evidence-based approach (including concepts and theories, methods and processes for generating and synthesis of evidence, and guidance for policy and practice).

Here we provide a summary and highlight some of the important arguments and issues relating to advancing the approach.

Public health challenges in the 21st century

A number of important themes underpin the search for effectiveness and efficiency in public health. These themes include the focus on the social determinants of health, how evidence interacts with policy, and ethical considerations. These themes are introduced in the first section and further explored throughout the volume.

Social determinants and public health challenges

The assessment of future public health challenges must be based on a much better understanding of the influence of the social determinants of health—how social conditions shape health behaviours and experiences to impact on health outcomes.

Bartley and Blane consider UK trends in social, demographic, economic, and technological developments over the last century and their relationship to different measures of health and disease. Patterns of social inequalities in health are also explored.

The analysis depicts a historical pathway of interrelated social changes that have led to marked overall health improvements. However, the widening gap in life expectancy between different social groups can be related to the greater rate of improvement among more well off groups. It is clear that behavioural risk factors only partially explain the social health inequalities.

The analysis raises questions relating to the scope of the evidence base, and the need to understand the implications for health of changing social norms and expectations, living standards, working conditions, and aging.

The interface between evidence and policy

Law considers opportunities and challenges involved in developing evidence for policy makers who are seeking effective ways to address important public health concerns.

The current limited nature of the evidence base on the effectiveness and cost-effectiveness of public health interventions does present major difficulties. Much of the research has focused on individual level interventions rather than complex interventions directed at the wider determinants of health. This reflects in part the difficulties involved in applying research designs and methods derived from evidence-based medicine to public health.

Furthermore, many of the answers 'to what works for whom in what circumstances' can only be derived from syntheses of studies. This involves bringing together a wide range of evidence and study designs. But the methodology for synthesis of the 'mixed economy' of evidence is underdeveloped.

There are also major problems in interpretation of evidence. For example, although the evidence base is incomplete, there are political imperatives for action to tackle the problem. 'But scientific work focuses on changing knowledge whereas policy making tries to change everyday lives…. but scientists and policy makers may place different burdens of proof before they are willing to take decisions.'

Despite such difficulties, much progress has been made in developing the evidence base; and stakeholders including policy makers and the public now expect evidence to be considered when making decisions about public health policy.

Ethical concerns in using evidence

There are important ethical issues involved in applying an evidence-based approach to public health. McQueen discusses the ethical issues and dilemmas relating to evidence in the field of health promotion.

For example, much of the search for evidence on effectiveness adopts a 'scientific' methodology, involving use of experimental designs. This fails to take account of underlying values and concepts of health promotion practice (equity, empowerment, participation). 'Insufficient' evidence means judgements need to be made—but how and who should make such judgements? Furthermore, the lack of evidence raises the question of an intervention doing harm to individuals and communities; or the harm relating to benefits foregone by not investing in alternative interventions.

Perhaps most importantly, health promotion practice is highly 'context-specific', and the importance of 'contextualism' defies definition of simple causal relationships and 'challenges the notion of universality, comparability and best practice'.

Evidence-based frameworks for design and evaluation of interventions

A range of conceptual and methodological frameworks can be used to inform the design of public health policies and interventions, and evaluate their effectiveness and cost-effectiveness.

Theory-driven approaches to evaluation

Pawson and Sridharan describe the use of theory-driven approaches in the evaluation of public health programmes. They define *programmes as theories*—a set of hypotheses stating why the programme will work and produce the desired changes. The explicit statement of the programme theory is important as it provides the underlying logic for the evaluation. Pawson and Sridharan point out that theory-driven evaluation can help create a road map that is often missing at the start of an intervention.

A range of techniques can be used to set out the hypotheses, usually in a diagrammatic form. A distinction may be made between 'theories of change' that set out the stepping stones of the programme; while a 'realistic hypothesis' focuses on the mechanism for change, and how outcomes might vary in different contexts and with different population groups.

Pawson and Sridharan stress that theory-driven analysis demands a multi-method evidence base. Qualitative methods are required to generate process data, quantitative approaches measure outputs and outcomes, and comparative observation and measurements are required for contextual information.

Equity, risk, and vulnerability

Three chapters consider the relationship between individuals' experiences and behaviours and social context, and consequences for health. The notions of risk, vulnerability, and equity are explored from different but complementary perspectives.

A life course perspective

At all stages of life there are marked differences in health according to socio-economic circumstances. Graham and Power present a model to help explain this pattern.

The model defines the 'interlocking pathways' that link childhood disadvantages to poor adult health. The pathways cover the development of physical and emotional health and health behaviours that have a direct influence on health. They also cover cognitive development and educational attainment and adoption of social identifies (such as early parenthood) which have impact on their adult circumstances.

The model provides a framework to inform policy aimed at reducing health inequalities. Graham and Power state that the life course approach argues for an integrated approach which includes both targeted programmes and the mainstream policies. Macro systems and policies (including social welfare, education, and health services) need to reduce the inequalities in children's circumstances. These wider systems can provide the conditions that ensure more targeted programmes (such as Sure Start) are reinforced and not diluted. The goal is to increase the life chances and health chances of children from poorer backgrounds.

Vulnerability, disadvantage, and sexual health

Ingham and Smith examine evidence on teenage pregnancy, to understand the pathways linking social circumstances to this outcome, with its associated increased risks for the health and well-being of the child and mother.

There is a marked social gradient in teenage pregnancy in the UK. This can be attributed to a combination of factors linked to social circumstances, and in particular the 'seemingly deep-seated community norms involving lack of education or employment aspirations, gender roles and expectations and stigma'. For example, qualitative research indicates that structural factors such as educational and occupational opportunities are very much influenced by the expectations and experiences of families and communities. These norms and expectations have been established over generations. In some deprived areas low educational attainment and lack of visible employment opportunities present teenage pregnancy as a viable alternative and accepted 'career route'.

Ingham and Smith state that evidence of effectiveness of interventions tends to be skewed towards studies based on the 'scientific' evaluation design, and directs attention to specific forms of intervention. But this may produce a simplistic view when a wide range of factors are probably operating together to create vulnerability. There is a danger that important issues that are less amenable to intervention evaluation such as educational and employment opportunities, and gender-based norms and aspirations may not be addressed.

Social relationships, power and youth health

Lynam uses Bourdieu's theory of social relations as the analytical framework to explore how societal structures and practices can marginalize young people and limit their health chances. The analysis of young people's experiences demonstrates Bourdieu's concepts of *habitus* (the way individuals make sense of their situations), *fields* (social worlds) and forms of *capital* (drawing on different resources).

The report of the different teenagers' experiences highlights the processes that create or mitigate access to resources that impact on their development and health. For example a student's exclusion from school results from symptoms of depression being misdiagnosed as 'bad' behaviour. Marginalizing practices result from unquestioned assumptions of stereotypical images (an act of symbolic violence). There are also examples of individuals (parents, teenagers themselves, and support workers) questioning the 'symbolic order' by mobilizing support or resources for teenagers.

Lynam states that the findings reveal the need to address the social structures that place groups at risk. Practitioners themselves need to critically reflect on their own practice to ensure they do not reproduce and sustain the processes that create privilege for some while disadvantaging others.

Health economics, public health and resource allocation

Three groups of health economists (Griffin et al; Morris et al; Cookson and Culyer) give their perspectives on the application of economic evaluation to public health: the theory and practice (including the 'basic arithmetic' of quality adjusted life years—QALYs), strengths and weaknesses, and areas for further development.

Economic evaluation has a crucial role in providing a transparent framework for assessing the impact of health care and public health programmes and informing public resource allocation decisions. Quality adjusted life years (QALYs) provide a single overall assessment of health impact that takes account of both changes in length of life and health-related quality of life. The use of cost-effectiveness analysis allows different proposals to be compared on an equivalent basis, in terms of their incremental cost per QALY gained. Furthermore, a benchmark or 'threshold' cost per QALY can be established, to enable judgements about whether a programme is cost-effective or not compared with other uses of public money to improve health.

Overall, while economic evaluation using QALYs has clear benefits for supporting resource investment decisions about improving health outcomes, certain public health issues are not fully addressed.

Griffin and colleagues point out that economic evaluation of health care programmes uses a framework which aims to maximize health outcomes subject to the health sector budget constraint (an 'Extra Welfarist' perspective). This framework however could be extended to encompass 'Welfarist' normative principles for the evaluation of public health interventions. This extension would enable inter-sectoral comparisons and a consideration of equity, as well as frameworks used in other areas of policy evaluation (eg cost–benefit analysis).

Morris and colleagues focus specifically on the notions of efficiency and equity and how QALYs might help make decisions that involve a trade-off between the two.

Situations of potential trade-offs between cost-effectiveness and reducing health inequality are explored. Some cost-effective public health interventions can increase socio-economic inequalities in health. For example, preventative programmes designed to detect and manage risk factors may widen inequalities as lower social groups may have least access to these services. However, some public health interventions both reduce health inequalities and are cost-effective. Fluoridation of the public water supply has been shown to be cost-effective and to reduce inequalities in dental health across social classes. Since fluoridation of the public water supply is universally accessible to a community, people in lower social classes who have higher levels of dental caries are therefore likely to obtain greater health benefits.

Cookson and Culyer identify three important areas for further methodological research:

- improving methods of measuring health-related quality of life in order to construct QALYs;
- developing methods for adjusting QALYs to accommodate equity concerns; and
- developing methods for bringing together and weighing both QALY and non-QALY outcomes, including private consumption as well as outcomes in other public policy sectors (eg education, employment, crime).

Such future research will need to be guided by underlying philosophical views about the nature and purpose of economic evaluation in terms of outcomes for 'individual well-being'. For example, the adoption of a 'capability' approach might involve constructing a new all-purpose index of well-being with multiple dimensions reflecting both health and non-health-related quality of life—a sort of 'super-QALY'.

However, Cookson and Culyer state that even if there are *no methodological developments* in this area, there is scope for a vast improvement in evidence-based public health policy making by applying existing standard QALY methods more extensively and more rigorously to public health.

Stewardship of public health

The relationship between the role of the state and individual freedoms are at the centre of efforts to improve public health. This is the subject of the Nuffield Council on Bioethics' Report *Public health: ethical issues* published in 2007. The report seeks to provide a framework for assessing the legitimate goals and constraints of liberal states in pursuing public health measures. A summary of the main findings are reported by Lord Krebs and Schmidt.

The 'stewardship model' is proposed as a way of assessing whether and how different types of interventions might be justified. The model sets out a number of principles concerned with providing the necessary conditions for people to live healthy lives, but also minimizing unnecessary intrusion. In addition the intervention ladder provides a tool that helps apply these principles. 'In general the higher the rung on the ladder at which the policy maker intervenes (involving restricting or eliminating choice through laws or regulation) the stronger the justification has to be, both in ethical terms, and with regard to the evidence about causes of good and ill health and about the potential of particular interventions to promote the former and reduce the later.'

Generating evidence on the effectiveness of public health interventions

The Medical Research Council guidance (2008) sets out advice on methods for the evaluation of complex interventions (Craig et al 2008). A summary of the main aspects are presented.

Evaluation needs to determine whether an intervention is effective in the 'real world', especially how and why the effect of an intervention varies across different settings and different groups. Ideally the evaluation process comprises the following elements: setting out a theoretical understanding of the likely process of change, piloting studies to refine the intervention and selection, and use of an appropriate evaluation study design to determine impact. Process evaluation can be used to assess the quality of implementation, clarify causal mechanisms, and how contextual factors influence outcomes.

The choice of evaluation approach needs to be based on the 'best available method'-given the potential ethical, political, and practical constraints.

The series of case studies in subsequent chapters illustrate the evaluation approaches and methods employed to determine the effectiveness of different types of complex public health interventions.

Smoking cessation interventions

The evidence base on the effectiveness and cost-effectiveness of different interventions designed to help smokers quit is advanced, in comparison to many other areas of public health. West and Shahab examine theory, evaluation methods, and the evidence that is currently available.

A simple 'route to quit' model can be used to show how *in theory* smoking cessation interventions can influence behavioural processes to achieve increases in the rate of quit attempts and/or the rate at which these attempts succeed.

West and Shahab point out that although it may be possible to conduct RCTs to determine efficiency, there are many conditions in which the RCT is not the appropriate design to evaluate the likely effect of a smoking cessation intervention, as too much is lost by way of generalizability. In reality, there is 'no such thing as hard evidence', and judgements are required on the likely effect of interventions given different contexts and different target groups. West and Shahab state 'this is not about a lack of scientific rigour but an application of a rigorous evaluation process to a real world inference'.

A summary of types of smoking cessation interventions, their effectiveness, and the nature of the evidence available is presented. Interventions directed at populations such as tax increases, measures to control smuggling, and smoking restrictions have potentially wide reach but evidence is mostly from observational studies, while interventions such as behavioural support and medications (such as nicotine replacement therapy) have strong evidence for efficiency but are currently used by only a minority of smokers.

Prevention of type 2 diabetes

Khunti and colleagues describe the evaluation approach involved in design and development of a lifestyle modification programme to help prevent type 2 diabetes in multi-ethnic populations with prediabetes.

The initial phase of evaluation involved establishing a robust theoretical model of behaviour change to underpin the lifestyle programme. A single model was constructed based on review of a number of behaviour change theories, and selection and integration of elements (such as risk perception, self-efficacy, and self-regulation) judged to be particularly relevant.

The research team used the theoretical model and findings of qualitative research with patients recently diagnosed with prediabetes to develop a group-based structured education programme. This was subsequently evaluated through randomized controlled trials.

The aim was then to adapt the programme and educator training protocols to reflect the needs of the South Asian population. The process of refining the curriculum, resources and training programmes involved two cycles of piloting, each using quantitative and qualitative research methods. The next step was to conduct a definitive randomized controlled trial in a primary care setting with progression to type 2 diabetes as the outcome measures.

Early intervention to enhance the health and well-being of disadvantaged children

The Sure Start Programme was established with the aim of improving the health and well-being of children from birth to four and their families in the most deprived areas of England. Melhuish and colleagues describe how the national evaluation of the Programme had a major role in developing policy and assisting programme design and implementation to improve effectiveness.

Sure Start Local Programmes (SSLPs) were set up in 1998, with over 500 planned by 2004 to reach one third of poor children under four. The national evaluation was designed to investigate the local context, implementation, and the economics and impact of the local programmes, and a range of methods were employed.

The first phase of the impact evaluation used a quasi-experimental design. It compared the functioning of 9- to 36-month-old children and their families living in 150 SSLP communities across England with counterparts living in 50 communities that were planned to become SSLP areas. This early impact evaluation showed relatively less disadvantaged families in the SSLP areas benefited from the programme, while the most disadvantaged three-year-olds and their families (including teenage parents, lone parents, workless households) experienced adverse effects.

The management of local programmes were assessed across a range of dimensions relating to systems and processes (including leadership, strategies for identifying families, training of staff). This showed variation in quality of implementation of local programmes. Furthermore, better implemented programmes were shown to produce greater benefits for children and families. The findings provided important guidance on the conditions necessary for programmes to generate benefits for children and their families.

The longitudinal phase of the impact evaluation compared children's outcomes in SSLP areas with those involved in the UK cohort study (Millennium Cohort Study) that were not living in SSLP areas. The results of this phase differed markedly from those of the early impact evaluation, showing positive effects across all population subgroups, including the most disadvantaged. The contrast in findings was explained in terms of the increased exposure of children and families to SSLPs that had become more effectively managed and delivered over time.

Promoting the emotional and behavioural well-being of young people in secondary education

The Gatehouse Project was a school-based programme undertaken in Victoria, Australia, designed to promote the emotional and behavioural well-being of secondary school students and also to reduce rates of substance use, that were known to be related to emotional well-being.

It was based on a theoretical framework that recognized the importance of healthy attachments and relationships as critical to emotional well-being, and therefore focused on promoting security, communication, and positive regard through valued participation. A whole school strategy approach was used as the operational framework. It employed curriculum based learning together with school-wide processes for promoting emotional well-being. The project was conceived as a process of building the local capacity of schools for continual review and improvement of their practices and policies.

Different evaluation methods were used at different stages of the project. Outcome evaluation was based on use of a cluster randomized controlled trial in 26 secondary schools (1997–2000). The findings indicated that the prevalence of any drinking, smoking, marijuana use and peers' drug use was between 3% and 5% lower for students in the intervention schools compared to those in the comparison schools. However Bond and Butler state that the explanatory mechanisms for change in students' behaviour remained unclear, as there was no change in students' reporting of increased connectedness to schools. They discuss some of reasons for this finding, as well as the challenges of evaluating school-based interventions.

The influence of the workplace on mental well-being

The workplace can be viewed as an important psychosocial environment that poses risks to health or can enhance health. It therefore is an important focus for improving public health.

The Whitehall II study is an observational study of 10,000 British civil servants followed up from 1985 onwards. The investigation of social and occupational influences on health and illness has been a central theme in repeated data collections over 20 years. Kivimaki and colleagues describe in detail how this study has been used to test the hypothesis that psychosocial factors at work affect employees' well-being.

Findings have shown an improvement in mental health by age, but the rate of improvement is slower for employees in lower occupational positions. Psychosocial work stressors, such as high job demands, lack of control over work, high-effort-low-reward conditions, and perceived unfairness, predict worse mental well-being across various measures in longitudinal analyses.

Periods of major organizational change provided the opportunity to conduct a 'natural experiment' of the impact of job security on mental well-being. It showed that compared to employees whose jobs are secure at baseline and follow-up, self-reported psychological morbidity is higher among those who lost job security.

Kivimaki and colleagues state that the study established associations between work stressors and poor mental well-being, but causality remained uncertain. But they also assert *that a true association exists that cannot be fully explained by bias and confounding.* Furthermore the main findings of the Whitehall II study have been replicated in other occupational cohorts. However randomized controlled trials are needed to confirm that interventions at work are able to reduce the risk of poor mental well-being among employees.

Area-based interventions addressing disadvantage

Cummins reports on the Glasgow Superstore Study—this was a quasi-experimental study of the impact on diet and psychological health of the opening of a major food superstore in one of the most socio-economically deprived areas of Glasgow.

The study compared changes in diet and self-reported psychological health in the area where the new supermarket was built (the intervention area), with a comparison area matched by deprivation, using a prospective 'before and after' postal survey. It was hypothesized that the increase in accessibility and affordability of local food would have a direct environmental influence on diet; and also that the increased opportunities for employment and the highly visible inward investment would influence social and psychosocial determinants of health. However, the evaluation itself found little evidence that the opening of the food supermarket had any overall major effect on self-reported fruit and vegetable consumption or other outcomes.

While the study findings were disappointing, Cummins highlights important lessons relating to the methodological and conceptual difficulties involved in evaluating complex area-based interventions. Clear and rigorous a priori specification of the underlying conceptual causal models and pathways that drive area-based interventions is crucial. Qualitative approaches could help design and refine the models. Use of multi-methods approaches (both quantitative and qualitative) enable triangulation of data in assessing impacts and exposures (such as the nature of 'local' shopping habits). Unforeseen changes in the timing and nature of the 'intervention' (such as those arising from local planning procedures) require flexibility in the evaluation plan. Adequate control groups are required in monitoring impacts, matching as far as possible, to take account of baseline differences in characteristics that might be related to outcomes.

Increasing physical activity through environment change

Policy makers now view improvements in the environment (such as urban infrastructure and facilities, access to open space, transport systems) as important policy options for increasing levels of physical activity, as well as meeting other policy goals.

Gebel and colleagues examine the nature of the evidence available and what is known about the impact of such environmental changes on physical activity. They consider primary studies and systematic reviews drawn from published and grey literature sources.

Evidence of determining causal relationships is rare, given the methodological and practical problems in conducting controlled experimental studies. Much of the evidence derives form cross-sectional analytic studies reporting associations between different types of environmental characteristics and physical activity. Longitudinal observational studies include, for example, 'relocation' studies that track changes in behaviour of residents that move between different types of neighbourhoods.

Overall, despite a substantial increase in research in this field, it is still in its 'infancy'. Many methodological issues and gaps remain. The researchers urge use of opportunistic studies and natural experiments to further evaluate the effectiveness of environmental changes on physical activity.

Use of fiscal policy to influence health behaviours

Fiscal policy has been used by governments to influence health behaviours particularly in the case of tobacco control, and to some extent with respect to alcohol.

Ludbrook considers the nature of evidence on the effect of fiscal policies on health behaviours (smoking, alcohol consumption, and diet), including the underpinning economic theory and methodological difficulties relating to evaluation.

The use of fiscal measures represents population-wide interventions, and evaluations are based on comparison with other populations (cross-sectional studies), or with the same population over time (time series analyses or cohort studies). However controlling for potential confounding factors (including differences in social or legislative context and interactions with other policy or economic changes) is a major difficulty.

Studies of estimates of price elasticity of demand for tobacco give estimates of the size of price effect. One review of the literature has indicated a wide range of estimates (for a 10% price increase demand may reduce by between 1.4% and 12.3%). The variability in effect sizes reflects in part contextual factors across different countries as well as differences in methodologies employed. Results also depend on the extent to which data can be adjusted to account for tax avoidance through (legal) cross-border purchasing and smuggling.

Analyses of the impact of taxation in the UK show that above-inflation rises in taxes ensured that prices remained high and contributed to declining smoking prevalence and aggregate consumption. However it is difficult to determine the relative contribution of taxation among other measures.

Synthesis of evidence and development of guidance

NICE (founded in 1999) has gained considerable experience in the development of evidence-based guidance on health care treatments and practices, and more recently (since 2005) on public health interventions. NICE principles, processes, and methods enable the development of guidance on effective ways to improve health and reduce health inequalities. The approach seeks to ensure that the guidance is relevant to policy makers and practitioners, is based on the best available evidence, and can be practically implemented in different local contexts.

A collection of chapters sets out NICE's approach to developing national guidance and standards on effective and cost-effective interventions for improving health and reducing health inequalities.

Assessing quality of evidence: studies and methods fit for purpose

Determining the 'best available evidence' on what works is fundamental to guiding policy decisions and investments. Petticrew considers the approaches and methods for assessing the quality of evaluation studies and evidence of effectiveness.

As discussed widely in this volume, the concept of a 'hierarchy' of evidence has been used as the basis for conventional methods for assessing the quality of evidence. This has randomized controlled trials (and meta-analysis of RCTs) at the apex. The RCT design emphasizes internal validity, ie minimizes the risk of bias of study estimates of intervention effects. However, the application of the hierarchical approach to assessing the quality of studies in public health (and other areas of social policy) has important limitations. Petticrew points out that the hierarchical approach is likely to exclude most complex public health interventions that have not as yet been subject to RCTs. Furthermore, the use of the RCT design is often not ethical, politically, or methodologically practical in many areas of public health.

Petticrew states that appraisal of evidence needs to consider 'fitness for purpose' of the study, ie the extent to which any study can provide meaningful evidence to address the range of review questions. 'Study design is often a crude indicator of study quality.' A broader framework is required that can incorporate different types of evidence and study designs while maintaining a formal assessment of the risk of bias posed by each study.

Assessing evidence the NICE way

How NICE applies the notion of 'best available evidence' is explained by Littlejohns and colleagues. It is acknowledged that the traditional hierarchical approach to evidence was originally designed primarily for assessing the effectiveness of therapeutic interventions. However the extended remit of NICE now ranges from prevention and health improvement to treatment and rehabilitation. This has required a more pluralistic approach to evidence and the critical appraisal process. It is important that interventions are not excluded inappropriately when evidence from observational studies is available, although they have not been evaluated by RCTs. Furthermore there are many questions such as 'generalizibilty' (external validity) as well as effectiveness and cost-effectiveness that must be addressed in guidance. 'The primary principle should be the extent to which the study design and analyses are fit for purpose, and to minimize the effect of bias and chance on the results.'

Making social value judgements

There are always levels of uncertainty and gaps relating to available evidence. Further recommendations about what interventions should be adopted cannot be based purely on scientific evidence, particularly as ethical issues and social values are important factors in decision making. Doyle describes how NICE has developed a framework of principles and methods for a systematic approach to considering social and ethical issues. This includes a Social Values Judgements guidance document. This framework was developed prior to the extension of NICE's remit to public health. The principles were mainly derived from traditional medical ethics and, while not inappropriate to public health guidance, do not take account of additional issues associated with public health—for example, commitments to tackling health inequalities (or inequity), multilateral action, participation, and empowerment, and to a focus on the social determinants of health.

Nevertheless, the social values relating to public health are being integrated within the NICE policy. The 'stewardship model' is being used as a valuable reference point (Nuffield Council on Bioethics, 2007) for the development of a more coherent approach for public health. This model is viewed as compatible with NICE's public health responsibilities: *to look after important needs of people both individually and collectively, and an obligation to provide conditions that allow people to be healthy, especially in relation to reducing health inequalities, and to take an active role in promoting the health of the public.*

NICE also seeks to 'actively consider reducing health inequalities including those associated with sex, age, race, disability and socioeconomic status'. This commitment requires all those involved in developing guidance to be proactive in identifying potentially negative impacts of guidance on equality and considering any measures that could lead to positive impacts.

Developing public health guidance

Three chapters document the development of NICE guidance for difference types of complex public health interventions. The authors describe the main stages involved in the guidance development process: the conceptual rationale, systematic review of evidence, development and testing of recommendations, and support to implementation. The three examples show:

- the positioning of guidance in the policy context;
- the importance of setting out the conceptual rationale for the intervention;
- what constitutes the 'best available evidence' in different topic areas; and
- how issues of equity and implementation are considered as well as the evidence on effectiveness and cost-effectiveness in making recommendations.

Guidance on changing the behaviour of individuals and populations to improve health (Swann et al)

For the purposes of this guidance, human behaviour was defined as: 'the product of individual or collective human actions, seen within and influenced by their structural, social and economic context'. A conceptual framework was developed to underpin the development of the guidance. This sought to explain how 'health' was experienced at individual, community, and population levels and across the life course.

Given the breadth and nature of this topic, the assembly and synthesis of the 'best available evidence' demanded consideration of a diverse set of literatures. These were drawn from a range of disciplines and were methodologically varied. The empirical evidence on effectiveness and cost-effectiveness interventions was limited and particular attention was given to theories, concepts, and accounts of behaviour and behaviour change, from the social and behavioural sciences. Psychological literature in particular was judged relevant for structuring and informing interventions.

The recommendations themselves presented a set of principles for planning, delivery and evaluation of interventions at population, community, and individual levels.

Guidance for schools on promoting the social and emotional wellbeing of children (Killoran et al)

NICE guidance examined the effectiveness and cost-effectiveness of primary school-based approaches in improving children's social and emotional well-being through universal and targeted interventions. Conceptually, the development of the guidance was based on the life course model. This indicates that the different aspects of social and emotional well-being are critical assets in determining a child's development and also future life chances. In principle schools have an important role in strengthening these assets (including self-esteem, communication, and social skills).

The reviews of the evidence of effectiveness showed substantial variation in the quality of the evaluation studies, reflecting in part the considerable methodological, ethical, and practical difficulties involved in conducting controlled trials in this area. The strongest evidence that universal and targeted interventions had positive effects was provided by a small number of good quality trials.

The guidance recommended that all primary schools should adopt a 'whole school' approach to promoting children's social and emotional well-being. The approach should comprise both universal and targeted interventions. The components of universal approaches were defined, covering curriculum, training and development of teachers and support staff, support to parents and carers, and wider activities. The provision of targeted inventions involved the identification and assessment of those children who were at risk (or already showing early signs) of anxiety, emotional distress, or behavioural problems, and the agreement of an action plan according to the child's needs.

Guidance on promoting physical activity through environmental changes (Crombie et al)

This NICE guidance focused on: What environmental interventions can increase levels of physical activity amongst the general population as part of daily life?

A logic model was used to make explicit what environmental features (and potential points of intervention) could in principle shape individuals' attitudes, experiences, and choices about physical activity and yield longer term health outcomes.

The effectiveness reviews covered five topics: policy, transport, urban planning, the built environment, and the natural environment. A range of different types of evidence, drawn from both published and grey literature sources, were considered. Experimental evaluation designs in this area are scarce, and the 'best available evidence' was derived mainly from observational studies.

Recommendations included the need to give the highest priority to active modes of transport and to develop networks of cycling and walking routes. Recommendations also proposed that open space and parks should be reached by active modes of transport; that stairs are signposted and attractive to use; and that playgrounds encourage active play.

Appraisal of health technologies

Health technologies versus public health provide contrasting pictures on what constitutes the 'best available evidence' and what evaluation and appraisal methods are 'fit for purpose'. Barnett and colleagues describe in detail the NICE processes and methods involved in appraisal of health technologies. This centres on the use of 'the reference case'—a template which defines the parameters for input into the 'model' for estimating cost-effectiveness (Cost Effectiveness Incremental Ratio, measured in terms of quality adjusted life years).

However, Barnett and colleagues point out that despite the availability of trial evidence, gaps and uncertainty about the evidence remain. Furthermore, judgements on what technologies should be recommended must take account of ethical, equity, and legal issues. For example the particular issues around end of life must now be explicitly considered when making recommendations on certain drugs.

Supporting implementation of guidance

The impact of the NICE guidance is clearly dependent on how it affects policy and practice. NICE's strategy to support implementation of the published guidance is concerned with securing its integration within the 'public health system' at national and local levels. Moore and colleagues describe the main elements of this support strategy.

Particular emphasis is placed on helping local agencies develop their own capacity to manage the process of implementing guidance, within the context of joint planning and management arrangements. A combination of consultancy support and range of support tools are offered to local authorities, schools, and businesses as well as health agencies. This work on supporting implementation of public health guidance is at a comparatively early stage, and a range of challenges remain.

Reflections on public health evidence: its creation, transfer, and impact on policy

Three chapters reflect on epistemological, practical, and historical issues relating to the development of an evidence-based approach to public health.

Understanding the social model of health as the basis for public health action

Kelly explores epistemological and methodological difficulties relating to creation of public health evidence. Kelly argues that there are two distinct analytic levels—the individual and the social—for defining and understanding the causal pathways that determine patterns of health and disease, and the potential for public health action.

Medical science is based on a 'reductionist' epistemology and a set of empirical methods and tools that focuses attention on the individual level. However this biomedical approach has limited utility for analysis of social processes and their impact on health. It is much more difficult to discern how societal structures operate, through such processes as social stratification, cultural norms, and individual 'life worlds', to impact on health. We lack the necessary 'realist' epistemology and methods of analysis.

However, Kelly points out that 'individual level interventions will not in themselves fundamentally transform the health of the public'. The scale of changes necessary for improving public health demands social level intervention. It is therefore vital that public health research pursues understanding of the causal relationships that operate at this social level.

Public health knowledge to policy action

Anderson and McQueen set out the need for an integrated approach to knowledge generation, synthesis, dissemination, uptake, and evaluation. While there is considerable acceptance of the value of evidence synthesis, as yet its systematic translation into policy and practice is lacking.

Anderson and McQueen point out that 'Creation of knowledge by itself doesn't change policy'. This requires investment in the 'knowledge to action cycle'. This is a complex, iterative process. It comprises the 'stages of knowledge creation; selection and adaptation to local context; assessment of barriers to knowledge use and implementation in policies or programs; monitoring knowledge use; and evaluating resulting outcomes to sustain the knowledge to action cycle'.

There are now a number of examples of initiatives and developments that provide models and lessons for creating an integrated approach to knowledge synthesis and translation. These include the Cochrane Collaboration Public Health Review Group, the US Task Force on Community Preventive Services, and the WHO Commission on the Social Determinants of Health.

The gaps and uncertainties in the evidence on the effectiveness and cost-effectiveness of interventions hinder the development of evidence-based guidance. Nevertheless, the work, for example, of the CSDH shows how different types of evidence can be systematically appraised and scrutinized to produce robust recommendations that address the problems relating to the social determinants of health. They spell out how to bring about improvements in daily living conditions and changes in the underpinning political processes that drive health inequalities.

Models of the evidence-policy interface

Policy making is a complex and messy process. A historical perspective provides valuable insights about policy making and the potential for getting public health evidence into policy. Berridge traces the different phases in the changing nature of health and health services research and its relationship to policy development. 'Evidence-based public health' is part of recent history.

Berridge identifies four schools of thought to categorize the relationship between research and policy. These 'schools' are:

- the evidence-based medicine approach: assumes a rational and technical model of evidence and policy;
- the enlightenment model: involves research feeding a climate of policy making. It is analogous to the journalist school which focuses the debate on issues of controversy (such as AIDS, BSE, smoking);
- sociology of scientific knowledge: views discovery of scientific facts as a social process. The strength of scientific claims depends on the research being sustained and supported by its proponents; and
- policy science perspective: involves the interaction of government departments and external groups as 'policy networks' (or 'policy communities') to formulate expert advice.

Application of this thinking to the case study of the Black Report on health inequalities shows that a combination of different models can operate simultaneously. It serves to demonstrate the highly complex nature of policy making. Berridge concludes that 'political and electoral concerns, the media, health activism, industrial interests, civil servants, expert communities and government agencies help determine the boundaries and the impact of evidence on policy'.

Index

NICE = National Institute for Health and Clinical Excellence (NICE)